INTRAOPERATIVE IMAGING IN
NEUROSURGERY

INTRAOPERATIVE IMAGING IN
NEUROSURGERY

Editors

Karanjit Singh Narang

Associate Director (Neurosurgery)
Institute of Neurosciences
Medanta—The Medicity
Gurugram, Haryana, India

Ajaya Nand Jha

Chairman
Institute of Neurosciences
Medanta—The Medicity
Gurugram, Haryana, India

Foreword
Michael Schulder

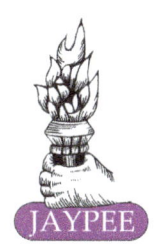

JAYPEE   *The Health Sciences Publisher*

New Delhi | London | Panama

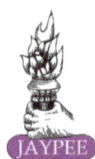

Jaypee Brothers Medical Publishers (P) Ltd.

Headquarters
Jaypee Brothers Medical Publishers (P) Ltd.
4838/24, Ansari Road, Daryaganj
New Delhi 110 002, India
Phone: +91-11-43574357
Fax: +91-11-43574314
E-mail: jaypee@jaypeebrothers.com

Overseas Offices

J.P. Medical Ltd.
83, Victoria Street, London
SW1H 0HW (UK)
Phone: +44-20 3170 8910
Fax: +44 (0)20 3008 6180
E-mail: info@jpmedpub.com

Jaypee-Highlights Medical Publishers Inc.
City of Knowledge, Bld 235, 2nd Floor
Clayton, Panama City, Panama
Phone: +1 507-301-0496
Fax: +1 507-301-0499
E-mail: cservice@jphmedical.com

Jaypee Brothers Medical Publishers (P) Ltd.
17/1-B, Babar Road, Block-B
Shaymali, Mohammadpur
Dhaka-1207, Bangladesh
Mobile: +08801912003485
E-mail: jaypeedhaka@gmail.com

Jaypee Brothers Medical Publishers (P) Ltd.
Bhotahity, Kathmandu, Nepal
Phone: +977-9741283608
E-mail: kathmandu@jaypeebrothers.com

Website: www.jaypeebrothers.com
Website: www.jaypeedigital.com

Inquiries for bulk sales may be solicited at: jaypee@jaypeebrothers.com

Intraoperative Imaging in Neurosurgery

First Edition: 2017

ISBN: 978-93-86322-90-6

Printed at

Dedicated to

My loving wife Dr Sherry Narang,
my kids Gurneet and Harjas and
my caring parents.
Over and above to all my patients who
have taught me and are still teaching me.

—**Karanjit Singh Narang**

Everyone who has made my life more worthwhile.
My wife Dr Urvashi Prasad Jha, who is my greatest motivator;
my children Ruchira and Siddharth Jha; son-in-law and daughter-in-law,
Dr Ashu Jadhav and Trudy Rebert, and of course, my mother, Mrs Sita Jha.

—**Ajaya Nand Jha**

Contributors

Aditya Gupta
Director Neurosurgery
Artemis Hospital
Gurugram, Haryana, India
aditya.gupta@artemishospitals.com

Ajaya Nand Jha
Chairman
Institute of Neurosciences
Medanta—The Medicity
Gurugram, Haryana, India
ajaya.jha@medanta.org

Alessandro Olivi
Direttore
Instiute id Neurochirurgia Resposabile
UOC di Neurochirurgia
Largo Gemelli 8, Roma
alessandro.olivi@policlinicogemelli.it

Alexandra J Golby
Director
Image-guided Neurosurgery
Professor (Neurosurgery)
Harvard Medical School
Brigham Health and Women's Hospital
75, Francis Street
Boston, MA 02115
Massachusetts, USA
agolby@partners.org

Ami Raval
Senior Neurosurgery Specialist
Boston, MA, Massachusetts, USA
Health Care Associates in Medicine, PC
1099 Tagree Street
Staten Island, NY 10304
New York, USA
araval1@nshs.edu

Andreas Unterberg
Professor, Director and Head
Department of Neurosurgery
Heidelberg University Hospital
Im Neuenheimer Feld 400 69120
Heidelberg, Germany
andreas.unterberg@med.uni-heidelberg.de

Anshu Mahajan
Associate Consultant Neurointerventional Surgery
Medanta—The Medicity
Gurugram, Haryana, India
anshu.mahajan@medanta.org

Christian Senft
Professor and Vice Chairman
Center of Clinical Neurosciences
Department of Neurosurgery
University Hospital Frankfurt
Frankfurt, Germany
c.senft@med.uni-frankfurt.de

Christopher Nimsky
Professor and Chairman
Department of Neurosurgery
The Philipps University of Marburg
Baldingerstrasse
35033 Marburg, Germany
nimsky@med.uni-marburg.de

Deepak Bhangale
Associate Consultant Neurosurgery
Medanta—The Medicity
Institute of Neurosciences
Gurugram, Haryana, India
deepak.bhangale@medanta.org

Gavin Quigley
Consultant Neurosurgeon
Royal Victoria Hospital
Belfast BT12 6BA, UK
gavin.quigley@belfasttrust.hscni.net

Gord Von Campe
Head Neurosurgery
Department of Neurosurgery
Medical University of Graz
Auenbruggerplatz 29
A-8036 Graz, Austria
gord.von-campe@medunigraz.at

Harsh Sapra
Director Neuroanesthesia
Medanta—The Medicity
Gurugram, Haryana, India
harsh.sapra@medanta.org

Ivan Ng Hua Bak
Senior Neurosurgeon
Fellow of the Royal College of Surgeons, Edinburgh
Fellow of Academy of Medicine (Neurosurgery), Singapore
Practices at Neurosurgery Partners, Brain + Spine Solutions
38 Irrawaddy Road, #10–60/62
Mount Elizabeth Novena Specialist Center
Singapore 329563
ivan_ng@nni.com.sg

Karanjit Singh Narang
Associate Director Neurosurgery
Institute of Neurosciences
Medanta—The Medicity
Gurugram, Haryana, India
karanjit.singh@medanta.org

Michael R Chicoine
Associate Professor
Department of Neurosurgery
Washington University School of Medicine
660 S Euclid Avenue, Campus Box 8057
St Louis, Missouri 63110, USA
chicoinem@wudosis.wustl.edu

Michael Schulder
Professor and Vice Chairman
Residency Program Director
Director, Brain Tumor Center
Department of Neurosurgery
Hofstra Northwell School of Medicine
Hofstra University
450, Lakeville Road
Lake Success, NY 11042, New York, USA
Vice President, World Society for
Stereotactic and Functional Neurosurgery
AANS Historian
mschulder@northwell.edu

Moritz Scherer MD
Resident of Neurosurgery and Research Fellow
Heidelberg University Hospital
Im Neuenheimer Feld 400
69120 Heidelberg, Germany
moritz.scherer@med.uni-heidelberg.de

Olutayo Olubiyi
Post-doctoral Research Fellow
Golby Lab Research Fund and
Neurosurgical Brain Mapping Lab
Department of Neurosurgery
Harvard Medical School
Boston, MA 02115, Massachusetts, USA
oolubiyi@partners.org

Pawan Goyal
Consultant Neurosurgery
Artemis Hospital
Gurugram, Haryana, India
pawan.goyal@artemishospitals.com

Peter Nakaji
Senior Neurosurgeon
Barrow Neurological Institute
St John's Hospital and Medical Center
2910 North Third Avenue
Phoenix, Arizona AZ 85013, USA
peter.nakaji@bnaneuro.net

Ratnadip Bose
Associate Consultant Neurosurgery
Institute of Neurosciences
Medanta—The Medicity
Gurugram, Haryana, India
ratnadip.bose@medanta.org

Richard Bucholz
Co-President of IOIS
St Louis University
St Louis, Missouri, USA
richard@bucholz.org

Rishabh Kedia
Associate Consultant Neurosurgery
Medanta—The Medicity
Institute of Neurosciences
Gurugram, Haryana, India
rishabh.kedia@medanta.org

Roy Torcuator
Senior Neurosurgeon and Neuro-oncologist
St Luke's Medical Center
32nd Street, Fort Bonifacio, Taguig
Manila, Philippines
c/o *agolby@partners.org*

Sudhir Dubey
Director Neurosurgery
Institute of Neurosciences
Medanta—The Medicity
Gurugram, Haryana, India
sudhir.dubey@medanta.org

Vipul Gupta
Director Neurointerventional Surgery
Artemis Hospital
Gurugram, Haryana, India
vipul.gupta@artemishospitals.com

Foreword

Intraoperative Imaging in Neurosurgery is testimony to the rapid pace of change in our world. When I presented preliminary work on the use of a low-field compact intraoperative MRI (iMRI) at the 2000 meeting of the Neurological Society of India (NSI), there were a handful of iMRI units around the world. This was a time of great excitement for us, where our idea of best and most detailed imaging method could be actually incorporated into our operating rooms. The general reaction at the NSI conference was that such luxuries were very nice in the United States or Western Europe, but Indian neurosurgeons would have to make do with much simpler technology at best, may be two-dimensional ultrasound.

How times have changed, for better and for worse. Many Indian neurosurgical centers now use the most sophisticated devices for intraoperative imaging, including iMRI, intraoperative computed tomography, and three-dimensional intraoperative ultrasonography. These have been joined in this work by neurosurgeons elsewhere in Asia and of course around the world. Many institutions have contributed peer-reviewed publications that demonstrate the utility of iMRI and meet the criteria for evidence-based medicine. Intraoperative imaging has been embraced by colleagues around the world.

On the other hand, this complex and expensive technology has been challenged as not being "cost-effective". Many neurosurgeons reject the extra time and work involved in imaging during surgery. Industrial partners have lost interest as hospital systems shy away from the necessary investment for iMRI implementation. About 45 years ago, the United States made trips to the moon and back routine. Now that expertise has been lost, because of a lack of political will and a collective insistence that we build on the early accomplishments of the Apollo astronauts. Will neurosurgery see the same thing happen with iMRI? Do we lack the political will to insist that we make intraoperative imaging a ubiquitous technology, another step forward in taking the guesswork out of brain surgery of all kinds?

I hope that the book will spur us to continue our efforts to ensure that we keep pushing forward with the development of iMRI and related technologies, so that they become as expected a part of neurosurgical routine as has been the case for diagnostic MRI and surgical navigation. Let us go forward and not backwards.

Michael Schulder MD
Professor and Vice Chairman
Residency Program Director
Director, Brain Tumor Center
Department of Neurosurgery
Hofstra Northwell School of Medicine
Hofstra University
450, Lakeville Road
Lake Success, NY 11042, New York, USA
Vice President, World Society for
Stereotactic and Functional Neurosurgery
AANS Historian
mschulder@northwell.edu

Preface

Our first exposure to neurosurgery during general surgery residency left us with an impression of unconscious patients with shaved heads, and the neurosurgeon drilling burr holes manually with Hudson's brace hoping to hit the spot, having blood under the bone. As general surgery residents, we never understood why they cannot do an exploratory craniotomy such as we used to exploratory laparotomy and look inside. The answer from the Chief of Neurosurgery was a bit snobbish, but very true—neurosurgery requires pin-point precision. We cannot sacrifice a millimeter of brain, unlike people who can get away by removing feet of intestines.

After entering neurosurgical residency, we fully understood the need for precision. From marking the skin incision to reaching the intraparenchymal pathology accurately in neurosurgery, required experience, training and a lot of luck. Post-operative scans would show residual tumor and re-exploration was not uncommon. Things changed when navigation was adopted. Accuracy in marking scalp incisions and reaching target pathology increased significantly.

Only after we started working in an institute with intraoperative MRI, did we realize what we were leaving behind after surgery. It was like a Lie Detector test. You do the surgery, and then think it was a good job done until the MRI picks up the fallacy!

Our strong motivation to compile the book was to spread awareness and education regarding the available technology today, that can help in making neurosurgery more safe and precise.

The book has valuable contributions from authors from all over the world who share their experiences with the specific technologies, they use for intraoperative imaging.

Karanjit Singh Narang
Ajaya Nand Jha

Acknowledgments

We sincerely thank:
- All our contributors for taking time out from their hectic schedules, to provide their chapters.
- Our families for putting up with us through all these years.
- Our colleagues for their persistent efforts to ensure completion of this book, especially Drs Rishabh Kedia and Ratnadip Bose and Ms Marion Gomes.
- Our long suffering publisher, M/s Jaypee Brothers Medical Publishers (P) Ltd, New Delhi, India.
- Most of all, our patients.

Contents

History of Neuroimaging

Karanjit Singh Narang, Rishabh Kedia, Ajaya Nand Jha

INTRODUCTION

Advances in the field of radiology and in turn modern neurosurgery have been so rapid that, it is almost impossible to recall the older techniques and still be abreast with the latest modalities at the same time. The obsolete modalities have become a part of theoretical textbooks only. The neurosurgical residents of this generation might not even know about the older techniques such as pneumoencephalography. These advances are not just useful in making the work of a neurosurgeon easier, but at the same time, it helps in reducing the mortality and morbidity in patients or aid in better outcomes.[1]

GENEALOGY OF NEUROIMAGING

X-ray

Sir Victor Horsley was the first neurosurgeon to use X-rays in neurosurgery way back in the late 19th century after their discovery.[2] Soon after the discovery of plain radiograph and its utility in clinical medicine, some specialists tried to X-ray of skull of patients in order to diagnose suspected lesions in the brain.[3-6] One of the most famous publications of its time was "Röntgen-diagnostik der Erkrankungen des Kopfes" by Arthur Schüller.[7] The same was later translated into English under the name "Radiology of Diseases of the Head". "Neuroradiology" was first used by Schüller describing pathologies of the brain using skull radiographs.[8] The modality gained such popularity in those times that Walter Dandy and George Heuer published a paper proving changes seen in 45 patients with brain tumors out of their enlisted 100 patients **(Figure 1.1)**.[9]

However, this modality had its own limitations namely long period of immobility to acquire image, soft tissue pathologies could not be detected, neoplasms without bony involvement or calcification were literally invisible. In reality, by the time actual pathologies were identified on skull radiographs, clinically, it was too late for the patient to undergo any intervention.[10] Despite of the advances over the centuries, spine radiograph is still an essential part of orthopedics and neurosurgery.

Ventriculography and Pneumoencephalography

Walter Dandy came up with an idea of somehow analyzing the changes in the morphology of the ventricles by injecting some contrast material, in order to localize lesions in the brain and diagnosing pathologies in a timely manner.[10] He failed with his experiments using different radiopaque contrast materials, until he accidentally noticed that air in the ventricles in head injury patients made the ventricles partially radiopaque.[10,11] This discovery resulted in further increase in detection capacity of brain tumors in his patients **(Figure 1.2)**.[12]

Pneumoencephalography was also discovered by him, when he further noticed that the air from the ventricles escaped into the subarachnoid space.[13] The procedure was then popularized in the form of drawing small amount of CSF during lumbar puncture and injecting air instead. This discovery paved the path for contrast studies of the brain.

However, these techniques proved to be associated with significant morbidity and mortality, especially with neurosurgeons other than Dandy.[8] Through the following years of discovery, refinement of the procedure led to the discovery of a skull table by Lysholm which helped with the movement of patient in some positions to enable the air to move to different parts of the brain as needed.[14]

Myelography with Contrast

Myelography was first done using air as contrast medium as was the case with ventriculography in the early 20th century.[15,16] By the same time, iodine was discovered to be a safe radiopaque contrast. Although initially iodine was used

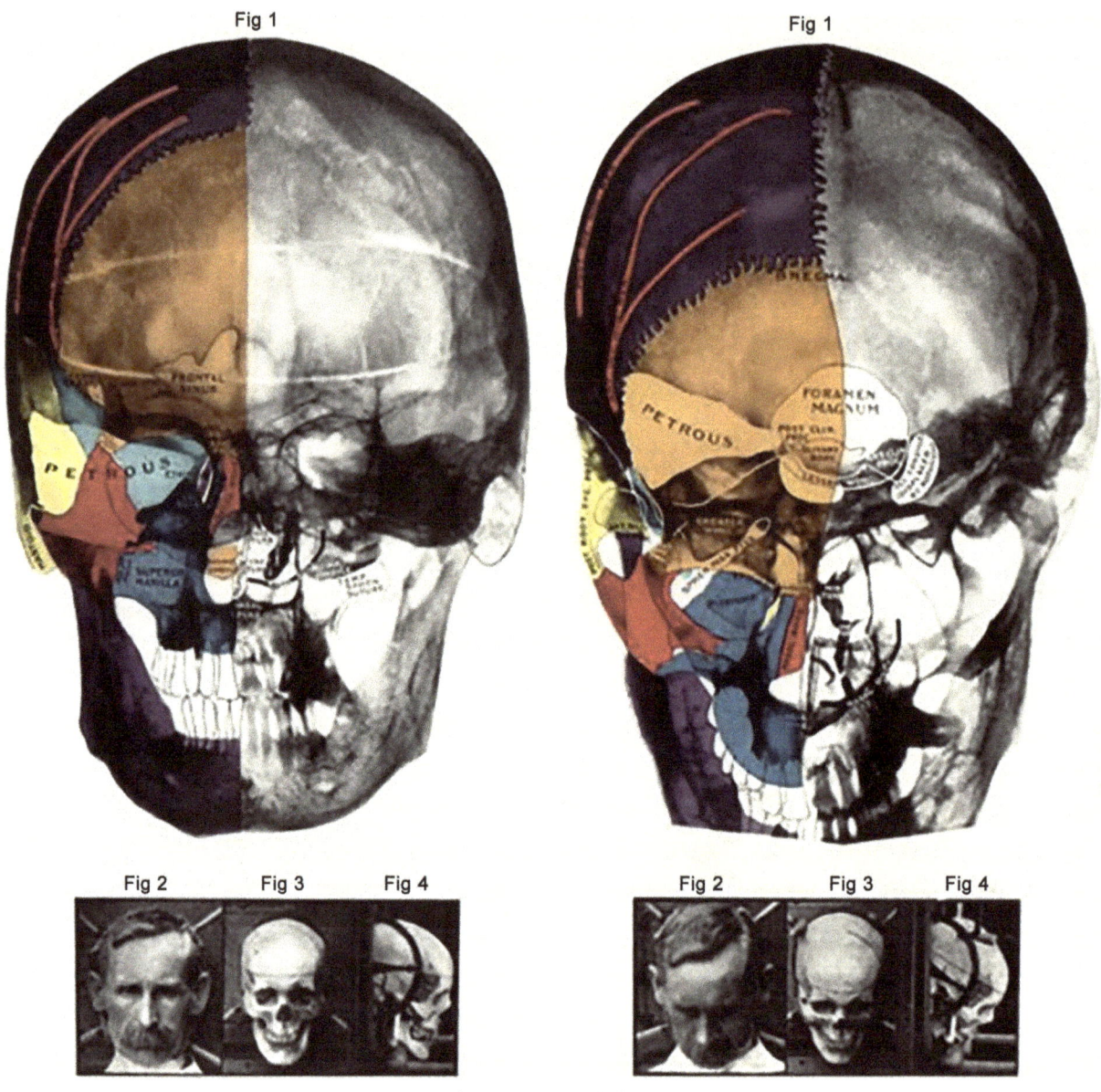

Figure 1.1 X-ray skull
Source: Adapted from www.archive.org.

with an oily medium, which led to cases of arachnoiditis and was later replaced by water soluble material over the next 50 years.[17] Lumbar discography came to be popular in the mid-20th century where injection of radiopaque material was done directly into the intervertebral disks.[18,19]

Angiography of the Intracranial and Spinal Vessels

Egas Moniz dreamt of making either the brain or the cerebral vessels opaque on imaging. His efforts led to the discovery of angiography of cerebral vessels.[20] In the early 20th century, he performed multiple experiments on animals and cadavers. Once confident of his method, he performed a "cutdown" to reach the carotid artery and injected contrast material directly into it making angiography possible. Loman and Myerson further refined the technique by allowing percutaneous access to the carotid artery and injecting contrast material without "'cutdown" procedure.[21] Angiography of the vertebral arteries was discovered approaching it through the brachial, subclavian, and vertebral arteries over the next few years.[22] The most famous Seldinger technique, using a catheter instead of a needle, was devised in 1953, but it took almost

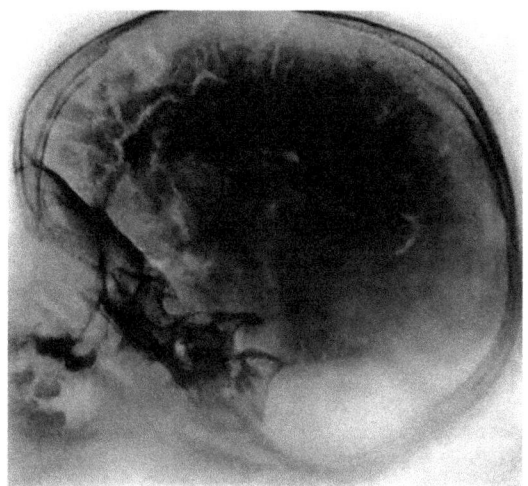

Figure 1.2 Roentgenography of the brain after the injection of air into the spinal canal
Source: Adapted from Dandy WE. Röntgenography of brain after the injection of air into the spinal canal. Ann Surg. 1919;70:397-403.

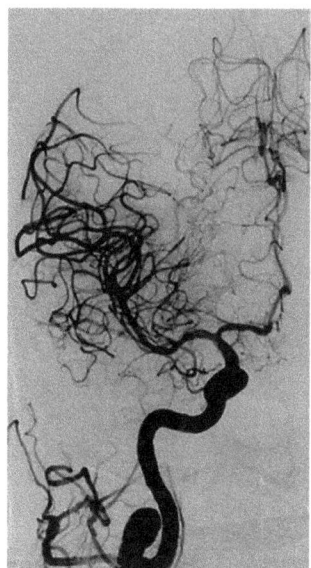

Figure 1.3 Digital subtraction angiography of intracranial vessel

10 years to be used in cerebral angiography.[23,24] The transfemoral approach was also developed along the same time and was accepted quite late. The technique kept improving with the help of technological advances such as digital subtraction, safer contrast agents, magnification technology, and multiple planes of imaging. Glue, particles, coils, and Onyx were discovered for intravascular procedures **(Figure 1.3)**.

The procedure has withstood the early complications[25] and the modern day cerebral angiography does not require any general anesthesia and takes much shorter time, thus reducing the incidence of the known complications.

Spinal angiography was developed almost four decades after cerebral angiography.[26,27] It is still considered the gold standard for diagnosing spinal vascular lesions.[28]

Computed Tomography

The development of computed tomography (CT) started with the ideas of William Oldendorf[29,30] and mathematically developed by physicist Allan Cormack.[31,32] A few years later, Geoffrey Hounsfield developed a cross-sectional scanner based on the same concept. The first patient to be scanned using CT was a woman with a suspected tumor in her brain in 1972.[33] This was followed by multiple patients and the first paper on CT imaging of the head was published in 1973.[34] This proved to be a ground-breaking discovery of its time. Hounsfield and Cormack were the most famous names in the medical community worldwide and even received the Nobel prize for their contribution in 1979. The initial versions of a CT scanner allowed only imaging of the head. Multiple improvements and advancements of the initial idea of CT scanner led to bigger and better machines which could scan the entire human body. Eventually, advancements were made in decreasing the total radiation dosage, time taken for scans and quality of images. Earlier scans used 8-13 mm slice thickness, thus their quality was poor based on current scans. It took a few hours for the first machines to process each scan. The market politics estimated that not many CT scanners would be sold worldwide at the time of its inception due to its high cost and fewer advantages.[35,36] This modality changed neurosurgery as we speak. It was beyond anyone's imagination that without cutting into the brain we would be able to see the contents of the brain. The initial advantages of a CT scan of brain helped in identifying bleeds, calcification, edema, and necrosis. With the introduction of intravenous contrast, CT angiography of cerebral vessels was also made possible. Once all this became a part of the routine practice, the age-old procedure of pneumoencephalography became obsolete **(Figure 1.4)**.[37,38]

The biggest advantage of CT scan in diagnosing many intracranial pathologies with one single scan turned down all concerns regarding scanners using high doses of ionizing radiation, high costs, etc. It started being called a "doctor's toy" and was leading to less skilled doctors.[39] All such skepticism has been proven wrong even decades after its discovery when it continues to be an indispensable tool even today.

Magnetic Resonance Imaging

Felix Bloch and Edward Purcell were the ones who developed the magnetic resonance imaging (MRI) based on nuclear magnetic resonance.[40,41] It was the first time that an imaging modality did not involve any nuclear radiation.[42] Raymond Damadian, a physician from the US, came up with the idea almost 25 years later that this modality could differentiate

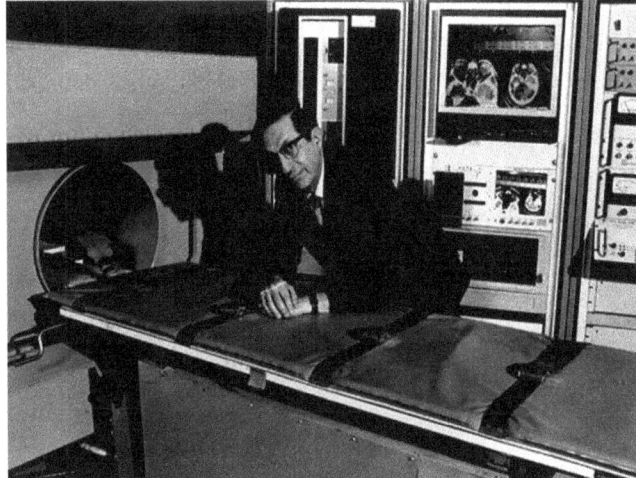

Figure 1.4 The first full body CT scanner
Source: Adapted from The Washington Post.

diseased tissue, especially tumors from normal tissue.[43] Herman Carr published his thesis based on MRI at Harvard University in the same year as Bloch and Purcell.[44] Paul Lauterbur was inspired by Carr's thesis and used it to devise a way of generating two-dimensional and three-dimensional MR images. The credit for constructing the first MRI machine goes to Damadian (1972). Lauterbur took out the first scan using MRI of a mouse a year later.[45,46] Peter Mansfield developed a new algorithm for MRI machines which greatly reduced the time required to acquire images and improve their quality too. In 1977, Damadian, Minkoff and Goldsmith were able to acquire the first human MRI scan.[47]

Publications started coming in during the 1980s using MRI for neuroimaging, especially in comparison to CT images.[48,49] The first MRI machine to be used in hospital set-ups commercially and contrast for MRI based on Gadolinium were also developed during the same time.[16,50] MRI ever since its inception has revolutionized neuroimaging.[51] It was earlier considered to be "extremely difficult, time-consuming, and often disappointing".[52] Its challenges still remain, especially in unstable patients and the ones who have a fear of closed spaces.[53]

Image-guided Neurosurgery and Stereotaxy

The ever-improving radiological modalities and technologies over the past few decades have led to improved diagnosis of neurosurgical diseases and also better treatment outcomes. All machines developed with the intention of accurately localizing intracranial structures based on landmarks on the surface were first devised using Broca's craniograph[54] and Kocher's craniometer.[55] They proved to be less than optimal and were not of much use clinically. Then came the "encephalometer" developed by Russian anatomist Zernov.

He developed a device which was based on an arc-shaped instrument attached to the skull.[56] Three-dimensional Cartesian coordinate system was used in experimental monkeys through orthogonal stereotactic frame by Victor Horsley and Robert Henry Clarke.[57]

In the early 20th century, Kirschner first used frame-based stereotaxy while injecting into the foramen ovale to treat trigeminal neuralgia.[58] Ernest Spiegel and Henry Wycis developed the "stereoencephalotome",[59] and Lars Leksell was the legendary neurosurgeon who first developed the most popular stereotactic device to be used in humans. Spiegel and Wycis were the first surgeons to perform stereotactic thalamotomy in humans using radiography in stereotaxy based on landmarks inside the brain such as calcified pineal gland and ventricles. Leksell based his system on the radius of the arc which was later used by the popular frame developed by Edwin Todd and Trent Wells. This led to the eventual development of Brown-Robert-Wells frame which used data from the computed tomographic scans into the surgical setting.[60] Jean Talairach devised a special frame used in epilepsy surgery for temporal lobe lesions and used the anterior and posterior commissure as basis of intracranial landmarks.[61]

Stereotactic neurosurgery for psychiatric and functional disorders lost their popularity soon after levodopa started being used as a treatment for Parkinson's disease.[62] Over the years, CT and MRI scans got integrated with stereotaxy and more accurate targeting of regions and lesions in the brain were made possible. This revived stereotactic neurosurgery as developed by Leksell in the form of deep brain stimulation, vascular neurosurgery, epilepsy, neuro-oncology, and radiation therapy.[63]

Rapid advances in technology have facilitated the development of frameless neuronavigation systems, which began with Roberts and colleagues in 1986.[64] Stealth Station and Vector Vision navigation systems have introduced technology and instruments that allow frameless stereotaxy, and have become popular with many neurosurgeons.[65] Intraoperative MRI (iMRI) has been proven to be more effective in achieving better resections and in turn better survival in patients with gliomas. Multiple papers have been published in international journals acknowledging the fact as at least a level 2 evidence of the same.[66] A recent study showed the use of iMRI for placement of ventricular catheters to prevent complications.[67]

During endovascular surgery, angiography can be used to provide regular updates. Plain X-ray image intensifiers are widely used in spinal surgery, for example, to ensure correct level localization and confirm screw position. Intraoperative ultrasound is also used in some centers, and may be particularly useful in the emergency setting to exclude hematoma collection.[1] The acquisition of more than just standard MRI intraoperatively, particularly, functional MRI (fMRI) and diffusion tensor imaging (DTI), may offer additional safety for complex tumor resections[68] and management of vascular lesions[69] but robust evidence in this regard is awaited. However, the equipment used to obtain this data is expensive and thus not widely available, and there are some important considerations, including that iMRI prolongs surgery and requires reconfiguration of the operating room. Certainly, wherever available, preoperative functional imaging and particularly fMRI can assist neurosurgical operation planning.[70]

REFERENCES

1. Kirkman M. The role of imaging in the development of neurosurgery. J Clin Neurosci. 2015;22:55-61.
2. Gunderman RB. X-ray vision: the evolution of medical imaging and its human significance. Oxford: Oxford University Press; 2013.
3. van Dijck J. X-ray vision in Thomas Mann's the magic mountain. In: van Dijck J (Ed). The Transparent Body. A Cultural Analysis of Medical Imaging. Seattle: University Of Washington Press; 2005. p. 84.
4. Proust M. Swann's way. Remembrance of things past, vol. 1. New York: Henry Holt and Company; 1922.
5. Church A. Cerebellar tumor: recognized clinically, demonstrated by X-ray—proved at autopsy. Am J Med Sci. 1899;177:125-30.
6. Pfahler GE. Cerebral skiagraphy: transactions of the American Roentgen Ray Society. In: Proceedings of the 5th Annual Meeting of the American Roentgen Ray Society, September 9, 10, 12, 13. Missouri: St. Louis; 1904;4:175-83.
7. Schüller A. Röntgen-diagnostik der erkrankungen des kopfes. Vienna: Holder; 1912.
8. Bull JW. The history of neuroradiology. Proc R Soc Med. 1970;63:637-43.
9. Heuer GJ, Dandy WE. Roentgenography in the localization of brain tumor, based on a series of one hundred consecutive cases. Bull Johns Hopkins Hosp. 1916;27:311-22.
10. Dandy WE. Ventriculography following the injection of air into the cerebral ventricles. Ann Surg. 1918;68:5-11.
11. Haschek E, Lindenthal O. A contribution to the practical use of photography according to Roentgen. Wien Chir Wochenschr. 1896;9:63.
12. Alper MG. Three pioneers in the early history of neuroradiology: the Snyder lecture. Doc Ophthalmol. 1999;98:29-49.
13. Dandy WE. Röntgenography of brain after the injection of air into the spinal canal. Ann Surg. 1919;70:397-403.
14. Lysholm E. Apparatus and technique for roentgen examination of the skull. Stockholm: PA Norstedt & Söner; 1931.
15. Wilderoe S. Uber die diagnostische bedeutung der interspinalen luftinjektioned bei Ruckenmarksleiden, besonders bei geschwulsten. Z Chir. 1921;48:394-7.
16. Jacobaeus HC. On insufflation of air into the spinal canal for diagnostic purposes in cases of tumors of the spinal canal. Acta Med Scand. 1921;55:555-64.
17. Taveras JM. Diamond jubilee lecture. Neuroradiology: past, present, future. Radiology. 1990;175:593-602.
18. Lindblom K. Diagnostic puncture of intervertebral disks in sciatica. Acta Orthop Scand. 1948;17:231-9.
19. Collis JS Jr, Gardner WJ. Lumbar discography: an analysis of one thousand cases. J Neurosurg. 1962;19:452-61.
20. Doby T. Cerebral angiography and Egas Moniz. Am J Roentgenol. 1992;159:364.
21. Loman J, Myerson A. Visualization of the cerebral vessels by direct intracarotid injection of thorium dioxide (Thoratrast). AJR Am J Roentgenol. 1936;35:188-93.
22. Schechter MM, de Gutiérrez-Mahoney CG. The evolution of vertebral angiography. Neuroradiology. 1973;5:157-64.
23. Greitz T. The history of Swedish neuroradiology. Acta Radiol. 1996;37:455-71.
24. Seldinger SI. Catheter replacement of the needle in percutaneous arteriography: a new technique. Acta Radiol. 1953;39:368-76.
25. Moniz E. L'encephalographie arterielle, son importance dans la localization des tumeurs cerebrales. Rev Neurol (Paris). 1927;2:72-90.
26. Di Chiro G, Doppman J, Ommaya AK. Selective arteriography of arteriovenous aneurysms of spinal cord. Radiology. 1967;88:1065-77.
27. Baker HL Jr, Love JG, Layton DD Jr. Angiographic and surgical aspects of spinal cord vascular anomalies. Radiology. 1967;88:1078-85.
28. Chen J, Gailloud P. Safety of spinal angiography: complication rate analysis in 302 diagnostic angiograms. Neurology. 2011;77:1235-40.
29. Goldman LW. Principles of CT and CT technology. J Nucl Med Technol. 2007;35:115-28; quiz 129-30.
30. Oldendorf WH. Isolated flying spot detection of radiodensity discontinuities: displaying the internal structural patterns of a complex object. Biomed Electron Ire Trans. 1961;8:68-72.
31. Cormack AM. Representation of a function by its line integrals, with some radiological applications. J Appl Phys. 1963;34:2722-7.
32. Cormack AM. Representation of a function by its line integrals, with some radiological applications. II. J Appl Phys. 1964;35:2908-13.
33. Bull J. History of computed tomography. In: Newton TH, Potts GD (Eds). Radiology of the Skull and Brain. St. Louis: CV Mosby Company; 1981.
34. Ambrose J, Hounsfield G. Computerized transverse axial tomography. Br J Radiol. 1973;46:148-9.
35. Hoeffner EG, Mukherji SK, Srinivasan A, et al. Neuroradiology back to the future: brain imaging. Am J Neuroradiol. 2012;33:5-11.
36. Oldendorf WH. The quest for an image of the brain. New York: Raven Press; 1980.
37. Huckman MS. Neuroradiology without benefit of computers: a memoir. Am J Neuroradiol. 2010;31:783-6.
38. Amundson P, Dugstad G, Noyes W. Cerebral angiography via the femoral artery with reference to cerebrovascular disease. Acta Neurol Scand. 1967;43:115.
39. Alker G. A great leap from tiny chips: computerization, 1960s and 1970s. In: Doby T, Alker G (Eds). Origins and Development of Medical Imaging. Springfield, IL: Southern Illinois University Press; 1997. p. 111.
40. Bloch F, Hanson WW, Packard M. Nuclear Induction. Phys Rev. 1946;69:127.
41. Purcell EM, Torrey HC, Pound RV. Resonance absorption by nuclear magnetic moments in a solid. Phys Rev. 1946;69:37-8.

42. Young IR. Significant events in the development of MRI. J Magn Reson Imaging. 2004;20:183-6.

43. Damadian R. Tumor detection by nuclear magnetic resonance. Science. 1971;171:1151-3.

44. Carr H. Free precession techniques in nuclear magnetic resonance [Ph.D. thesis]. Harvard University; 1952.

45. Lauterbur PC. Image formation by induced local interactions: examples employing nuclear magnetic resonance. Nature. 1973;242:190-1.

46. Lauterbur PC. Magnetic resonance zeugmatography. Pure Appl Chem. 1974;40:149-57.

47. Damadian R, Goldsmith M, Minkoff L. NMR in cancer: XVI. FONAR image of the live human body. Physiol Chem Phys. 1977;9:97-100, 108.

48. Holland GN, Moore WS, Hawkes RC. Nuclear magnetic resonance tomography of the brain. J Comput Assist Tomogr. 1980;4:1-3.

49. Runge VM, Carollo BR, Wolf CR, et al. Gd DTPA: a review of clinical indications in central nervous system magnetic resonance imaging. Radiographics. 1989;9:929-58.

50. Teasdale GM, Hadley DM, Lawrence A, et al. Comparison of magnetic resonance imaging and computed tomography in suspected lesions in the posterior cranial fossa. BMJ. 1989;299:349-55.

51. Hoeffner EG, Mukherji SK, Srinivasan A, et al. Neuroradiology back to the future: spine imaging. Am J Neuroradiol. 2012;33:999-1006.

52. Geva T. Magnetic resonance imaging: historical perspective. J Cardiovasc Magn Reson. 2006;8:573-80.

53. Singer OC, Sitzer M, du Mesnil de Rochemont R, et al. Practical limitations of acute stroke MRI due to patient-related problems. Neurology. 2004;62:1848-9.

54. Broca P. Memoir on the craniograph and some of its applications. Mémoires De La Société d'Anthropologie; 1863.

55. Schültke E. Theodor Kocher's craniometer. J Neurosurg. 2009;64:1001-4; discussion 1004-5.

56. Zernov DN. L'encéphalometrie. Rev Gen Clin Ther. 1890;19: 302.

57. Horsley V, Clarke RH. The structure and function of the cerebellum examined by a new method. Brain. 1908;31:45-124.

58. Kirschner M. Die Punktionstechnik und die Elektrokoagulation des Ganglion Gasseri. Arch Klin Chir. 1933;176:581-620.

59. Spiegel EA, Wycis HT, Marks M, et al. Stereotaxic apparatus for operations on the human brain. Science. 1947;106:349-50.

60. Heilbrun MP, Roberts TS, Apuzzo ML, et al. Preliminary experience with Brown-Roberts-Wells (BRW) computerized tomography stereotaxic guidance system. J Neurosurg. 1983;59:217-22.

61. Talairach J, Hecaen H, David M, et al. Recherches sur la coagulation thérapeutique des structures sous-corticales chez l'homme. Rev Neurol . 1949;81:4-24.

62. al-Rodhan NR, Kelly PJ. Pioneers of stereotactic neurosurgery. Stereotact Funct Neurosurg. 1992;58:60-6.

63. Leksell L. A stereotaxic apparatus for intracerebral surgery. Acta Chir Scand. 1950;99:229-33.

64. Roberts DW, Strohbehn JW, Hatch JF, et al. A frameless stereotaxic integration of computerized tomographic imaging and the operating microscope. J Neurosurg. 1986;65:545-9.

65. Orringer DA, Golby A, Jolesz F. Neuronavigation in the surgical management of brain tumors: current and future trends. Expert Rev Med Devices. 2012;9:491-500.

66. Kubben PL, ter Meulen KJ, Schijns OE, et al. Intraoperative MRI-guided resection of glioblastoma multiforme: a systematic review. Lancet Oncol. 2011;12:1062-70.

67. Janson CG, Romanova LG, Rudser KD, et al. Improvement in clinical outcomes following optimal targeting of brain ventricular catheters with intraoperative imaging. J Neurosurg. 2014;120:684-96.

68. Nimsky C. Intraoperative acquisition of fMRI and DTI. Neurosurg Clin N Am . 2011;22:269-77.

69. Campbell PG, Jabbour P, Yadla S, et al. Emerging clinical imaging techniques for cerebral cavernous malformations: a systematic review. Neurosurg Focus. 2010;29:E6.

70. Belyaev AS, Peck KK, Brennan NM, et al. Clinical applications of functional MR imaging. Magn Reson Imaging Clin N Am. 2013;21:269-78.

2

Intraoperative Imaging in Neurosurgery

Michael Schulder, Ami Raval

INTRODUCTION

History of Neuroimaging and Stereotaxy

For the past century and half, neurosurgeons have been attempting to localize lesions within the brain using various techniques. Given its intricate and delicate nature, the ability to noninvasively understand the anatomical and functional regions within the nervous system was essential to neurosurgeons. While the field of neuronavigation has developed significantly due to the parallel strides made in neuroradiology, the ability to find tumors, and other intracranial targets was present even earlier when Zernov developed the encephalometer, a device that fixed onto the skull in order to localize structures intracranially based on surface landmarks using an arc device.[1]

Imaging of the skull and its contents began shortly after Roentgen discovered the X-ray in 1895.[2] Calcified areas, such as the pineal gland, choroid plexus, and basal ganglia could now be identified, and even certain pathologies such as craniopharyngiomas and calcified meningiomas could be localized. The next revolutionary development in neuroimaging was air ventriculography, which was described by Walter Dandy after he demonstrated that injection of air into the lateral ventricles or into the spinal canal could provide even further information. Shortly thereafter, Egas Moniz introduced cerebral angiography, in order to diagnose vascular pathologies, but also to demonstrate large intracranial lesions causing sufficient mass effect that they displaced cerebral blood vessels.[1-3] Combining ventriculography and stereotaxis, neurologists and neurosurgeons learned that certain periventricular regions such as the basal ganglia and thalamus could be localized due to their association to stable deep structures such as the third ventricle. Using the fundamentals of this technique, the first frame to treat trigeminal neuralgia was applied onto a human, and subsequently, Ernest A Spiegel

and Henry T Wycis attached a frame to a patient's head, and then performed a pneumoencephalogram. Using a brain atlas along with major internal landmarks that were identified using pneumoencephalography, the first human thalamotomy was performed. Following this pioneering work, Lars Leksell developed an arc-centered stereotactic frame, which used pins in order to fixate the frame to the skull, and used polar coordinates.[4,5] Since then, many other variations of the stereotactic frame system have been developed for intracranial surgery using different devices in order to fixate the frame to the skull **(Figure 2.1)**.[6-12]

The early 1980s were a fruitful time for technology in general, with strides made in radiology, imaging, robotics, and computers. After the development of computed

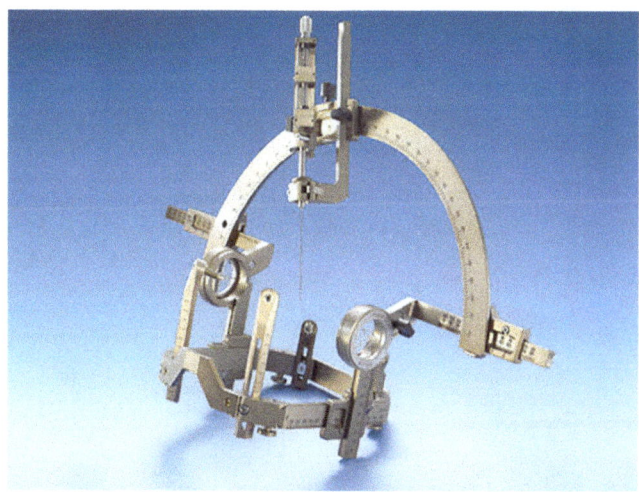

Figure 2.1 Modern version of a Leksell stereotactic frame for intracranial biopsy
Courtesy: Elekta AB Publication, Stockholm, Sweden.

tomography (CT) scans by Hounsfield and Cormack, Shalit was one of the first to describe the use of intraoperative CT scans for brain tumors.[13,14] In 1987, Young et al. demonstrated that stereotactic coordinates could be derived from CT images, and then translated into a CT robotic stereotactic system; this allowed direct utilization of the CT images in the operating room for localization and targeting of deep intracranial structures.[9] Unfortunately, despite its potential applicability, use of the intraoperative CT was not common initially, mainly because of its cost and the difficulties of incorporating it into the operating room infrastructure.[15] Today, it mainly continues to be used for spinal and functional neurosurgery **(Figure 2.2)**.[15-19]

While frame-based stereotaxy was found to be highly accurate, the frame itself limited the range of surgical approaches. Additionally, early on, only one type of imaging data set could be used for localization and of course, required the physical placement of a frame onto a patient's skull, which does cause discomfort to the patient **(Figure 2.1)**. In response to these constraints, the "frame-based" stereotactic system started to evolve into frameless ones. Roberts et al. was one of the first to describe utilizing an operating microscope with ultrasound emission and recording microphones that can allow the surgeon to correlate his microscope location with that of predefined targets on CT or magnetic resonance (MR) using a sonic digitizer. Using this concept of emission of signals from a variety of sources and then processing the data using digitizers so that the "source of the signal emission" can be localized with reference to a three-dimensional (3D) reconstructed imaging study, others created various neuronavigation systems utilizing ultrasonic, magnetic, and infrared-based sources.[20]

Once it was demonstrated that intraoperative imaging was logistically possible, it was imperative to be able to combine that with frameless stereotaxy in order to allow "real-time" intraoperative localization. In 1995, Black et al. performed the first neurosurgical procedure using an [intraoperative magnetic resonance imaging (MRI) (ioMRI)].[21] This revolutionized the field of neuronavigation in that by combining intraoperative imaging with neuronavigation, updated images could be acquired and then incorporated into the navigation dataset, thereby allowing surgeons access to "near real-time" imaging. With this technology, two neurosurgeons had the ability to operate in the same room with the ioMRI without mobilizing the patient or the magnet. Imaging, surgical and stereotactic spaces were unified in this device.

Initial disadvantages of the ioMRI, however, included a small working space of 56 cm between the coils, lower quality images due to lower magnetic field strength and increased costs of obtaining new MRI compatible equipment.[22] Since then, many more models of ioMRI have been introduced, including ones where the machine can be moved in and out of the operative field **(Figures 2.3 and 2.4)**. Conversely, an ioMRI operating suite can be constructed where patients can be wheeled into and out of an MRI that has been built into the operating room **(Figure 2.5)**. These systems have varying ergonomic and imaging advantages, although none achieve the unity of concept that the original double donut design provided.

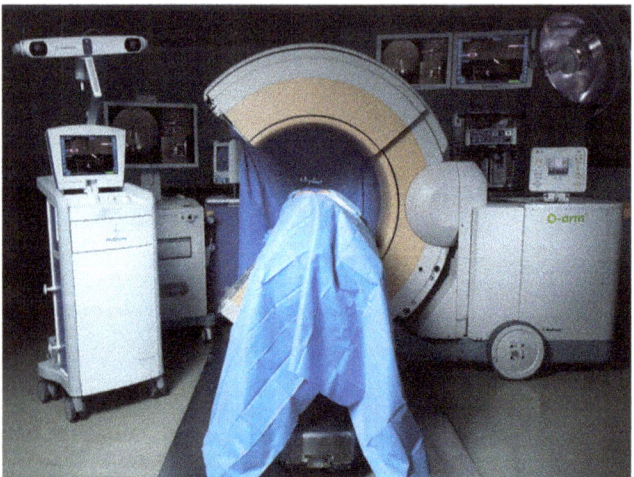

Figure 2.2 Intraoperative cone-beam computed tomography (CT) scanner. Patients can be positioned on a standard operating room table, with the scanner moved under and around the patient without significant interruption of operating room workflow. This can be utilized for both cranial and spinal neurosurgical procedures
Courtesy: O-arm® Surgical imaging with StealthStation® navigation system, Medtronic Inc,. Minneapolis, MN.

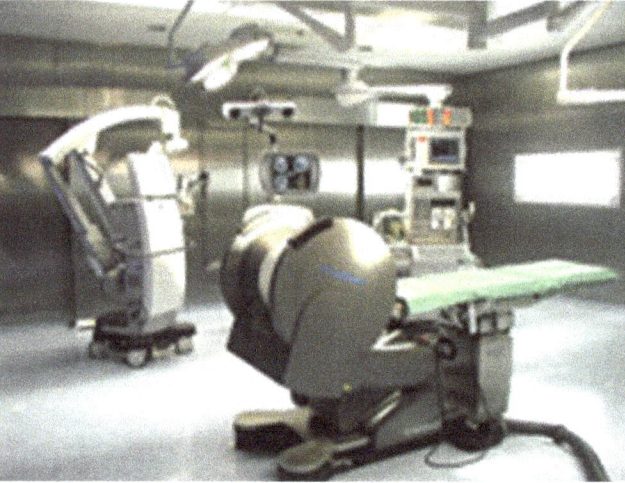

Figure 2.3 Operating room set-up with microscope and navigational camera in background with intraoperative low field magnetic resonance imaging (MRI). Magnet is elevated up on both sides of the head that is resting on a standard operating room table
Courtesy: PoleStar® Surgical MRI system, Medtronic Inc., Minneapolis, MN.

Perhaps with the introduction of the ioMRI, the concept of intraoperative imaging came to a forefront in neurosurgery, and served as an impetus for the development of not only other advanced modalities of intraoperative imaging, but also for higher quality technological improvements in the existing ones. Software systems for intraoperative CT (iCT) became significantly faster, more user friendly, and less expensive than the ioMRI systems so that image acquisition was better and more rapid. Therefore, intracranial hemorrhages could be detected sooner than ioMR imaging. Additionally, it provided

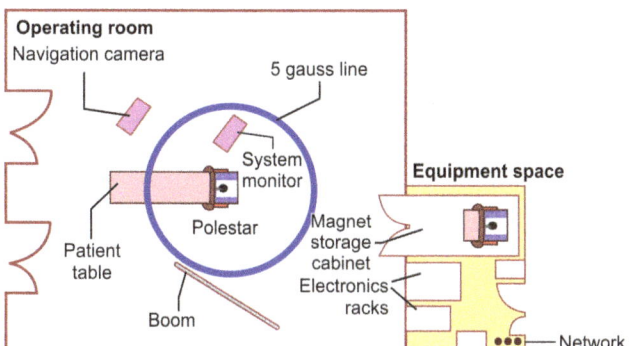

Figure 2.4 Architectural setup of operating using low field intraoperative magnetic resonance imaging (MRI). When not in use, the MRI is kept in a storage cabinet and brought out to behind and under the head when needed
Courtesy: PoleStar® Surgical MRI system, Medtronic Inc., Minneapolis, MN.

better bony resolution than MRI and its use was expanded to complex spinal, orthopedic, and sinus surgeries.[23]

Other methods of utilizing intraoperative neuroimaging with neuronavigation include fusing preoperative images with 3D ultrasonography. This bypasses much of the logistical limitations of the ioMRI and offers a quick and useful way of pinpointing a lesion and visualizing it prior to durotomy and brain tumor resection. It can also be used by the surgeon to account for brain shift and other anatomic changes that may have occurred during surgery **(Figure 2.6)**. While it has been shown to be less effective in assessing the extent of tumor resection, it provides an inexpensive, more accessible means for surgeons to compare anatomic data before and after tumor resection. Interactive neuronavigation systems have now been developed that utilize not only CT and MR images, but can incorporate intraoperative 3D ultrasonography data, functional MRI (fMRI), and diffusion tensor imaging (DTI) mapping data so that the surgeon has the maximal information possible when approaching a brain tumor **(Figures 2.6 to 2.8)**.[24-27] Additionally, in the past 15 years, frameless neuronavigation has expanded to incorporating intraoperative MRI with other operative tools, such as a navigational microscope, so that margins of tumor, the planned surgical approach and functional data can all be displayed within the surgeon's microscope viewing field. Surgical instruments can also be registered to the neuronavigation dataset so that the distal tips of catheters and endoscopes can be tracked.

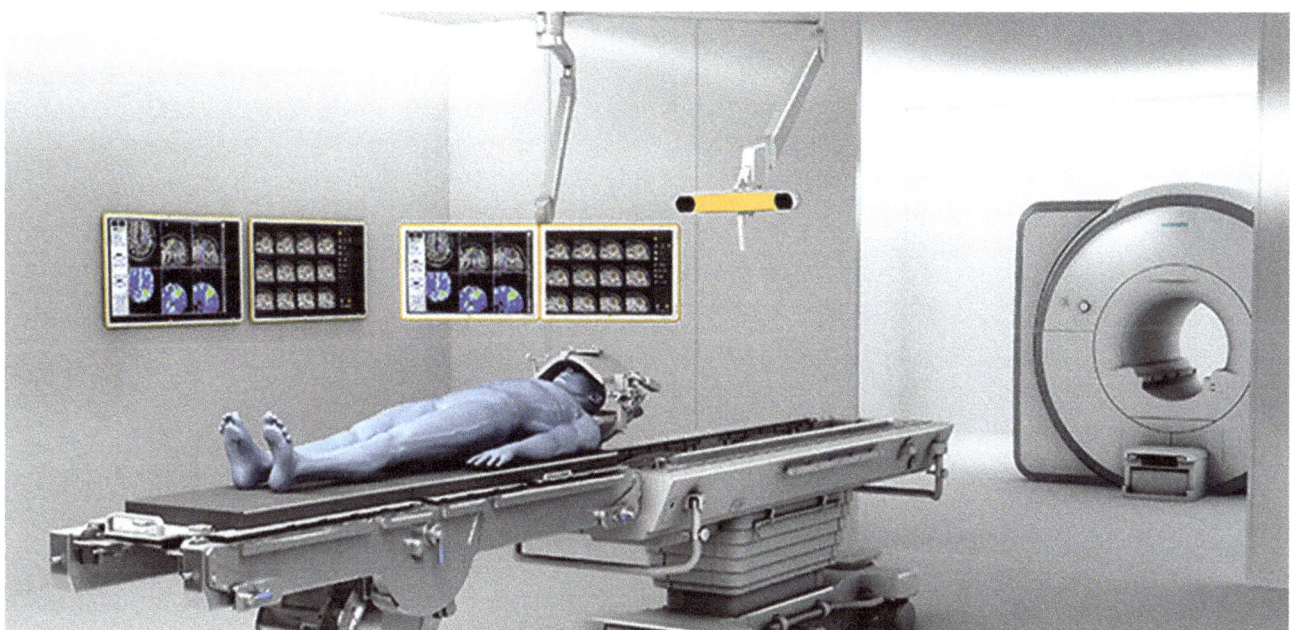

Figure 2.5 Intraoperative magnetic resonance imaging (MRI) suite. During surgery, patients can be moved into and out of a fixed MRI unit that was constructed directly within the operative suite or in an alcove adjacent to the operating suite
Courtesy: Brainlab® Inc., Westchester, IL.

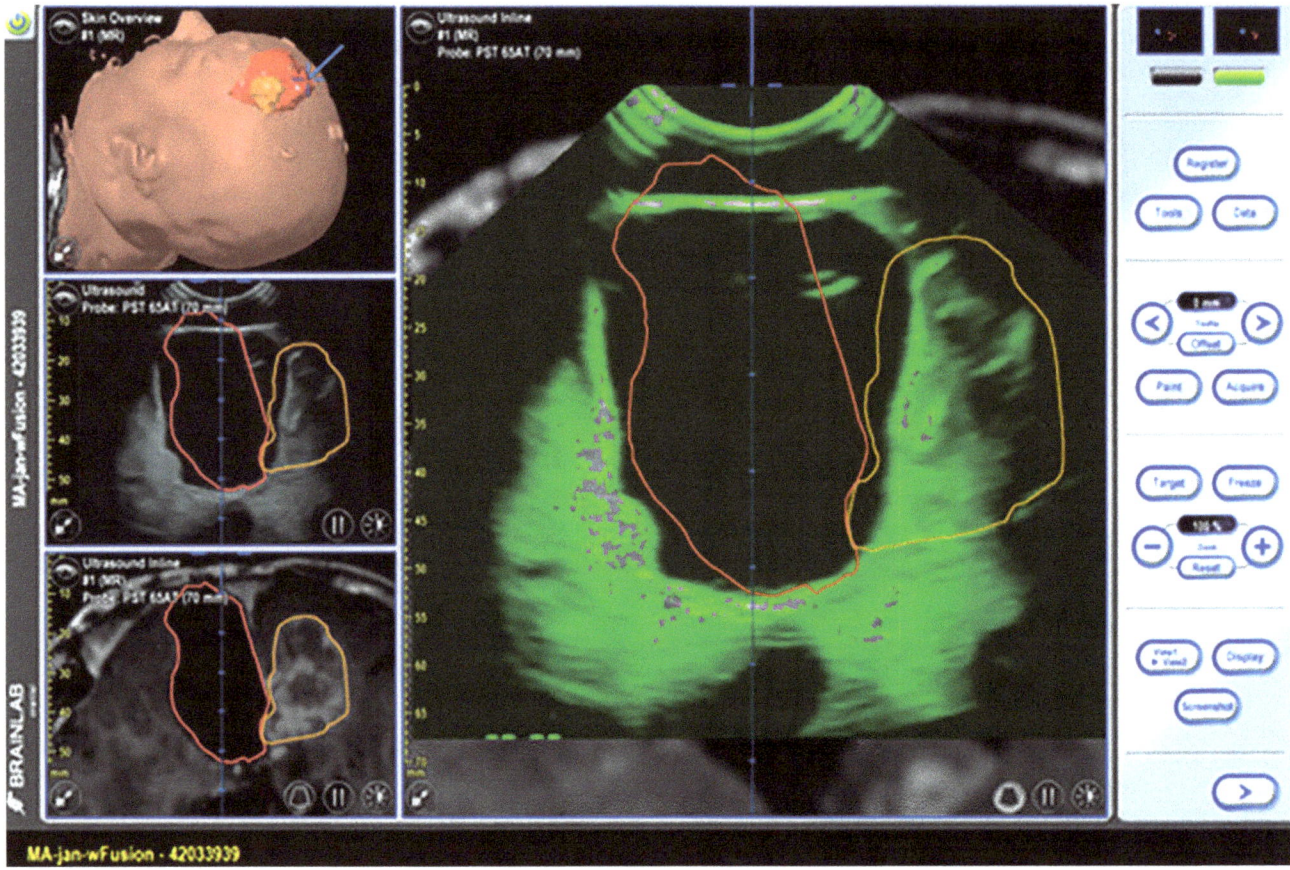

Figure 2.6 Preoperative magnetic resonance imaging (MRI) images have been integrated with the brainlab intraoperative ultrasound neuronavigational platform that can allow for real-time high resolution 3D ultrasound data
Courtesy: Brainlab® Inc., Westchester, IL.

CLINICAL BENEFITS OF INTRAOPERATIVE NEURONAVIGATION

Until the 1980s, cranial localization of the lesion, surgical planning of the extents of the craniotomy and incision were done using measurements taken from standard preoperative CT and MR images. This inevitably led to larger craniotomies, longer incisions and increased operative time. With the advent of neuronavigation, surgeons were able to identify where the intracranial lesion should be, thereby making a shorter incision, smaller craniotomy and thus, decreasing the overall surgical time for the patient.[1,28,29]

Multiple studies have shown the benefit of surgical navigation in intracranial surgery. In 2006, Willems et al. compared the patients that underwent surgery using intraoperative navigation with patients that underwent standard surgery using preoperative images alone. Outcomes they looked at included the duration of surgery, extent of resection and patient's functional status. In this study, it was demonstrated that the number of patients that had

residual tumor postoperatively was approximately half of those patients that underwent standard surgery.[30,31] In 2000, Paleologos published a study evaluating the clinical utility of patients that underwent image-guided craniotomy compared with conventional craniotomy.[29] While this study cited similar "operative times" between standard surgery and intraoperative image-guided surgery, there was a statistically significant shorter "surgical time" for the latter group ($p = 0.02$). In this study, "operative time" included the time from which the patient was under anesthesia to reversal of anesthesia while "surgical time" was from incision time to reversal of anesthesia. Likely, the reason operative times were similar in both cohorts was the increased surgical time in the standard surgery group due to longer incisions, larger craniotomies and increased time needed for surgeons to cautiously perceive and avoid anatomic structures was in exchange for the time needed to set up and register the image guidance system prior to incision time.

The aforementioned study showed that image-guided neurosurgery leads to decreased overall patient morbidity

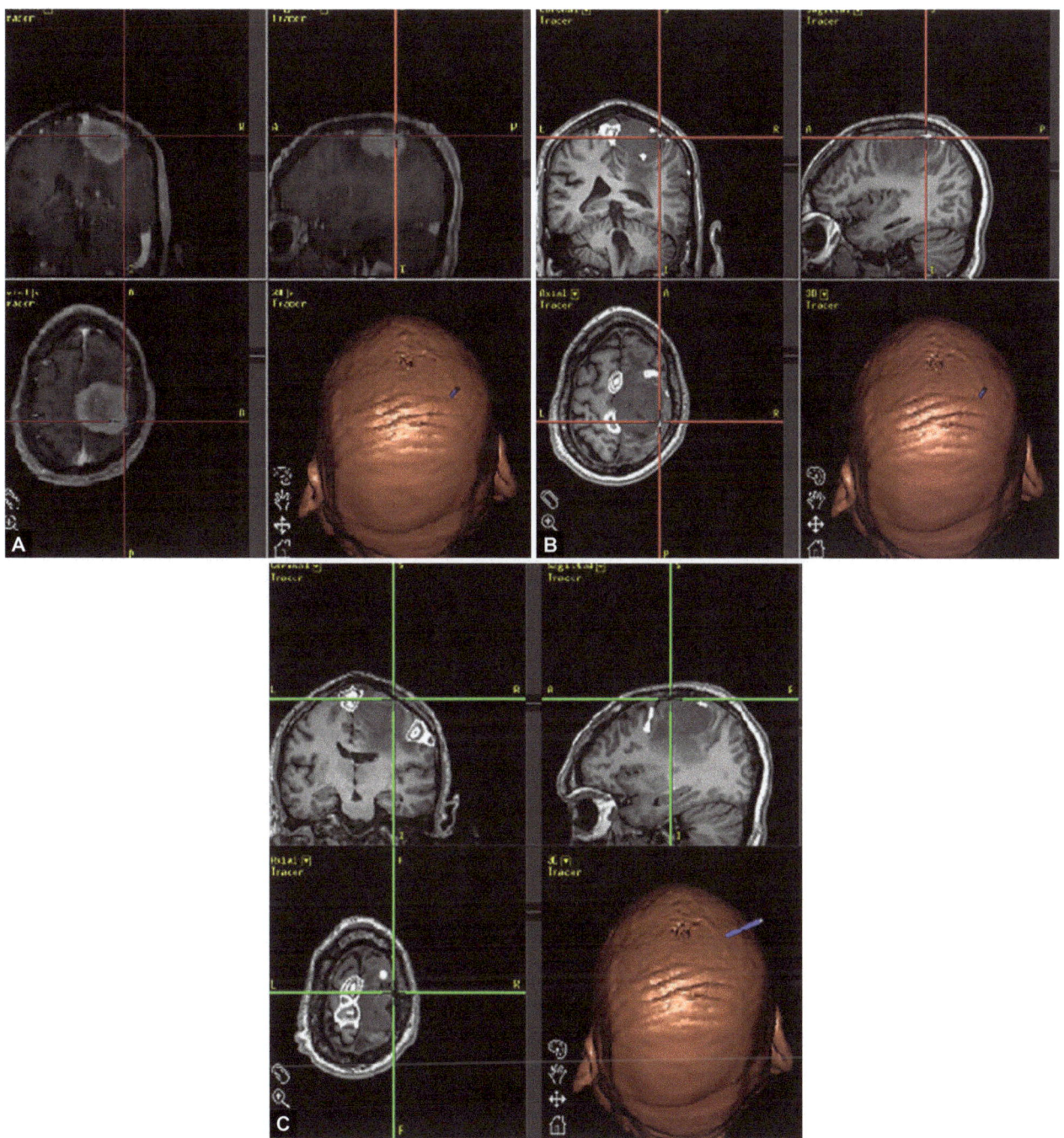

Figures 2.7A to C Series of medtronic stealth neuronavigation screenshot images that demonstrate a left frontoparietal mass. (A) The exact margins of the tumor can be visualized with a three-dimensional model reconstructed from thin cut magnetic resonance (MR) images; (B and C) Functional magnetic resonance imaging (fMRI) data has been incorporated into the neuronavigational plan in order to visualize areas of eloquence in relationship to the mass

and shorter postoperative inpatient hospital stays.[29,32,33] Complication rates in cases of standard surgery were significantly higher than that of cases where intraoperative image guidance was used (14% vs 6%, P = 0.019). Mean hospital stays were also reduced from 13.5 days to 8.5 days in cases where intraoperative image guidance was utilized (P = 0.017). Lastly, more cases of standard surgery patients required blood transfusions perioperatively than intraoperative image

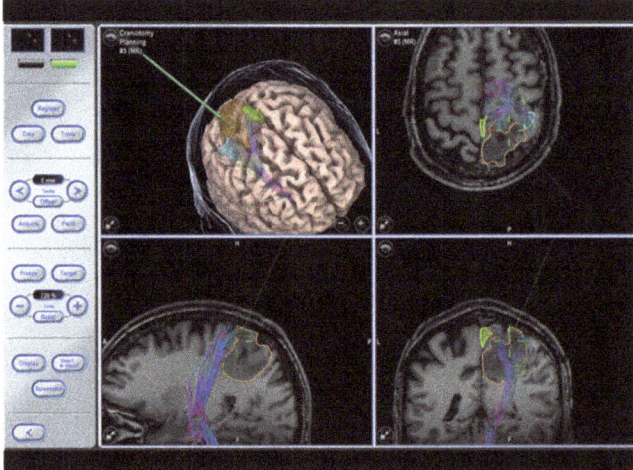

Figure 2.8 Cranial navigation software demonstrating tumor outlined and adjacent diffusion tensor imaging (DTI) fiber tracts of eloquent areas
Courtesy: Brainlab® Inc., Westchester, IL.

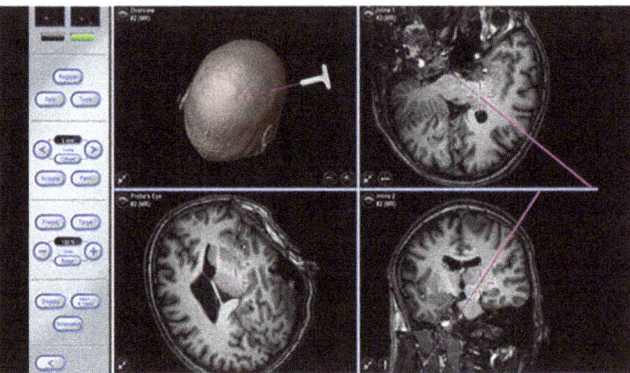

Figure 2.9 Computer screen shot taken during a frameless intracranial stereotactic biopsy using three-dimensional reconstructions from preoperative magnetic resonance imaging (MRI) images. The exact trajectory of the planned biopsy to a left thalamic lesion can be visualized in three-dimensional planes so that eloquent structures may be avoided *Courtesy:* Brainlab® Inc., Westchester, IL.

guidance system (P = 0.03). In another British study from the same year that looked mainly at the use of image guidance in patients undergoing craniotomy for meningioma resection. These results also demonstrated statistically significant shorter surgical times, shorter postoperative times in the intensive care unit and shorter overall length of hospital stay for patients in whom image-guided surgery was performed compared with standard surgery.[32,34]

Another benefit of neuronavigation is the ability to display 3D locations of instruments, with their orientations and trajectories in a precise manner **(Figure 2.9)**. For example, being able to plan a direct approach to a tumor or a catheter pass into a dysmorphic ventricle not only decreases overall operative time, but also decreases patient morbidity by decreasing brain manipulation and trauma. Vital structures such as dural venous sinuses and cranial nerves can also be avoided as 3D reconstructions of imaging data give precise feedback to the surgeon regarding their location. This, in turn, increases surgeon confidence and perception of safety, and thereby shortens surgical time.[29,35,36]

Interestingly, Schackert et al. retrospective analysis demonstrated neuronavigational devices allow not only a targeted approach, but allow multiple tumors to be excised in one session without increasing the patient's hospital stay.[33] Therefore, it is feasible that if a patient presents with multiple metastases that could be accessible via one single craniotomy, using intraoperative neuronavigation allows the surgeon to be able to resect more than a single lesion, and thereby decrease tumor burden and avoid the patient further invasive treatments, which may include additional craniotomies.

LIMITATIONS OF INTRAOPERATIVE NEURONAVIGATION

As with learning any new technique, there is a learning curve that is encountered when initially using neuronavigation. For the generation of neurosurgeons that were trained prior to age of neuronavigation, this learning curve is more apparent than perhaps with recently trained neurosurgeons and current neurosurgical residents. As neuronavigational techniques and system platforms become increasingly sophisticated, so does the time needed in order to learn how to use the navigational operating system, software and its updates. Even so, as neurosurgeons and the various technicians gain experience in the systems and its various features, the learning curve becomes easier and ultimately, the time spent in preoperative registration and planning is made up by the potential time taken in order to localize a lesion intraoperatively without guidance.[22,32] Therefore, as surgeons become comfortable with a particular navigational system and have foresight to counter the various nuances that each system has, they can utilize the navigational system to their benefit in the operating room.

One of the main limitations is intraoperative brain distortion, or brain shift. Studies have cited that brain shift can occur up to much as 2.4 cm during tumor resection.[37,38] Even subtle shifts in the brain can compromise placements of probes into deep intracranial structures or even inaccurate biopsies of deep lesions. In addition, older patients with cerebral atrophy have larger extra-axial cerebrospinal fluid (CSF) spaces and patients that have undergone previous surgery and/or radiation can increase scarring requiring more brain manipulation at the time of surgery.[39] Several papers have addressed this issue, and recommended techniques aimed to minimize brain distortion by minimizing use of mannitol, hypertonic saline and CSF drainage as well as the avoidance of pneumocephalus.[29,40-43] In addition, tracing around tumor margins with neuronavigation and subsequent dissection around cystic tumors without breaching the cyst wall, whenever possible, may help to decrease brain shift.[39] However, the most obvious way to avoid intraoperative errors in navigation due to shift is with updated imaging with ioMR, iCT, or intraoperative ultrasound (iUS), as will be discussed here.

The use of neuronavigation in surgery for the posterior fossa has been debated. Given the size and well-defined borders of the posterior fossa, some would argue against the necessity for it.[32] The limitations encountered with acquiring an adequate 3D registration model can be overcome by using surface fiducial markers that can be placed over the occiput prior to obtaining the preoperative images. In these cases, neuronavigation is invaluable when trying to access a deep-seated cerebellar arteriovenous malformation (AVM), a pineal tumor, or a small, deep cerebellar metastasis.

Lastly, the concept of intraoperative neuronavigation relies on adequate imaging capabilities. Thin cut preoperative CT images or MRI images must be acquired and in order to construct a 3D model, the technique with which they are acquired must be of good quality, with no significant movement of the patient, appropriate timing of contrast injection, and avoidance of gantry tilt.

OVERALL COSTS WITH NEURONAVIGATION

Neuronavigation systems are expensive and costs of acquiring one, including software, equipment, operative instruments ranges anywhere from $250,000 to just under $1 million dollars.[29] Based on one study, approximately 200 image-guided craniotomies would need to be performed in order to recover the cost of acquiring a neuronavigation system. The mean total cost per procedure was approximately 20% less for patients that underwent image-guided surgery compared with standard surgery, i.e. $14.480 versus $17, 360, P = 0.03. This includes additional preoperative scans needed for the neuronavigation system.[29] Additionally, Paleologos' study also demonstrated that increased hospital stays in cohorts that underwent standard surgery reflected the higher complication rates of these patients. Therefore, lower complication rates in patients that undergo image-guided surgery, and subsequent lower hospital stays for patients would lead to lower overall costs of the treatment. It must also be recognized that added costs of prolonged hospitalization secondary to increased complications ultimately translate to increased healthcare costs both for the patient and for society in general, in that these patients have a faster recoveries with

earlier return to work time, decreased morbidities, shorter follow-up time with decreased chance of needing adjuvant therapy.

INTRAOPERATIVE IMAGING

Intraoperative Ultrasonography

Intraoperative ultrasound (iUS) has been used in neurosurgery for many years.[27,44,45] While there is an abundance of evidence that ioMRI increases the extent of resection and improves overall outcomes, it is mainly available at larger tertiary care centers and therefore, is not widely available. Intraoperative ultrasonography, therefore, offers a more practical and cost-efficient alternative when iCT and ioMRI systems are not available. While conventional 2D-US have their inherent limitations, advances in the field of ultrasonography now allow 3D images to be integrated with neuronavigation platforms that can allow for high-resolution 3D ultrasound data that some authors claim is comparable to image quality of ioMRI **(Figure 2.6)**.[46] Also, because ultrasonographic devices are less expensive than iCT and ioMRI, their use does not necessitate any special requirements or place any restrictions in an operative room.

The largest reported experience with 3D ultrasonography has been in Norway, where Unsgaard et al. evaluated biopsies performed from tumor margins that were visible in US images and compared them with preoperative MR T1 and MR T2 images that were registered on neuronavigation. In their cohort of patients with low-grade gliomas (LGGs), biopsy results done using navigated 3D US correlated had equivalent results to those done using navigated preoperative T1 images.[46] While this study reported a high specificity and positive predictive value for resection of gliomas, there was a low negative predictive value as well; that is, even when iUS was negative, there was a possibility of tumor still present within the margins of the surgical cavity. The results of this study indicated that US does underestimate the extent of glioma infiltration, but that prior to resection, reformatted 3D US images are as helpful as MR images in localizing and delineating solid components of tumors and metastases.[46]

Additional studies demonstrated that image fusion between preoperative MR imaging and intraoperative 3D ultrasonography into an ultrasonography neuronavigation system is also possible **(Figure 2.6)**.[47,48] Solheim et al. looked at the use of the SonoWand system in their cohort of patients with high-grade gliomas. Their rate of gross total resection (GTR) was 63% in patients in whom the tumor was deemed "resectable". This indicates that while there is a learning curve as with most technologies, iUS is a relatively "user-friendly" and widely applicable technology.[49] Moiyadi et al. also reviewed their series of patients that underwent surgery using 3D navigable iUS for gliomas. In their cohort of malignant gliomas, GTR was achieved in 47% of the cases, with a GTR rate of 88% for the resectable group. In 59% of their cases, further resection was prompted by intraoperative images.[50]

Ultrasonography can also be used in conjunction with advanced image processing, such as DTI or functional MR data. In order to visualize fiber tracts and their relationship to tumors during resection, Coenen et al. described their technique of fusing preoperative DTI data with MR T1 data. This data was then coregistered into a 3D ultrasonography navigation system and used simultaneously with intraoperative 3D US images to visualize brain shift during tumor resection and associated deformation of the fiber tracts. Using fixed and shifting landmarks near fiber tracts adjacent to tumors, image data was sequentially updated during surgery, allowing for intraoperative identification and avoidance of eloquent intracranial areas.[24]

Rasmussen et al. reported on their series of 12 patients where preoperative fMRI and DTI images were obtained and imported into an US-based navigation system. iUS was used to update preoperative fMRI and DTI data. Navigation based on fMRI data was found to be beneficial for preoperative planning in all 12 cases. In five of the cases, DTI data was found to be useful for planning with the navigation system and in two cases, was important during the resection. The authors felt that while fMRI is beneficial for preoperative planning, DTI was helpful during the resection itself. This study demonstrated that the ability to update preoperative MRI data for brain shift using iUS-based neuronavigation was feasible and advantageous during surgery.[27]

In addition to intra-axial tumors, ultrasonography can be used for spinal surgery such as syrinx surgery, spinal tumors, hemangioblastomas, vascular malformations and even for pituitary surgery.[51-55] The Doppler capability of the US allows surgeons to obtain significant angiographic data intraoperatively, such as verifying complete resection of vascular lesions and visualization of major vessels in the vicinity of the tumor.[55] Using specific probes, it can also be used to guide catheters into ventricles as well as cystic lesions such as abscesses, metastases and arachnoid cysts.

Limitations of the iUS include the learning curve involved in getting oriented to US imaging. The inability to visualize the entire cranium can lead to difficulties with orientation. Additionally, as the Unsgaard group demonstrated, imaging artifacts created by blood products, hemostatic agents implanted within the resection cavity, and even the handling of the adjacent tissue can decrease the image quality and ultimately, its usefulness during surgery. Meticulous attention to these details can overcome these obstacles.[56] Moiyabi et al. suggest that using the merged images initially with both preoperative MR scans and iUS images initially facilitates the limitations encountered when initially learning the technology. Once the user becomes proficient with maneuvering the US, direct intraoperative ultrasonography can be used.[50]

Thus, while ioMRI may ultimately be better in terms of image quality, ioUS is a practical, cost-efficient modality of intraoperative imaging that can be utilized in a versatile manner. It can be used by both trained surgeons and residents, and does not require any significant changes to operative workflow or operating room infrastructure. When one becomes adept at the capabilities of the technology, ultrasonography offers a cost-efficient method to ioMRI in settings where resources are limited. With future improvements in image resolution and increasing the variety of different imaging modalities with which to merge ultrasonography data to, the scope of this technique can continue to expand.

Intraoperative Angiography

The question of performing intraoperative angiography remains a controversial one in that while it does allow for early identification of residual AVM, stenosis or occlusion of critical vessels, confirms aneurysm obliteration, it does increase operative time, and imaging quality is suboptimal in most cases.[57-59] Studies have shown that injection of intraoperative fluorescein during aneurysm surgery provided significant clinical utility by demonstration flow within the parent vessels and more importantly, in perforating vessels, thereby ultimately preventing unexpected stroke postoperatively.[60] Limitations in using intraoperative fluorescein are that it demonstrates visualization of vascular anatomy only that which has been dissected and exposed. Therefore, in cases where clipping of an aneurysm has been performed where the dome of aneurysm has not been completely exposed, intraoperative fluorescein is less useful in providing sufficient information as to whether the flow in the dome of the aneurysm has stopped. Nevertheless, intraoperative angiography is a simple method that provides real-time information in detecting the patency of parent, branching, perforating arteries and residual aneurysm and may be used in adjunct to other modalities such as Doppler US in order to prevent any unforeseen complications or avoid further surgery.[61,62]

Intraoperative Computed Tomography

The first iCT was used in early 1980s. With this first model, the gantry was immobile and patients had to be positioned on the scanner table and moved into the gantry. Therefore, only certain positions were possible and patients could not be placed in a head clamp during the scan. In the early 1990s, a mobile CT scanner was developed, where the scanner was installed on a gantry carrier and therefore, the scan could be performed with the patient on a regular operating table with the CT being moved over the patient.[63-65] Given the image quality of the early scanners, along with the cost, modification to the operating room workflow, and the novelty of the concept, it was mainly used in stereotactic and functional neurosurgery initially.

Today, the modern iCT scanner has the spatial resolution that surpassed most ioMRI systems. The same scanner hardware inside the gantry as a standard non-intraoperative scanner is used so that high quality, multiplanar, 3D reconstructions can be obtained and these images can also be coregistered with preoperative MR images in order to gain better resolution of the soft tissue contrast (Figure 2). Most importantly, the radiation exposure can be filtered and reduced for both the patient and staff using special automated dose modulation software.[63,66] Additionally, it can be argued that the overall radiation exposure is not increased because both the usual pre and postoperative CT scans are replaced by the iCT scan.[63]

One of the major advantages of iCT over ioMRI is that with neuronavigational software, cranial as well as spinal neurosurgery can be performed, with continuous updates available for navigation. Because virtually any part of the body can be scanned, it can be used by a number of surgical subspecialties and therefore increases its applicability and cost-effectiveness for the institution purchasing the scanner **(Figure 2.2)**. Normal operating room tables and surgical instruments can be used without significant interruption of operating room workflow. It is particularly useful for complex spinal instrumentations and spinal trauma. Intraoperative scans can be obtained once the patient is in the final position, after correction of the subluxation and bony decompression has been achieved, prior to and after placement of instrumentation, reducing the rate of misplaced hardware and revision surgery.[63,67]

While iCT has demonstrated to be beneficial in contrast enhancing lesions, it has been proven to be less helpful in non-contrast enhancing lesions, such as low-grade gliomas as well as tumors at the skull base. Margins of the tumor cannot be readily identified with these tumors due to similar contrast density compared to normal brain parenchyma or bony artifacts. Additionally, while the radiation dose of iCT can be modulated, it must still be used with caution in children. Lastly, similarly to ioMRI, specific head holders and pins must be utilized in order to minimize metal imaging artifact.[63]

Intraoperative Magnetic Resonance Imaging

Neurosurgeons have long been using some form of intraoperative imaging, both for spine and cranial surgery. Since the advent of X-ray, fluoroscopy has been used for both spinal and cranial neurosurgery. Intraoperative CT scans provided much needed real-time feedback that surgeons often needed.[12] However, performing repeated CT scans for a patient undergoing craniotomy not only exposed the patient to significant ionizing radiation, but the quality of the images

acquired were not ideal when operating on lesions that were not well visualized on CT imaging to begin with, such as LGGs, cortical dysplasias, or hamartomas.

The ability to update the stereotactic neuronavigation system with the newly acquired, high quality intraoperative imaging is the most salient feature of the ioMRI system. Given that the ioMRI system can acquire such standard sequences as T1, T2 and post-contrast T1 weighted scans, surgeons are able to obtain highly sensitive images that can not only account for the brain shift that has occurred during surgery, but also can allow surgeons to determine their tumor margins and extent of resection **(Figures 2.10A to D)**.[21,22]

Initial ioMRI systems were low field units with a 0.5 Tesla (T) magnet with a "double donut" design. Patients are positioned and fixed inside the scanner and the surgeons had to stand between the coils in order to access the patient and more importantly, they had a limited operative field, with a 56 cm space between the coils of the magnet. With this ioMRI unit, an infrared LED-based neuronavigational system was also integrated within the vertical space between the coils.[21] Newer models allowed the magnet to be "mobile"; the MRI unit could either be moved away from the patient when not scanning **(Figures 2.3 and 2.4)** or the patient could be moved into and out of a fixed MRI unit that was constructed directly within the operative suite or in an alcove adjacent to the operating suite **(Figure 2.5)**. Studies have demonstrated that movement of either entity did not risk surgical sterility or affect patient safety.[68]

Generally, low-field strength refers to ioMRI systems of 0.5 T or less, but other unique "ultra-low field" models emerged in order to overcome the obstacles of size, restrictive operative access and minimizing patient movement. These systems were 0.2 T strength or less and can usually be used with a regular operating room staff team **(Figures 2.3 and 2.4)**.[69] The benefits of the compact nature of the model are counterbalanced by the reduced image quality and limited imaging modalities available such as spectroscopy, angiography, or diffusion-weighted imaging when comparing with higher strength systems. On the other hand, while the high-field systems (1.5 T and greater) enable acquisition of higher quality images with more "advanced" techniques, these systems come at higher costs and the work of integrating the system not only into the operating room workflow, but also involve reorganizing the operating suite's infrastructure **(Figure 2.5)**. In addition, additional instruments and especially trained personnel may be needed. Lastly, the extent to which this affects the neurosurgeon's overall routine and overall surgical time varies between the different systems.

Low-field Intraoperative MRI for Resection of High-grade Glioma

While ioMRI has multiple applications, many studies have demonstrated that one of the main benefits of using ioMRI has

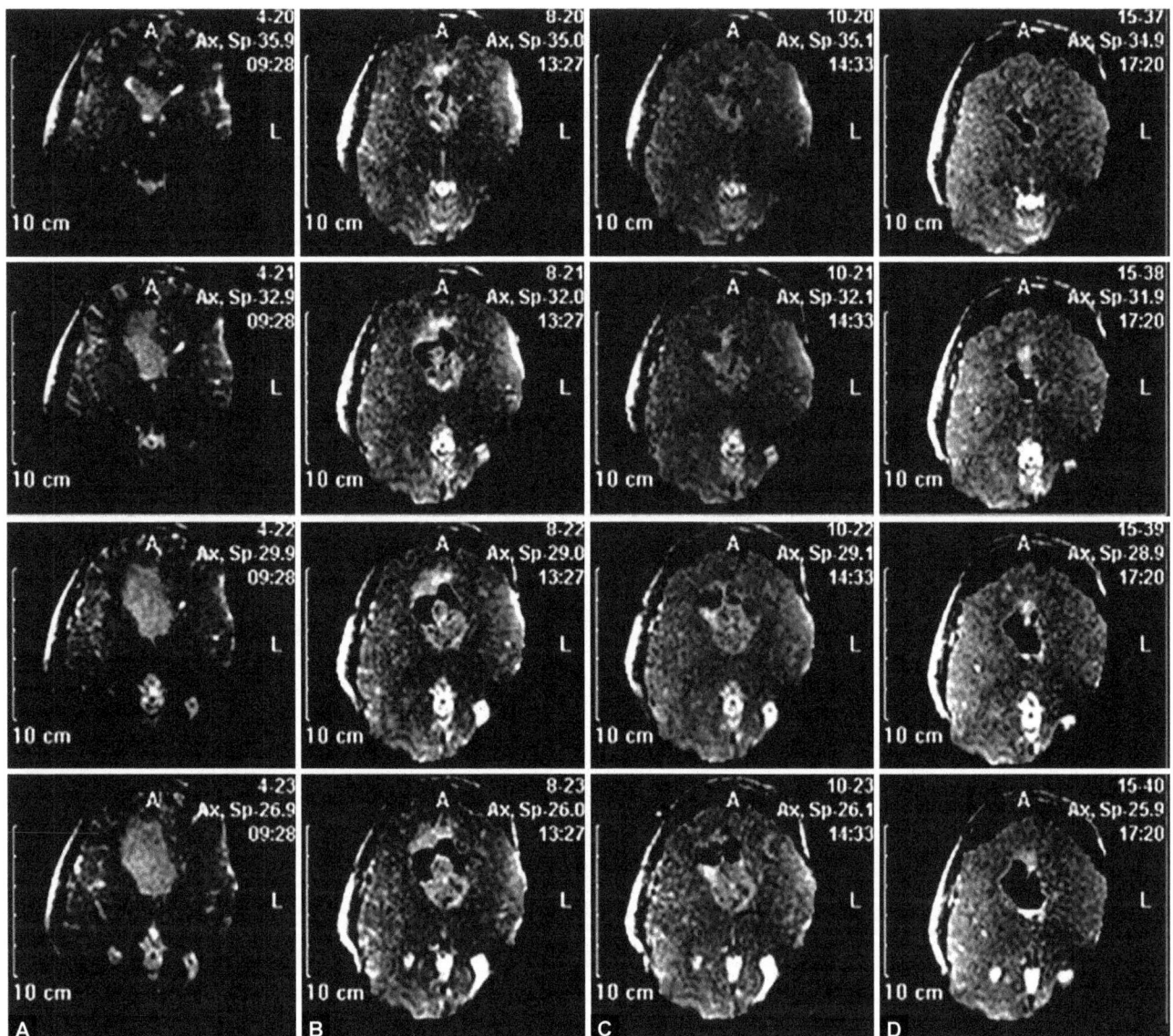

Figures 2.10A to D Intraoperative MRI (ioMRI) images obtained on a patient with an intraventricular mass using low field ioMRI. (A) Preoperative axial T1 postcontrast images; (B) First intraoperative magnetic resonance (MR) images performed demonstrating partial resection of mass; (C) Second intraoperative MR images demonstrating residual tumor; (D) Final intraoperative MR images confirming gross total resection of tumor
Courtesy: Odin PoleStar® N-20 ioMRI system.

been to increase the extent of resection of glial tumors.[38,70-72] In 2011, Kubben and colleagues performed a systemic review evaluating the added value of ioMRI in surgical resection of high-grade gliomas.[73] They reviewed 12 non-randomized cohort studies that matched selection criteria from 1999–2010. In this meta-analysis, they compared extent of tumor resection, quality of life and survival within these studies. Knauth et al. was one of the first groups to evaluate, in 1999, whether low-field ioMRI with neuronavigation use increased the extent of tumor resection in patients with high-grade gliomas compared with neuronavigation alone. In 22/38 cases (53.7%), ioMRI use demonstrated residual tumor. In 17

of the 22 cases, resection of residual tumor was resumed after updating the neuronavigation system. Early postoperative imaging demonstrated that eight patients had residual tumor, which had been seen on intraoperative imaging as well. Therefore, 14 of the 22 patients ultimately had GTRs using ioMRI, increasing the GTR rate from 36.6% to 75.6% (P = 0.004).[70]

Shortly, thereafter, two additional studies were published looking at extent of resection in high grade gliomas. Wirtz and colleagues report on 66 cases of high-grade glioma that underwent surgery. Intraoperative scans demonstrated residual enhancing tumor in 41/66 patients (62.1%), no contrast enhancement in 18/66 patients (27.2%), and inconclusive in 7/66 patients (10.6%). For 43 of these cases, there was additional resection of tumor based on intraoperative MR imaging. Early postoperative imaging demonstrated GTR in 37 of the 66 patients (56%), and residual tumor in 22/66 patients (33%). This study indicated that ioMRI use increased the GTR rate from 27.2% to 56%. The median survival for patients that underwent GTR was 13.3 months compared to those that underwent subtotal resection, which was 9.2 months; these results were statistically significant (P = 0.0035).[71] Bohinski and colleagues also reported on their cohort of 30 patients with high-grade glioma. Nine patients did not require additional resection, and ultimately had GTR on postoperative imaging. About 17 patients had intraoperative scans for which additional resection was needed after ioMRI. Of the patients who had additional resection, 13 ultimately had GTR, significantly increasing the GTR rate from 30% to 73%.[68]

Schneider and colleagues performed a retrospective analysis on 31 primary glioblastoma multiforme (GBM) patients on a 0.5 T scanner. They performed volumetric analysis of tumor preoperatively and postoperatively. First ioMRI scan demonstrated GTR in two of the 31 patients while last ioMRI scan demonstrated GTR in 11 of the 31 patients, thereby increasing the GTR rate from 6.5% to 35.5%. Median survival for patients with subtotal resection was 237 days compared with 537 days for patients that underwent GTR (P = 0.004).[73,74] Lenaburg et al. in their retrospective analysis of 35 GBM cases using a 0.2 T scanner, cite that 25 of the 35 cases led to additional resection, and last ioMRI scan in 27 of the 35 cases showed tumor resection of greater than 95%.[73,75]

Senft et al. published a study in 2010 (Technol Canc Res Treat) that retrospectively examined 41 primary GBM cases on a 0.15 T scanner. Ten patients underwent surgery with ioMRI where 31 patients underwent conventional surgery with neuronavigation. All 10 cases that utilized ioMRI demonstrated GTR on postoperative MRI performed within 72 hours of surgery, whereas 19 of the 31 cases that underwent conventional surgery had evidence of GTR. In addition, median survival for the ioMRI group was 88 weeks compared to 68 weeks in the cohort that underwent conventional surgery (P = 0.07).[76]

This report was followed up by the same authors with a prospective, randomized and controlled trial in 2011. In this study, patients were randomized to a treatment arm that underwent ioMRI-assisted surgery while those in the control group had surgery with neuronavigation only. The primary endpoint was extent of resection on early postoperative MRI within 72 hours of surgery; secondary endpoints were volume of residual tumor on postoperative MRI and progression-free survival at 6 months. Gross total resections were achieved in 23 (96%) of the 24 patients that had ioMRI assisted surgery compared to 17 (68%) of 25 patients in the control group (P = 0.023). Median postoperative volume of contrast enhancing tumor was 0 cm^3 in the intraoperative MRI group and 0.03

cm^3 in the conventional group (P = 0.0015). At 6 months, 16/24 (67%) patients in the ioMRI group had stable disease compared to 9/25 (36%) (P = 0.046). Lastly, the ioMRI group had a median progression free survival of 226 days compared to 154 days in the conventional surgery group, but this was not statistically significant (P = 0.083). This study was the first Level I evidence that demonstrated that ioMRI improved the extent of resection of high-grade gliomas.[77]

Senior Author's Experience

In the senior author's experience with low-field ioMRI (PoleStar N20), 531 neurosurgical procedures were performed using the ioMRI between the years of 2000 and 2013. Of these cases, 162 cases (31%) were for glioma and 102 cases (19%) were for resection of pituitary adenoma. In the LGG cohort (n = 68), use of the ioMRI affected the course of surgery in 44 patients (64.7%). 35 of the 44 patients' tumors (79.5%) were deemed to be "resectable", given its location and relationship to eloquent cortex and vital structures, and therefore, had a craniotomy for either intended subtotal resection or GTR. Nine patients had an "unresectable" tumor and therefore, underwent a stereotactic biopsy. In the patients that underwent a craniotomy for LGG resection, ioMRI affected the course of surgery in 24 patients (69%) by demonstrating residual tumor, which led to additional tumor resection. In 10 patients (23%), ioMRI confirmed that the surgical goals had been reached, thereby avoiding further dissection and surgery that could have led to new neurological deficit. In one patient, a post-resection hemorrhage was demonstrated within the surgical bed, which led to evacuation of the hematoma intraoperatively. Intraoperative MRI was helpful in patients that underwent stereotactic biopsy in that it confirmed the cannula placement within radiographically lesional tissue, and therefore avoided further passes of the stereotactic cannula. In three patients, intraoperative MRI led to change in position of the cannula as neuronavigation from preoperative images was inaccurate. In the high-grade glioma cohort, intraoperative MRI affected surgery in 56/94 patients (60%). About 49 patients underwent craniotomy while seven underwent a stereotactic biopsy given the location of the tumor. In the patients who underwent resection for HGG, intraoperative MR imaging led to additional tumor resection in 37 patients (39%) **(Figure 2.10)**. In 12 patients, ioMRI confirmed intended extent of resection, avoided further dissection, and/or demonstrated the surgical bed's relationship to eloquent brain (13%). In five of the seven patients that underwent stereotactic biopsy, cannula placement was readjusted either based on ioMR images demonstrating less optimal placement of cannula or due to inconclusive or negative frozen biopsy.

One hundred and nine patients underwent surgery for resection of pituitary adenoma. In this cohort, ioMRI affected surgery in 53 cases (49%). In 37/53 (70%) patients, ioMRI led to additional tumor removal and dissection. In 13 patients, ioMRI demonstrated adequate decompression of the optic chiasm with no evidence of residual tumor. Therefore, in these patients, further dissection was avoided (25%). In one case, ioMRI demonstrated that the initial transphenoidal approach was too low given abnormal transnasal anatomy; trajectory was then redirected more superiorly afterwards. In three additional cases, ioMRI guidance was utilized to drain a multilobulated cyst associated with craniopharyngioma, place a ventricular catheter in another large cyst within a craniopharyngioma and lastly, to confirm decompression of the optic chiasm from a suprasellar cyst.

High-field Intraoperative MRI for Resection of High-grade Glioma

Much less data is available regarding the use of high-field ioMRI, likely due to the fact that their utilization and incorporation into surgery is much less compared to the lower field ioMRI systems given the increased costs and required changes to operating room infrastructure. In 2006, Nimsky et al. reviewed their cohort of 137 patients that underwent resection of tumors using intraoperative high-field MRI in an operative suite utilizing functional neuronavigation. Utilization of the ioMRI increased the GTR rate from 27% to 40%.[38]

In 2009, Hatiboglu and colleagues published one of the first series looking at volumetric measurement of extent of resection of gliomas using high-field ioMRI (1.5 T). 21 patients in their cohort of 44 underwent further resection of residual tumor based on ioMRI results, with resultant complete resection of tumor in 15 (70%) of the 21 patients. GTR for the entire cohort as a result of utilizing ioMRI was achieved in 15 (24%) of the 44 patients. In patients with GBM, extent of resection increased from 83% to 98% after ioMRI scan, with resultant GTR in 12 (92%) of 13 patients (P <0.001).[72]

Most recently, Haydon et al. reported their results of resection of glioma using high-field 1.5 T ioMRI. Preoperative, intraoperative and postoperative volumetric extents of resection were determined using manual segmentation. Use of ioMRI resulted in further extent of resection in 113 (60%) of their glioma cases, with higher frequency of additional resection in their high-grade glioma group compared with their LGG group (65% vs 54%). In the high-grade glioma cohort, the number of complete resections increased from 24% to 57% with use of ioMRI leading to additional resection. The additional resection after ioMRI led to increased mean extent of resection from 94% to 98%.[78]

Intraoperative MRI for Resection of Low-grade Glioma

In the past, surgical management for LGGs has been under debate. Management of patients with presumed LGGs would be to perform a biopsy and then treat with radiation. However, several large prospective studies have demonstrated that

chemotherapy and radiation have been unsuccessful as primary treatment for these tumors.[79]

Claus et al. reviewed their series of patients at Brigham and Women's Hospital, evaluating the utilization of ioMRI for patients with gliomas. Complete resection was achieved in 56 (36%) of 156 patients with LGGs. In this study, patients who underwent partial resection of tumor were 1.4 times more likely than patients with total resection to develop recurrence. Additionally, patients who underwent partial resection were at 4.9 times the risk of death as patient who underwent total resection. This was one of the first studies to suggest an association between surgical resection and survival for patients who underwent surgery for LGG with ioMRI.[80] Following this study, additional retrospective studies have demonstrated that surgical resection increased survival in patients with LGGs.[81-83]

In the Hatiboglu et al. study from MD Anderson Cancer Center, extent of resection (EOR) of LGGs was examined using high-field 1.5 T ioMRI. The EOR increased from 63% to 100% for patients with nonenhancing World Health Organization (WHO) grade I gliomas. In the group that had nonenhancing tumors that were WHO grade II glioma on pathology, performing an ioMRI scan led to an increase in the percentage of tumor resected from 69% to 78%. While these results were not statistically significant due to limited number of patients in both cohorts, these implied that for low-grade nonenhancing tumors, ioMRI did lead to increased tumor resection.[72]

Pamir et al. published their series of patients using an ultra-high field ioMRI with a 3 T magnet utilizing MR spectroscopy. In this study, 56 patients underwent surgery using the ioMRI. At first ioMRI imaging, GTR was achieved in 31 (55.4%) of cases, with residual tumor remaining in 25 (44.6%). What was interesting about this study was that intraoperative sonography was also used to localize tumor, and then concurrently with the ioMRI scans to detect residual tumor. Only in four (16%) of the 25 cases was sonography able to detect the residual tumor. This was compared to 21 (37.5%) patients that had tumor that was not appreciated by gross examination or via ultrasonography that was picked up via ioMRI. There was additional surgical resection of tumor in 21 of the 25 cases, with ultimately, GTR achieved in 41 (73.2%) of the 56 patients, increasing the overall GTR rate from 55.4% to 73.2%. This study also showed that while intraoperative ultrasonography is useful for localization of tumor and determination of EOR, it has decreased sensitivity for detecting residual tumor when compared with ioMRI. In addition, proton MR spectroscopy was a capability that was used intraoperatively with the high-field ioMRI in order to differentiate residual tumor tissue from peritumoral changes that would not be possible with ultrasonography or even low-field ioMRI.[84,85]

While the aforementioned study used high-field ioMRI, Senft et al. evaluated their results for gliomas using low-field MRI and compared contrast-enhancing tumors with nonenhancing tumors. In this cohort of 21 cases with nonenhancing tumors, 14 (66.7%) patients' intraoperative scans demonstrated residual tumor, leading to further resection in 10 patients (47.6%). In this cohort of 10 patients with residual tumor, the intended goal for GTR was in two patients and this was achieved using ioMRI. In the remaining eight patients, additional resection was continued until the surgeon deemed it not possible due to relationship of tumor to eloquent cortex. Therefore, while the GTR rate was not as high for the cohort of patients with nonenhancing lower grade tumors compared with enhancing tumors, the surgical goal of maximal subtotal tumor resection could be achieved utilizing ioMRI. While there was an increased rate of complete tumor resection in patients with contrast enhancing tumors, the authors noted that intraoperative visualization of complete resection is less specific with non-contrast enhancing tumors. They suggested that when using low-field ioMRI systems, sequences such as intraoperative T2 or fluid attenuation inversion recovery (FLAIR) sequences may more helpful in delineating tumor margins for nonenhancing tumors. To date, there has not been any study that has directly compared low-field ioMRI with high-field ioMRI in EOR for gliomas.[69]

Intraoperative MRI for Transphenoidal Surgery

Intraoperative MRI has been used for transphenoidal surgery to treat sellar and suprasellar tumors since 2000.[86-95] The ability to detect residual tumor via ioMRI can increase the rate of complete tumor removal, and prevent injury to vital structures such as optic chiasm and carotid arteries. For nonfunctioning macroadenomas, ioMRI has demonstrated to be useful as once the tumor has been partially decompressed, anatomical shifts may occur such as the bowing down of the diaphragm sella and CSF leak and egress which can prove preoperative imaging used for neuronavigation less sensitive. Wu et al. study demonstrated that low-field ioMRI use resulted in additional tumor resection in 17 (49%) of 55 cases, and increased the rate of complete resection from 58% to 84%.[95] Nimsky et al. also looked at their cohort of nonfunctioning macroadenomas and using a high-field ioMRI, showed that their rate of complete tumor resection increased from 58% to 82%.[92] Both these studies demonstrated that while ioMRI does increase the rate of complete resection, the strength of the magnetic field was not a factor in transphenoidal surgery for nonfunctioning macroadenomas.

Berkmann et al. evaluated the correlation between visual improvement and optic nerve decompression detected by ioMRI in patients that underwent transphenoidal resection of pituitary lesions. Intraoperative MR imaging was performed after the surgeon felt that complete resection or surgical goals, (i.e. decompression of optic chiasm) had been achieved, if complete tumor removal was not safely possible. About 32 patients underwent surgery, and complete resection was achieved in 17 patients (53%), as demonstrated by initial ioMRI scan. Eight patients (25%) of the total cohort underwent further resection, and in four of these eight patients, suprasellar remnants of tumor were detected with subsequent decompression of the optic chiasm. Improvement of visual acuity was noted in 24 of the 32 patients (86%) one month postoperatively. In addition, ioMRI demonstrated residual tumor in the suprasellar or parasellar region in two patients that required transcranial procedures at a later time. This study implied that use of ioMRI may allow for early detection of symptomatic, compressive suprasellar remnants that may not otherwise detected until postoperatively.[96]

For functioning pituitary adenomas, ioMRI use has been less reported. This may be because most functioning adenomas present earlier, and are often smaller at diagnosis. For functioning adenomas, complete tumor resection is crucial for long-term endocrine remission.[86,97-99] In Fahlbusch et al. study, high-field ioMRI increased the rate of endocrine remission from 33% to 44% during the first 3 months postoperatively while ultra-low-field ioMRI increased the remission rate by 5.1% during the first postoperative month.[87,100] While the aforementioned studies demonstrated a relatively small increase in the remission rate and short term follow up, Tanei et al. study evaluating the use of high-field 1.5 T ioMRI for transphenoidal surgery for functioning adenomas with a follow up of 13–54 months demonstrated a long-term remission rate increase from 57% to 79%.[86] Additionally, postoperative imaging is difficult to interpret many times given that postoperative changes, including sellar floor reconstruction may distort anatomy.[99] Utilization of ioMRI may detect tumor remnants that may otherwise be difficult to appreciate on standard postoperative MRI.[86]

Adjunctive Techniques with Intraoperative MRI

While intraoperative imaging provides real-time anatomical information, what is at least equally important is the ability to identify functional tissue so that neurological function may be preserved during surgery. Studies evaluating cortical mapping for glioma surgery have demonstrated that infiltrative tumors can have functional tissue contained within the tumor substance.[101] Therefore, being able to obtain a complete resection may be at the expense of causing a catastrophic neurological deficit. Utilizing other techniques such as intraoperative monitoring, awake cortical mapping and subcortical mapping can provide significant information about the relationship of the tumor and its margins to functional brain. Hatiboglu et al. study from MD Anderson Cancer Center demonstrated that intraoperative cortical mapping is feasible with intraoperative MR imaging, providing the capability of maximizing extent of resection and minimizing postoperative neurological deficit.[26]

Leuthardt et al. described their technique of performing awake craniotomies with intraoperative cortical mapping and high-field ioMRI .They performed 12 awake craniotomies and demonstrated 11 of the 12 ioMRI scans demonstrated residual tumor. Five of the tumors were in eloquent areas, while in six cases, further surgical resection was performed, with an ultimate GTR in five of the 12 patients.[102] Weingarten et al. also report their series of patients that underwent awake cortical mapping and ioMRI. Their GTR rate was 70%, with no patients having a permanent postoperative deficit.[103] These studies demonstrate that using both techniques proved to be complementary as it maximized tumor resection while identifying those patients in which further surgery would have caused a neurological deficit.

Other functional imaging modalities such as fMRI, positron emission tomography (PET), magnetic source imaging, cortical and subcortical mapping, and using DTI are now being used in order to identify these functional areas so that they can be avoided during surgery (**Figures 2.7 and 2.8**).[84,104] Nimsky et al. performed fMRI intraoperative DTI sequences using high-field ioMRI in 37 patients undergoing glioma surgery. Using intraoperative MR tractography, the authors were able to show that white matter tracts shift from −8 mm to +15 mm and that their position in relation to the tumor resection cavity margin also changed. In deep-seated tumors near eloquent areas of the brain, intraoperative DTI plays a valuable role (**Figure 2.8**).[104]

A more recently used method for intraoperative tumor visualization is utilizing fluorescence guidance and 5-aminolevulenic acid (5-ALA). 5-ALA is orally administered preoperatively, and is systemically metabolized and promotes accumulation of fluorescent protoporphyrin IX into high-grade gliomas. Studies have demonstrated that higher grade gliomas accumulate more protoporphyrin IX compared to lower grade gliomas because of increased proliferation and blood-brain barrier permeability.[105-108] Given the selective accumulation of this agent into tumors, using an operating microscope with the appropriate filter allows the surgeon to delineate normal tissue and tumor tissue. Initial studies by Stummer et al. and Koc et al. demonstrated significant differences in rates of GTR between 5-ALA fluorescein-guided resection versus control.[107-111] While there was a statistically significant increase in progression free survival for the 5-ALA group compared with the control group, there was no significant difference in overall survival times between the two groups.

Tsugu and colleagues published a study in 2011 that compared ioMRI-guided resection with resection guided by 5-ALA and ioMRI. Of the 21 patients that were 5-ALA induced fluorescence positive, surgery with ioMRI was performed in 10 with an average resection rate of 92.6% versus 92.8% in patients who underwent surgery without ioMRI. 5-ALA fluorescence was not detected in 12 patients with gliomas, and in this cohort, surgery with ioMRI was performed in nine, with the average resection rate of 89.2% versus 68.7% average resection rate in patients without ioMRI. Therefore, in patients that were 5-ALA fluorescence negative, ioMRI was beneficial for achieving a better resection rate. It must be noted, however, that the group that was 5-ALA negative had greater percentage of patients with WHO grade II and III gliomas (75%) compared with the group that was 5-ALA positive, of which the majority was WHO grade IV (81%).[112]

Eyupoglu et al. also evaluated ioMRI in combination with 5-ALA, with superimposed functional neuronavigation. Tumor resection was carried out using the 5-ALA signal with functional neuronavigation guidance in order to avoid eloquent areas. Once 5-ALA signal was no longer seen, an ioMRI was performed. If residual tumor was identified on ioMRI scans, decision to continue with additional resection was made if functional neuronavigation demonstrated a good margin between residual tumor and functional brain tissue. In all cases, the 5-ALA signal was redetected once surgery was continued. In their cohort of 37 patients, all of whom had WHO grade III or IV gliomas, 21 ioMRI scans confirmed complete resection performed with 5-ALA fluorescence. In the remaining subgroup where patients that had tumors adjacent, but not within eloquent brain areas, the combination of 5-ALA, and ioMRI increased the extent of tumor resection from 61.7% to 100%. Only one patient had a decrease in their postoperative Karnofsky performance score by 20%. Additionally, in patients that had tumors within eloquent brain areas, ioMRI in combination with functional neuronavigation proved to be superior to 5-ALA resection technique.[113]

OPTIMIZATION OF COSTS OF INTRAOPERATIVE NAVIGATION AND IMAGING

Given the mounting need for delivery of "cost-effective" medical care, well-designed studies assessing the value of integrating intraoperative imaging and neuronavigation will need to be conducted. The biggest obstacle in the implementation of these technologies is the cost. A modern high-field ioMRI system costs approximately US $3,000,000. In addition, surgical and anesthetic equipment used in the operating room, shielding of the operating room, and software and MR equipment upgrades and maintenance ultimately costs the hospital over US $3,000,000. If this cost cannot be matched by the number of cases for which it is used for, centers now have justified the cost by using the high-field (1.5 T) MRI for generalized diagnostic purposes for the hospital during operating room "off-time".[114]

There is sufficient evidence at this point that the use of neuronavigation and intraoperative imaging can reduce costs by decreasing reoperation rates, increasing patient safety and decreasing neurological morbidity. Furthermore, by increasing the extent of resection of tumors while preserving neurological function, these technologies are decreasing not only the likelihood of recurrence but also overall survival. Hall et al. published a study in 2003 comparing the costs and benefits of brain tumor resection in a conventional operating room versus ioMRI suite. In this study, ioMRI surgery had a shorter length of stay, lower total hospital costs and lower cost-to-charge ratio compared to conventional operating room surgery, suggesting that ioMRI surgery was correlated with improved net health outcomes. This study, however, was a retrospective, nonrandomized, case-controlled study with a small patient cohort.[115]

Makary et al. recently compared the clinical effectiveness and costs of using a low-field ioMRI compared with a conventional MRI for brain tumor surgery. Intraoperative MRI patients tended to have shorter hospital length of stay (LOS) compared with the conventional surgery group; however, this was not statistically significant. Patients undergoing ioMRI-guided surgery had fewer postoperative complications than the conventional cohort. While EOR was not analyzed between the two cohorts, repeat resection occurred at a longer time interval than for the conventional group (P = 0.02). This study also performed a feasibility analysis for a low-field ioMRI system and concluded that the ioMRI had substantially greater capital costs compared to the average capital cost of ultrasonography and CT. Based on the author's institutional experience, the total implementation and operation cost for a low-field ioMRI's 5 year useful life was over $3.8 million while the depreciation cost per ioMRI procedure increased threefold over the machine's lifetime because its usage actually decreased over this same time period. On the other hand, their cost effectiveness analysis demonstrated that ioMRI was increasingly cost-effective for each added repeat "resection free year" for the patient when compared with a conventional MRI. Even though both ioMRI and conventional MRI patients had similar repeat resection rates, the longer resection-free postoperative interval for the ioMRI cohort was associated with a more cost-effective outcome.[116]

So, why is the utilization of ioMRI not increasing more rapidly in an age when technological advances in medicine and society are readily embraced in other ways? Perhaps it is because neurosurgeons are learning that this technology is more useful for subsets of patients with certain tumors such as LGGs, a disease with a relatively low incidence. Much data have been published about the role of ioMRI in surgery for infiltrative glioma and pituitary adenoma; however, its role in other neoplasm types has not been fully clarified.[116,68,71,88,117-120] In comparison to high-field ioMRIs, intraoperative low-field systems have longer scanning times, with lower resolution due the low signal to noise ratio obtainable. The imaging quality secondary to image artifacts has led to misinterpretation of intraoperative imaging with a high false-positive rate of up to 16%. This can lead to incomplete resections or unnecessary resections with an increasing risk of neurological morbidity. Also, low-field ioMRI is limited to basic T1, T2 and FLAIR-weighted imaging, thereby limiting the ability to acquire such "advanced" studies as fMRI, DTI, and MR spectroscopy. These systems are, however, much more compact, mobile and open bore, allowing the surgeon the greatest access to patients with limited OR modifications and less disruption to workflow.[121] High-field ioMRI systems offer shorter scanning time and better image quality with the ability to perform the above-mentioned advanced studies, but their use requires special infrastructural modifications in order to allow better imaging quality and improve surgical access.[69,122]

In today's era of evidence and outcomes-based medicine, the ioMRI must be able to significantly affect LOS, repeat resection rates and overall increased institutional utilization, the latter likely being most significant in term of justifying its high "up-front" financial cost. Hall's study, among others evaluating the economic feasibility of high-field ioMRI has demonstrated that the ability to offset the high capital costs of a high-field ioMRI is by utilizing it for routine diagnostic imaging.[68,72,115,116,123-125] Ultimately, the feasibility of incorporating intraoperative MR imaging into a practice for brain tumor surgery may require well-designed studies that analyze the medical outcomes and economic value of implementation of these technologies into day-to-day neurosurgical practice. However, as technological advances in the fields of neurosurgery and neuroradiology continue to mount, the field of neurosurgery must embrace the incorporation of these advances into routine practice, so that ultimately, just as neuronavigational systems have now become a standard of practice, utilization of intraoperative imaging will become customary and current obstacles encountered will be overcome by striving to improve the current systems.

REFERENCES

1. Enchev Y. Neuronavigation: geneology, reality, and prospects. Neurosurg Focus. 2009;27(3):E11.
2. Leeds NE, Kieffer SA. Evolution of diagnostic neuroradiology from 1904 to 1999. Radiology. 2000;217(2):309-18.
3. Dandy WE. Rontgenography of the brain after the injection of air into the spinal canal. Ann Surg. 1919;70(4):397-403.
4. Spiegel EA, Wycis HT, Marks M, et al. Stereotaxic apparatus for operations on the human brain. Science. 1947;106(2754):349-50.
5. Leksell L. The stereotaxic method and radiosurgery of the brain. Acta Chir Scand. 1951;102(4):316-9.
6. Riechert T, Wolff M. A new directive apparatus for the coagulation of the ganglion Gasseri and other intracerebral procedures. Acta Neurochir (Wien). 1952;2(3-4):405-7.
7. Wells TH, Cosman ER, Ball RE. The Brown-Roberts-Wells (BRW) arc: its concept as a spatial navigation system. Appl Neurophysiol. 1987;50(1-6):127-32.
8. Heilbrun MP, Roberts TS, Apuzzo ML, et al. Preliminary experience with Brown-Roberts-Wells (BRW) computerized tomography stereotaxic guidance system. J Neurosurg. 1983;59(2):217-22.
9. Young RF. Application of robotics to stereotactic neurosurgery. Neurol Res. 1987;9(2):123-8.
10. Benabid AL, Lavallee S, Hoffmann D, et al. Potential use of robots in endoscopic neurosurgery. Acta Neurochir. Suppl (Wien). 1992;54:93-7.

11. Apuzzo ML, Chen JC. Stereotaxy, navigation and the temporal concatenation. Stereotact Funct Neurosurg. 1999;72(2-4):82-8.
12. Apuzzo ML, Sabshin JK. Computed tomographic guidance stereotaxis in the management of intracranial mass lesions. Neurosurgery. 1983;12(3):277-85.
13. Hounsfield GN. Computerized transverse axial scanning (tomography). 1. Description of system. Br J Radiol. 1973;46(552):1016-22.
14. Shalit MN, Israeli Y, Matz S, et al. Intra-operative computerized axial tomography. Surg Neurol. 1979;11(5):382-4.
15. Gasiński P, Zieliński P, Harat M, et al. Application of intraoperative computed tomography in a neurosurgical operating theatre. Neurol Neurochir Pol. 2012;46(6):536-41.
16. Holly LT, Foley KT. Intraoperative spinal navigation. Spine (Phila Pa 1976). 2003;28(15):S54-61.
17. Hum B, Feigenbaum F, Cleary K, et al. Intraoperative computed tomography for complex craniocervical operations and spinal tumor resections. Neurosurgery. 2000;47(2):374-80.
18. Beck M, Mittlmeier T, Gierer P, et al. Benefit and accuracy of intraoperative 3D-imaging after pedicle screw placement: a prospective study in stabilizing thoracolumbar fractures. Eur Spine J. 2009;18(10):1469-77.
19. Tormenti MJ, Kostov DB, Gardner PA, et al. Intraoperative computed tomography image-guided navigation for posterior thoracolumbar spinal instrumentation in spinal deformity surgery. Neurosurg Focus. 2010;28(3):E11.
20. Roberts DW, Strohbehn JW, Hatch JF, et al. A frameless stereotaxic integration of computerized tomographic imaging and the operating microscope. J Neurosurg. 1986;65(4):545-9.
21. Black PM, Moriarty T, Alexander E, et al. Development and implementation of intraoperative magnetic resonance imaging and its neurosurgical applications. Neurosurgery. 1997;41(4):831-42.
22. Liang D, Schulder M. The role of intraoperative magnetic resonance imaging in glioma surgery. Surg Neurol Int. 2012;3(4):S320-7.
23. Lee CC, Lee ST, Chang CN, et al. Volumetric measurement for comparison of the accuracy between intraoperative CT and postoperative MR imaging in pituitary adenoma surgery. Am J Neuroradiol. 2011;32(8):1539-44.
24. Coenen VA, Krings T, Weidemann J, et al. Sequential visualization of brain and fiber tract deformation during intracranial surgery with three-dimensional ultrasound: an approach to evaluate the effect of brain shift. Neurosurgery. 2005;56(1):133-41.
25. Gasco J, Tummala S, Mahajan NM, et al. Simultaneous use of functional tractography, neuronavigation-integrated subcortical white matter stimulation and intraoperative magnetic resonance imaging in glioma surgery: technical note. Stereotact Funct Neurosurg. 2009;87(6):395-8.
26. Hatiboglu MA, Weinberg JS, Suki D, et al. Utilization of intraoperative motor mapping in glioma surgery with high-field intraoperative magnetic resonance imaging. Stereotact Funct Neurosurg. 2010;88(6):345-52.
27. Rasmussen IA, Lindseth F, Rygh OM, et al. Functional neuronavigation combined with intra-operative 3D ultrasound: initial experiences during surgical resections close to eloquent brain areas and future directions in automatic brain shift compensation of preoperative data. Acta Neurochir (Wien). 2007;149(4):365-78.
28. Orringer DA, Golby A, Jolesz F. Neuronavigation in the surgical management of brain tumors: current and future trends. Expert Rev Med Devices. 2012;9(5):491-500.
29. Paleologos TS, Wadley JP, Kitchen ND, et al. Clinical utility and cost-effectiveness of interactive image-guided craniotomy: clinical comparison between conventional and image-guided meningioma surgery. Neurosurgery. 2000;47(1):40-7.
30. Willems PW, Taphoorn MJ, Burger H, et al. Effectiveness of neuronavigation in resecting solitary intracerebral contrast-enhancing tumors: a randomized controlled trial. J Neurosurg. 2006;104(3):360-8.
31. Willems PW, van der Sprenkel JW, Tulleken CA, et al. Neuronavigation and surgery of intracerebral tumours. J Neurol. 2006;253(9):1123-36.
32. Garber ST, Jensen RL. Image guidance for brain metastases resection. Surg Neurol Int. 2012;3(2):S111-7.
33. Schackert G, Steinmetz A, Meier U, et al. Surgical management of single and multiple brain metastases: results of a retrospective study. Onkologie. 2001;24(3):246-55.
34. Weiss L, Gilbert HA, Posner JB. Brain metastasis. Boston: GK Hall; 1980.
35. Wadley J, Dorward N, Kitchen N, et al. Pre-operative planning and intra-operative guidance in modern neurosurgery: a review of 300 cases. Ann R Coll Surg Engl. 1999;81(4):217-25.
36. Roessler K, Ungersboeck K, Dietrich W, et al. Frameless stereotactic guided neurosurgery: clinical experience with an infrared based pointer device navigation system. Acta Neurochir (Wien). 1997;139(6):551-9.
37. Nabavi A, Black PM, Gering DT, et al. Serial intraoperative magnetic resonance imaging of brain shift. Neurosurgery. 2001;48(4):787-97.
38. Nimsky C, Ganslandt O, Buchfelder M, et al. Intraoperative visualization for resection of gliomas: the role of functional neuronavigation and intraoperative 1.5 T MRI. Neurol Res. 2006;28(5):482-7.
39. Benveniste RJ, Germano IM. Correlation of factors predicting intraoperative brain shift with successful resection of malignant brain tumors using image-guided techniques. Surg Neurol. 2005;63(6):542-8.
40. Dorward NL, Alberti O, Velani B, et al. Postimaging brain distortion: magnitude, correlates, and impact on neuronavigation. J Neurosurg. 1998;88(4):656-62.
41. Golfinos JG, Fitzpatrick BC, Smith LR, et al. Clinical use of a frameless stereotactic arm: results of 325 cases. J Neurosurg. 1995;83(2):197-205.
42. Sipos EP, Tebo SA, Zinreich SJ, et al. In vivo accuracy testing and clinical experience with the ISG viewing wand. Neurosurgery. 1996;39(1):194-202.
43. Yamasaki T, Moritake K, Takaya M, et al. Intraoperative use of doppler ultrasound and endoscopic monitoring in the stereotactic biopsy of malignant brain tumors. Technical note. J Neurosurg. 1994;80(3):570-4.
44. Gronningsaeter A, Kleven A, Ommedal S, et al. SonoWand: an ultrasound-based neuronavigation system. Neurosurgery. 2000;47(6):1373-9.
45. Koivukangas J, Louhisalmi Y, Alakuijala J, et al. Ultrasound-controlled neuronavigator-guided brain surgery. J Neurosurg. 1993;79(1):36-42.
46. Unsgaard G, Selbekk T, Brostrup Müller T, et al. Ability of navigated 3D ultrasound to delineate gliomas and metastases:

comparison of image interpretations with histopathology. Acta Neurochir (Wien). 2005;147(12):1259-69.

47. Lindseth F, Kaspersen JH, Ommedal S, et al. Multimodal image fusion in ultrasound-based neuronavigation: improving overview and interpretation by integrating preoperative MRI with intraoperative 3D ultrasound. Comput Aided Surg. 2003;8(2):49-69.

48. Lindseth F, Langø T, Bang J, et al. Accuracy evaluation of a 3D ultrasound-based neuronavigation system. Comput Aided Surg. 2002;7(4):197-222.

49. Solheim O, Selbekk T, Jakola AS, et al. Ultrasound-guided operations in unselected high-grade gliomas: overall results, impact of image quality and patient selection. Acta Neurochir (Wien). 2010;152(11):1873-86.

50. Moiyadi AV, Shetty PM, Mahajan A, et al. Usefulness of three-dimensional navigable intraoperative ultrasound in resection of brain tumors with a special emphasis on malignant gliomas. Acta Neurochir (Wien). 2013;155(12):2217-25.

51. Bonsanto MM, Metzner R, Aschoff A, et al. 3D ultrasound navigation in syrinx surgery: a feasibility study. Acta Neurochir (Wien). 2005;147(5):533-40.

52. Gläsker S, Shah MJ, Hippchen B, et al. Doppler-sonographically guided resection of central nervous system hemangioblastomas. Neurosurgery. 2011;68(2):267-75.

53. Kolstad F, Rygh OM, Selbekk T, et al. Three-dimensional ultrasonography navigation in spinal cord tumor surgery. Technical note. J Neurosurg. Spine. 2006;5(3):264-70.

54. Solheim O, Selbekk T, Løvstakken L, et al. Intrasellar ultrasound in transsphenoidal surgery: a novel technique. Neurosurgery. 2010;66(1):173-85.

55. Unsgaard G, Ommedal S, Rygh OM, et al. Operation of arteriovenous malformations assisted by stereoscopic navigation-controlled display of preoperative magnetic resonance angiography and intraoperative ultrasound angiography. Neurosurgery. 2005;56(2):281-90.

56. Selbekk T, Jakola AS, Solheim O, et al. Ultrasound imaging in neurosurgery: approaches to minimize surgically induced image artefacts for improved resection control. Acta Neurochir (Wien). 2013;155(6):973-80.

57. Barrow DL, Boyer KL, Joseph GJ. Intraoperative angiography in the management of neurovascular disorders. Neurosurgery. 1992;30(2):153-9.

58. Derdeyn CP, Moran CJ, Cross DT, et al. Intraoperative digital subtraction angiography: a review of 112 consecutive examinations. Am J Neuroradiol. 1995;16(2):307-18.

59. Payner TD, Horner TG, Leipzig TJ, et al. Role of intraoperative angiography in the surgical treatment of cerebral aneurysms. J Neurosurg. 1998;88(3):441-8.

60. Suzuki K, Kodama N, Sasaki T, et al. Confirmation of blood flow in perforating arteries using fluorescein cerebral angiography during aneurysm surgery. J Neurosurg. 2007;107(1):68-73.

61. Li J, Lan Z, He M, et al. Assessment of microscope-integrated indocyanine green angiography during intracranial aneurysm surgery: a retrospective study of 120 patients. Neurol India. 2009;57(4):453-9.

62. Ma CY, Shi JX, Wang HD, et al. Intraoperative indocyanine green angiography in intracranial aneurysm surgery: Microsurgical clipping and revascularization. Clin Neurol Neurosurg. 2009;111(10):840-6.

63. Uhl E, Zausinger S, Morhard D, et al. Intraoperative computed tomography with integrated navigation system in a multidisciplinary operating suite. Neurosurgery. 2009;64(5 Suppl 2):231-9.

64. Okudera H, Kobayashi S, Sugita K. Technical note: mobile CT scanner gantry for use in the operating room. Am J Neuroradiol. 1991;12(1):131-2.

65. Okudera H, Kobayashi S, Kyoshima K, et al. Development of the operating computerized tomographic scanner system for neurosurgery. Acta Neurochir (Wien). 1991;111(1-2):61-3.

66. Hundt W, Rust F, Stäbler A, et al. Dose reduction in multislice computed tomography. J Comput Assist Tomogr. 2005;29(1):140-7.

67. Kosmopoulos V, Schizas C. Pedicle screw placement accuracy: a meta-analysis. Spine (Phila Pa 1976). 2007;32(3):E111-20.

68. Bohinski RJ, Kokkino AK, Warnick RE, et al. Glioma resection in a shared-resource magnetic resonance operating room after optimal image-guided frameless stereotactic resection. Neurosurgery. 2001;48(4):731-42.

69. Senft C, Seifert V, Hermann E, et al. Usefulness of intraoperative ultra low-field magnetic resonance imaging in glioma surgery. Neurosurgery. 2008;63(4 Suppl 2):257-66.

70. Knauth M, Wirtz CR, Tronnier VM, et al. Intraoperative MR imaging increases the extent of tumor resection in patients with high-grade gliomas. Am J Neuroradiol. 1999;20(9):1642-6.

71. Wirtz CR, Knauth M, Staubert A, et al. Clinical evaluation and follow-up results for intraoperative magnetic resonance imaging in neurosurgery. Neurosurgery. 2000;46(5):1112-20.

72. Hatiboglu MA, Weinberg JS, Suki D, et al. Impact of intraoperative high-field magnetic resonance imaging guidance on glioma surgery: a prospective volumetric analysis. Neurosurgery. 2009;64(6):1073-81.

73. Kubben PL, ter Meulen KJ, Schijns OE, et al. Intraoperative MRI-guided resection of glioblastoma multiforme: a systematic review. Lancet Oncol. 2011;12(11):1062-70.

74. Schneider JP, Trantakis C, Rubach M, et al. Intraoperative MRI to guide the resection of primary supratentorial glioblastoma multiforme: a quantitative radiological analysis. Neuroradiology. 2005;47(7):489-500.

75. Lenaburg HJ, Inkabi KE, Vitaz TW. The use of intraoperative MRI for the treatment of glioblastoma multiforme. Technol Cancer Res Treat. 2009;8(2):159-62.

76. Senft C, Franz K, Blasel S, et al. Influence of iMRI-guidance on the extent of resection and survival of patients with glioblastoma multiforme. Technol Cancer Res Treat. 2010;9(4):339-46.

77. Senft C, Bink A, Franz K, et al. Intraoperative MRI guidance and extent of resection in glioma surgery: a randomised, controlled trial. Lancet Oncol. 2011;12(11):997-1003.

78. Haydon DH, Chicoine MR, Dacey RG. The impact of high-field-strength intraoperative magnetic resonance imaging on brain tumor management. Neurosurgery. 2013;60 Suppl 1:92-7.

79. Shaw EG, Wisoff JH. Prospective clinical trials of intracranial low-grade glioma in adults and children. Neuro Oncol. 2003;5(3):153-60.

80. Claus EB, Horlacher A, Hsu L, et al. Survival rates in patients with low-grade glioma after intraoperative magnetic resonance image guidance. Cancer. 2005;103(6):1227-33.

81. Berger MS, Deliganis AV, Dobbins J, et al. The effect of extent of resection on recurrence in patients with low grade cerebral hemisphere gliomas. Cancer. 1994;74(6):1784-91.

82. Keles GE, Lamborn KR, Berger MS. Low-grade hemispheric gliomas in adults: a critical review of extent of resection as a factor influencing outcome. J Neurosurg. 2001;95(5):735-45.

83. Smith JS, Chang EF, Lamborn KR, et al. Role of extent of resection in the long-term outcome of low-grade hemispheric gliomas. J Clin Oncol. 2008;26(8):1338-45.

84. Pamir MN, Ozduman K, Dincer A, et al. First intraoperative, shared-resource, ultrahigh-field 3-Tesla magnetic resonance imaging system and its application in low-grade glioma resection. J Neurosurg. 2010;112(1):57-69.

85. Pamir MN, Özduman K, Yildiz E, et al. Intraoperative magnetic resonance spectroscopy for identification of residual tumor during low-grade glioma surgery: clinical article. J Neurosurg. 2013;118(6):1191-8.

86. Tanei T, Nagatani T, Nakahara N, et al. Use of high-field intraoperative magnetic resonance imaging during endoscopic transsphenoidal surgery for functioning pituitary microadenomas and small adenomas located in the intrasellar region. Neurol Med Chir (Tokyo). 2013;53(7):501-10.

87. Bellut D, Hlavica M, Schmid C, et al. Intraoperative magnetic resonance imaging-assisted transsphenoidal pituitary surgery in patients with acromegaly. Neurosurg Focus. 2010;29(4):E9.

88. Bohinski RJ, Warnick RE, Gaskill-Shipley MF, et al. Intraoperative magnetic resonance imaging to determine the extent of resection of pituitary macroadenomas during transsphenoidal microsurgery. Neurosurgery. 2001;49(5):1133-43.

89. Gerlach R, du Mesnil de Rochemont R, Gasser T, et al. Feasibility of Polestar N20: an ultra-low-field intraoperative magnetic resonance imaging system in resection control of pituitary macroadenomas: lessons learned from the first 40 cases. Neurosurgery. 2008;63(2):272-84.

90. Martin CH, Schwartz R, Jolesz F, et al. Transsphenoidal resection of pituitary adenomas in an intraoperative MRI unit. Pituitary. 1999;2(2):155-62.

91. Pergolizzi RS, Nabavi A, Schwartz RB, et al. Intra-operative MR guidance during trans-sphenoidal pituitary resection: preliminary results. J Magn Reson Imaging. 2001;13(1):136-41.

92. Nimsky C, von Keller B, Ganslandt O, et al. Intraoperative high-field magnetic resonance imaging in transsphenoidal surgery of hormonally inactive pituitary macroadenomas. Neurosurgery. 2006;59(1):105-14.

93. Schwartz TH, Stieg PE, Anand VK. Endoscopic transsphenoidal pituitary surgery with intraoperative magnetic resonance imaging. Neurosurgery. 2006;58(1):ONS44-51.

94. Vitaz TW, Inkabi KE, Carrubba CJ. Intraoperative MRI for transphenoidal procedures: short-term outcome for 100 consecutive cases. Clin Neurol Neurosurg. 2011;113(9):731-5.

95. Wu JS, Shou XF, Yao CJ, et al. Transsphenoidal pituitary macroadenomas resection guided by PoleStar N20 low-field intraoperative magnetic resonance imaging: comparison with early postoperative high-field magnetic resonance imaging. Neurosurgery. 2009;65(1):63-70.

96. Berkmann S, Fandino J, Zosso S, et al. Intraoperative magnetic resonance imaging and early prognosis for vision after transsphenoidal surgery for sellar lesions. J Neurosurg. 2011;115(3):518-27.

97. Campbell PG, McGettigan B, Luginbuhl A, et al. Endocrinological and ophthalmological consequences of an initial endonasal endoscopic approach for resection of craniopharyngiomas. Neurosurg Focus. 2010;28(4):E8.

98. Minniti G, Jaffrain-Rea ML, Esposito V, et al. Evolving criteria for post-operative biochemical remission of acromegaly: can we achieve a definitive cure? An audit of surgical results on a large series and a review of the literature. Endocr Relat Cancer. 2003;10(4):611-9.

99. Zirkzee EJ, Corssmit EP, Biermasz NR, et al. Pituitary magnetic resonance imaging is not required in the postoperative follow-up of acromegalic patients with long-term biochemical cure after transsphenoidal surgery. J Clin Endocrinol Metab. 2004;89(9):4320-4.

100. Fahlbusch R, Keller Bv, Ganslandt O, et al. Transsphenoidal surgery in acromegaly investigated by intraoperative high-field magnetic resonance imaging. Eur J Endocrinol. 2005;153(2):239-48.

101. Ojemann JG, Miller JW, Silbergeld DL. Preserved function in brain invaded by tumor. Neurosurgery. 1996;39(2):253-8.

102. Leuthardt EC, Lim CC, Shah MN, et al. Use of movable high-field-strength intraoperative magnetic resonance imaging with awake craniotomies for resection of gliomas: preliminary experience. Neurosurgery. 2011;69(1):194-205.

103. Weingarten DM, Asthagiri AR, Butman JA, et al. Cortical mapping and frameless stereotactic navigation in the high-field intraoperative magnetic resonance imaging suite. J Neurosurg. 2009;111(6):1185-90.

104. Nimsky C, Ganslandt O, Hastreiter P, et al. Preoperative and intraoperative diffusion tensor imaging-based fiber tracking in glioma surgery. Neurosurgery. 2007;61(1):178-85.

105. Krammer B, Plaetzer K. ALA and its clinical impact, from bench to bedside. Photochem Photobiol Sci. 2008;7(3):283-9.

106. Panciani PP, Fontanella M, Schatlo B, et al. Fluorescence and image-guided resection in high grade glioma. Clin Neurol Neurosurg. 2012;114(1):37-41.

107. Stummer W, Pichlmeier U, Meinel T, et al. Fluorescence-guided surgery with 5-aminolevulinic acid for resection of malignant glioma: a randomised controlled multicentre phase III trial. Lancet Oncol. 2006;7(5):392-401.

108. Stummer W, Reulen HJ, Novotny A, et al. Fluorescence-guided resections of malignant gliomas--an overview. Acta Neurochir Suppl. 2003;88:9-12.

109. Stummer W, Novotny A, Stepp H, et al. Fluorescence-guided resection of glioblastoma multiforme by using 5-aminolevulinic acid-induced porphyrins: a prospective study in 52 consecutive patients. J Neurosurg. 2000;93(6):1003-13.

110. Stummer W, Stepp H, Möller G, et al. Technical principles for protoporphyrin-IX-fluorescence guided microsurgical resection of malignant glioma tissue. Acta Neurochir (Wien). 1998;140(10):995-1000.

111. Koc K, Anik I, Cabuk B, et al. Fluorescein sodium-guided surgery in glioblastoma multiforme: a prospective evaluation. Br J Neurosurg. 2008;22(1):99-103.

112. Tsugu A, Ishizaka H, Mizokami Y, et al. Impact of the combination of 5-aminolevulinic acid-induced fluorescence with intraoperative magnetic resonance imaging-guided surgery for glioma. World Neurosurg. 2011;76(1-2):120-7.

113. Eyüpoglu IY, Hore N, Savaskan NE, et al. Improving the extent of malignant glioma resection by dual intraoperative visualization approach. PLoS One. 2012;7(9):e44885.

114. Ramina R, Coelho Neto M, Giacomelli A, et al. Optimizing costs of intraoperative magnetic resonance imaging. A series of 29 glioma cases. Acta Neurochir (Wien). 2010;152(1):27-33.

115. Hall WA, Kowalik K, Liu H, et al. Costs and benefits of intraoperative MR-guided brain tumor resection. Acta Neurochir Suppl. 2003;85:137-42.

116. Makary M, Chiocca EA, Erminy N, et al. Clinical and economic outcomes of low-field intraoperative MRI-guided tumor resection neurosurgery. J Magn Reson Imaging. 2011;34(5):1022-30.

117. Darakchiev BJ, Tew JM, Bohinski RJ, et al. Adaptation of a standard low-field (0.3-T) system to the operating room: focus on pituitary adenomas. Neurosurg Clin N Am. 2005;16(1):155-64.

118. Fahlbusch R, Ganslandt O, Buchfelder M, et al. Intraoperative magnetic resonance imaging during transsphenoidal surgery. J Neurosurg. 2001;95(3):381-90.

119. Oh DS, Black PM. A low-field intraoperative MRI system for glioma surgery: is it worthwhile? Neurosurg Clin N Am. 2005;16(1):135-41.

120. Jolesz FA. Future perspectives for intraoperative MRI. Neurosurg Clin N Am. 2005;16(1):201-13.

121. Ronkainen J, Tervonen O. Cost analysis of an open low-field (0.23T) MRI unit: effect of procedure shares in combined imaging, interventional, and neurosurgical use. Acta Radiol. 2006;47(4):359-65.

122. Blanco RT, Ojala R, Kariniemi J, et al. Interventional and intraoperative MRI at low field scanner: a review. Eur J Radiol. 2005;56(2):130-42.

123. Nimsky C, Ganslandt O, Von Keller B, et al. Intraoperative high-field-strength MR imaging: implementation and experience in 200 patients. Radiology. 2004;233(1):67-78.

124. Hall WA, Liu H, Martin AJ, et al. Safety, efficacy, and functionality of high-field strength interventional magnetic resonance imaging for neurosurgery. Neurosurgery. 2000;46(3):632-41.

125. Lewin JS, Metzger A, Selman WR. Intraoperative magnetic resonance image guidance in neurosurgery. J Magn Reson Imaging. 2000;12(4):512-24.

3

Intraoperative Magnetic Resonance Imaging

Christopher Nimsky

INTRODUCTION

Intraoperative imaging has gained increasing interest in the last two decades. If intraoperative imaging depicts that a resection is incomplete, tumor residues that were initially missed can be removed during the same operation. In contrast to the subjective estimation by the neurosurgeon, intraoperative imaging allows an objective evaluation of the intraoperative situation, thus acting as quality control during surgery.[1-8]

Intraoperative imaging should be accompanied by a close integration of navigation.[7,9,10] Navigation allows the visualization of the essentials of pre- and intraoperative imaging in the surgical field, so that the image data provides an immediate intraoperative feedback. The most important aspect is to prevent increased neurological deficits despite increased resections that might result from the attempt to remove initially overlooked tumor remnants that are detected by intraoperative imaging.

In standard navigation, the physical space of the surgical field is registered to the three-dimensional (3-D) image space, which is based on anatomical data from magnetic resonance imaging (MRI) or computed tomography (CT). In microscope-based navigation the segmented extent and localization of a tumor is superimposed on the microscope field of view through contours using the heads-up display technology of modern operating microscopes. Standard navigation is based on anatomical information only, which has become a routine tool in neurosurgical departments. This technique was developed further by the integration of additional information obtained by other modalities resulting in the so-called multimodal navigation.

An initial step in establishing multimodal navigation was the development of functional navigation in which preoperative data from magnetoencephalography (MEG)[11-13] and functional magnetic resonance imaging (fMRI)[14,7] define localizations of cortical eloquent brain areas, such as the motor and speech areas. This method of functional navigation allowed more thorough resections of tumors in risk zones with low morbidity. Integration of diffusion tensor imaging (DTI) data delineating the course of major white matter tracts extended this concept also to subcortical areas,[15-18] while the co-registration of positron emission tomography (PET) data and information from MR spectroscopy (MRS) added metabolic information leading to true multimodal navigation.[19-23]

Combining intraoperative high-field MRI and microscope-based navigation enables an intraoperative possibility to compensate for the effects of brain shift by an immediate updating the image information. Updated navigation with intraoperative image data allows a reliable identification of tumor remnants. Microscope-integrated heads-up displays visualize the segmented tumor remnant in the surgical field facilitating the precise localization and orientation in the resection cavity.[24-28]

However, these updates typically are updates of anatomical data only, so that functional data that were integrated in the preoperative navigation planning are lost. Intraoperative high-field MRI does not only allow standard anatomical imaging by measuring T1- and T2-weighted sequences, with high-field MR settings intraoperative fMRI, as well as, intraoperative DTI, which is clinically more important, become feasible.

INTRAOPERATIVE MAGNETIC RESONANCE IMAGING BEYOND STANDARD IMAGING

Intraoperative Diffusion Tensor Imaging

Pre- and intraoperative DTI for tractography of major white matter tracts in glioma surgery can be performed using a 1.5 Tesla MR scanner.[17,18,29,30] Intraoperative fiber tract visualization using a software solution that was running on the MR scanner platform needed less than 1 minute, so that the whole evaluation could be performed during surgery. The interactive 3-D display with co-registered b0 diffusion images gave a quick and intuitive overview of the position of major white matter tracts. Thus, fiber tracking is not only a method for preoperative neurosurgical visualization but also for further intraoperative planning. Only in one patient of the initial investigation series a neurological aggravation (2.7%) was observed; it was probably not related to a misinterpretation of fiber tracking. The measured extent of shifting of the major white matter tracts in glioma surgery corresponded well to previous data on brain shift of the so-called deep tumor margin which was reported to be up to more than one centimeter.[27,31] Furthermore, the individually unpredictable direction and great interindividual variability of white matter tract shifting confirmed these previous data.[26,27,32] The absolute amount of shifting correlated with the tumor volume, i.e. that in larger tumors greater deformations were likely to occur. However, the direction of white matter tract shifting, whether in the outward or inward direction in respect to the craniotomy opening seemed to be unpredictable. Even the opening of the ventricular system was no reliable parameter to predict inward shifting due to the loss of cerebrospinal fluid.

The knowledge of the actual position of major white matter tracts during glioma resection helps to prevent too extensive resections that could potentially damage major white matter tracts and subsequently result in postoperative neurological deficits. When data from fiber tracking are integrated into a navigational setup, preferably with the simultaneous application of fMRI, serving as seed regions for DTI fiber tracking algorithms, it is essential that the effects of brain shift, which clearly effect the spatial position of major white matter tracts, are compensated for. In contrast to mathematical models,[33-36] which still have great restrictions simulating the brain-shift behavior for deep brain structures, intraoperative DTI is a reliable possibility to obtain actual data for fiber tracking representing the intraoperative situation after substantial parts of a glioma are removed and further guidance is needed.

The implementation of a DTI tracking algorithm in the navigation software allows to perform an intraoperative update of the navigation system with the intraoperative DTI data in less than 5–10 minutes, thus compensating for the effects of brain shift not only for standard 3-D anatomical data but also for the position of major white matter tracts.[16] This update possibility delineating the course of major white matter tracts based on intraoperative data is a prerequisite for a real electrophysiological validation of the white matter tract data. Reports on comparisons between subcortical electrical stimulations and preoperative DTI data showed some inconsistencies, which were probably due to the effects of brain shift.[37,38]

Maximal safety may require combining electrophysiological brain mapping with functional navigation that integrates fMRI or MEG-data and DTI-based fiber tracking acquired before or during surgery. Intraoperative electrophysiological mapping can identify cortical eloquent brain areas; subcortical electrical stimulation helps to identify major white matter tracts during surgery. Recent studies emphasize that functional navigation and subcortical stimulation are complementary methods that may facilitate the preservation of pyramidal tracts.

Future research will have to be in the field of quantification and reduction of spatial inaccuracies of the raw DTI data,[39] as well as to improve sequence design, tracking parameters, and algorithms. Besides progress in sequence development with reduced image distortion, de-noising increased number of diffusion directions, and higher resolution of the raw data, further progress will also relate to a more accurate reconstruction of neural connectivity patterns. Correct identification of areas of fiber crossings is not possible by standard DTI because of its inability to resolve more than a single axon direction within each imaging voxel. Techniques, that can resolve multiple axon directions within a single voxel, may solve the problem of white matter fiber crossings, as well as white matter insertions into the cortex.

Further challenges relate to the effects of edema surrounding a tumor where fiber tracking is performed. Effects of edema, the resection cavity, and tumor remnants directly may impede the correct tracking, so that either existing fibers are not visualized at all or even erroneous tracking may result. There are various technical attempts to approach the limitations of DTI-based tractography; an agreed standard, or ideal solution is not yet defined.[40-42] It will be important to compare the different approaches especially in respect to their reliability and also clinical applicability.[43]

A recent study investigated differences in the metabolism of fiber tract alterations between gliomas grade II to IV by correlation of fiber density values with metabolite concentrations measured by fiber density mapping and MR spectroscopic imaging. Structural integrity of fiber tracts was assessed as the fiber density ipsilateral-to-contralateral ratio (FD-ICR). Metabolite concentrations for choline-containing compounds and N-acetyl-aspartate were computed and correlated to FD-ICR values after co-registration with anatomic MR imaging. In tumor areas, choline-containing compound concentrations of altered fiber tracts were significantly different between low- and high-grade glioma and showed different courses for the correlations of FD-ICR and choline-containing compounds. In high-grade glioma, increasing fiber destruction was associated with a massive progression in cell membrane proliferation. Peritumor fiber structures showed significantly decreased N-acetyl-aspartate concentrations for all patients, but only patients with glioblastoma multiforme had significantly decreased fiber density compared with the contralateral side. Glioma grades II and III had significantly higher peritumor FD-ICR than glioblastoma multiforme. A multiparametric MR imaging strategy that provides information about both structural integrity and metabolism of the tumor is required for detailed assessment of glioma-related fiber tract alterations.[44]

Intraoperative Functional Magnetic Resonance Imaging

To implement intraoperative fMRI a passive stimulation paradigm with shielded electrical peripheral nerve stimulation of the median and tibial nerve was applied in a setting with a 1.5T intraoperative magnet. For electrical stimulation an electromagnetically shielded coaxial lead was developed, while shielding was achieved by connecting the conductor's shielding-mesh to the MRI cage. The impulse generator was located outside the radiofrequency-shielded cabin and the conductor was threaded through a waveguide array into the actual operating theater. After induction of anesthesia and patient positioning, the stimulation electrodes were attached and the motor threshold was defined. After an initial anatomical and functional MR scans, two further data sets were acquired during and at the end of the surgical procedure. The block-design stimulation paradigm alternated four rest and four activation periods. For functional imaging, slices parallel to the anterior-posterior commissural plane were acquired as T2-weighted echo planar imaging sequences. The fMRI data were analyzed during acquisition by an online statistical evaluation package installed on the MR scanner console. In addition, phase reversal of somatosensory evoked potentials was used for verification of intraoperative fMRI. In four anesthetized patients with lesions in the vicinity of the central region a total of eleven fMRI measurements were successfully acquired and analyzed online. Activation was found in the somatosensory cortex, which could be confirmed by intraoperative phase reversal for each measurement. No neurological deteriorations or complications due to the stimulation technique were observed. Thus, intraoperative fMRI is technically feasible allowing a real time identification of eloquent brain areas despite brain shift.[45] Similar results could also be reproduced applying a sophisticated setup with a low-field (0.3T) scanner.[46]

In a recent publication, a new technique that combines awake surgery and i-fMRI, named "awake" i-fMRI (ai-fMRI) was proposed. Ai-fMRI was applied to the real-time localization of sensor motor areas during awake craniotomy in seven patients. The results showed that ai-fMRI could successfully detect activations in the bilateral primary sensor motor areas and supplementary motor areas for all patients, indicating the feasibility of this technique in eloquent area localization. The reliability of ai-fMRI was further validated using intraoperative stimulation mapping in two of the seven patients. Comparisons between the pre-fMRI-derived localization result and the ai-fMRI derived result showed that the former was subject to a heavy brain shift and led to incorrect localization, while the latter solved that problem.[47]

Nevertheless, the clinical necessity for intraoperative fMRI is debatable, since the position of cortical eloquent brain areas can be identified and marked after dural opening when applying preoperative data-based functional navigation. The shifting of the cortical eloquent areas during a procedure can be observed by the surgeon without much guesswork, so that a time-consuming fMRI update procedure might only be of interest in very selected cases, where the updated fMRI information is used as seed regions for fiber tracking algorithms to reconstruct the arcuate fasciculus[48,49] applying intraoperative DTI to update reconstructed language fibers.

Intraoperative Magnetic Resonance Spectroscopy and Other Techniques

Intraoperative MR spectroscopy (MRS) still has its limitations due to the brain air interface, so that there remain some distinct challenges for updating also the MRS information during surgery. Applying chemical shift imaging (CSI) using a 1.5T system we were not able to get reliable data, due to the close air interface in the vicinity of the resection cavity. Measurements on the healthy hemisphere on the other hand were possible, however had no clinical relevance. Maybe some surgical means like better covering the surgical field may be a possibility to allow also for intraoperative MRS measurements. In the literature, there are some reports about single voxel measurements that were applied with the attempt to differentiate between tumor tissue and surgically-induced changes at the resection border.[50,51] There are also only rare reports on the intraoperative application of perfusion measurements[52] to delineate tumor remnants, as well as example the application of techniques like arterial spin labeling in visualization of vasculature.

CONCLUSION

Multimodal functional navigation enables removing a tumor close to eloquent brain areas with low postoperative deficits, while additional intraoperative imaging ensures that the maximum extent of the resection can be achieved. Intraoperative imaging allows updating the preoperative image data compensating for the effects of brain shift. Intraoperative imaging beyond standard anatomical imaging adds further safety for complex tumor resections.

REFERENCES

1. Black PM, Moriarty T, Alexander III E, et al. Development and implementation of intraoperative magnetic resonance imaging and its neurosurgical applications. Neurosurgery. 1997;41:831-45.
2. Hall WA, Kowalik K, Liu H, et al. Costs and benefits of intraoperative MR-guided brain tumor resection. Acta Neurochir. 2003;85:137-42.
3. Hall WA, Liu H, Martin AJ, et al. Safety, efficacy, and functionality of high-field strength interventional magnetic resonance imaging for neurosurgery. Neurosurgery. 2000;46:632-42.

4. Kubben PL, terMeulen KJ, Schijns OE, et al. Intraoperative MRI-guided resection of glioblastoma multiforme: a systematic review. Lancet Oncol. 2011;12:1062-70.

5. Nimsky C. Intraoperative MRI in glioma surgery: proof of benefit? Lancet Oncol. 2011;12:982-3.

6. Nimsky C, Ganslandt O, Fahlbusch R. Comparing 0.2 tesla with 1.5 tesla intraoperative magnetic resonance imaging analysis of setup, workflow, and efficiency. Acad Radiol. 2005;12:1065-79.

7. Nimsky C, Ganslandt O, Von Keller B, et al. Intraoperative high-field-strength MR imaging: implementation and experience in 200 patients. Radiology. 2004;233:67-78.

8. Sutherland GR, Kaibara T, Louw D, et al. A mobile high-field magnetic resonance system for neurosurgery. J Neurosurg. 1999;91:804-13.

9. Nimsky C, Ganslandt O, Kober H, et al. Intraoperative magnetic resonance imaging combined with neuronavigation: a new concept. Neurosurgery. 2001;48:1082-91.

10. Steinmeier R, Fahlbusch R, Ganslandt O, et al. Intraoperative magnetic resonance imaging with the magnetom open scanner: concepts, neurosurgical indications, and procedures: a preliminary report. Neurosurgery. 1998;43:739-48.

11. Ganslandt O, Buchfelder M, Hastreiter P, et al. Magnetic source imaging supports clinical decision making in glioma patients. Clin Neurol Neurosurg. 2004;107:20-6.

12. Ganslandt O, Fahlbusch R, Nimsky C, et al. Functional neuronavigation with magnetoencephalography: outcome in 50 patients with lesions around the motor cortex. J Neurosurg. 1999;91:73-9.

13. Ganslandt O, Steinmeier R, Kober H, et al. Magnetic source imaging combined with image-guided frameless stereotaxy: a new method in surgery around the motor strip. Neurosurgery. 1997;41:621-8.

14. Nimsky C, Ganslandt O, Kober H, et al. Integration of functional magnetic resonance imaging supported by magnetoencephalography in functional neuronavigation. Neurosurgery. 1999;44:1249-56.

15. Nimsky C, Ganslandt O, Fahlbusch R. 1.5 T: intraoperative imaging beyond standard anatomic imaging. Neurosurg Clin N Am. 2005;16:185-200.

16. Nimsky C, Ganslandt O, Fahlbusch R. Implementation of fiber tract navigation. Neurosurgery. 2006;58:ONS-292-304.

17. Nimsky C, Ganslandt O, Hastreiter P, et al. Preoperative and intraoperative diffusion tensor imaging-based fiber tracking in glioma surgery. Neurosurgery. 2005;56:130-8.

18. Nimsky C, Ganslandt O, Merhof D, et al. Intraoperative visualization of the pyramidal tract by diffusion-tensor-imaging-based fiber tracking. Neuroimage. 2006;30:1219-29.

19. Ganslandt O, Stadlbauer A, Fahlbusch R, et al. Proton magnetic resonance spectroscopic imaging integrated into image-guided surgery: correlation to standard magnetic resonance imaging and tumor cell density. Neurosurgery. 2005;56:291-8.

20. Stadlbauer A, Ganslandt O, Buslei R, et al. Gliomas: histopathologic evaluation of changes in directionality and magnitude of water diffusion at diffusion-tensor MR imaging. Radiology. 2006;240:803-10.

21. Stadlbauer A, Moser E, Gruber S, et al. Integration of biochemical images of a tumor into frameless stereotaxy achieved using a magnetic resonance imaging/magnetic resonance spectroscopy hybrid data set. J Neurosurg. 2004;101:287-94.

22. Stadlbauer A, Nimsky C, Buslei R, et al. Proton magnetic resonance spectroscopic imaging in the border zone of gliomas: correlation of metabolic and histological changes at low tumor infiltration--initial results. Invest Radiol. 2007;42:218-23.

23. Stadlbauer A, Prante O, Nimsky C, et al. Metabolic imaging of cerebral gliomas: spatial correlation of changes in O-(2-18F-fluoroethyl)-L-tyrosine PET and proton magnetic resonance spectroscopic imaging. J Nucl Med. 2008;49:721-9.

24. Ferrant M, Nabavi A, Macq B, et al. Serial registration of intraoperative MR images of the brain. Med Image Anal. 2002;6:337-59.

25. Hastreiter P, Rezk-Salama C, Soza G, et al. Strategies for brain shift evaluation. Med Image Anal. 2004;8:447-64.

26. Nabavi A, Black PM, Gering DT, et al. Serial intraoperative magnetic resonance imaging of brain shift. Neurosurgery. 2001;48:787-98.

27. Nimsky C, Ganslandt O, Cerny S, et al. Quantification of, visualization of, and compensation for brain shift using intraoperative magnetic resonance imaging. Neurosurgery. 2000;47:1070-80.

28. Nimsky C, von Keller B, Schlaffer S, et al. Updating navigation with intraoperative image data. Top Magn Reson Imaging. 2009;19:197-204.

29. Nimsky C, Ganslandt O, Hastreiter P, et al. Intraoperative diffusion tensor imaging: shifting of white matter tracts during neurosurgical procedures: initial experience. Radiology. 2005;234:218-25.

30. Nimsky C, Ganslandt O, Keller v B, et al. Intraoperative high-field strength MR imaging: implementation and experience in 200 patients. Radiology. 2004;233:67-78.

31. Dorward NL, Alberti O, Velani B, et al. Postimaging brain distortion: magnitude, correlates, and impact on neuronavigation. J Neurosurg. 1998;88:656-62.

32. Keles GE, Lamborn KR, Berger MS. Coregistration accuracy and detection of brain shift using intraoperative sononavigation during resection of hemispheric tumors. Neurosurgery. 2003;53:556-64.

33. Chen I, Coffey AM, Ding S, et al. Intraoperative brain shift compensation: accounting for dural septa. IEEE Trans Biomed Eng. 2011;58:499-508.

34. Miga MI, Roberts DW, Kennedy FE, et al. Modeling of retraction and resection for intraoperative updating of images. Neurosurgery. 2001;49:75-84; discussion 84-75.

35. Roberts DW, Miga MI, Hartov A, et al. Intraoperatively updated neuroimaging using brain modeling and sparse data. Neurosurgery. 1999;45:1199-206; discussion 1206-1197.

36. Soza G, Grosso R, Labsik U, et al. Fast and adaptive finite element approach for modeling brain shift. Comput Aided Surg. 2003;8:241-6.

37. Kamada K, Todo T, Masutani Y, et al. Combined use of tractography-integrated functional neuronavigation and direct fiber stimulation. J Neurosurg.2005;102:664-72.

38. Kinoshita M, Yamada K, Hashimoto N, et al. Fiber-tracking does not accurately estimate size of fiber bundle in pathological condition: initial neurosurgical experience using neuronavigation and subcortical white matter stimulation. Neuroimage. 2005;25:424-9.

39. Merhof D, Soza G, Stadlbauer A, et al. Correction of susceptibility artifacts in diffusion tensor data using non-linear registration. Med Image Anal. 2007;11:588-603.

40. Farquharson S, Tournier JD, Calamante F, et al. White matter fiber tractography: why we need to move beyond DTI. J Neurosurg. 2013;118:1367-77.

41. Fernandez-Miranda JC. Editorial: Beyond diffusion tensor imaging. J Neurosurg. 2013;118:1363-5.

42. Tournier JD, Mori S, Leemans A. Diffusion tensor imaging and beyond. Magn Reson Med. 2011;65:1532-56.

43. Nimsky C. Fiber tracking-we should move beyond diffusion tensor imaging. World Neurosurg Epub. 2013/09/07:2014.

44. Stadlbauer A, Hammen T, Buchfelder M, et al. Differences in metabolism of fiber tract alterations in gliomas: a combined fiber density mapping and magnetic resonance spectroscopic imaging study. Neurosurgery. 2012;71:454-63.

45. Gasser T, Ganslandt O, Sandalcioglu E, et al. Intraoperative functional MRI: implementation and preliminary experience. Neuroimage. 2005;26:685-93.

46. Gasser T, Szelenyi A, Senft C, et al. Intraoperative MRI and functional mapping. Acta Neurochir Suppl. 2011;109:61-5.

47. Lu JF, Zhang H, Wu JS, et al. "Awake" intraoperative functional MRI (ai-fMRI) for mapping the eloquent cortex: Is it possible in awake craniotomy? Neuroimage Clin. 2012;2:132-42.

48. Kuhnt D, Bauer MH, Becker A, et al. Intraoperative visualization of fiber tracking based reconstruction of language pathways in glioma surgery. Neurosurgery. 2012;70:911-9; discussion 919-920.

49. Kuhnt D, Bauer MH, Egger J, et al. Fiber tractography based on diffusion tensor imaging compared with high-angular-resolution diffusion imaging with compressed sensing: initial experience. Neurosurgery. 2013;72(Suppl 1):165-75.

50. Pamir MN, Ozduman K, Yildiz E, et al. Intraoperative magnetic resonance spectroscopy for identification of residual tumor during low-grade glioma surgery: clinical article. J Neurosurg. 2013;118:1191-8.

51. Roder C, Skardelly M, Ramina KF, et al. Spectroscopy imaging in intraoperative MR suite: tissue characterization and optimization of tumor resection. Int J Comput Assist Radiol Surg. 2013.

52. Roder C, Bender B, Ritz R, et al. Intraoperative visualization of residual tumor: the role of perfusion-weighted imaging in a high-field intraoperative magnetic resonance scanner. Neurosurgery. 2013;72:ons151-8; discussion on158, 2013.

4

Intraoperative Magnetic Resonance Imaging: Changing Face of Neurosurgery

Anshu Mahajan, Vipul Gupta

INTRAOPERATIVE MAGNETIC RESONANCE IMAGING AND ITS ORIGIN

The first intraoperative magnetic resonance imaging (iMRI) for neurosurgical operations was installed in Boston (1994), Harvard Medical School which was a 0.5 Tesla (T) system. The intraoperative magnetic resonance used for first brain tumor removal was done in 1996. Since then, multiple modification has been made in magnet strength of MRI and operating room (OR) suite setup.[1] iMRI systems have been subdivided into low-field (0.12–0.5 T), mid-field (0.5–1T), and high-field (1.5–3.0T) systems. High-field systems have the advantage of superior image quality and various advance applications like diffusion tensor imaging (DTI) and functional MRI (fMRI), but they compromise with surgical access or time required in patient transportation. Whereas, patient movement is not required in low-field systems and at the same time, it also maintains the surgical access and real-time imaging, but image quality is limited. High-field iMRI systems are very expensive and available at few select neurosurgical centers. Low-field iMRI systems are the ones which are predominantly used all over the world.

Low-field Intraoperative Magnetic Resonance Imaging Systems

These include the magnets with strength of less than 0.5T. The vertical gap or biplanar system are the two major design in low-field iMRI. The vertical-gap iMRI system (0.2 T) was developed by combined efforts of Toronto Western Hospital and the University of Toronto. Here, two flat magnetic poles (25–40 cm in diameter) are used and the patient is placed in between the poles. A concept of twin operating system was introduced by researchers group at the University of Cincinnati Medical Center where they had employed 0.3T imager facility for both surgical procedures and for routine diagnostic imaging. A different concept by Bohinski et al.[77]

presented the Cincinnati system where a compact 0.12T intraoperative magnetic resonance imager is placed under the surgical table (not in use), hence standard instruments can be allowed to use.[3] A modification of this concept using local radiofrequency (RF) shielding and 0.15T imager has also been introduced. A horizontally open moveable iMRI (0.23T) was introduced at Oulu University Hospital, Finland having the easy and fast shut-down possibility. Hence, operation could be performed next to the scanner without the need of patient being shifted to the magnetic fringe fields.

Mid-field Intraoperative Magnetic Resonance Imaging Systems

Magnetic fields of 0.5–1.0T are included in mid-field iMRI. The "double doughnut"- shaped 0.5T magnet, a first interventional MRI used consists of two parallel vertical magnets and a 56 cm wide gap between the poles for patient access.[4,5]

High-field Intraoperative Magnetic Resonance Imaging Systems

Three different concepts of high-field iMRI have been introduced:

1. The concept of University of Calgary, the mobile imager was primarily developed for intraoperative use. Here the magnet is moved on ceiling-mounted track beams from parking alcove where it is housed to the surgical area whenever imaging is required.
2. The high-field concept (by University of Erlangen-Nürnberg) had utilized microscope-based navigation system in the fringe fields of a general-purpose 1.5T imager. Here, the patient rotates from the operating position into the scanner of imaging with the help of rotating operating table. The advantage of using intraoperative DTI has been reported by Nimsky et al.[6,7] whereas the benefit of

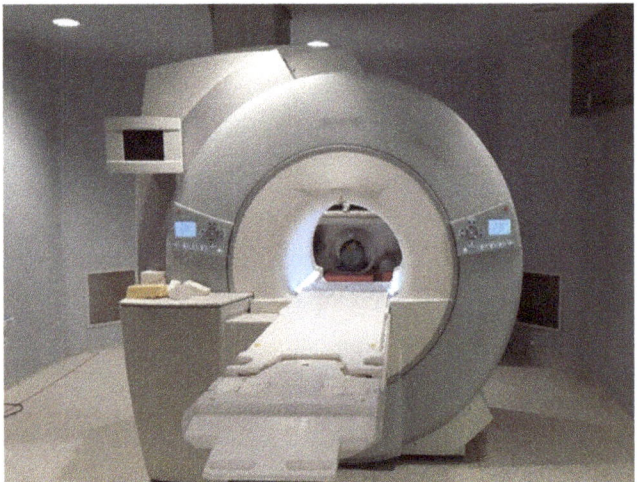

Figure 4.1 Siemens intraoperative magnetic resonance imaging system

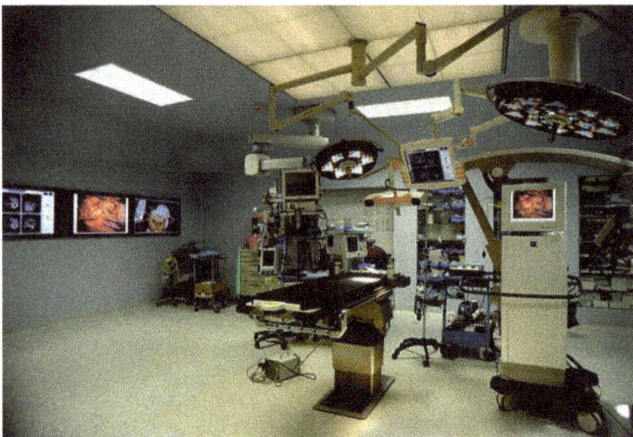

Figure 4.2 Operating room at Medanta—the Medicity

magnetic resonance spectroscopy (MRS) and fMRI has been demonstrated by Liu H et al. and Martin AJ et al.[8,9] Rapid and repetitive multiple imaging, which is required during brain biopsies can be performed using MR compatible instruments at the bore entrance.[10]

3. Very high-field iMRI systems using 3T magnets have also been launched in past few years offering high-quality imaging capabilities. High-strength magnetic field systems though highly desirable, their installation and maintenance are very expensive in addition to the technical manpower and personal costs.

The MRI suite **(Figure 4.1)** and OR in our institute have been shown in **Figures 4.1 and 4.2**.

ANESTHESIA FOR INTRAOPERATIVE MAGNETIC RESONANCE IMAGING

The anesthesia has a major role in iMRI-guided surgery including preoperative evaluation and management of anesthesia. The anesthesiologist must have training and knowledge of specific complications pertaining to iMRI and is responsible for identifying limitations associated with the iMRI. The preoperative anesthesia evaluation include exploration of history of ferromagnetic objects implanted in patient including surgical clips, cochlear implants, stents, bullet, pacemakers implanted fusion pumps, implanted defibrillators, etc. which are contraindicated to MRI. These ferromagnetic objects are subjected to displacement or dislodgment and there is also risk of heating of these objects which can cause burns. Artifacts caused by dentures may significantly degrade iMRI images. Surgical clips that contain mostly nickel are not considered dangerous. The equipment for iMRI have filtered electrical current which does not interfere with the performance of the magnet **(Figure 4.3)**.[11,12]

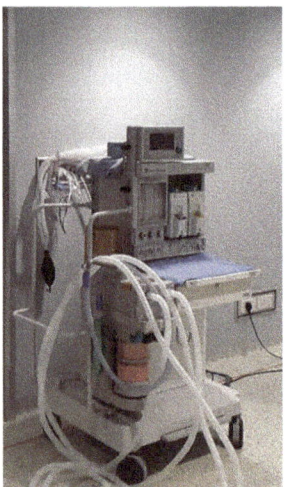

Figure 4.3 Magnetic resonance safe anesthesia machine and vaporizers

Blood Pressure

Minimal adaptations are required with the use of standard blood pressure monitoring techniques. Arterial line should be used for blood pressure monitoring in major craniotomies. Nonferrous transducers should be used.[13]

Electrocardiogram

Magnetic resonance safe electrodes and cables should be used. Some changes in electrocardiogram (ECG) waveform are usually present even in filtered system. ECG wires can cause distortion of MR images and ECG signals but telemetric ECG eliminates the need for wires. There are risks of burns, thermal injuries, and shock hazards to the patient during ECG monitoring. These risks can be minimize by placing the ECG leads near the center of the scanner, keeping the electrode close to each other and avoiding the loops of the cables. Noise free view of ECG wave form during the procedures should be achieved by adjusting the electronic filters on ECG monitors. If any cardiac event is encountered or suspected during the procedure, patient should be immediately removed from the high-field MRI.[14-16]

Acoustic Noise

Ear plugs can be used as effective barrier against sound but at the same time it should not affect the commands from physician and respond to emergency.

Temperature Control

Temperature monitoring should be done in all cases. Heat generated by magnetic field can increase body temperature and contrarily, cool MRI environment required in MR room may decrease body temperatures.[16]

Pulse Oximetry

Magnetic resonance compatible nonferrous and fiber optic oximeters are available. The oximeter machine should remain 2 meters away from the MR scanners to prevent migration. The oximeter probe should be kept on a distal extremity as far from the magnetic field as possible. Oxygen in the MRI is supplied by wall outlet extending to the hospital central supply or aluminum cylinder.[16]

Capnography

Capnography monitoring should be used in all cases requiring general anesthesia. The anesthesiologist uses end-tidal CO_2 monitors with elongated sampling tube for monitoring. Delay in gas sampling readings is likely because the analyzer is located far from the magnet.[14,15]

General Anesthesia Consideration

Proper functioning of the anesthesia machine should be evaluated prior to their clinical use. Patient is to be induced in an adjacent area outside of the magnetic field on MRI table that will be used during the surgery. After induction, additional monitors are utilized that include arterial line, central venous line and urinary catheters.

For ventilation maintenance and drug administration, an extended anesthetic circuit is required. So, there is increased dead space which causes delay in expected anesthetic effect. An intravenous (IV) anesthetic with volatile agents combination is preferred. Desflurane is a preferred volatile agent. It allows rapid return of the consciousness, thus allowing prompt neurological examination. The preferential IV anesthetic agents for the management of neurosurgeries are remifentanil and dexmedetomidine.[17,18]

SAFETY OF CONTRAST AGENT

Gadolinium-based contrast agents (GBCAs) use are associated with increase incidence to cause fatal disease called nephrogenic systemic fibrosis (NSF). A boxed warning and new warnings about risk of NSF for all GBCAs has been advised by the Food and Drug Administration (FDA). The boxed warning states that exposure to GBCAs increases the NSF risk in patients who have acute or chronic severe renal failure [glomerular filtration rate (GFR) less than 30 mL/min/1.73 m^2]. The anesthesiologist must be aware of this warning and should screen all the patient for renal dysfunction.[19]

SAFETY OF INTRAOPERATIVE MAGNETIC RESONANCE IMAGING

Three major components of MR system include: (1) the static magnetic field (B0); (2) the RF electromagnetic field (B1); and (3) the gradient magnetic field (dB/dt).[20,21]

1. Static magnetic field is created with either permanent or superconducting magnets. Its main function is to align the protons. To date, there have been no firmly established biological adverse effects of magnetic fields of up to 3T, however, mechanical effects are extremely dangerous. The magnetic isocenter has very high and homogeneous magnetic field and magnetic field decays over the distance from the magnet. There is a MR safe line defined at 5G (1T–10,000G). All MR installations have a unique gauss plot to define the area around the device **(Figure 4.4)**. An important transitional zone occurs as you close to the magnet, as the magnetic field increases rapidly, there will be faster acceleration of ferrous objects and, so the higher potential energy delivery to healthcare workers or the patient near the iMRI.

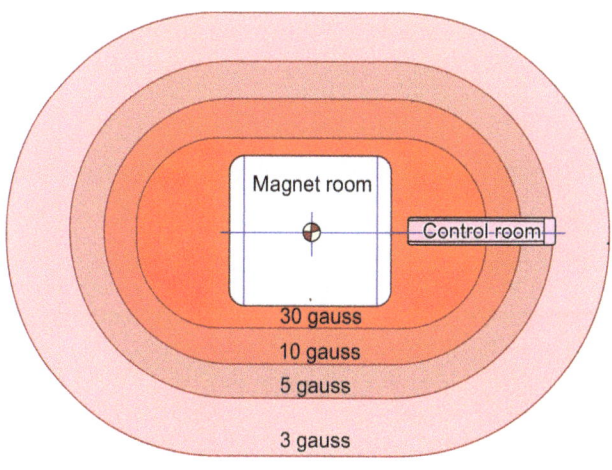

Figure 4.4 Gauss plot

2. The second major component in MR is the dB/dt. Its main function is the localization of protons. It can cause neural and muscular activation and can cause induced voltage in conductive objects (e.g. pacemaker), instrument movement or failure and spatial artifacts in the images. It is the major source of noise in the MR environment and create heat within the tissues. All scanners are optimized to function at low dB/dt to limit its risk.
3. The third physical force in MRI is the B1. Its main function is excitation of protons. The main risk of the RF field is heating. The danger of RF is addressed by limiting the specific absorption rate (SAR), avoiding looped wires near the patient or staff and individually screening equipment for compatibility with the RF field in the ranges use for iMRI cases.[22]

INFECTION CONTROL IN THE INTRAOPERATIVE MAGNETIC RESONANCE IMAGING SUITE

It is achieved with autoclave, a decontaminator and instrument packaging facilities within the iMRI department. Ninety-five percent of instruments used in the iMRI suite are color-coded and grouped together for cleaning and sterilization. The iMRI suite is cleaned and prepared under the same standard practices as other ORs. The patient is moved into the operating environment, within the confines of the two coils. A specially designed sterile drape is used to create a sterile barrier between the physician and the coils. The physicians wear sterile vests that promote sterility of the properly gowned physicians' backs. The final sterile field is created once the patient has been placed in the correct operating position and the physician is properly gowned and the coils properly draped.[23,24]

AMERICAN COLLEGE OF RADIOLOGY: MRI SAFE PRACTICE GUIDELINES

American College of Radiology (ACR) proposed a blue ribbon panel regarding safety of MRI to provide guidance and standards for safe MRI examination. These guidelines were initially published in 2002 and are regularly revised since then.[23,25,26]

According to ACR standard, there is concept of different zones in facilities with MRI scanners:
- *Zone 1:* A non-restricted area that is accessible to all individuals, with no restriction to any material and equipment.
- *Zone 2:* A semi-restricted area in which MRI personnel obtain patients answers to MRI screening questions, take patient histories and perform the final MRI safety patient screening.
- *Zone 3:* A restricted area that should be constantly supervised by trained MR personnel and secured against unauthorized entry.
- *Zone 4:* A restricted area that contains the MRI unit. This zone is always within the 5 G line and is only be accessed by trained personnel, screened staff, patient, and equipment.

This zone approach requires approximately designed MRI suites with access controls that are enforced and adhered by staff.

Patient and personnel screening are the integral part to the ACR guidelines which relies on trained MR personnel.

Device and equipment screening must be done to see for compatibility with MRI.

INTRAOPERATIVE USE OF CONTRAST AGENTS

Sometimes, due to leakage of contrast agents into the resection cavity it may mimic like residual tumor.[27-30] Enhancement becomes more pronounced at the resection margins with increased elapsed time after contrast injection. This can be minimized by immediate administration of contrast prior to iMR and restricting image sequence.[28,30] Intraoperative use of ultrasound aspiration and electrocoagulation may also cause intraparenchymal enhancement.[31] A way out to leakage of contrast has been suggested as monocrystalline iron oxide nanoparticles (MIONs). In animal models, MIONs are specifically taken up by malignant glioma cells which cause increase signal intensities in T1-weighted sequences.[32] Even after surgical manipulation, MIONs remain stable, which is reported by Hunt et al. in two patients.[33] Glioma tumor manipulation causes release of angiogenic active molecules and parenchymal tumor infiltration leads to susceptible blood brain barrier. This enhancing zone has been found histologically positive for tumor.[34] Compared to 1.5T MRI image the same lesion-to-white matter contrast can be obtained using low-field (0.2T) MRI with double dose of contrast medium.[35] To differentiate the recurrent tumor site from reactive changes caused by radiotherapy, dynamic contrast study has been successfully used in iMRI.[36]

SURGICAL DEVICES AND INSTRUMENTS

When surgical instruments which are made of ferromagnetic iron alloys are brought into the magnetic field may become projectiles which may interfere with MRI functioning.[37,38] There are MRI compatible and safe instruments which can be used.[38]

INTRAOPERATIVE IMAGING AND NEURONAVIGATION

In most of the iMRI centers, neuronavigation technology has been implemented. It helps in imaging and resection of residual tumor tissue visible in iMR images. Multiple different neuronavigation technologies are available, also known as frameless stereotaxy systems.[39-42] One of the most commonly used neuronavigation systems is optical navigation. fMRI and magnetoencephalography (MEG) data have also been incorporated into a neuronavigation system.[43,44] In burr hole procedures, there are devices for proper placement of biopsy needles, drainage catheters or other instruments under iMR guidance. They can function independently without the help of other navigation system or can use optical navigation system for alignment of the trajectory plane with the imaging plane.[45]

IMPACT ON LENGTH OF OPERATION

There is lengthening of operation time with the use of iMRI. In a comparative study by Hall et al. comprising 12 pediatric and 35 adult patients, they looked for the mean time interval between first and repeat resections in iMRI suite and conventional OR. The mean time interval in the iMRI group was 18 months and 11.3 months for pediatric and adult patients, respectively whereas in the conventional OR group it was 13.3 months and 9.3 months, respectively.[45]

INTRAOPERATIVE MAGNETIC RESONANCE IMAGING-GUIDED NEUROSURGERY APPLICATION

The major goal of iMRI is to provide near real-time image guidance for interventional and surgical procedures. This is basically provided for catheter based or endoscopic procedures. iMRI is mainly implicated for multiple surgical and interventional procedures including biopsies, craniotomies for image-guided resection of intracranial tumor, epileptogenic foci, intracranial cyst drainage, placement of electrodes and thermal ablation of tumors. Its use in glioma surgery is to achieve complete resection as much as possible. Conventional imaging techniques including T1W, T2W, and fluid-attenuated inversion recovery (FLAIR) images are mainly used for anatomic assessment of brain lesions. In FLAIR images, cerebrospinal fluid (CSF) bright signal is suppressed and is thus used especially for detection of periventricular white matter lesion. T2W images are especially useful for detecting posterior fossa lesion. The integration of fMRI and DTI into planning of surgery and intraoperative guidance system will increase the chance of complete resection of tumor and preservation of functioning brain tissue. DTI and fMRI images provide information regarding the white matter tracts and eloquent cortical areas. MR spectroscopy provides metabolic information, so it can be used to differentiate normal brain tissue and pathologic lesion. The use of molecular imaging techniques may also improve the detection of tumor margins.[46,47]

IMAGING IN INTRAOPERATIVE MAGNETIC RESONANCE IMAGING

Basic Principle of Magnetic Resonance Imaging

Magnetic resonance imaging uses the phenomenon of nuclear magnetic resonance (NMR), discovered by Bloch et al.[48] and Purcell et al.[49]

Basically, it is based on electromagnetic activity of atomic nuclei with odd number nucleons. The best target for in vivo MRI is hydrogen nuclei (1H) which has following advantages: (a) it produces the greatest NMR signal among all nuclei present in tissues; (b) it achieves excellent contrast between different tissues.

On exposure to magnetic field, hydrogen nuclei precess around the particular magnetic field axis with a frequency called as Larmor frequency **(Figure 4.5)**.[50] When a patient is placed in a magnetic field, a small fraction of hydrogen nuclei in the body align themselves along the magnetic field to attain the lowest energy level producing a net magnetization Z–axis direction known as longitudinal magnetization (LM) **(Figure 4.6)**.

After the application of excitation RF pulse, there is realignment of portion of the LM in a plane perpendicular to it (XY plane) **(Figure 4.7)**.

When the RF pulse is switched off, there is realignment of magnetic field from transverse to LM and it induces a current in a receiver coil. This current becomes MR signal **(Figure 4.8)**.

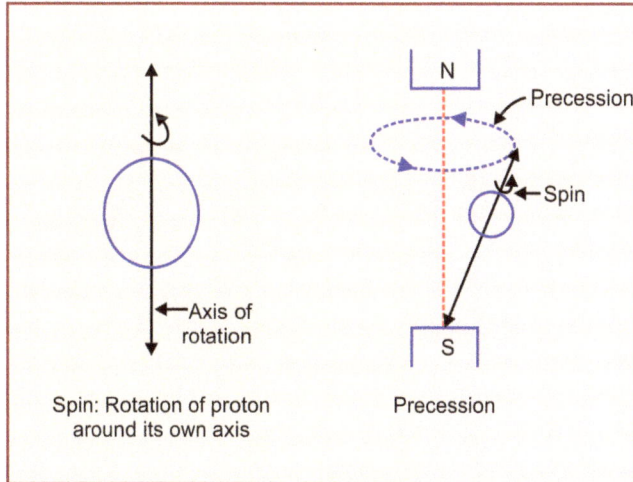

Figure 4.5 Precession of proton around the axis of the magnetic field

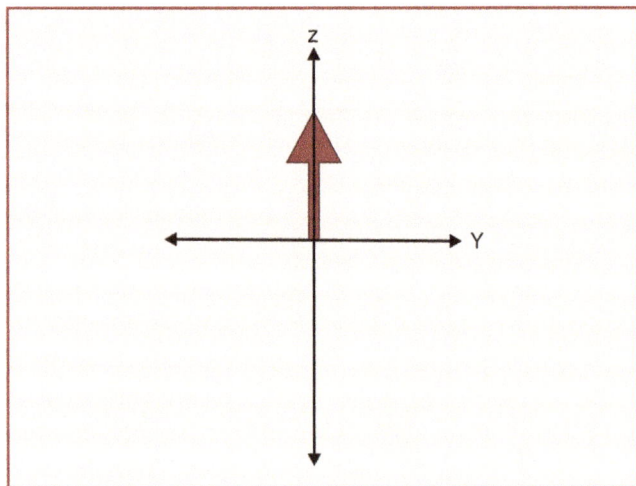

Figure 4.6 Formation of longitudinal magnetization

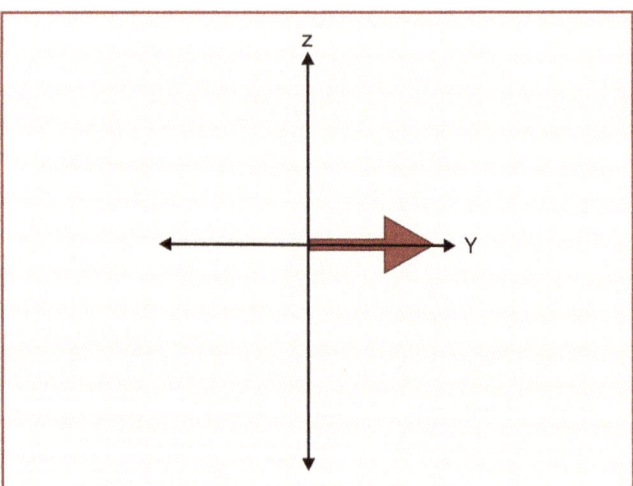

Figure 4.7 Formation of transverse magnetization

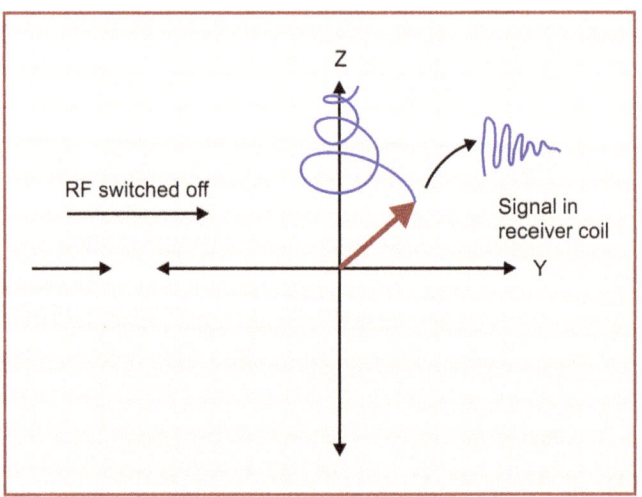

Figure 4.8 Realignment of magnetic field

Longitudinal Relaxation Time

The time taken by LM to recover after RF pulse is switched off is known as longitudinal relaxation time (T1). This is the time when LM reaches back to 63% of its original value. T1 depends upon tissue composition, structure, and surroundings. If surrounding matter has magnetic field which fluctuates at Larmor frequency, energy transfer from protons to the surrounding is easy and fast. Water molecules move rapidly, the proton in water takes long time to transfer their energy, thus water has long T1. On the other hand, in fatty acids fluctuating magnetic field have frequency near Larmor frequency, there is fast energy transfer from fat protons to the surrounding, so fatty acids have short T1.[51,52]

Transverse Relaxation Time

It is the time taken by transverse magnetization (TM) to disappear or to reduce to 37% of its maximum value. It depends inhomogenicity of local magnetic fields within the tissue. Water molecules move very fast, their magnetic fields fluctuate fast. These fluctuating magnetic fields cancel each other. So, because of lack of inhomogenicity, protons stay in phase for a long–time resulting into long transverse relaxation time (T2) for water. On the other hand, in fat tissue because of inhomogenicity of magnetic field within the tissue, proton go out of the phase very fast, therefore fat has short T2.[52]

LOCALIZATION OF THE SIGNAL

To obtain the final MR image, imaging volume of interest is divided into subdivisions called voxels (volumetric regions) by using gradient coils in three directions (x-, y-, and z-axis). So, magnetic fields are superimposed upon the main magnetic field along X-, Y-, and Z-axis to localize from where the signals are coming. These magnetic fields have different strength in varying location hence, these fields are called gradient fields. These gradients are produced by coils called as gradient coils. The three gradients are: (1) slice selection gradient (z-axis), (2) phase encoding gradient (y-axis), and (3) frequency encoded gradient (x-axis).

Information from all three axes is sent to computers to get the particular point in that slice from which the signal is coming. Coordinates provided by these three gradients aid in exact localization of signal to a particular voxels and this information is stored in K-space. K-space is a matrix where the acquired data is stored. Fourier transformation of data are then performed to get the final image.

- *TE (Echo time):* It is the time interval between the application of the excitation RF pulse and the peak of the corresponding detected signal.
- *TR (Repetition time):* It is the time interval between the application of two successive excitation RF pulses.

By varying the TR and TE of pulse sequences, different weightings can be provided to the acquired MR images.

T1WI is obtained using shorter values of TR and TE. T2WI is obtained by using longer values TE and TR.[51-53]

NORMAL SIGNAL INTENSITY

Signal intensity depends on density of protons in the tissue, T1, T2 and flow and diffusion effect. Water has long T1 and long T2 and it appears dark on T1-weight imaging (T1WI) and bright on T2-weight imaging (T2WI). Fat has short T1 and T2 and it appears bright on T1WI and less bright on T2WI. Inspite of its short T2, fat does not appears dark on T2WI because of its high proton content.

- Air is dark on all pulse sequences because of very low proton content
- Cortical bone is also dark on both T1 and T2W images because of the very low mobile protons
- Appearance of medullary bone depends upon the degree of fat replacement
- Circulating blood in the vessels appear flow void (dark) on spin echo sequences and bright on gradient echo sequences
- Calcification is usually dark on both T1WI and T2WI with some exception. Lesions having high content of proteinaceous material, methemoglobin and cholesterol debris appear bright on T1WI
- The normal white matter is bright on T1WI as compared to gray matter. It is because of the myelin content of white matter.[53,54]

SELECTION OF SEQUENCE IN OPEN NEUROSURGERY

Intraoperative magnetic resonance imaging is useful for brain tumor resection, pituitary tumor surgeries, skull base resections and excision of refractory epileptic areas.

T1WIs, T2WI, and FLAIR are used for anatomic assessment of the brain lesions. Periventricular white matter lesions are better detected on FLAIR images. For posterior fossa lesion, it is less sensitive than T2WI to detect the pathology. Most of the diseases are associated with increased T1 and T2 relaxation times with edema hence, appear bright on T2WI images.

T2WIs are also used for calculation of T2 and volume ratio of hippocampus for the diagnosis of hippocampal sclerosis.

T1 magnetization-prepared rapid acquisition gradient-echo (MP-RAGE) is used to obtained 3D reference image for navigation purposes after fixation of the head with MRI compatible head holder.[53-55]

Intravenous Gadolinium

Intravenous gadolinium injection is essential for the evaluation of brain tumors. Tumor enhancement suggest break in blood brain barrier and it does not necessarily represent tumor vascularity. Tumor vascularity is assessed with MR perfusion.[54]

Susceptibility-weighted Imaging

Susceptibility-weighted imaging (SWI) shows high sensitivity to magnetic susceptibility differences of various substances particularly calcification, blood calcification and slow flow in vascular structures.

It provides information in variety of disorders including the cerebral hemorrhage and petechial hemorrhage in diffuse axonal injury, infarct, neoplasm, and various neurodegenerative disorders which are associated with iron deposition or intracranial calcification. Various studies has shown that SWI is more sensitive than conventional T2WI gradient–echo sequences.[55]

Four sets of images are obtained: (1) SWI, (2) SWI [minimum intensity projection (mIP)], (3) magnitude, and (4) phase image. The mIP images are very helpful for demonstration of cortical veins and their tubular nature, thereby differentiating from focal lesions.

For left-handed system (e.g. in Siemens MRI machine), calcium will be dark on both SWI and phase image and hemorrhage will be dark on SWI and bright on phase image as depicted in case study of high-grade glioma **(Figures 4.9A to D)**.

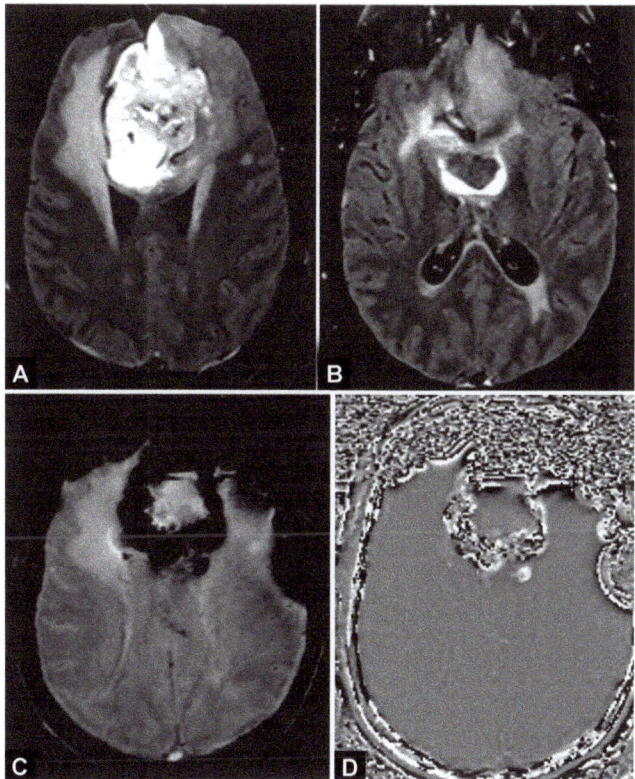

Figures 4.9A to D (A and B) Preoperative T2W FLAIR scan shows high-grade bifrontal glioma and (C and D) SWI and phase image acquired postoperatively showing hyperacute bleed at the tumor resection margins
Abbreviations: FLAIR, fluid-attenuated inversion recovery; SWI, susceptibility-weighted imaging

The main limitation for the use of SWI intraoperatively is the susceptibility artifacts arising at the air tissue interface at the craniotomy site which may mask the visualization of small superficial hemorrhages at the operative site. Artifacts may also be related to operative instrument and operative bed debris.[56,57]

Diffusion-weighted Images

Diffusion-weighted images (DWIs) can used to assess ischemic infarct which arises during the surgery. In routine, diffusion is performed with echo-planar imaging (EPI) sequence and the acquisition time is less than a minute. With preset postprocessing, a few sets of images are available for viewing after the acquisition. These include images with b value 0, higher b value and apparent diffusion coefficient (ADC) map. DWIs are high b value images. DWI can detect early ischemic lesion as early as minutes to hours. Infarct will be seen bright on DWI and dark on ADC maps **(Figures 4.10A to D)**.[53,54]

Magnetic Resonance Spectroscopy

Magnetic resonance spectroscopy is employed to obtain metabolic information so as to differentiate boundary between a pathologic lesion and normal brain tissue. Metabolic information regarding the glioma is used for selection of stereotactic biopsy sites, treatment planning and the assessment of residual tumor. It can be acquired both preoperatively and intraoperatively. Three methods have been employed for intraoperative acquisition of MRS data in neurosurgery: (1) Single voxel spectroscopy (SVS), (2) Turbo-spectroscopic imaging (TSI), and (3) Chemical shift imaging (CSI). CSI and TSI are commonly used. SVS is used only if data are inconclusive. MRS detects only those metabolites with a concentration greater than 0.5 mM/IL.

Spectral lines of N-acetylaspartate (NAA, at 2.0 ppm), choline (Cho-containing compounds at 3.2 ppm), total creatinine (Cr, at 3.0) and phosphocreatine (at 3.9 ppm), myoinositol (at 3.6 ppm), lactate (at 1.3 ppm), a mixture of glutamine and glutamate (overlapping multiplates at 2.0–2.5 ppm, and 3.75 ppm, respectively) and lipids (broad lines between 0.9 and 1.3 mm) can be observed in MRS spectra of brain. High-grade tumor shows increase in choline and decrease in NAA and also shows lipid peak. Lactate is not seen in normal brain and is a marker of anaerobic metabolism. Extra-axial tumors such as meningioma are characterized by absence of NAA and high alanine or creatine ratio. Metastases shows increase in choline but can be differentiated from high-grade glioma by their increase lipid levels. MRS has been combined with MR perfusion, DWIs for tumor grading and differentiating the tumor recurrence from the radiation necrosis.[58,59]

DYNAMIC SUSCEPTIBILITY-WEIGHTED CONTRAST-ENHANCED PERFUSION-MRI

Dynamic susceptibility-weighted contrast-enhanced perfusion-MRI (DSC-MRI) utilizes the contrast agent (gadolinium-based) susceptibility effect within the intravascular compartment and thus, allowing the measurement of blood flow in the desired brain region. DSC-MRI can be performed using any of the two sequences: (1) status epilepticus-EPI (SE-EPI) and (2) gradient echo-EPI (GRE-EPI). Three perfusion parameters commonly employed in neurosurgery include: (1) relative peak height (rPH), (2) relative cerebral blood volume (rCBV), and (3) percentage of signal intensity recovery. DSC–MRI uses gadolinium-based contrast agent administration for image acquisition which changes the relaxation parameters in its distribution. As the contrast agent passes through the microvasculature in high concentration, there is decrease in the signal in surrounding tissues which is due to magnetic susceptibility-

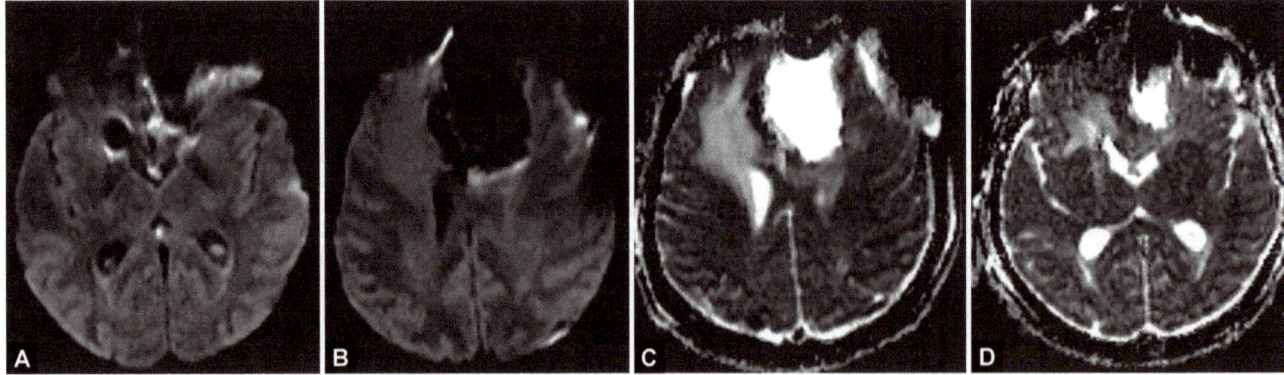

Figures 4.10A to D (A and B) DWI and (C and D) ADC maps acquired postoperatively show resection cavity with no evidence of any diffusion restriction
Abbreviations: ADC, apparent diffusion coefficient; DWI, diffusion-weighted images

induced shortening of T2 relaxation time. This drop in signal is proportional to the perfusion. More the number of vessels per voxel of the tissue, more will be the signal drop if considering the concentration of contrast agent constant. Recurrent tumor can be distinguish from the tumor necrosis based on high rCBV in recurrent tumor. Higher rCBV values from more malignant regions of glioma (due to increase cellularity and microvascular density) can be exploited for biopsy site localization. It is also used to differentiate necrotic tumor from a pyogenic brain abscess. Solitary metastases can also be differentiated from glioma based on differences in the measurement of peritumoral rCBV.[54,60,61]

"Diffusion tensor imaging and fMRI" can be further employed to obtain information regarding eloquent cortical areas and white matter tracts. The combined use of both techniques helps localize twice as many functional areas as fMRI alone can.

Diffusion Tensor Imaging

Diffusion tensor imaging is a unique non-invasive MRI technique which quantifies change in neural tissue microstructure. It is used for detecting anisotropic water diffusion. Water molecules diffusion is greatest along the longitudinal direction of neural sheath. The degree of anisotropy allows data profiling based upon white matter tract position, orientation and white matter tracts integrity with respect to adjacent tumor.[62] In DTI, images are acquired in at least six usually 12–24 directions instead of three in usual trace diffusion. Pure ADC for each pixel is calculated from these images in multiple direction which is known as principal eigenvalue. This value is calculated along the true axis of diffusion called as eigenvector. The image formed with principal eigenvalue is called as diffusion tensor image which gives orientation of fiber tracts. The two main parameters derived from DTI data are (1) mean diffusivity (MD) or in other term ADC and (2) fractional anisotropy (FA). FA reflects the directionality of molecular displacement by diffusion and vary between 0 (isotropic diffusion) and 1 (infinite anisotropic diffusion). FA value of CSF is 0. MD reflects the average magnitude of molecular displacement by diffusion. The more the MD value, the more the isotropic is the medium. Color-coded maps of FA are generated to depict white matter tracts. White matter tracts with orientation in anterior-posterior, left-right and superior to inferior direction are coded as green, red, and blue, respectively.[63,64] Fiber tractography is a 3D reconstruction technique to access neural tracts using data collected by DTI. It also provide information regarding edema, infiltration, disruption and displacement of white matter tracts by adjacent lesions. It allows the detection of white matter tracts involvement by gliomas which is helpful in planning the extent of tumor resection and predict the recurrence of postoperative tumor **(Figure 4.11)**.[65]

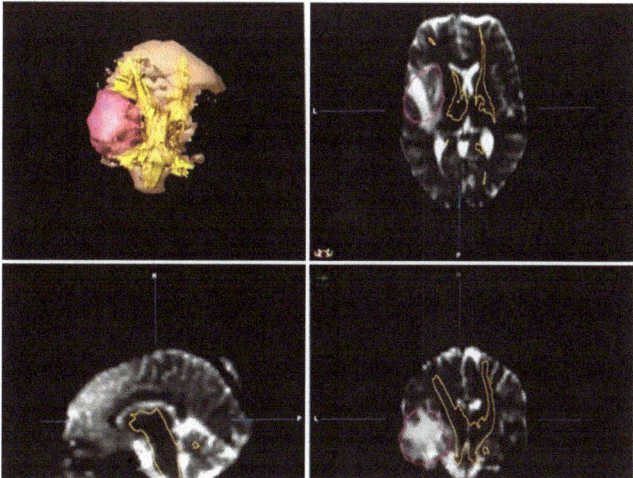

Figure 4.11 Diffusion tensor imaging (DTI) fiber tracking showing peri-insular glioma and its relation with pyramidal tracts

Functional Magnetic Resonance Imaging

Functional magnetic resonance imaging provides functional information by assessing cortical activity of brain. This method provides the information regarding the anatomical location of eloquent areas close to the pathology and thus helps in minimizing postoperative morbidity and attaining best functional outcome. fMRI uses the method of blood oxygen level dependent (BOLD) imaging and detects slight variation in flow of the blood in response to actions and stimuli. When any brain area is excited by particular task, blood flow to that area increases. The increase in blood flow is much more than the metabolic demand with resultant increased amount of oxyhemoglobin and relatively less deoxyhemoglobin in that area which is then detected on T2*WI GRE sequences. A resultant BOLD map is usually superimposed on a T1WI image. Protocol of fMRI on 1.5 T is a single shot EPI [repetition time (TR)/echo time (TE): 300 ms/40 ms; field of view (FOV): 210 mm; matrix: 64 × 64; slice thickness: 7 mm; intersection gap: 1mm; repetitions: 72] with a scan time of ~ 4 minute passive stimulation techniques or patient is asked to perform specific task by controlled awakening from anesthesia for stimulating a particular area in brain. A block design of passive stimulation paradigms in which block of neural stimulation are alternate by rest is commonly employed. Propofol is considered best anesthetic agent for iMRI acquisition as stimulus evoked cortical activity is not interfered by it below the limit of fMRI data acquisition. Thus, fMRI is very helpful in surgical planning of the tumor, thereby providing crucial information regarding positioning of craniotomy sites, margins of surgical excision, and surgical approach to the lesions and also enable the surgeon to demarcate borders between eloquent areas and tumor.[66-68]

SCAN PROTOCOL

There are three sets of scans which are acquired for tumor resection. First is acquired before the start of the surgery. The second set is acquired intraoperatively to evaluate tumor resection extent. Third set is acquired after the completion of craniotomy to exclude the presence of hematoma developed during the surgery closure. Coronal, sagittal T2WI, and 3D coronal T1WI are employed for transsphenoidal surgeries. Sometimes, it may vary with surgeon preference and circumstances.

BRAIN SHIFT

The brain shift and the deformed intracranial structures can be detected by iMRI. The most important factor in tumor resection is movement of the tumor margins rather than the cortical shift. iMRI offers the advantage of brain shift

compensation, which may be crucial for gross total resection of tumors.[47] The data from repeat scanning need to imported into the neuronavigation device **(Figure 4.12)**.

Brain Biopsy

Precision of biopsy needle placement within the lesion can be directly confirmed using iMR. Using different trajectories of iMR, multiple lesions can be sampled through the same burr hole. iMR helps in alignment and stabilization of the biopsy needle, an important step in obtaining samples.[34]

Prospective Stereotaxy

Prospective stereotaxy is helpful in determining the trajectory of the biopsy needle. The target, proposed and actual trajectory can be displayed using this high-field imaging which eludes the problems associated with brain shift.[69]

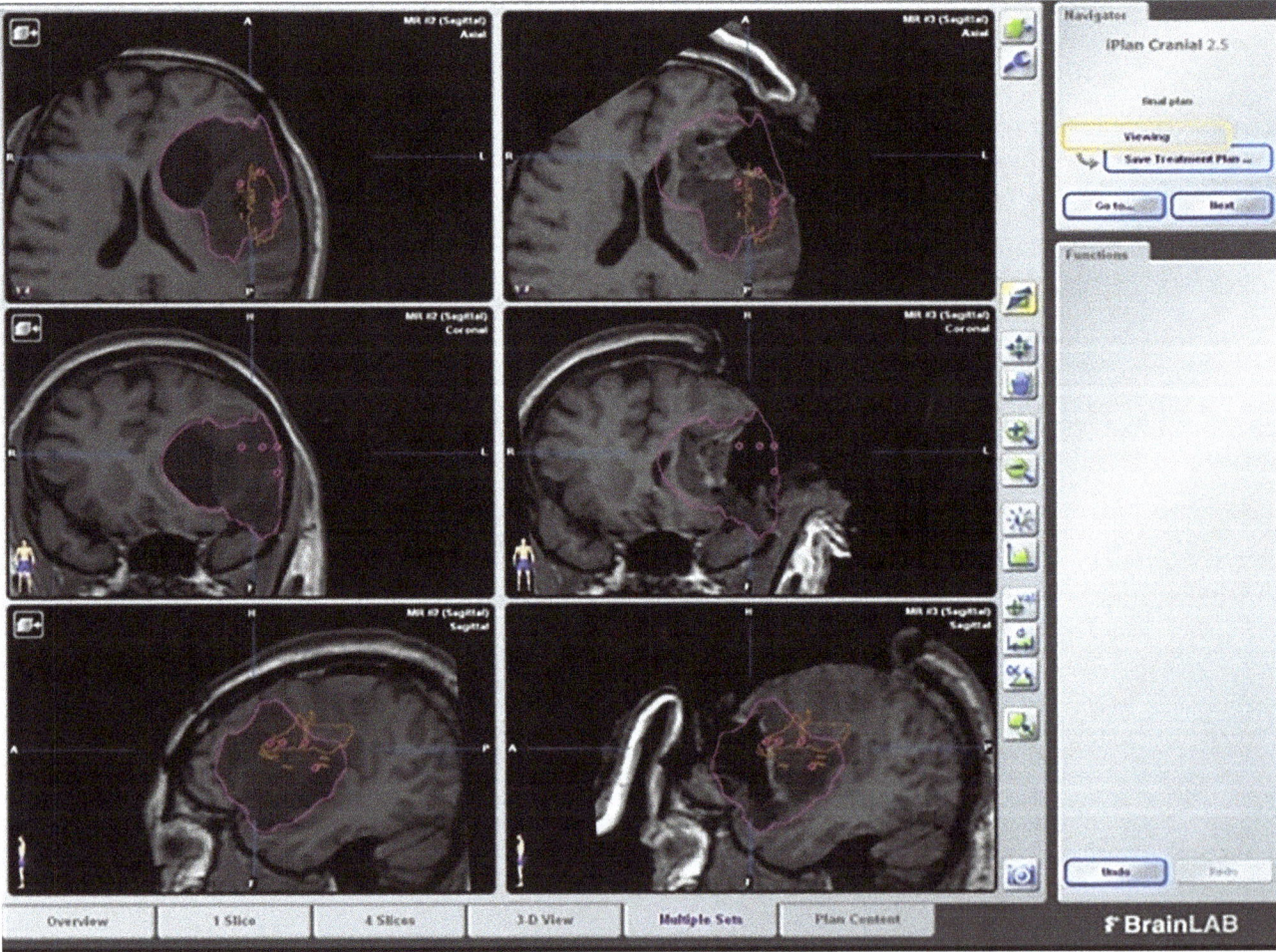

Figure 4.12 Navigation screen showing coregistered preoperative and intraoperative T1-weighted images depicting segmented tumor remnant

MAGNETIC RESONANCE SPECTROSCOPY–GUIDED BRAIN BIOPSY

With high field strength MRI, MRS helps in assessing the chemical metabolites of the tumor. MRS can detect high choline and decreased NAA levels in tumor, thus reflecting the high cell membrane turnover. Radiation necrosis and recurrent tumor can be differentiated using MRS. So, it can be used to direct the biopsy to the area thought to possess the highest diagnostic yield in a heterogeneous tumor.[70,71]

INTRAOPERATIVE MAGNETIC RESONANCE IMAGING GUIDANCE TO VENTRICLE AND CYST

Intraoperative magnetic resonance (iMR) is mainly difficult situation such as with varying skull geometries, ventricular shapes, congenital anomalies and in small or pediatric anatomy. iMRI imaging allows for visualization of smaller fluid-filled spaces as well as catheter trajectory determination. Nimsky et al. indicate that among the iMR pediatric cases at their institution, it was monitoring of catheter placement and consecutive cyst alteration which proved to be the most beneficial application of this technology.[47]

ROLE OF INTRAOPERATIVE MAGNETIC RESONANCE IMAGING IN DEEP BRAIN STIMULATION

Deep brain stimulation (DBS) is a procedure which involves neurostimulator (electrode) implantation that sends electrical impulses, to a specified brain area, commonly used for treatment of different movement and affective disorders like Parkinson's disease, essential tremor, dystonia, and obsessive–compulsive disorder. Depolarization blockade, synaptic inhibition and desynchronization of abnormal neuron oscillatory activity has been proposed as different mechanism of action of DBS. DBS has also been found beneficial in patients having refractory epilepsy not responding to antiepileptic drugs or after surgical resection and also in patients where epilepsy surgery is contraindicated **(Figures 4.13 and 4.14)**.

The subthalamic nucleus (STN), anterior and central-medial thalamic nucleus, and hippocampus are common stereotactic targets for DBS. In traditional DBS surgery, microelectrode recording (MER) is used to map the STN and localized its center of motor region. With iMRI, the surgeons can see this region directly and can place the DBS electrode without the need for MER. This real-time iMRI is very useful for guiding DBS electrode placement to the STN, with the help of skull-mounted aiming device. This is done under local anesthesia utilizing preoperative imaging, implantation device and postimplantation MRI.[72,73]

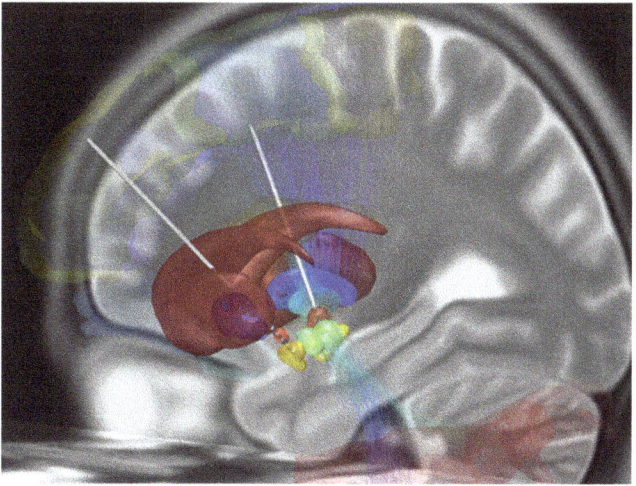

Figure 4.13 Deep brain stimulation (DBS) electrodes reconstruction image. Substantia nigra (yellow), red nucleus (green), subthalamic nucleus (orange), the striatum (red), the internal pallidum (cyan) and external pallidum (blue). Cortical regions in which the tracts terminate are shown as translucent colors and fiber tracts are shown as color-coded fibers[74]

INTRAOPERATIVE MAGNETIC RESONANCE IMAGING

For Transsphenoidal Surgery

Intraoperative magnetic resonance imaging improves the visualization of intrasellar and parasellar compartments and acts as an immediate second look, thus facilitating increase in the percentage of tumor removal. However, even with high-field imaging, tumor remnants could not be detected in every case. To differentiate residual tumor from normal tissue and postoperative changes, dynamic contrast-enhanced MRI (CEMRI) is used. Gadolinium soaked cotton pledgets have been used to identify residual tumor. Also, iMRI and endoscopic transsphenoidal surgery can be complementary to each other providing more information and, thus facilitate the complete resection of tumor.[75]

For Primary Brain Tumor

Intraoperative helps in achieving more complete tumor removal and at the same time increase the chance of preserving the functioning brain tissue. However, even with the use of iMRI, postoperative deficit can results as some functioning brain tissue may exists within the tumor because edematous and infiltrative tissue which is functioning may be seen as hypointense areas on T1WI and hyperintense on T2WI. With the help of DTI, the relationship of the tumor with white matter tracts can be traced. The primary aim of using intraoperative imaging is to look for the remnants of tumor and to plan for exact area of surgical resection. Upgradation of image data is also an important aspect of intraoperative imaging for navigation purpose. Case studies are described in **Figures 4.15 and 4.16** shown further.

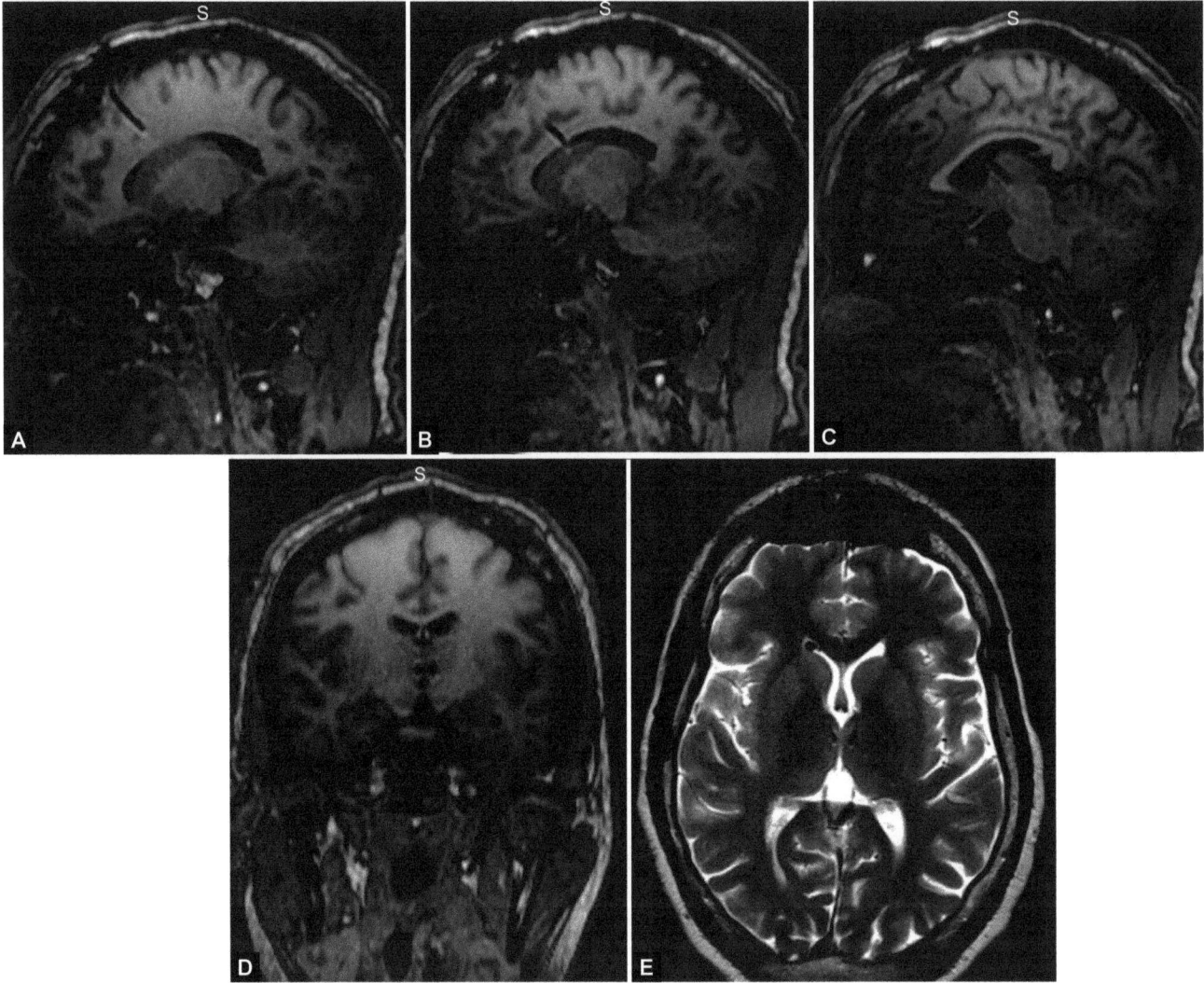

Figures 4.14A to E (A to C) Magnetic resonance imaging (MRI) sagittal T1 MP-RAGE showing safe electrode trajectory to the target (anterior nucleus of thalamus); and (D and E) T1WI coronal image and T2WI axial image showing final electrode position into the anterior nucleus of thalamus
Abbreviations: MP-RAGE, magnetization-prepared rapid acquisition gradient-echo

For Vascular Neurosurgery

Intraoperative magnetic resonance imaging is useful for the complete resection of small vascular lesions like cavernoma. Intraoperative diffusion or perfusion MRI can diagnose acute occlusion of intracranial vessel and can also assessed real-time condition of the brain.[44] Magnetic resonance angiography (MRA), magnetic resonance venography (MRV) and diffusion can identify the vascular structure and function which may prevent injury during the surgery. It can also obviate the need for second surgery in arteriovenous malformation (AVM) resections by identifying the feeding arteries, nidus and draining vein. For deep-seated lesion, navigation approach is less accurate due to intraoperative

brain shift and retraction.[46] Intraoperative angiography role in aneurysm clipping is reserved for complex lesion due to availability indocyanine green (ICG) and micro-Doppler flow probes.

For Spine Surgery

The procedures which have been performed with iMRI include cervical laminectomy, cervical foraminotomies, cervical vertebrectomies with fusion, and cervical and lumbar discectomies with or without fusion. In case of cervical fractures requiring reconstruction, iMRI is a useful tool but not an alternative of plain radiographs as there is

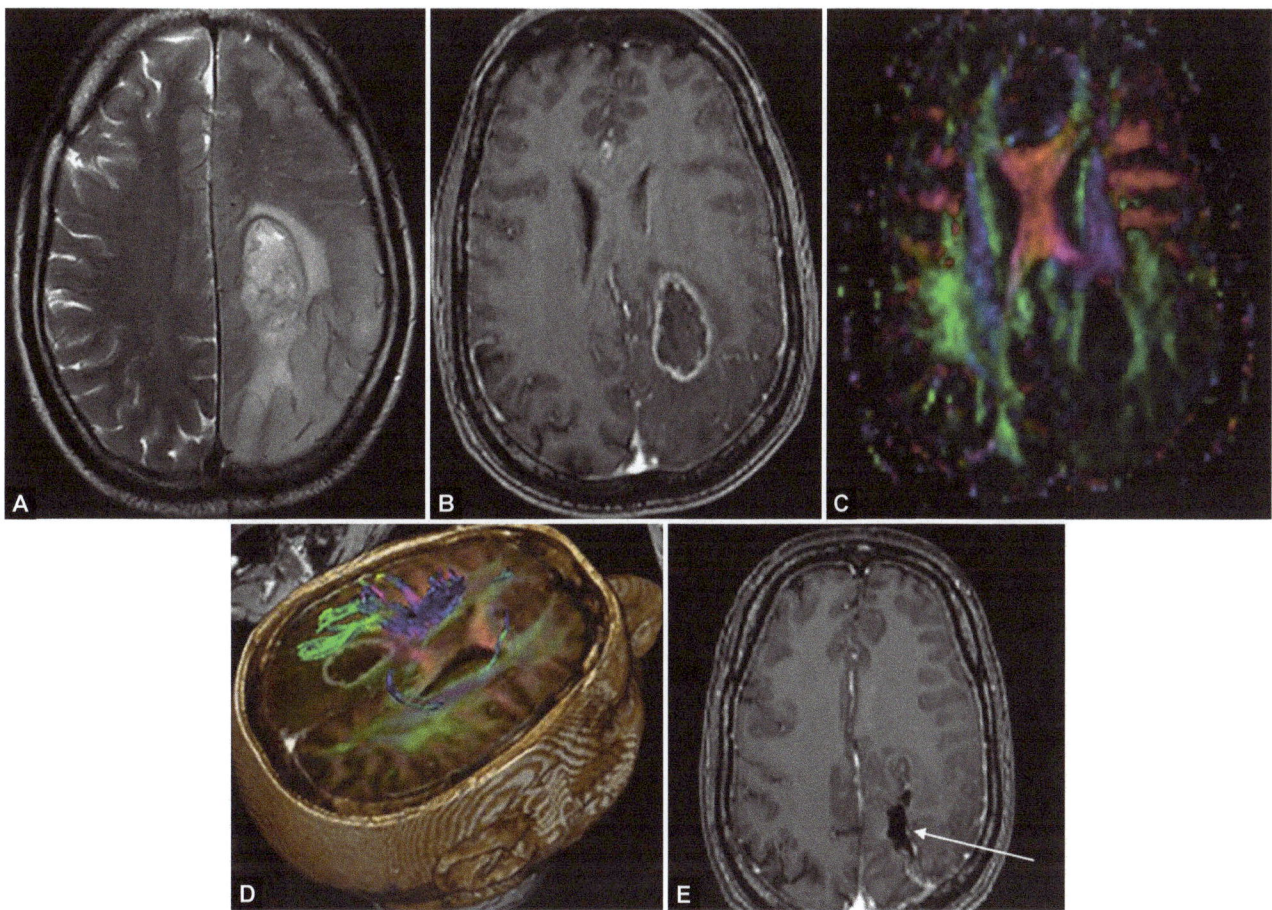

Figures 4.15A to E Left frontoparietal high-grade glioma. (A to D) Preoperative axial T2 FSE, axial postcontrast and coregistered FA maps from DTI; and (E) Postoperative axial postcontrast images at the end of resection, showing resection cavity
Abbreviations: DTI, diffusion tensor imaging; FA, functional anisotropy; FSE, fast spin-echo

significant image artifacts in surgical area despite the use of MR compatible materials, thus impairing to assess the proper placement of instrumentation. The advantage of iMRI is in cervical spine surgery because of the capability of providing high-resolution images to visualize the osteolytic lesion and soft tissue pathology. Other application of iMRI also include spinal cord tumor resection and screw fixation or spinal endoscopy trajectory planning.[76,46]

REFERENCES

1. Black PM, Moriarty T, Alexander E, et al. Development and implementation of intraoperative magnetic resonance imaging and its neurosurgical applications. Neurosurgery. 1997;41(4):831-42.
2. Hall WA, Kowalik K, Liu H, et al. Costs and benefits of intraoperative MR-guided brain tumor resection. Acta Neurochir Suppl. 2002;85:137-42.
3. Hall WA, Liu H, Truwit CL. Navigus trajectory guide. Neurosurgery. 2000;46(2):502-4.
4. Hushek SG. Design of a mid-field intraoperative MR system at 0.5 Tesla. In: Lufkin RP (Ed). Interventional MRI. St. Louis: Mosby; 1999. pp. 15-28.
5. Schenck JF, Jolesz FA, Roemer PB, et al. Superconducting open-configuration MR imaging system for image-guided therapy. Radiology. 1995;195(3):805-14.
6. Nimsky C, Ganslandt O, Hastreiter P, et al. Intraoperative diffusion-tensor MR imaging: shifting of white matter tracts during neurosurgical procedures--initial experience. Radiology. 2005;234(1):218-25.
7. Nimsky C, Ganslandt O, von Keller B, et al. Preliminary experience in glioma surgery with intraoperative high-field MRI. Acta Neurochir Suppl. 2003;88:21-9.
8. Liu H, Hall WA, Truwit CL. The roles of functional MRI in MR-guided neurosurgery in a combined 1.5 Tesla MR-operating room. Acta Neurochir Suppl. 2003;85:127-35.
9. Martin AJ, Liu H, Hall WA, et al. Preliminary assessment of turbo spectroscopic imaging for targeting in brain biopsy. AJNR Am J Neuroradiol. 2001;22(5):959-68.
10. Tummala RP, Chu RM, Liu H, et al. Optimizing brain tumor resection high-field interventional MR imaging. Neuroimaging Clin N Am. 2001;11(4):673-83.

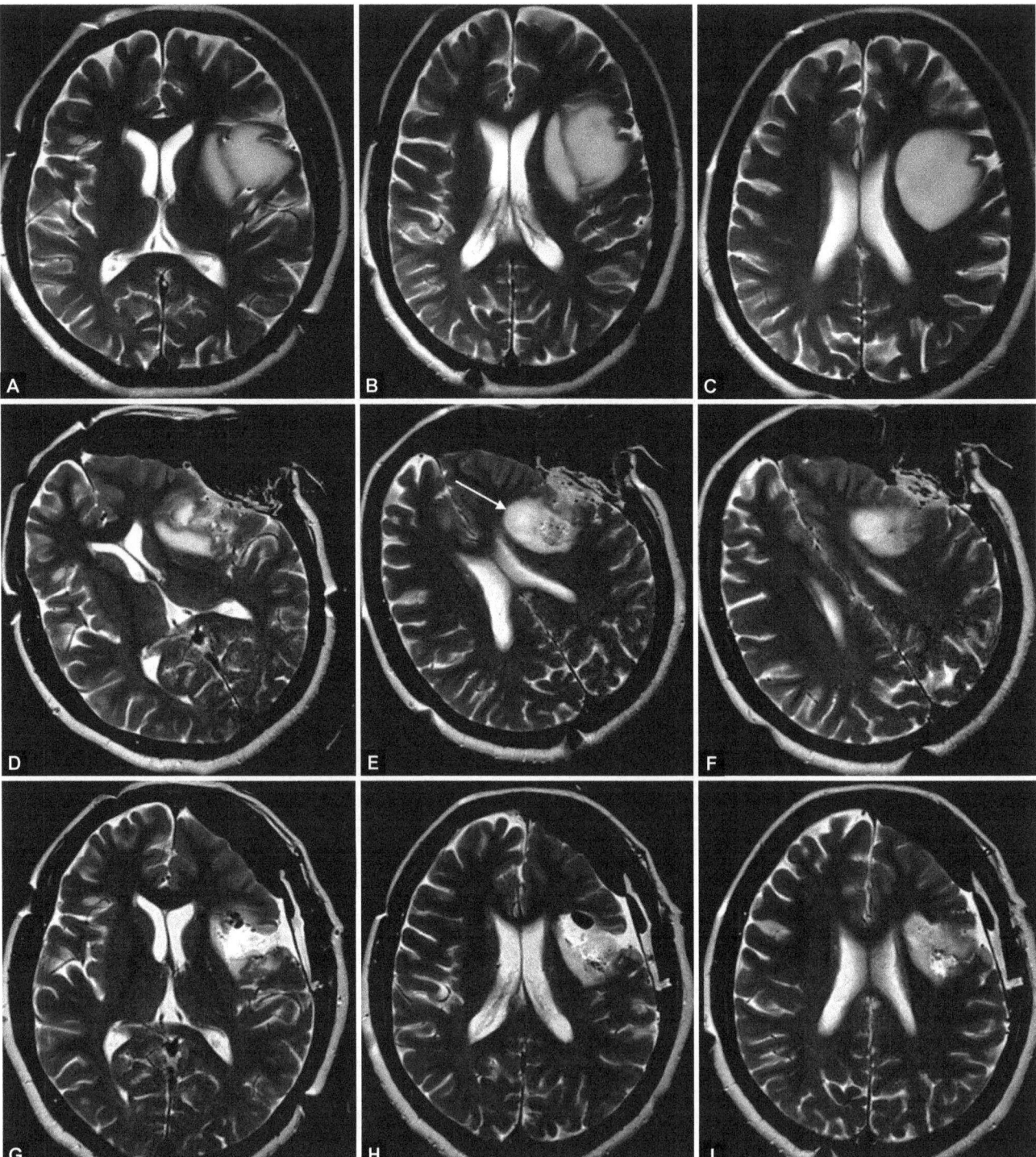

Figures 4.16A to I (A to C) Preoperative scan shows World Health Organization (WHO) grade III left peri-insular astrocytoma; (D to F) Intraoperative scan obtained after debulking of the tumor and shows a small remnant of tumor (white arrow); and (G to I) Postoperative scan showing satisfactory resection cavity with punctate hemorrhages at resection margins. Comparison can be done with the preoperative images shown in Figures 16A to C

11. Bergese SD, Puente EG. Anesthesia in the intraoperative MRI environment. Neurosurg Clin N Am. 2009;20(2):155-62.

12. Barua E, Johnston J, Fujii J, et al. Anesthesia for brain tumor resection using intraoperative magnetic resonance imaging (iMRI) with the Polestar N-20 system: experience and challenges. J Clin Anesth. 2009;21(5):371-6.

13. Patteson SK, Chesney JT. Anesthetic management for magnetic resonance imaging: problems and solutions. Anesth Analg. 1992;74(1):121-8.

14. Bell C, Conte AH. Monitoring oxygenation and ventilation during magnetic resonance imaging: a pictorial essay. J Clin Monit. 1996;2:71-4.

15. Gooden CK. Anesthesia for magnetic resonance imaging. Curr Opin Anaesthesiol. 2004;17(4):339-42.

16. Roth JL, Nugent M, Grey JE, et al. Patient monitoring during magnetic resonance imaging. Anesthesiology. 1985;62(1):80-3.

17. Mackenzie RA, Southron PA, Stensrud PE. Anesthesia at remote locations. In: Miller RD (Ed). Anesthesia, 5th edition. Philadelphia: Churchill Livingstone; 2000. pp. 2241-69.

18. Bergese SD, Khabiri B, Roberts WD, et al. Dexmedetomidine for conscious sedation in difficult awake fiberoptic intubation cases. J Clin Anesth. 2007;19(2):141-4.

19. Kanal E, Barkovich AJ, Bell C, et al. ACR guidance document for safe MR practices: 2007. AJR Am J Roentgenol. 2007; 188(6):1447-74.

20. Shellock FG. Magnetic resonance procedures: health effects and safety. Boca Raton (FL): CRC Press; 2000.

21. Shellock FG, Kanal E. Magnetic resonance: bioeffects, safety, and patient management. Philadelphia: Lippincott-Raven; 1996.

22. Johnston T, Moser R, Moeller K, et al. Intraoperative MRI: safety. Neurosurg Clin N Am. 2009;20(2):147-53.

23. Hushek SG, Russell L, Moser RF, et al. Safety protocols for interventional MRI. Acad Radiol. 2005;12(9):1143-8.

24. Black PM, Moriarty TM, Eben A, et al. Development and implementation of intraoperative magnetic resonance imaging and its neurosurgical applications. Neurosurgery. 1997;41(4):831-45.

25. The Joint Commission. Preventing accidents and injuries in the MRI suite. Sentinel Event Alert. 2008;38.

26. Kanal E, Borgstede JP, Barkovich AJ, et al. American College of Radiology White Paper on MR Safety. AJR Am J Roentgenol. 2002;178(6):1335-47.

27. Nimsky C, Ganslandt O, Hastreiter P, et al. Intraoperative compensation for brain shift. Surg Neurol. 2001;56(6):357-64.

28. Steinmeier R, Fahlbusch R, Ganslandt O, et al. Intraoperative magnetic resonance imaging with the magnetom open scanner: concepts, neurosurgical indications, and procedures: a preliminary report. Neurosurgery. 1998;43(4):739-47.

29. Tuominen J, Yrjänä SK, Katisko JP, et al. Intraoperative imaging in a comprehensive neuronavigation environment for minimally invasive brain tumour surgery. Acta Neurochir Suppl. 2003;85:115-20.

30. Wirtz CR, Knauth M, Staubert A, et al. Clinical evaluation and follow-up results for intraoperative magnetic resonance imaging in neurosurgery. Neurosurgery. 2000;46(5):1112-20.

31. Knauth M, Aras N, Wirtz CR, et al. Surgically induced intracranial contrast enhancement: potential source of diagnostic error in intraoperative MR imaging. AJNR Am J Neuroradiol. 1999;20(8):1547-53.

32. Knauth M, Egelhof T, Roth SU, et al. Monocrystalline iron oxide nanoparticles: possible solution to the problem of surgically induced intracranial contrast enhancement in intraoperative MR imaging. AJNR Am J Neuroradiol. 2001;22(1):99-102.

33. Hunt MA, Bagó AG, Neuwelt EA. Single-dose contrast agent for intraoperative MR imaging of intrinsic brain tumors by using ferumoxtran-10. AJNR Am J Neuroradiol. 2005;26(5):1084-8.

34. Sutherland GR, Kaibara T, Louw DF. Intraoperative MR at 1.5 Tesla--experience and future directions. Acta Neurochir Suppl. 2003;85:21-8.

35. Knauth M, Wirtz CR, Aras N, et al. Low-field interventional MRI in neurosurgery: finding the right dose of contrast medium. Neuroradiology. 2001;43(3):254-8.

36. Schwartz RB, Hsu L, Kacher DF, et al. Intraoperative dynamic MRI: localization of sites of brain tumor recurrence after high-dose radiotherapy. J Magn Reson Imaging. 1998;8(5):1085-9.

37. Fried PM, Hsu L, Topulos GP, et al. Image-guided surgery in a new magnetic resonance suite: preclinical considerations. Laryngoscope. 1996;106(4):411-7.

38. Jolesz FA, Morrison PR, Koran SJ, et al. Compatible instrumentation for intraoperative MRI: expanding resources. J Magn Reson Imaging. 1998;8(1):8-11.

39. Barnett GH. Surgical navigation for brain tumors. In: Winn HR (Ed). Youman's neurological surgery, 5th edition. Philadelphia: Saunders; 2004. pp. 941-9.

40. Bernadete EA, Leonard MA, Weiner HL. Comparison of frameless stereotactic systems: accuracy, precision, and applications. Neurosurgery. 2001;49(6):1409-15.

41. Koivukangas J, Louhisalmi Y, Alakuijala J, et al. Ultrasound-controlled neuronavigator-guided brain surgery. J Neurosurg. 1993;79(1):36-42.

42. McInerney J, Roberts DW. Frameless stereotaxy of the brain. Mt Sinai J Med. 2000;67(4):300-10.

43. Bernstein M, Al-Anazi AR, Kucharczyk W, et al. Brain tumor surgery with the Toronto open magnetic resonance imaging system: preliminary results for 36 patients and analysis of advantages, disadvantages, and future prospects. Neurosurgery. 2000;46(4):900-7.

44. Gralla J, Ganslandt O, Kober H, et al. Image-guided removal of supratentorial cavernomas in critical brain areas: application of neuronavigation and intraoperative magnetic resonance imaging. Minim Invas Neurosurg. 2003;46(2):72-7.

45. Bernays RL, Kollias SS, Khan N, et al. A new artifact-free device for frameless, magnetic resonance imaging-guided stereotactic procedures. Neurosurgery. 2000;46(1):112-6.

46. Mamata Y, Mamata H, Nabavi A, et al. Intraoperative diffusion imaging on a 0.5 Tesla interventional scanner. J Magn Reson Imaging. 2001;13(1):115-9.

47. Chu RM, Tummala RP, Hall WA. Intraoperative magnetic resonance imaging-guided neurosurgery. Neurosurgery Quarterly. 2003;13(4):234-50.

48. Bloch F, Hansen WW, Packard M. Nuclear induction. Phys Rev. 1946;69:127.

49. Purcell EM, Torrey HC, Pound RV. Resonance absorption by nuclear magnetic moments in a solid. Phys Rev. 1946;69:37-8.

50. Curry TS, Dowdey JE, Murray RC. Fluoroscopic imaging. In: Curry TS, Dowdey JE, Murray RC (Eds). Christensen's Physics of diagnostic radiology, 4th edition. Philadelphia: Lea and Febiger; 1990.

51. Bushberg JT, Seibert JA, Leidholdt EM, Boone JM. Nuclear magnetic resonance. In: The essential physics of medical imaging, 2nd edition. Philadelphia: Lippincott-Williams and Wilkins; 2002. pp. 373-413.
52. Mitchell DG. MRI principles. Philadelphia: Saunders; 1999.
53. Hendee WR, Ritenour ER. Fundamentals of magnetic resonance. In: Medical imaging physics, 4th edition. New York: Wiley-Liss; 2002. pp. 355-65.
54. Chavhan GB. MRI made easy, 2nd edition. New Delhi: Jaypee Brothers Medical Publishers (P) Ltd; 2013.
55. Haacke EM, Mittal S, Wu Z, et al. Susceptibility-weighted imaging: technical aspects and clinical applications, part 1. AJNR Am J Neuroradiol. 2009;30(1):19-30.
56. Hingwala D, Kesavadas C, Thomas B, et al. Clinical utility of susceptibility-weighted imaging in vascular diseases of the brain. Neurol India. 2010;58(4):602-7.
57. Mittal S, Wu Z, Neelavalli J, et al. Susceptibility-weighted imaging: technical aspects and clinical applications, part 2. AJNR Am J Neuroradiol. 2009;30(2):232-52.
58. Ross BD, Coletti P, Lin A. Magnetic resonance spectroscopy of the brain: neurospectroscopy. In: Edelman RR, Hesselink JR, Zlatkin MB and Crues JV (Eds). Clinical magnetic resonance imaging, 3rd edition. Philadelphia: Saunders-Elsevier; 2006. pp. 1840-907.
59. Brandao L, Domigues R. MR spectroscopy of the brain. Philadelphia: Lippincott-Williams and Wilkins; 2003.
60. Rosen BR, Belliveau JW, Chien D. Perfusion imaging by nuclear magnetic resonance. Magn Reson Q. 1989;5(4):263-81.
61. Jezzard P. Advances in perfusion MR imaging. Radiology. 1998;208(2):296-9.
62. Nimsky C, Ganslandt O, Hastreiter P, et al. Preoperative and intraoperative diffusion tensor imaging-based fiber tracking in glioma surgery. Neurosurgery. 2005;56(1):130-7.
63. Mukherjee P, Chung SW, Berman JI, et al. Diffusion tensor MR imaging and fiber tractography: technical considerations. AJNR Am J Neuroradiol. 2008;29(5):843-52.
64. Le Bihan D, Mangin JF, Poupon C, et al. Diffusion tensor imaging: concepts and applications. J Magn Reson Imaging. 2001;13(4):534-46.
65. Yu CS, Li KC, Xuan Y, et al. Diffusion tensor tractography in patients with cerebral tumors: a helpful technique for neurosurgical planning and postoperative assessment. Eur J Radiol. 2005;56(2):197-204.
66. Hall WA, Truwit CL. Intraoperative magnetic resonance imaging. Acta Neurochir Suppl. 2011;109:119-29.
67. Gasser T, Ganslandt O, Sandalcioglu E, et al. Intraoperative functional MRI: implementation and preliminary experience. Neuroimage. 2005;26(3):685-93.
68. Parmar H, Sitoh YY, Yeo TT. Combined magnetic resonance tractography and functional magnetic resonance imaging in evaluation of brain tumors involving the motor system. J Comput Assist Tomogr. 2004;28(4):551-6.
69. Truwit C, Liu H. Prospective stereotaxy for intraoperative MR- and CT-guided procedures. Eur Radiol. 2000;10:C37.
70. Hall WA, Martin A, Liu H, et al. Improving diagnostic yield in brain biopsy: coupling spectroscopic targeting with real-time needle placement. J Magn Reson Imaging. 2001;13(1):12-5.
71. Hall WA, Liu H, Martin AJ, et al. Brain biopsy sampling by using prospective stereotaxis and a trajectory guide. J Neurosurg. 2001;94(1):67-71.
72. Starr PA, Martin AJ, Larson PS. Implantation of deep brain stimulator electrodes using interventional MRI. Neurosurg Clin N Am. 2009;20(2):193-203.
73. McIntyre CC, Thakor NV. Uncovering the mechanisms of deep brain stimulation for Parkinson's disease through functional imaging, neural recording, and neural modeling. Crit Rev Biomed Eng. 2002;30(4-6):249-81.
74. Horn A, Kühn A. Lead-DBS: a toolbox for deep brain stimulation electrode localizations and visualizations. Neuroimage. 2015;107:127-35.
75. Pergolizzi RS, Nabavi A, Schwartz RB, et al. Intraoperative MR guidance during transsphenoidal pituitary resection: preliminary results. J Magn Reson Imaging. 2001;13(1):136-41.
76. Duprez TP, Jankovski A, Grandin C, et al. Intraoperative 3T MR imaging for spinal cord tumor resection: feasibility, timing, and image quality using a "twin" MR-operating room suite. AJNR Am J Neuroradiol. 2008;29(10):1991-4.
77. Bohinski RJ, Kokkino AK, Warnick RE, Gaskill-Shipley MF, Kormos DW, Lukin RR, et al. Glioma resection in a shared-resource magnetic resonance operating room after optimal image-guided frameless sterotactic resection. Neurosurg. 2001;48:731-44.

Low-Field Intraoperative Magnetic Resonance Imaging

Christian Senft

GLIOMA SURGERY AND NEURONAVIGATION

Microsurgical resection has been the first step in the treatment of gliomas for many years. Aside from obtaining tissue samples for histopathology, resection of brain tumors may relieve mass effect and reduce symptoms caused by the compression of neural structures. There has been a long scientific debate regarding the value of cytoreductive surgery in gliomas after the introduction of radiation therapy and chemotherapy,[1,2] but many contemporary reports suggest that the extent of tumor resection is an independent prognostic factor in both high- and low-grade gliomas.[3,4] Although, gliomas are infiltrative tumors that cannot be cured by surgery (Sahm, Arch Neurol 2012), increasing evidence suggests that despite advances in chemotherapy, radical removal of the tumor, i.e. of the visible part on magnetic resonance imaging (MRI) scans, corresponds with better patient prognosis. In 2001, Lacroix et al. reported better outcomes for patients with malignant gliomas if at least 97% of the tumor volume could be removed.[5] In 2008, Pichlmeier et al. confirmed that complete removal of the contrast-enhancing tumor, part of a glioblastoma, is an independent prognostic factor.[6] Partial removal does not necessarily bring survival benefits, and experimental data indicate that particularly cells at the tumor margin are fate-determining.[7] In addition to extent of resection and the biological signature of the tumor, the clinical patient status as determined by the Karnofsky performance scale has often been shown to be a strong prognostic factor in glioma patients.[2,8] Therefore, tumor resections must not be undertaken at the cost of neurological deterioration.

In order to avoid surgically-induced neurological deficits and clinical deterioration, eloquent structures, especially the motor cortex and the corticospinal tract, need to be identified and spared during tumor resection. Eloquent structures such as motor or speech cortical areas may be identified either anatomically or, due to anatomical variety regarding the cortical representation of language and speech areas in particular, with the help of intraoperative neurophysiological monitoring techniques.[9]

The introduction of neuronavigation systems in the 1990s has dramatically influenced brain tumor surgery. Being a technology similar to global positioning system (GPS), they allow neurosurgeons to transfer preoperative neuroimaging data, e.g. anatomical as well as functional MRI, into a computer workstation in the operating room. After matching points on the patient's head with corresponding points on the images, a navigational tool is depicted on a screen in its corresponding anatomic location along with the preoperative data. As a result, neuronavigation assists in cranial neurosurgery to confirm the exact localization of anatomic structures or lesions in an online fashion. Neuronavigation has become a standard part of modern neurosurgical operating rooms, helping to plan skin incisions, tailor craniotomies, and make approaches to intraparenchymal lesions less invasive.[10] The usefulness of neuronavigation, however, is limited during the dissection of brain tissue due to anatomical alterations caused by leakage of cerebrospinal fluid, brain edema, or removal of tissue itself. These alterations, called brain shift, cause significant inaccuracy of the neuronavigation because it relies on preoperative images.[11]

THE NEED FOR INTRAOPERATIVE IMAGING

Low-grade gliomas in particular, but to lesser extent also high-grade gliomas, are often difficult to distinguish from healthy brain parenchyma, which needs to be spared during surgery. This renders tumor resections guided by (even microscopic) vision incomplete in many cases, even if the surgeon believes to have achieved a complete resection.[12] Further, the above-mentioned phenomenon of brain shift requires an intraoperative update of the imaging data if neuronavigation shall not be inaccurate. Thus, intraoperative imaging was developed in order to overcome the limitations of neuronavigation based on preoperative images and to visualize tumor remnants that might have been left otherwise unrecognized by the neurosurgeon.[13,14]

Magnetic resonance imaging is the standard imaging modality of the brain and therefore, it is regarded the ideal means of intraoperative imaging. Although, ultrasound provides good depiction of intraparenchymal lesions when the skull is opened before opening the dura, imaging by ultrasound becomes unreliable with regard to assessing the extent of resection and identification of tumor remnants during or after tumor resection.[15] Consequently, MRI devices were developed for intraoperative neurosurgical use. The first intraoperative MRI (iMRI) unit was installed in 1994 at the Brigham and Women's Hospital in Boston.[16] For technical reasons, it was designed as a low magnetic field strength device with 0.5 Tesla (Signa SP, GE Medical Systems, Milwaukee, WI).

In today's iMRI-guided brain tumor surgery, there is a wide variety of different MRI setups. The field strength of devices in use ranges from ultra-low-field (0.15 Tesla) to high-field (3.0 Tesla),[17-22] and they require different adjustments of OR infrastructure, e.g. ferromagnetic shielding or the need for special instruments. Also, the costs for the installation of an iMRI vary significantly between the currently available systems, ranging from $1.5 million to well above $5 million, especially for high-field (1.5 or 3.0 Tesla) devices. Today, low-field iMRI units are still those predominantly in use.

Also in the mid 1990s, Siemens Corporation developed a C-shaped resistive MRI scanner with a static magnetic field with a strength of 0.2 Tesla (Magnetom Open). In contrast to the Signa SP which marked the center of the operating theater, the Magnetom Open was setup at the one end of the operating room, separated from the surgical area by radiofrequency shielding, thus allowing for the use of standard instrumentarium during surgery. The patient had to be transferred to the magnet which featured a 240° opening, allowing for safe placement of the anesthetized patient's head into the scanner's field of view.[23,24] However, image acquisition necessitated transferring the patient from the operating site to the scanner, which is time-consuming.

The AIRIS II MRI scanner (Hitachi Corporation), which was developed primarily as a conventional diagnostic tool employing a magnetic field strength of 0.3 Tesla, has also been used for intraoperative scanning.[18,25] It is an open MRI unit with two horizontally-oriented magnets with a vertical opening of 17 inches. Surgeries can be performed either in the adjacent operating room, or with the patient positioned on the scanner's table.

The PoleStar by Odin or Medtronic Inc. is one of the most frequently used low-field systems today with a static magnetic field strength of 0.12 (Model N-10) or 0.15 Tesla (Models N-20, N-30), respectively. It was developed to overcome the necessity of using special, MRI-compatible instruments and surgical devices, demanded by other iMRI systems, yet avoiding cumbersome patient transfer to the scanner. The PoleStar was designed as a mobile MRI unit with two vertical magnets spaced 25 or 27 cm apart, respectively. During surgery, the magnet is parked underneath the operating table, so that conventional instruments can be used **(Figure 5.1)**, whereas for intraoperative scanning it is moved upwards.[26,27]

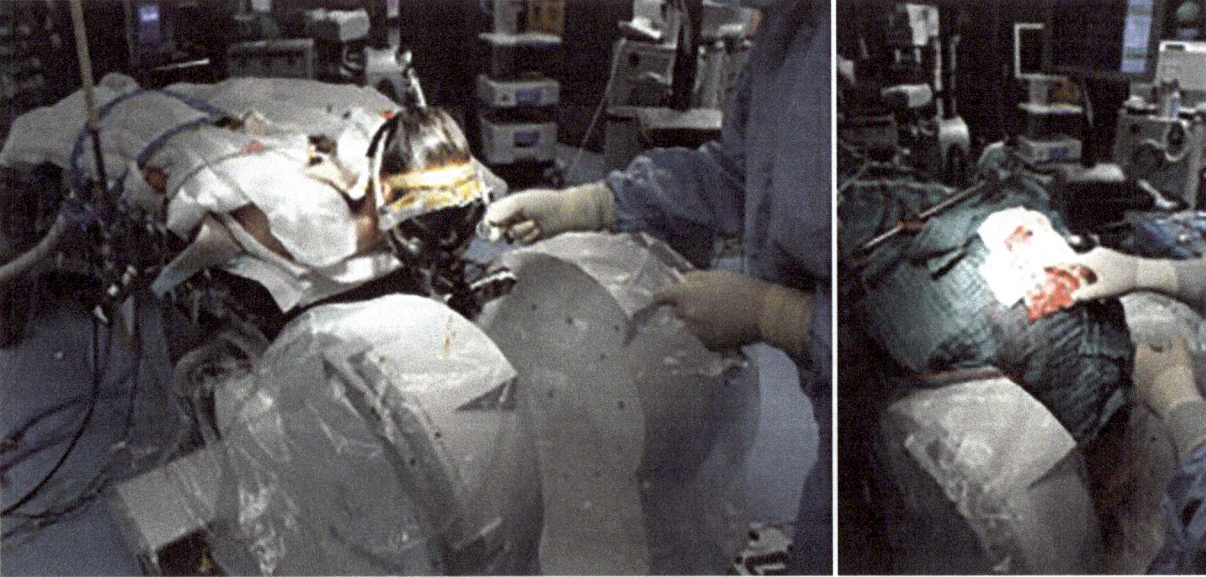

Figure 5.1 Intraoperative setup of surgery with the PoleStar low-field intraoperative magnetic resonance imaging (iMRI). The patient is in supine position, the magnet is parked underneath the patient's head and can be elevated for scanning during surgery

In order to minimize interference induced by electromagnetic currents, etc. the PoleStar can be used in a shielded room, or the device and the patient need to be covered by a shielding tent during the scanning periods.

INFLUENCE OF INTRAOPERATIVE MAGNETIC RESONANCE IMAGING

Despite this heterogeneity of systems, all investigators who reported on the influence of iMRI on the course of surgery stated that intraoperative scanning had revealed residual tumor tissue in a significant number of cases, resulting in extended resections due to intraoperative imaging ranging between 10% and 70%.[21,24,25,28-33] **Figures 5.2A to E** give an example of detection of residual tumor tissue. As a result, the rates of complete resection have thus, increased by usually greater than 20%.[34,35] It becomes clear that, although arguably not all imaging sequences might have been performed at the point when the surgeon was convinced to have resected the initially intended amount of tumor, iMRI has had a major influence on the course of surgery in a large number of patients.[36] With the use of iMRI, the rate of tumor remnants left behind unintentionally can be reduced to almost 0%.

INTEGRATION OF INTRAOPERATIVE MAGNETIC RESONANCE IMAGING INTO THE NEUROSURGICAL ROUTINE

Following the initial years of its use, it has become clear that iMRI does not represent a fancy neurosurgical tool, but that it has well been incorporated into the daily neurosurgical routine. All other tools and techniques that neurosurgeons have adopted to facilitate safe brain tumor surgery can be applied in an iMRI setup.[37] There are no reports of direct patient harm because of (low-field) iMRI use. To prevent patient injury and neurological deterioration due to overly aggressive resection, iMRI can also be combined with intraoperative monitoring techniques, such as motor or sensory-evoked potentials during surgery, even when applied in the fringe field.[38,39] Further, intraoperative diffusion-weighted imaging to depict white matter tracts a feasible in both, high-field and low-field iMRI systems.[40-42]

As a result, it can be concluded that, after careful patient selection, surgical resection of gliomas can be increased to a maximum extent with acceptable risks for the patients, given the proven benefit of maximum resection. Complication rates have been reported to lie between 5% and 18% directly, postoperatively.[14,17,25,32,43] Permanent deficits occurred in

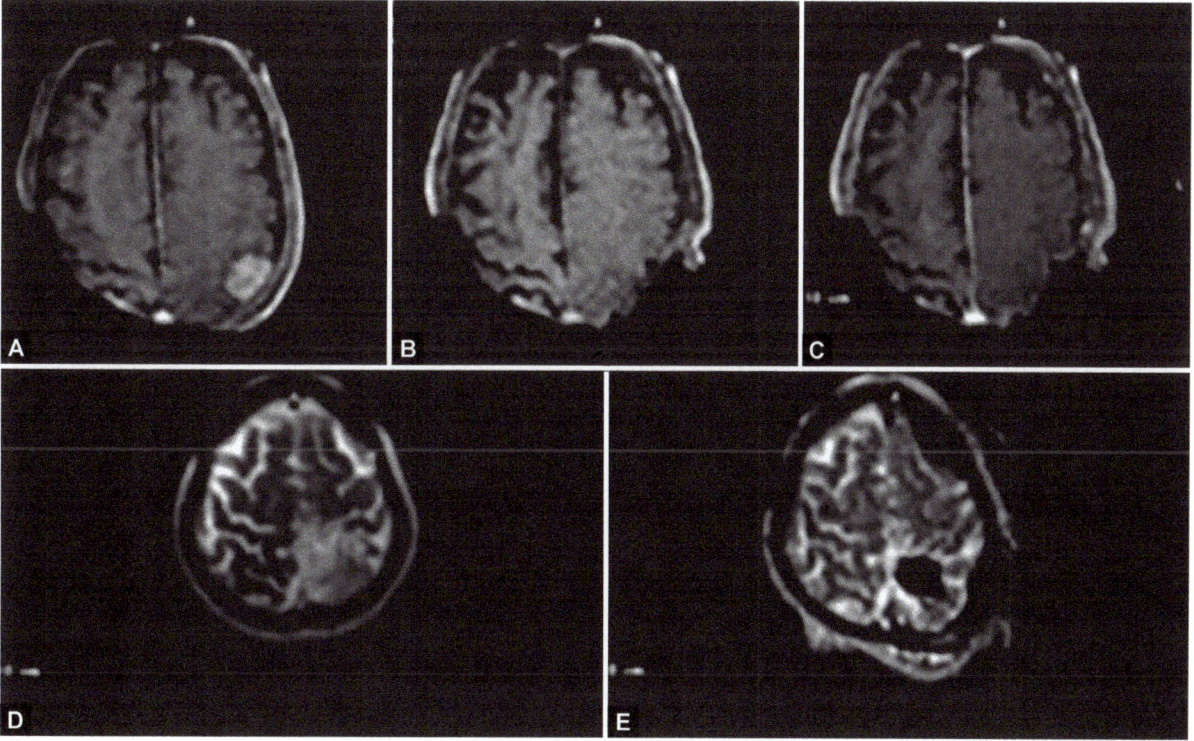

Figures 5.2A to E Screenshots of images taken intraoperatively with a low-field intraoperative magnetic resonance imaging (iMRI) at 0.15 Tesla. (A) Axial T1-weighted images of a contrast-enhancing glioblastoma before tumor resection; (B) Represent images after tumor resection without contrast agent; (C) With contrast agent, showing complete removal of enhancing tissue; (D) Corresponding axial T2-weighted images of a patient with a non-enhancing before tumor removal; and (E) After tumor removal, indicating gross total resection

constantly less than 10% of patients, which is comparable to the complication rates in conventional glioma surgery. In two own series of patients, an extended resection after iMRI scans revealed that residual tumor did not correlate with postoperative morbidity.[21,39]

EVIDENCE OF INTRAOPERATIVE MAGNETIC RESONANCE IMAGING USE

Only few studies on iMRI in neurosurgery have aimed to evaluate the influence of iMRI on the clinical course of glioma patients, while early reports focused on the feasibility, safety and influence on the course of surgery in the application of iMRI in glioma surgery. Their results added to the growing evidence that extent of resection translates into prolonged survival in glioma patients. However, none of these studies compared patients treated under iMRI-guidance with a control group of patients. Conflicting retrospective analyses concerning the benefit of iMRI in malignant glioma surgery[30,44] eventually prompted the conduction of prospective studies.

In 2011, Kubben et al. published a review on the scientific evidence of published papers on iMRI, thus far and concluded that there was only level two evidence at best.[45] In the same issue, we reported the results of a prospective trial that had been conducted at our institution for which patients harboring contrast-enhancing gliomas were randomized to undergo either iMRI-guided or conventional microsurgical tumor resection.[46] The use of a neuronavigation system in the control group was at the discretion of the attending surgeon. Comparable to the results of the 5-aminolevulinic acid (5-ALA) study of Stummer and colleagues,[47] we observed a significantly higher rate of complete tumor resections in the group of patients who were operated with the use of an iMRI compared to the control group; we also found that complete tumor removal was associated with longer progression-free survival.[46] This study provides high-class scientific evidence to use iMRI in glioma surgery. In a post-hoc analysis of the study data, we could also confirm previous reports on the limited value of neuronavigation. There was no benefit of neuronavigation use in terms of extent of resection, which emphasizes the need to update neuronavigation data intraoperatively. While we performed this study with a low-field system featuring a limited field of view and lower resolution than diagnostic high-field MRI, it can be expected that high-field iMRI systems will essentially be equally effective in improving extent of resection in malignant gliomas.[48]

FUTURE PERSPECTIVES

The aforementioned studies[46,47] raise the question whether one should rely on 5-ALA-induced fluorescence or iMRI in the resection of malignant gliomas. One obvious advantage over the administration of fluorescent porphyrins to visualize tumor tissue intraoperatively is the usability of iMRI also in low-grade gliomas and the lack of anatomical or functional information provided by 5-ALA. A few groups have thus, far tried to combine both techniques, with no clear superiority of one method over the other.[49,50]

While there is increasing interest in the neurosurgical community to use high-field systems for intraoperative use, there still is a preponderance of low-field systems. Image quality of the latter is sufficient for intraoperative needs and their installation and maintenance costs are tremendously lower than those of high-field systems. With an acceptable interruption of the surgical workflow, they are likely to continue to be part of the neurosurgical armamentarium. It remains to be seen whether ultimately high-field systems will prevail over low-field systems due to superior image quality and/or additional imaging opportunities, e.g. magnetic resonance (MR) spectroscopy. The use of both clearly leads to better surgical results.

Despite radical surgical approaches, glioma patients will not be cured by neurosurgical intervention, but meticulous and radical function-preserving neurosurgical tumor removal is one of the strongest prognostic factors. In contrast to patient age or molecular tumor biology, it is the one factor that can be directly influenced by neurosurgeons. The use of modern tools such as iMRI will continue to translate into patients' benefit. However, because of the enormous costs associated with iMRI systems, we expect the formation of specialized, leading centers, where all technology is gathered to provide optimum patient care.

REFERENCES

1. Curran WJ, Scott CB, Horton J, et al. Does extent of surgery influence outcome for astrocytoma with atypical or anaplastic foci (AAF)? A report from three Radiation Therapy Oncology Group (RTOG) trials. J Neurooncol. 1992;12(3):219-27.
2. Tortosa A, Viñolas N, Villà S, et al. Prognostic implication of clinical, radiologic, and pathologic features in patients with anaplastic gliomas. Cancer. 2003;97(4):1063-71.
3. Sanai N, Berger MS. Glioma extent of resection and its impact on patient outcome. Neurosurgery. 2008;62(4):753-64.
4. McGirt MJ, Chaichana KL, Gathinji M, et al. Independent association of extent of resection with survival in patients with malignant brain astrocytoma. J Neurosurg. 2009;110(1):156-62.
5. Lacroix M, Abi-Said D, Fourney DR, et al. A multivariate analysis of 416 patients with glioblastoma multiforme: prognosis, extent of resection, and survival. J Neurosurg. 2001;95(2):190-8.
6. Pichlmeier U, Bink A, Schackert G, et al. Resection and survival in glioblastoma multiforme: an RTOG recursive partitioning analysis of ALA study patients. Neuro Oncol. 2008;10(6):1025-34.
7. Glas M, Rath BH, Simon M, et al. Residual tumor cells are unique cellular targets in glioblastoma. Ann Neurol. 2010;68(2):264-9.

8. Laws ER, Parney IF, Huang W, et al. Survival following surgery and prognostic factors for recently diagnosed malignant glioma: data from the Glioma Outcomes Project. J Neurosurg. 2003;99(3):467-73.

9. Berger MS, Ojemann GA, Lettich E. Neurophysiological monitoring during astrocytoma surgery. Neurosurg Clin N Am. 1990;1(1):65-80.

10. Wirtz CR, Albert FK, Schwaderer M, Heuer C, Staubert A, Tronnier VM, et al. The benefit of neuronavigation for neurosurgery analyzed by its impact on glioblastoma surgery. Neurol Res. 2000;22(4):354-60.

11. Roberts DW, Hartov A, Kennedy FE, et al. Intraoperative brain shift and deformation: a quantitative analysis of cortical displacement in 28 cases. Neurosurgery. 1998;43(4):749-58.

12. Albert FK, Forsting M, Sartor K, et al. Early postoperative magnetic resonance imaging after resection of malignant glioma: objective evaluation of residual tumor and its influence on regrowth and prognosis. Neurosurgery. 1994;34(1):45-60.

13. Ram Z, Hadani M. Intraoperative imaging--MRI. Acta Neurochir Suppl. 2003;88:1-4.

14. Nimsky C, Ganslandt O, Buchfelder M, et al. Glioma surgery evaluated by intraoperative low-field magnetic resonance imaging. Acta Neurochir Suppl. 2003;85:55-63.

15. Rygh OM, Selbekk T, Torp SH, et al. Comparison of navigated 3D ultrasound findings with histopathology in subsequent phases of glioblastoma resection. Acta Neurochir (Wien). 2008;150(10):1033-41.

16. Black PM, Moriarty T, Alexander E, et al. Development and implementation of intraoperative magnetic resonance imaging and its neurosurgical applications. Neurosurgery. 1997;41(4):831-42.

17. Black PM, Alexander E, Martin C, et al. Craniotomy for tumor treatment in an intraoperative magnetic resonance imaging unit. Neurosurgery. 1999;45(3):423-31.

18. Muragaki Y, Iseki H, Maruyama T, et al. Usefulness of intraoperative magnetic resonance imaging for glioma surgery. Acta Neurochir Suppl. 2006;98:67-75.

19. Pamir MN, Peker S, Ozek MM, et al. Intraoperative MR imaging: preliminary results with 3 tesla MR system. Acta Neurochir Suppl. 2006;98:97-100.

20. Jha AN, Rahmathulla G, Vaishya S, et al. Intraoperative high field magnetic resonance imaging in neurosurgery: our initial experience with the brain suite. Neurol India. 2007;55(2):169-72.

21. Senft C, Seifert V, Hermann E, et al. Usefulness of intraoperative ultra low-field magnetic resonance imaging in glioma surgery. Neurosurgery. 2008;63(4 Suppl 2):257-66.

22. Leuthardt EC, Lim CC, Shah MN, et al. Use of movable high-field-strength intraoperative magnetic resonance imaging with awake craniotomies for resection of gliomas: preliminary experience. Neurosurgery. 2011;69(1):194-205.

23. Tronnier VM, Wirtz CR, Knauth M, et al. Intraoperative diagnostic and interventional magnetic resonance imaging in neurosurgery. Neurosurgery. 1997;40(5):891-900.

24. Wirtz CR, Bonsanto MM, Knauth M, et al. Intraoperative magnetic resonance imaging to update interactive navigation in neurosurgery: method and preliminary experience. Comput Aided Surg. 1997;2(3-4):172-9.

25. Bohinski RJ, Kokkino AK, Warnick RE, et al. Glioma resection in a shared-resource magnetic resonance operating room after optimal image-guided frameless stereotactic resection. Neurosurgery. 2001;48(4):731-42.

26. Schulder M, Sernas TJ, Carmel PW. Cranial surgery and navigation with a compact intraoperative MRI system. Acta Neurochir Suppl. 2003;85:79-86.

27. Schulder M, Salas S, Brimacombe M, et al. Cranial surgery with an expanded compact intraoperative magnetic resonance imager. Technical note. J Neurosurg. 2006;104(4):611-7.

28. Nimsky C, Ganslandt O, Tomandl B, et al. Low-field magnetic resonance imaging for intraoperative use in neurosurgery: a 5-year experience. Eur Radiol. 2002;12(11):2690-703.

29. Knauth M, Wirtz CR, Tronnier VM, et al. Intraoperative MR imaging increases the extent of tumor resection in patients with high-grade gliomas. AJNR Am J Neuroradiol. 1999;20(9):1642-6.

30. Hirschberg H, Samset E, Hol PK, et al. Impact of intraoperative MRI on the surgical results for high-grade gliomas. Minim Invasive Neurosurg. 2005;48(2):77-84.

31. Wirtz CR, Knauth M, Staubert A, et al. Clinical evaluation and follow-up results for intraoperative magnetic resonance imaging in neurosurgery. Neurosurgery. 2000;46(5):1112-20.

32. Schneider JP, Trantakis C, Rubach M, et al. Intraoperative MRI to guide the resection of primary supratentorial glioblastoma multiforme--a quantitative radiological analysis. Neuroradiology. 2005;47(7):489-500.

33. Maesawa S, Fujii M, Nakahara N, et al. Clinical indications for high-field 1.5 T intraoperative magnetic resonance imaging and neuro-navigation for neurosurgical procedures. Review of initial 100 cases. Neurol Med Chir (Tokyo). 2009;49(8):340-9.

34. Oh DS, Black PM. A low-field intraoperative MRI system for glioma surgery: is it worthwhile? Neurosurg Clin N Am. 2005;16(1):135-41.

35. Kuhnt D, Ganslandt O, Schlaffer SM, et al. Quantification of glioma removal by intraoperative high-field magnetic resonance imaging: an update. Neurosurgery. 2011;69(4):852-62.

36. Hall WA, Liu H, Maxwell RE, et al. Influence of 1.5-Tesla intraoperative MR imaging on surgical decision making. Acta Neurochir Suppl. 2003;85:29-37.

37. Seifert V, Senft C. Utilization of low-field intraoperative MRI in glioma surgery – An overview. In: Hall W, Nimsky C, Truwit C (Eds). Intraoperative MRI-guided neurosurgery. New York: Thieme; 2011. pp. 99-107.

38. Hatiboglu MA, Weinberg JS, Suki D, et al. Utilization of intraoperative motor mapping in glioma surgery with high-field intraoperative magnetic resonance imaging. Stereotact Funct Neurosurg. 2010;88(6):345-52.

39. Senft C, Forster MT, Bink A, et al. Optimizing the extent of resection in eloquently located gliomas by combining intraoperative MRI guidance with intraoperative neuro-physiological monitoring. J Neurooncol. 2012;109(1):81-90.

40. Schulder M, Azmi H, Biswal B. Functional magnetic resonance imaging in a low-field intraoperative scanner. Stereotact Funct Neurosurg. 2003;80(1-4):125-31.

41. Nimsky C, Ganslandt O, Hastreiter P, et al. Preoperative and intraoperative diffusion tensor imaging-based fiber tracking in glioma surgery. Neurosurgery. 2005;56(1):130-7.

42. Ozawa N, Muragaki Y, Nakamura R, et al. Intraoperative diffusion-weighted imaging for visualization of the pyramidal tracts. Part II: clinical study of usefulness and efficacy. Minim Invasive Neurosurg. 2008;51(2):67-71.

43. Zimmermann M, Seifert V, Trantakis C, et al. Open MRI-guided microsurgery of intracranial tumours. Preliminary experience using a vertical open MRI-scanner. Acta Neurochir (Wien). 2000;142(2):177-86.

44. Senft C, Franz K, Blasel S, et al. Influence of iMRI-guidance on the extent of resection and survival of patients with glioblastoma multiforme. Technol Cancer Res Treat. 2010;9(4):339-46.

45. Kubben PL, ter Meulen KJ, Schijns OE, et al. Intraoperative MRI-guided resection of glioblastoma multiforme: a systematic review. Lancet Oncol. 2011;12(11):1062-70.

46. Senft C, Bink A, Franz K, et al. Intraoperative MRI guidance and extent of resection in glioma surgery: a randomised, controlled trial. Lancet Oncol. 2011;12(11):997-1003.

47. Stummer W, Pichlmeier U, Meinel T, et al. Fluorescence-guided surgery with 5-aminolevulinic acid for resection of malignant glioma: a randomised controlled multicentre phase III trial. Lancet Oncol. 2006;7(5):392-401.

48. Nimsky C. Intraoperative MRI in glioma surgery: proof of benefit? Lancet Oncol. 2011;12(11):982-3.

49. Tsugu A, Ishizaka H, Mizokami Y, et al. Impact of the combination of 5-aminolevulinic acid-induced fluorescence with intraoperative magnetic resonance imaging-guided surgery for glioma. World Neurosurg. 2011;76(1-2):120-7.

50. Eyüpoglu IY, Hore N, Savaskan NE, et al. Improving the extent of malignant glioma resection by dual intraoperative visualization approach. PLoS One. 2012;7(9):e44885.

6

Two Room vs Single Room Intraoperative Magnetic Resonance Imaging Setup

Karanjit Singh Narang, Ratnadip Bose, Ajaya Nand Jha

INTRODUCTION AND HISTORICAL BACKGROUND

Accurate targeting of region of interest in the brain plays a pivotal role in determining the success of any neurosurgical procedure. Safety and accuracy of tumor resection depends on exact determination of tumor location and margin; accurate resection of epileptic focus depends on coregistration of anatomic and functional information; stereotactic target localization demands sub-millimetric accuracy.

Last 20–25 years have seen continuous quest for better neuronavigational tool. Intraoperative magnetic resonance imaging (MRI) has revolutionized neuronavigation since its discovery. Brain shift has been nagging problem in intraoperative localization. After craniotomy, burr hole, cerebrospinal fluid (CSF) drainage, or resection of lesion, the brain anatomy undergoes dynamic change, which makes it difficult to localize normal or pathological structures in the brain by using the set of images used preoperatively.[1-4] Gliomas, especially low-grade gliomas, have indistinct margins. They pose a difficult challenge even to well-experienced neurosurgeons, who often face the dilemma of leaving a part of tumor behind for fear of damaging normal brain tissue. Only intraoperatively acquired images provide updated anatomical information and help the neurosurgeon to perform real-time image-guided surgery.

The margin between normal brain tissue and some brain tumors is difficult to determine intraoperatively under a microscope. Modalities like functional MRI, diffusion tensor images, and cortical maps once superimposed with intraoperatively acquired images helps to minimize the risk of causing damage beyond the boundaries of a tumor especially to eloquent areas. Thus, the surgeon is equipped to achieve maximal resection of any lesion simultaneously avoiding unnecessary damage to viable neural structures.[5-14]

The first commercial intraoperative MRI machine was installed at Brigham and Women's Hospital, Boston USA in 1994. General Electric (GE) Medical System provided the 0.5T (tesla) open-configuration MRI scanner for intraoperative image-guidance. The open-configuration system has the highest magnetic field in the space between the double donuts, allowing the surgeon to operate on the patient with concurrent use of intraoperative MRI. The design of closed-configuration MRI scanners during those times prevented surgeons to have direct access to the patient. Major upgradations in the design and physics of the magnetic coils were required before optimum realization of the concept of intraoperative MRI.

Gronemeyer and colleagues were the earliest users of open MRI system with a low-field scanner for interventional procedure.[15,16] The greatest impediment that they faced was limited access to the patient and hence open surgeries were totally impossible. Further research led way to the "double-donut" open-configuration magnet design, which gave more working space to the surgeon with better approach to the surgical candidate in the operating room (OR). The one installed at Brigham and Women's hospital belonged to such a system.[17-20] The double-donut design provides vertical gap between the coils where the surgeon and assistant can stand while operating on the patient. The table on which the patient lies is relocated into the magnet "side docked" and "end docked" (orthogonal axes). This allows imaging of different areas with ease. Its open configuration allowed the operating surgeons to integrate it into various procedures including endoscopic, percutaneous, open surgical, and interventional. However, few more technological challenges were yet to be surmounted, like the invention of instruments used during that were MRI compatible and the display panels used in the OR and audio-visual communication between surgical team members. Initial problem was to develop a nonferromagnetic headholder akin to Mayfield. Once this hurdle was surpassed, next came the problem of drill. Till then, only biopsy procedures could be done, as it was not possible to raise a flap. Midas Rex Corporation (Medtronic, Minneapolis,

Minnesota) came up with an operating microscope with nonferromagnetic parts and joints. Next major milestone was development of nonferromagnetic bipolar cautery, which was safe to use in the presence of an electromagnet. It took each of them 6–12 months to be developed.

Meanwhile Gering and colleagues[21] developed a volumetric display software to make a quantitative analysis of brain shift.

However, the logistics associated with setting up such an iMRI system, such as, coolant, continuous power consumption, room-shielding and special instruments escalated the cost, and only a few neurosurgical centers could practically install such a set-up. Several neurosurgeons came up with pragmatic solutions. Moshe Hadani et al.[22] in 2001 came up with a new design, the PoleStar (Medtronic Navigation, Louisville, Colorado) N-10 iMRI system. This compact 0.12T- MRI system left very little electromagnetic foot print and hence required minimal modifications in the OR. More recently, PoleStar has come up with 0.15T N20 system,[23] which has been adopted by several centers without need for extensive remodeling the operation suite. The Hitachi 0.3T open-configuration MRI, installed at the University of Cincinnati,[24] has a higher field MRI; however, it allows only diagnostic procedures and is not suitable to maintain sterility during neurosurgical interventional procedures.

One major shortfall of the open-configuration MRI scanners has been low field magnets, which cannot yield high quality image comparable to 1.5 or 3T magnets. For a decade or so, the open-configuration scanners ruled as neurosurgeons saw in this a benefit that the patient did not have to be moved for intraoperative scanning. The first decade of the 21st century saw a gradual paradigm shift and neurosurgeons started moving patients in and out of MRI scanners for intraoperative imaging and OR protocols were developed for fast and smooth wheeling patients in and out of MRI scanners. As a natural next step in evolution came the high-field 1.5–3T closed bore MRI scanners, which yielded much better quality images.[25,26] Overhead camera for navigation or special markers fixed on patients were used to maintain the navigation registration data during the procedure.

The iMRIS system was developed by Dr Sutherland of Canada that used special rail track mounted on the ceiling to bring the 70 cm bore 1.5T-MRI scanner from an adjacent room into the OR during intraoperative scanning. During other times the MRI scanner is lodged in the adjacent room, which has radiofrequency- and sound-shielded doors. In this manner the same scanner can be used for multiple operating rooms and when not in use for intraoperative imaging, it can be used for other diagnostic purposes. This system includes an OR table which is MRI compatible, radiofrequency coils with 8-channels, special fixation devices for the head designed to fit into the iMRIs **(Figs 6.1A and B)**.

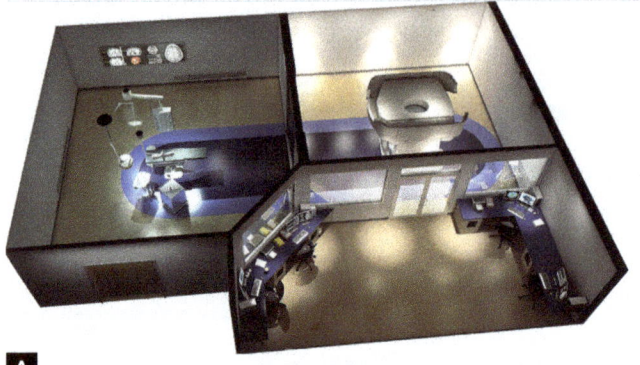

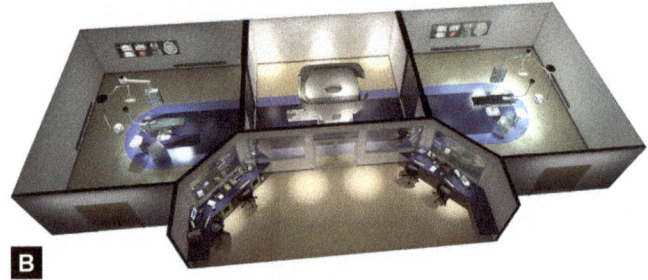

Figures 6.1A and B (A) Single room iMRIs setup;
(B) Two room iMRIs setup
Source: IMRIS.com

Using the same scanner for intraoperative use as well as for other diagnostic purposes had definite advantage from the point of maximum utilization of resources and hence more cost effective. This led BrainLab to come up with two-room iMRI system where one room contained the MRI scanner and one adjacent room had the operating theater. Keeping the MRI scanner in a separate room allows high-field scanners like 3T-MRI system to be used, which gives better image quality with improved resolution and with the flexibility of several specialized MRI sequences. Another major advantage of this two-room concept is that the MRI scanner does not interfere with the surgical workflow, allowing the surgical team more flexibility. Now, in a two-room iMRI system either the MRI scanner can be moved to the patient on the operating table, or the patient on the table can be moved to the scanner. Gradually, it was found that moving the patient to the scanner is safe and has advantages from room construction and logistical points of view and more cost effective too. Studies have shown that moving the patient to the scanner taken an average of 1.5 minutes and routine MRI sequences take another 6–8 minutes.[27] Thus, such a two-room system can be efficiently used for intraoperative scanning and for other diagnostic purposes as well, without any significant time constraint, nor does the OR is blocked totally for such cases (which require iMRI) only **(Figs 6.2A to C)**.

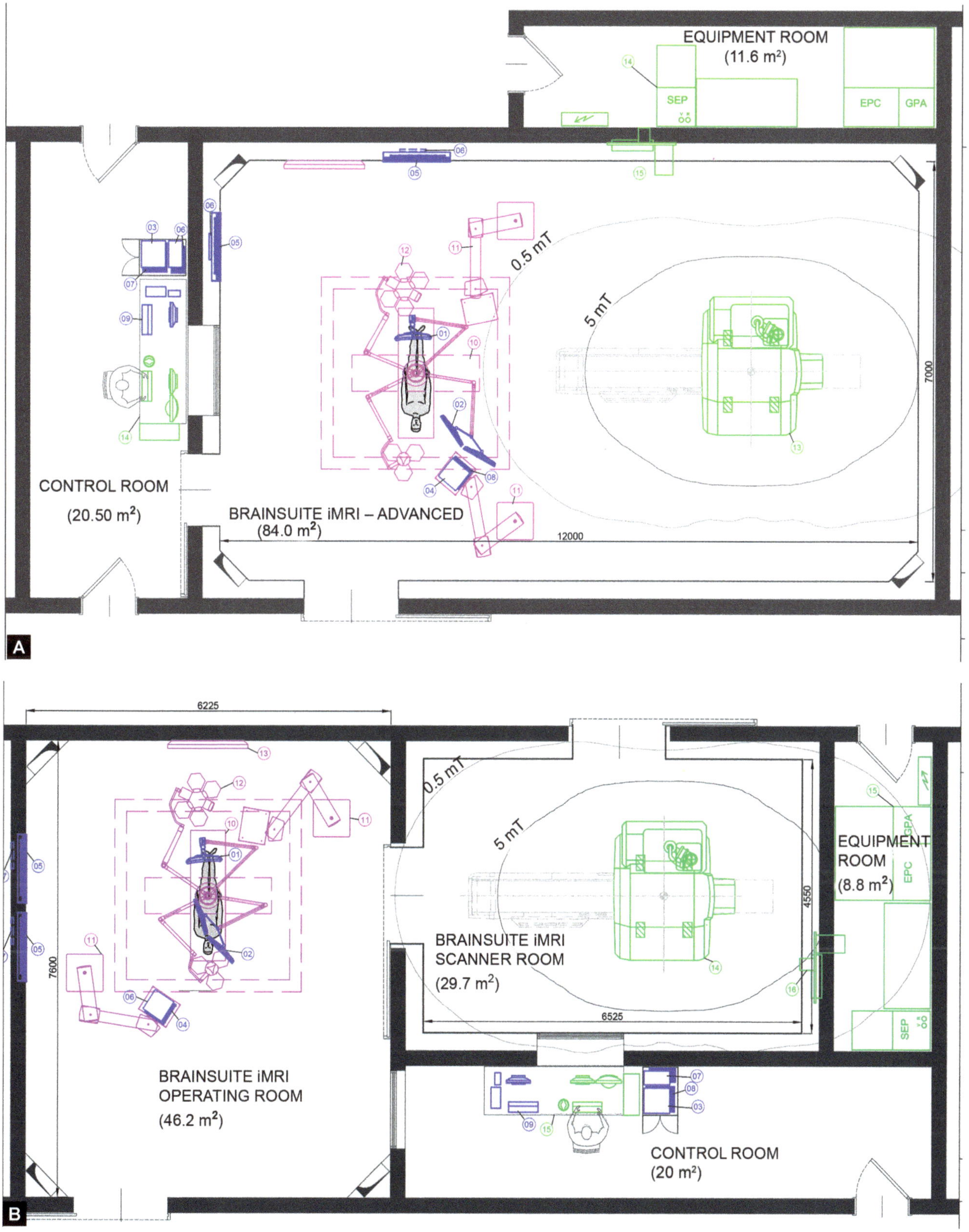

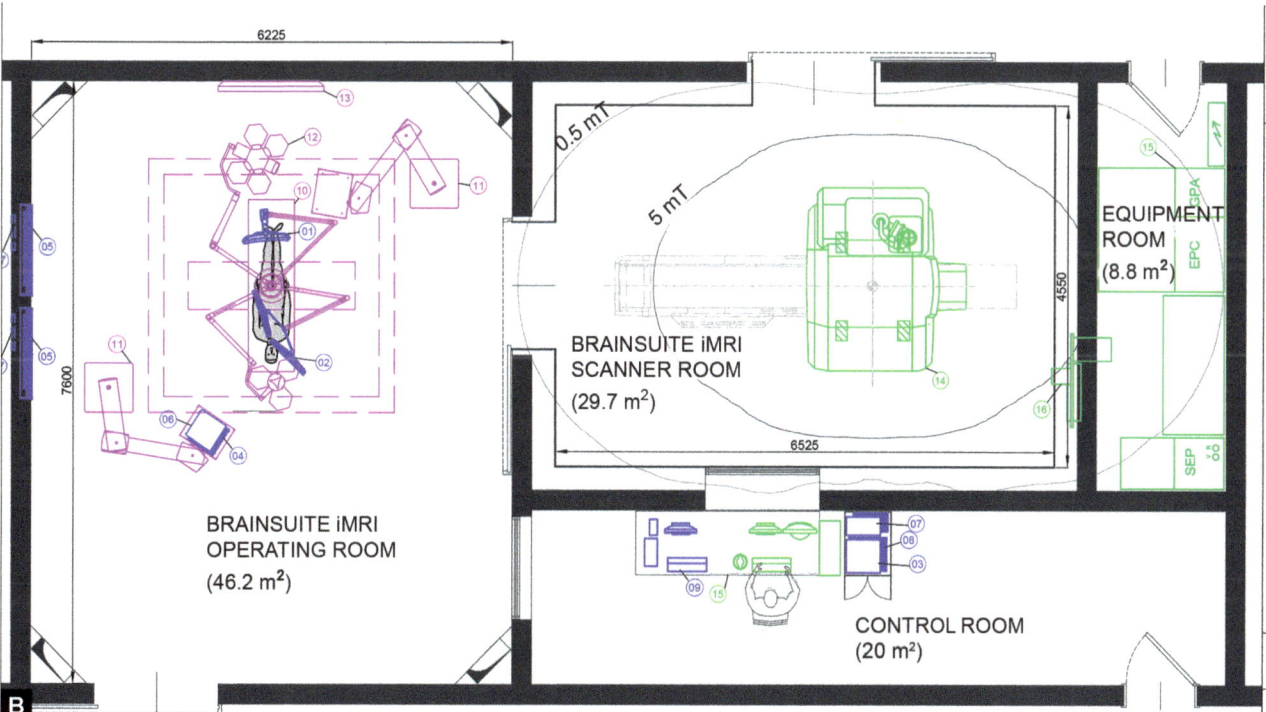

Figures 6.2A and B (A) iMRI—1 room setup; and (B) iMRI—2 room setup

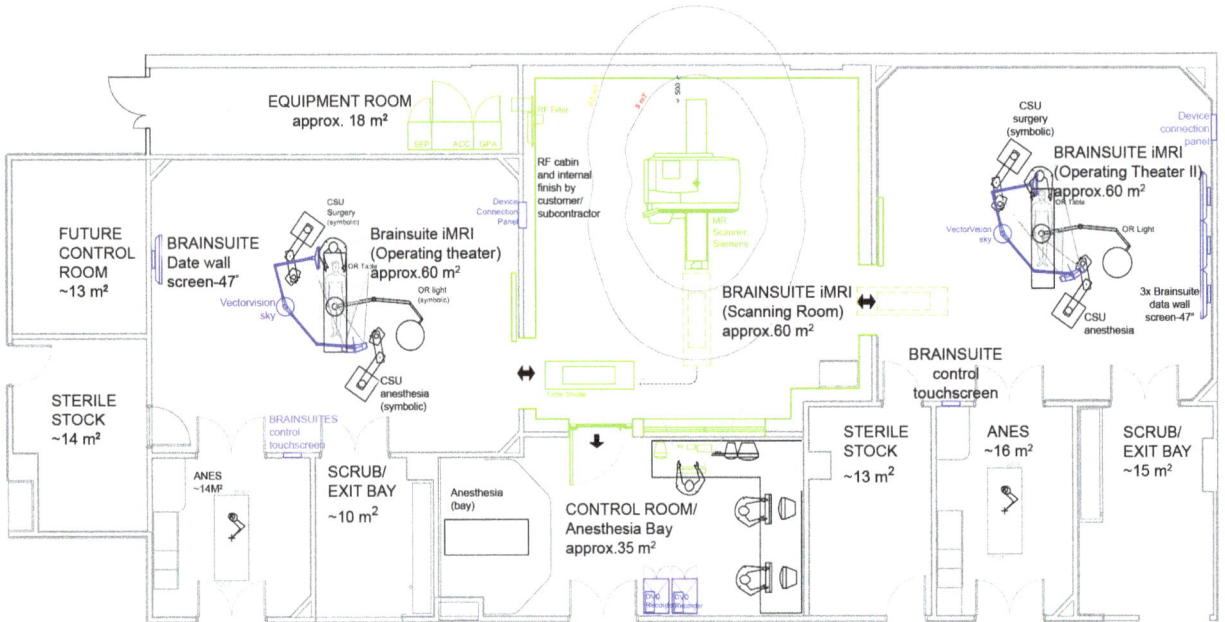

Figure 6.2C iMRI 3 room setup

ADVANTAGES OF TWO-ROOM INTRAOPERATIVE MRI SYSTEM OVER ONE-ROOM IMRI SYSTEM

As the technology of intraoperative MRI evolved, further refinements were made to make it more cost effective and to achieve maximum utilization of the resources, with simultaneous improvement in imaging quality.

The present decade has seen the donut open-configuration system MRI giving way to closed-configuration MRI systems to allow high-field (1.5–3 tesla) MRI scanners to be used which give better image quality with improved resolution and also allow multiple MRI sequences. Also this allows more room for the surgical team to maintain smooth surgical workflow.

These days, in a single-room iMRI brain suite, the closed-configuration MRI scanner is placed inside the operation theater and the operating table is placed outside the 5-gauss magnetic activity radius, which is usually marked by a colored line on the floor. During intraoperative scanning, the patient is wheeled inside the MRI scanner and after the scan patient is wheeled out back beyond the 5-gauss radius.

In a two-room iMRI suite, one room is setup for the surgery and the MRI scanner is setup in another adjacent room, which has radiofrequency- and sound-shielded sliding doors. For intraoperative scanning, the patient is wheeled to the adjacent MRI room.

In a two-room iMRI system either the MRI scanner can be moved to the patient on the operating table, or the patient on the table can be moved to the scanner. Gradually, it was found that moving the patient to the scanner is safe and has advantages from room construction and logistical points of view and more cost effective too. Studies have shown that moving the patient to the scanner taken an average of 1.5 minutes and routine MRI sequences take another 6–8 minutes.[27]

The major advantage of two-room suite is that one OR need not be dedicated for cases requiring intraoperative MRI. All varieties of neurosurgical cases can be performed and even the operating table can also be changed as per requirement. Only in cases requiring iMRI the door connecting to the MRI room is opened while transporting the patient to the scanner and back.

Further, the MRI scanner need not be dedicated for iMRI only. Intraoperative MRI takes only a few minutes and at other times it can very well be used for several other diagnostic purposes. A single-room suite would engage the scanner all throughout, whereas the actual need for iMRI takes only a few minutes.

Neurosurgical centers have come up with more innovative ideas. One room containing the MRI scanner is connected to multiple operation rooms, thereby allowing multiple surgeries, requiring intraoperative MRI, to be performed at a time.

All these modifications have played significant role in enhancing cost effectiveness. Otherwise the setting up of a brain suite with iMRI is a costly affair. Resource strain and expense have been the major deterrents across several centers. With newer innovative ideas, like the two-room set up, the concept of iMRI is getting more widely accepted worldwide.

Questions have been raised regarding the risk of infection during transport of patient to the scanner. However, no significant increase in infection rate, as compared to conventional neurosurgical procedures, has been found in such two-room iMRI systems.

In 2009, Brigham and Women's hospital at Boston developed the AMIGO suite (Advanced Multimodality Image Guided Operating). This was another advancement in intraoperative imaging. The AMIGO allows the operating surgeons to integrate MR images (3T), images from positron emission tomography–computed tomography (PET-CT), ultrasound, operating microscope, fluoroscopy in order to update the preoperative images used for guidance.

REFERENCES

1. Tronnier VM, Wirtz CR, Knauth M, et al. Intraoperative diagnostic and interventional magnetic resonance imaging in neurosurgery. Neurosurg. 1997;40(5):891-900.
2. Wirtz CR, Tronnier VM, Bonsanto MM, et al. Image-guided neurosurgery with intraoperative MRI: update of frameless stereotaxy and radicality control. Stereotact Funct Neurosurg. 1997;68(1–4 Pt 1):39-43.
3. Maurer CR, Jr, Hill DL, Martin AJ, et al. Investigation of intraoperative brain deformation using a 1.5-T interventional MR system: preliminary results. IEEE Trans Med Imaging. 1998;17(5):817-25.
4. Nimsky C, Ganslandt O, Hastreiter P, et al. Intraoperative compensation for brain shift. Surg Neurol. 2001;56(6):357-64.
5. Berger MS, Deliganis AV, Dobbins J, et al. The effect of extent of resection on recurrence in patients with low grade cerebral hemisphere gliomas. Cancer. 1994;74(6):1784-91.
6. Claus EB, Horlacher A, Hsu L, et al. Survival rates in patients with low-grade glioma after intraoperative magnetic resonance image guidance. Cancer. 2005;103(6):1227-33.
7. Keles GE, Anderson B, Berger MS. The effect of extent of resection on time to tumor progression and survival in patients with glioblastoma multiforme of the cerebral hemisphere. Surg Neurol. 1999;52(4):371-9.
8. Lacroix M, Abi-Said D, Fourney DR, et al. A multivariate analysis of 416 patients with glioblastoma multiforme: prognosis, extent of resection, and survival. J Neurosurg. 2001;95(2):190-8.
9. Berger MS, Rostomily RC. Low grade gliomas: functional mapping resection strategies, extent of resection, and outcome. J Neurooncol. 1997;34(1):85-101.
10. Fernandez-Hidalgo OA, Vanaclocha V, Vieitez JM, et al. High-dose BCNU and autologous progenitor cell transplantation given with intra-arterial cisplatinum and simultaneous radiotherapy in the treatment of high-grade gliomas: benefit for selected patients. Bone Marrow Transplant. 1996;18(1):143-9.
11. Johannesen TB, Langmark F, Lote K. Progress in long-term survival in adult patients with supratentorial low-grade gliomas: a population-based study of 993 patients in whom tumors were diagnosed between 1970 and 1993. J Neurosurg. 2003;99(5):854-62.
12. McGirt MJ, Chaichana KL, Gathinji M, et al. Independent association of extent of resection with survival in patients with malignant brain astrocytoma. J Neurosurg. 2008;110:156-62.
13. Sakata K, Hareyama M, Komae T, et al. Supratentorial-astrocytomas and oligodendrogliomas treated in the MRI era. Jpn J Clin Oncol. 2001;31(6):240-5.
14. Wirtz CR, Knauth M, Staubert A, et al. Clinical evaluation and follow-up results for intraoperative magnetic resonance imaging in neurosurgery. Neurosurg. 2000;46(5):1112-20.
15. Gronemeyer D, Seibel R, Erbel R, et al. Equipment configuration and procedures: preferences for interventional microtherapy. J Digit Imaging. 1996;9(2):81-96.
16. Gronemeyer DH, Seibel RM, Schmidt A, et al. Two- and three-dimensional imaging for interventional MRI and CT guidance. Stud Health Technol Inform. 1996;29:62-76.
17. Schenck JF, Jolesz FA, Roemer PB, et al. Superconducting open-configuration MR imaging system for image-guided therapy. Radiology. 1995;195(3):805-14.
18. Alexander E, 3rd, Moriarty TM, Kikinis R, et al. The present and future role of intraoperative MRI in neurosurgical procedures. Stereotact Funct Neurosurg. 1997;68(1–4 Pt 1):10-7.
19. Alexander E, 3rd, Moriarty TM, Kikinis R, et al. Innovations in minimalism: intraoperative MRI. Clin Neurosurg. 1996;43:338-52.
20. Moriarty TM, Kikinis R, Jolesz FA, et al. Magnetic resonance imaging therapy: intraoperative MR imaging. Neurosurg Clin N Am. 1996;7(2):323-31.
21. Gering DT, Nabavi A, Kikinis R, et al. An integrated visualization system for surgical planning and guidance using image fusion and an open MR. J Magn Reson Imaging. 2001;13(6):967-75.
22. Hadani M, Spiegelman R, Feldman Z, et al. Novel, compact, intraoperative magnetic resonance imaging-guided system for conventional neurosurgical operating rooms. Neurosurg. 2001;48(4):799-807.
23. Ntoukas V, Krishnan R, Seifert V. The new generation Polestar N20 for conventional neurosurgical operating rooms: a preliminary report. Neurosurg. 2008;62(3 Suppl 1):82-9.
24. Nimsky C, Ganslandt O, Fahlbusch R. 1.5 T: intraoperative imaging beyond standard anatomic imaging. Neurosurg Clin N Am. 2005;16(1):185-200.
25. Hushek SG, Martin AJ, Steckner M, et al. MR systems for MRI-guided interventions. J Magn Reson Imaging. 2008;27(2):253-66.
26. Hall WA, Truwit CL. Intraoperative MR-guided neurosurgery. J Magn Reson Imaging. 2008;27(2):368-75.
27. Pamir MN. 3 T ioMRI: the Istanbul experience. Acta Neurochir Suppl. 2011;109:131-7.

7

Anesthesia for Intraoperative Magnetic Resonance Imaging

Harsh Sapra

INTRODUCTION

Magnetic resonance imaging (MRI) is the use of extremely high magnetic fields and radiofrequency (RF) modulation in order to produce two and three-dimensional scans without the use of any ionizing radiation. Anesthesia in the MRI suite was first described in 1984.[1] Since then MRI has become increasingly common, and the demand for anesthetic services in this challenging environment has climbed. Intraoperative magnetic resonance imaging (iMRI) was first performed in 1993.[2] The principle behind iMRI is that the surgeon can do repeated scans during tumor resection to ensure that the greatest amount of tumor can be resected while the patient is still in the operating room, with the least amount of harm to normal tissue.

PHYSICS BEHIND MAGNETIC RESONANCE IMAGING

Magnetic resonance imaging units generally use hydrogen nuclei to generate images. When hydrogen nuclei are exposed to a static magnetic field, the orientation of their spinning axes will be aligned with that of the static field. Exposure to a second, transient magnetic field at right angles to the static field will cause the nuclei to "flip" orientation and rotate in alignment with the second magnetic field. This is an energy consuming process. When the second magnetic field is removed, the nuclei resume their original alignment releasing energy in the process. The characteristics of this energy release is captured and analyzed to create an image.

In MRI units, electric current is passed through a coil of wire which creates a magnetic field orientated along the alignment of the coil. MRI unit creates the static magnetic field (Bo). The wire in the coil creating the Bo field is typically several kilometers long, and the field strength is approximately 1.5 Tesla [1 Tesla (T)=10,000 Gauss]. For comparison, it may be worthwhile to note that the magnets used to pick up car wrecks in scrap metal yards are about 1.5T, while the earth magnetic field is about 0.5 Gauss.

SUPERCONDUCTIVITY

If the coil's wire is cooled to almost absolute zero kelvin (K), the wire's resistance becomes negligible. Under these conditions, current generated in the coil will continue to flow indefinitely with no energy input. The coil is then called a "superconductor". In an MRI unit, this is achieved by bathing the wire (copper embedded with a niobium or titanium alloy) in liquid helium at 4.22 K (–269°C). Therefore, the electromagnet created by this superconductor is always "on", day or night, regardless of whether a patient is being scanned or not. To turn the magnet off requires the helium to be allowed to evaporate, called a "quench". The helium is vented to the atmosphere via a "quench pipe". This is only done to allow maintenance, as to reinstate the magnet requires several days and is a very costly affair. An uncontrolled release of helium can create a hypoxic environment creating a medical emergency.

The primary coil creates a tunnel in which the patient lies. This tunnel is approximately 2 m long, with an inner core diameter of approximately 0.6 m. An MRI unit also contains RF coils, which provide "RF pulses" to produce the intermittent fields at right angles to Bo. The scanner also contains receiving coils, which receive the energy released by nuclei. Signals from hydrogen ions in different tissues can be distinguished by the variable concentration of protons in those tissues.

The field strength from the scanners fall away rapidly so that, beyond a relatively short distance (say, at the door to the scanning suite), the fringe fields are negligible. Conversely, the field strength rises rapidly as one nears the scanner and care must be taken not to inadvertently bring ferromagnetic objects dangerously dose to the magnet. Some suites have "Gauss lines" (e.g. 30 Gauss and 5 Gauss lines) drawn on the floor to act as a warning. RF waves from electronic equipment in adjacent offices must be excluded from the scanning suite to prevent interference. This is done by enclosing the scanner in a "Faraday cage", a copper sheet in the walls of the suite.

The rapidly changing currents in the gradient coils cause a loud-banging noise. This may be of concern where the patient's head and torso will be within the magnet's core.

Positioning of head within the tunnel may be an issue of concern for claustrophobic patients. "Open MRI" units are those in which the patient lies between two flat plates (rather than within a tunnel), thereby reducing claustrophobia. These operate at lower magnetic fields (approximately 0.2–0.5T).

EQUIPMENT CLASSIFICATION [AMERICAN SOCIETY FOR TESTING AND MATERIALS (ASTM) INTERNATIONAL, 2006]

- *MR-safe:* The device or implant is completely non-magnetic, non-electrically conductive and non-RF reactive, eliminating all of the primary potential threats during an MRI procedure.
- *MR-conditional:* A device or implant that may contain magnetic, electrically conductive or RF-reactive components that is safe for operations in proximity to the MRI, "provided the conditions for safe operation are defined and observed" (such as "tested safe to 1.5T" or "safe in magnetic fields below 500 Gauss in strength").
- *MR-unsafe:* Objects that are significantly ferromagnetic and pose a clear and direct threat to persons and equipment within the magnet room.

ANESTHETIC IMPLICATIONS

- *Remote location:* Even if iMRI takes place adjacent to the operating theater (OT), the scanner is located outside it, so all the issues of anesthesia in the remote location apply. These include the necessity to take adequate drugs, equipment, and assistance.
- *Conduct of anesthesia and patient transport:* The MRI table cannot be tilted so the patient is induced in an anesthetic room on a trolley that can be tilted. The patient is then shifted onto the MRI table (still in an anesthetic room) and then the patient's head is fixed with non-magnetic pin fixation. In order to optimize the image a "head box" containing an RF antenna is put over the patient's head and the patient is then carefully moved into theater for the initial scan. The head box is removed for surgery and replaced before each scan. Prior to patient transport in or out of the MRI suite, a mental checklist should be run with the following consideration:
  - Patient's airway, breathing and circulation
  - Patient's depth of anesthesia and muscle relaxation
  - Ferromagnetic substances on the patient (prostheses, implants, wire-reinforced endotracheal tubes, cautery grounding pads, etc.)
  - Ferromagnetic substances on the accompanying OT staff (e.g. stethoscopes, spectacles with metal frame, digital watches, mobile phones, credit cards, hair clips, etc.)
  - Whether monitors used are MRI compatible
  - Care of the patient's appendages and tubings which may get caught at the edges of the table while sliding the patient from one table to the other
  - Maintain sterility of the surgical field during iMRI
  - Ideally plug the patient's ears prior to shifting to MRI suite
  - Provide adequate padding at the patient's shoulders as the bottom of the coil can butt up against the patient's shoulders
  - Strap the patient well prior to leaving the MRI suite.
- *Limited access to the patient:* Most of the times, the anesthetist is barely able to see the patient inside the tunnel, let alone access the patient's airway. He can, thus, also miss any movement occurring inside the tunnel should the patient be coming out of anesthesia. Hence, a camera should be positioned so as to provide a view inside the tunnel from the console room. Furthermore, the patient's arms may be inaccessible, necessitating long intravenous (IV) tubing.
- *Ferromagnetism:* "Ferromagnetic" refers to an element that can become magnetized when exposed to an external magnetic field. The term can cause confusion, as not all ferromagnetic objects contain iron, and not all iron-containing (or ferrous) objects are ferromagnetic. Iron is the most common example of ferromagnetism, hence the name, but other ferromagnetic elements include nickel, cobalt, and some of the rare earth metals (e.g. gadolinium). Conversely, stainless steel is mostly iron, but the chromium, nickel, and carbon in the alloy alter its magnetic properties. The most common form of stainless steel is called "austenitic" and is non-ferromagnetic. Ferromagnetic objects will be drawn to the magnet, and can become dangerous missiles for staff and patients. Ferromagnetic items must be kept outside the 30 Gauss lines or, ideally, excluded from the MRI suite.[3] Only aluminum gas cylinders are acceptable. Most jewellery is safe (at least if it is real gold!). If unsure, remove it or test it with a magnet. Non-ferromagnetic metals will not be drawn to the magnet, but, when exposed to the magnetic fields, can have electric currents generated in them, causing heating or malfunctioning of electronic equipment. They can also cause image artifact.

The effects of the MRI on anesthesia equipment:
  - *Intravenous cannula needles:* These are made from stainless steel and are safe.[3]

– *Monitors:* MRI compatible monitors are commercially available but are expensive. These may include a master monitor and a slave monitor. The slave monitor can sit in the MRI control room and receive information wirelessly from the master, which stays in the MRI suite. Care should be taken to consult the product specifications before equipment labeled "MRI compatible" is purchased or used as some such items may still contain ferromagnetic components and will have a maximum magnetic field to which they can be exposed.[4]

– *Noninvasive blood pressure cuffs:* If the tubing connectors are made of plastic, not metal, these will function normally and are safe.

– *Invasive blood pressure transducers:* These are not ferromagnetic, and are safe to use. Transducer cables should be kept out of the magnet bore, so as to avoid image distortion.

– *Pulse oximeters:* Standard pulse oximeters can malfunction in the MRI suite and can cause patient burns due to overheating. MRI compatible pulse oximeters utilize fiberoptic cables. These function well but are fragile and expensive to repair, so great care must be taken with their use.

– *Electrocardiogram (ECG) monitoring:* The ECG is useful in the MRI suite only to demonstrate a rhythm, as artifactual ST and T wave changes are common, precluding any meaningful assessment of myocardial ischemia. Any conductor moving through a magnetic field will have a current induced in it. This is especially so for objects moving at right angles to the orientation of the magnetic field. For this reason, blood flowing through the aortic arch will generate a small current that will be detected by the ECG. This manifests as peaked T waves, predominantly in leads I, II, VI, and V2.[3] V5 displays the least ECG change. The intermittent fields cause artifact spikes. Standard ECG cables are insulated copper, and generate heat in the MRI scanner. This is especially so if the cables are allowed to loop. Carbon fiber leads have less potential to heat. All leads should be kept as close as possible to the center of the magnet bore and should all run in a straight line from the precordium towards the patient's feet. They should not lie directly on the patient's skin, because of the risk of burns. Braiding the leads to make one thick cable prevents one lead from forming a large loop. The ECG dots must be MRI compatible, again to avoid burns. Some MRI scanners have inbuilt ECG monitoring using wireless transmission of a signal from chest leads. However, this is only to allow cardiac gating for thoracic scans, not for diagnostic purposes.

– *Capnography:* Long sampling tubing may result in mixing of end-tidal gas with dead space gas. As a result, end-tidal measurements may not be accurate, although they are adequate for apnea monitoring and for trends. Long tubing also gives rise to a long lag time.

– *Temperature probes:* Thermistor probes are not practical because of the ferromagnetic content of their cables.

– *Anesthetic machines:* Standard Boyle machines and non-MRI compatible anesthesia workstations are unsuitable for use in the MRI. Datex makes an MRI compatible version of the Aestiva workstation. The Datex workstation has an alarm when the machine is exposed to a greater than 300 Gauss. Drager make an MRI compatible version of the Fabius workstation and it includes an MRI compatible ventilator that provides pressure support. At least one portable MRI-compatible anesthesia machine is available, at about the same cost as a standard machine (Magmedix portable anesthetic machine for MRI, model 2200). This incorporates a ventilator, sodalime canister and vaporizer, resembling a machine for military use.

– *Gas cylinders:* Standard oxygen and nitrous oxide cylinders have an aluminum body with brass fittings. Hence, they can be used in the MRI suite. However, they should be ideally checked with a strong hand magnet before being bought into the theater.

– *Breathing circuits:* Care should be taken to exclude positive end-expiratory pressure (PEEP) valves that contain metal springs.

– *Laryngoscopes:* Although laryngoscopes may be non-ferrous, the batteries are highly ferromagnetic and cannot be used in close proximity to the magnet. A technique has been described for substituting lithium batteries and aluminum spacers; allowing appropriate laryngoscope to be used anywhere in the MRI suite.[3]

– *Endotracheal tubes (ETT) and laryngeal masks (LMA):* The spring in the pilot balloon of a standard ETT can cause artifact. If this interferes with the area being scanned, the pilot balloon tubing can be knotted and the spring cut-off. Reinforced tubes will cause significant artifact due to the metal coil. Reinforced LMAs or FastTrachs are unsuitable for use in MRI as they cause excessive artifact. Classic LMAs are suitable.

– *Vaporizers:* Early generation vaporizers are not accurate in the MRI suite, due to malfunctioning of the bimetallic strip temperature compensation. Modern generation vaporizers (e.g. Datex Ohmeda Tec 7) are MRI compatible. Regardless, as in the operating theater, Australian, and New Zealand College of Anesthetists (ANZCA) guidelines mandate the use of agent monitoring.

– *Syringe pumps:* Common syringe pumps are not compatible with MRI. They function accurately up to 100 Gauss,[5] but pose a missile risk. They should, therefore be placed outside the scanning suite, with long minimum volume tubing running through a wall port. This leaves a large amount of dead space in the line, leading to drug wastage.

FERROMAGNETISM: MAGNETIC RESONANCE IMAGING AND IMPLANTED METALLIC DEVICES

- *Pacemakers:* A permanent pacemaker constitutes a contraindication to MRI scanning. Currents generated in the pacemaker circuitry, even at low-field strengths can cause serious malfunctions. Reports exist of patients with pacemakers being scanned in low-field strength scanners (0.5 T),[6] but the risk-benefit ratio needs to be seriously considered.
- *Cochlear implants:* These devices contain a magnet that holds the external component to the subcutaneous receiver and is also involved in signal transmission. This magnet may move and cause injury. If it is known at the time of cochlear implant insertion that future MRIs will be required, the internal magnet can be omitted and the external component secured with adhesive patches. In such a case, an MRI could be performed, although significant artifact could be expected in head scans.
- *Orthopedic prostheses:* The metal components of these prostheses are generally titanium or chromium or cobalt. Screws and plates are stainless steel. While these implants may cause some image artifact, they are safe in the MRI scanner. External fixation devices often contain iron, so are contraindicated.
- *Prosthetic heart valves:* These valves and annuloplasty rings undergo minimal heating and torque and are safe in MRI,[7,8] although some artifact may be caused.
- *Aneurysm clips:* Most modern clips are non-ferromagnetic and are safe in MRI. Manufacturers' specifications should be checked.
- *Tattoos and make-up:* Some tattoos and make-up contain metal pigments. These can cause image artifact or heat, causing skin discomfort.

MISCELLANEOUS ISSUES

- *Noise:* The noise is due to the rising electrical current in the wires of the gradient magnets being opposed by the main magnetic field. The stronger the main field, the louder the gradient. Noise levels in the magnet core approximate 95 dB or more.[9] Earplugs may assist in patient comfort. The staff members usually leave the theater whilst scanning occurs but provided they have ear protection there is no other reason they have to leave.
- *Quenches:* Sudden evaporation of the liquid helium due to a rise in temperature can lead to a dangerously hypoxic environment in the MRI suite. This may not be noticed as helium is colorless and odorless. A controlled quench will allow the gas to escape to the atmosphere via quench pipes, but damage to the casing of the scanner could allow helium directly into the room. As helium is lighter than air it will rise, so oxygen analyzers should be positioned high in the room.
- *Magnetic media:* Exposure to greater than 30 Gauss can cause corruption or memory loss with credit cards, computer discs, digital watches, and personal electronic organizers inadvertently brought near the magnet.
- *Contrast:* The most common agent, dimeglumine gadopentetate has a high therapeutic index compared to iodinated agents. Anaphylactoid reactions have been reported as having an incidence of approximately 1:100,000. The dose (0.2 mL/kg) should be injected over one minute to minimize pain on injection, as the preparation is hyperosmolar.

  There have been reports of patients with renal failure developing a rare, potentially life-threatening condition with gadolinium-contrast agents (Gd-CAs) called nephrogenic systemic fibrosis or nephrogenic fibrosing dermopathy (NSF or NFD). The glomerular filtration rate (GFR) should be estimated in all patients with kidney disease to identify those at risk of developing NSF/NSD. If the GFR is less than 30 mL/min/1.73 m^2, the risk of Gd-CAs should be balanced against benefit, and a minimal dose of Gd-CAs only administered if an unenhanced scan proves insufficient. The Gd-CA should not be administered again for at least 7 days.[10] Od-CAs may be classified as high-risk, e.g. gadopentelic acid, medium-risk, e.g. gadobenic acid and low-risk, e.g. gadoteridol.[10] The use of high-risk agents is contraindicated in neonates and during the perioperative period in patients undergoing liver transplantation. The Gd-CAs are not recommended in pregnancy unless absolutely necessary.
- *Cardiac arrest:* We cannot bring a defibrillator into the theater. The patient will have to be moved out of the theater into the anesthetic room should a defibrillator be needed.

CONCLUSION

Intraoperative magnetic resonance imaging undoubtedly improves surgical outcomes as it allows the surgeon to accurately determine whether additional resection is needed while the patient is still in the operating room, or to determine whether the surgical approach will impinge upon a critical area of the brain. It, however, does expose the patient and surgical personnel to significant hazards. The use of iMRI impacts all aspects of anesthesia care, but following safety procedures, constant training, and an understanding of the physics and physiology of strong magnetic fields can mitigate the hazards of working in this unique environment.

REFERENCES

1. Geiger RS, Cascorbi H. Anesthesia in an NMR scanner. Anesth Analg. 1984;63(6):622-3.
2. Black PM, Moriarty T, Alexander E, et al. Development and implementation of intraoperative magnetic resonance imaging and its neurosurgical applications. Neurosurgery. 1997;41(4):831-42.
3. Peden CJ, Menon DK, Hall AS, et al. Magnetic resonance for the anaesthetist. Part II: Anaesthesia and monitoring in MR units. Anaesthesia. 1992;47(6):508-17.
4. Farling P, McBrien ME, Winder RJ. Magnetic resonance compatible equipment: read the small print! Anaesthesia. 2003;58(1):86-7.
5. Bradley PG, Harding SG, Reape MK, et al. Evaluation of infusion pump performance in a magnetic resonance environment. Eur J Anaesthesiol. 2004;21(9):729-33.
6. Sommer T, Vahlhaus C, Lauck G, et al. MR imaging and cardiac pacemakers: in-vitro evaluation and in-vivo studies in 51 patients at 0.5 T. Radiology. 2000;215(3):869-79.
7. Menon DK, Peden CJ, Hall AS, et al. Magnetic resonance for the anaesthetist. Part I: Physical principles, applications, safety aspects. Anaesthesia. 1992;47(3):240-55.
8. Shellock FG. Prosthetic heart valves and annuloplasty rings: assessment of magnetic field interactions, heating, and artifacts at 1.5 Tesla. J Cardiovasc Magn Reson. 2001;3(4):317-24.
9. Patteson SK, Chesney JT. Anesthetic management for magnetic resonance imaging: problems and solutions. Anesth Analg. 1992;74(1):121-8.
10. Farling PA, Flynn PA, Darwent G, et al. Safety in magnetic resonance units: an update. Anaesthesia. 2010;65(7):766-70.

8

Intraoperative Computed Tomography

Alessandro Olivi

INTRAOPERATIVE IMAGING

Imaging tools for use in neurosurgical operating rooms have proven to be important in the optimization of surgical procedures. Several modalities including magnetic resonance imaging (MRI), ultrasonography (US), digital subtraction angiography (DSA), fluoroscopy and computed tomography (CT), among others, have successfully been employed for procedures ranging from brain tumor resection, vascular surgery and skull-base surgery to screw placement and tumor resection in spinal procedures.[1-6] The appeal of these tools lies in the ability to enhance the neurosurgeon's understanding of the neuroanatomy of individual patients for optimal preoperative planning as well as better intraoperative assessment of the success of particular surgical procedures. Traditionally, preoperative imaging with MRI or CT was acquired and merged with neuronavigational systems to allow for visualization of the brain or spine structures during surgery. Even though these have provided critical data; however, there have been increasing interest in the intraoperative use of these imaging modalities. A number of reasons have been given for the need for intraoperative imaging including accounting for intraoperative brain shift that might render preoperative data inaccurate; better real-time intraoperative monitoring of possible complications such as intracerebral hemorrhage, diffuse cerebral edema, infarct or neurovascular compromise; better intraoperative assessment of the positioning of hardware in the brain and spine as well as for improved resection of brain and spine tumors, among other applications.[7] Intraoperative CT (iCT) in particular has proven to be quite useful in this intraoperative imaging. iCT was pioneered in the 1980s but was somewhat limited in its application due to poor image quality as well as cumbersome, time consuming interruptions in the operative work flow.[5] Advances in technology over time have however led to marked improvement in the utility of iCT with enhanced image quality, decreased acquisition time coupled with software that allow for merging of CT and MRI images. This revolution in CT imaging has thus led to its application in a myriad of neurosurgical procedures with improved patient outcomes.

Availability and Cost

Limited data is available concerning the exact cost of equipping an operating suite with a CT scanner **(Figure 8.1)**. There is high cost associated with the initial set-up of the operating suite, which may be prohibitive for small volume hospitals to incorporate into routine care. However, a few studies have noted decreased cost associated with iCT use compared to the use of postoperative imaging. A recent study of the use of iCT in pedicle screw placement in spine surgery revealed less cost associated with iCT compared to

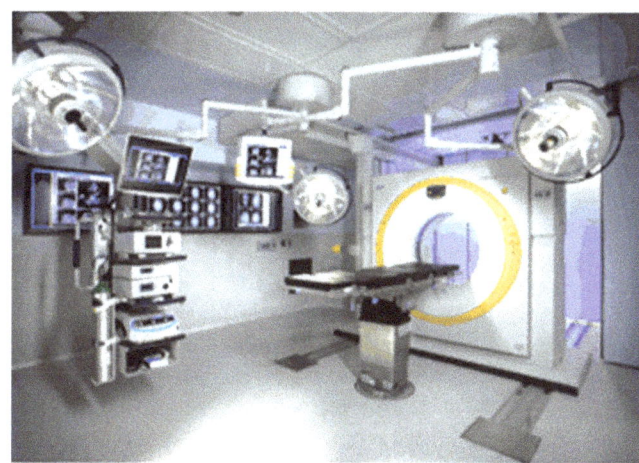

Figure 8.1 Intraoperative CT scanner setup

postoperative imaging ($233.35 ± 24.93 vs. $483.26 ± 17.74) or intraoperative neuromonitoring ($725.94 ± 1:158.96).[8] It is expected that the costs associated with such additions to the operating room will be reduced secondary to widespread use of the technology, particularly, in multidisciplinary setting where the technology may be shared among various surgical teams.[1,2] In addition, new advanced portable CT scan machines have become recently available to overcome, with acceptable quality and versatility, the financial challenges of a still preferable dedicated suite in small medical centers.

Advantages or Disadvantages

There have been a number of noted advantages with the use of iCT including better image quality with short acquisition times, particularly of osseous structures and high sensitivity for acute blood (which is critical during vascular interventions). Additionally, there is improved assessment of the placement of hardware during neurosurgical procedures such as fur, the placement of electrodes in the brain parenchyma as well as the placement of screws in spine surgeries and intraventricular catheters. Such assessment then allows for intraoperative repositioning of misplaced hardware before closure, thus obviating the need for reoperation potentially decreasing hospital stay while protecting patients from possible harmful neurologic sequelae from improperly placed hardware as well as minimizing the need for routine postoperative imaging.[1-6]

Disadvantages for the use of iCT include high cost associated with the construction of operating suites with the capabilities of iCT, steep learning curve for the surgical team, poor image quality for soft tissue structures, potential disruption of workflow and possible break in the sterile field during image acquisition.[4] Another theoretical disadvantage, particularly in the placement of vertebral body or pedicle screws, involves the increased number of intraoperative revisions of radiographically suboptimal but possibly clinically silent screws resulting in potentially unnecessary procedures and lengthening of the operative time.[9] While there has been concerns for increasing radiation exposure among patients who undergo iCT, a number of studies have revealed that radiation exposure is not significantly increased compared to patients who had not undergone iCT. Radiation exposure to operating room personnel is also markedly reduced as they exit the operating room before image acquisition begins.[10] Finally, even though there have been concerns about longer operative times, a number of studies have revealed minimal increases to the time with a range of 10–30 minutes.[1-6] It is conceivable that increasing incorporation of this imaging modality in routine care would result in the development of better workflow strategies that would further minimize the added operative time, resulting in a seamless experience for improved patient outcomes.

INTRAOPERATIVE COMPUTED TOMOGRAPHY INSTEAD OF FLUOROSCOPY, MRI AND ULTRASONOGRAPHY

As previously noted, there are a number of other modalities that can be employed for intraoperative imaging during neurological surgeries including MRI, fluoroscopy, US and X-rays. While US is affordable and can be easily replicated with increased sensitivity for assessing tumor resection and brain shift as well as Doppler assessment of vascular patency, it requires an experienced user and is limited in its applicability, especially in spine and complex skull base and vascular surgery.[5,11-13] Fluoroscopy has proven to be a valuable tool for spinal instrumentation, pituitary surgery and intraoperative angiography.[5,14] However, image quality is not as good as those provided by iCT, its range is limited to 3–4 vertebrae and is limited in its use in cranial pathology. MRI is an excellent intraoperative imaging tool, particularly for soft tissue structures. Its use in brain tumor resection has been well-documented and several studies have shown its superiority to iCT for the resection of low-grade tumors.[15,16] However, the use of intraoperative MRI is limited by high set-up and maintenance cost as well poor imaging of osseous structures.[5]

CLINICAL USES

Craniotomy

Stereotactic Procedures

The use of iCT for stereotactic procedures has been noted in several studies, both for frame-based and frameless stereotactic techniques. The most common use of iCT has been with stereotactic brain biopsies where CT imaging allows for the localization of lesions with subsequent modeling of needle trajectory for the acquisition of the biopsy specimen. Again, the preoperative merging of CT and MRI imaging modalities and the subsequent verification of CT images to rule out hemorrhagic complications have given a distinct advantages to the iCT technology. Indeed, it is well established that complications associated with CT-guided stereotactic biopsy include intracranial hemorrhage infection, seizure, post-procedure headache and non-diagnostic biopsies resulting in subsequent craniotomy for an open biopsy of the lesion.[17-21] Stereotactic procedures have also been used in conjunction with CT imaging for the placement of electrodes in the brain for deep brain stimulation (DBS) and for shunt placement.[22,23] iCT in conjunction with stereotaxy allows for optimized care by providing improved anatomic localization for the procurement of tissue specimen, the placement of electrodes and shunt placement, among other applications.

Tumor Resection

It is well recognized that the extent of turn or resection has implications for the long-term outcomes of patients with brain tumors including glioblastoma multiforme, astrocytomas and oligodendrogliomas, among others. As such, it is valuable to the neurosurgical team to be able to assess the extent of tumor resection intraoperatively. Current neuronavigational tools rely on preoperative imaging, which while useful, can be limited intraoperatively once resection has begun with resultant brain shifts. However, the use of iCT for intracranial tumor resection has been limited due to poor soft tissue image quality compared to MRI.[7,15,16] Newer CT scanners may yet result in enhanced soft tissue image quality leading to increasing use of iCT for brain tumors.[5] Nevertheless, iCT images merged with MRI images, in conjunction with neuronavigational tools have proven useful in the assessment of tumor localization as well as the extent of tumor resection.[23-25]

Skull Base Surgery

The complex architecture of the skull base renders intraoperative imaging invaluable for various surgical procedures. These include revision or primary endoscopic sinonasal surgery, endoscopic benign or malignant tumor resection, endoscopic mucocele drainage, and endoscopic tumor biopsy.[26-32] iCT has the advantage of identifying the osseous anatomy of the skull base allowing for technical optimization, i.e. more complete tumor resection or drainage of mucoceles as well as avoidance of complications such as vascular injury during these procedures.[30,32] A few studies utilizing iCT in skull base surgery have noted prompt intraoperative revisions, decreasing the need for a second operation based on postoperative imaging.[30,31]

Vascular Surgery

The use of iCT during intracranial vascular procedures has proven to be useful in the localization of vascular pathology, especially in the identification and repair of aneurysms, arteriovenous malformations and dural arteriovenous fistulae as well as in intracerebral hemorrhage. iCT coupled with angiography allows for the evaluation of vascular anatomy after repair of various pathologies.[11,33,34] During aneurysm repair, iCT allows, in some cases particularly when intraoperative angiography is not available, the surgical team to determine the proper placement of the aneurysmal clip helping to avoid potential ischemia, infarcts, unintended vessel occlusion, clip-related stenosis

or incomplete aneurysm clipping.[11] iCT also allows for intraoperative correction of suboptimally placed clips and rapid identification and possible correction of complications thus averting the need for a return to the operating room and these should be identified on postoperative imaging.[11,33,34]

Craniomaxillofacial Surgery

A number of studies have shown the utility of iCT during craniomaxillofacial surgery. This modality is particularly useful for complex craniofacial fractures, restoration of occlusive pathologies, mastication, and anatomic reconstruction of a symmetric facial skeleton.[35-38] These studies have indicated that iCT allows for immediate assessment of reduction and fixation of craniofacial fractures before the patient leaves the operating room, which may lead to decreased reoperation rates, with improved technical outcomes.[36,37]

Ventriculoperitoneal Shunt Placement

The placement of ventriculoperitoneal (VP) shunts is critical for the management of hydrocephalus and pseudotumor cerebri. However, incidence of shunt failure has been reported to be as high as 40% with subsequent need for revision.[39] A number of imaging modalities have been used intraoperatively for the determination of proper shunt placement including ultrasound, fluoroscopy, CT coupled with other neuronavigational tools.[39-41] iCT, coupled with fluoroscopy, has been noted in one recent study to result in better positioning of shunt with decreased shunt failure rates and improved neurologic outcomes for patients.[41] As improvements in the technology continue, it is conceivable that iCT will continue to play an important role in assisting the neurosurgical team in the placement of VP shunts.

Electrode Implantation for Deep Brain Stimulation and Seizure Focus Localization

Intraoperative CT has been used extensively in the neurosurgical operating room for the implantation of electrodes during DBS procedures and also for seizure focus localization operations.[1,5,23] These techniques rely on the precise placement of electrodes for optimal technical and clinical outcome for patients. Several studies have noted that iCT serves to ensure accurate placement of electrodes with the possibility of intraoperative correction of ill-placed electrodes.[23] Similar to the utility of iCT in other procedures, this avoids the need for a second surgery for revision of suboptimally placed electrodes while reducing the need for postoperative CT imaging and associated radiation as well as decreasing length of hospital stay.[5,23] Potential neurologic sequelae resulting from poorly placed electrodes will likewise be avoided.

Spine

Pedicle Screw

Intraoperative CT is particularly exquisite for the determination of the accuracy of pedicle screw placement in spinal surgeries due to the excellent delineation of the osseous anatomy with identification of relevant neurovasculature.[8-10,42-44] A number of studies have reported varying pedicle wall breach rates using anatomical landmarks for the placement of screws, with rates as high as 14.3%.[2,4,8,9] An assessment of pedicle placement with postoperative imaging and the identification of suboptimally placed screws can necessitate taking the patient back to the operating room for revision. However, intraoperative assessment allows for more rapid identification of the ill-placed hardware with proper correction before the patient leaves the operating room. Several studies have compared the postoperative breach rates of patient who underwent surgery with iCT versus those who had postoperative imaging, with data largely showing less breach rates for the former.[2] One study identified increased revision among patients who underwent pedicle screw placement with iCT.[9] This has the added concern of potential revisions of radiographically suboptimal but clinically silent screw placement that would have otherwise been observed in the patient if they had undergone imaging postoperatively. The impact of these revisions has yet to be characterized in terms of increased cost, neurologic complications, instrumentation failures and/or added radiation from use of iCT in comparison to secondary confirmation after intraoperative revision. While these potential drawbacks will need to be addressed, iCT will continue to serve as a critical adjunct to these procedures.

Tumor Resection

Spinal tumor resection has similarly benefited from the use of iCT. Optimal tumor resection, as in the brain, has implications for long-term patient outcomes. iCT not only allows for the optimal resection of tumors, but also allows for proper identification of the neurovascular structures, particularly the vertebral arteries in tumors of the cervical region, such that they are not placed at increased risk for inadvertent injury with resultant poor neurological outcomes.[45-48] A few studies have shown better resection of tumors during decompression of the anterior cervical spine cord along with symmetrical tumor resections after iCT revealed inadequate tumor resection.[46,47] With continued use, further strides will be made in the use of iCT for spine tumor resections.

Vertebroplasty

Vertebroplasty is successfully used for the treatment of vertebral compression fractures among patients with osteoporosis and/or metastatic lesions to the vertebral column.[49] These procedures can be performed under fluoroscopy and/or intraoperative CT imaging. Such imaging has the advantage of allowing for proper localization of the fractures as well as to aid in determining whether there has been extravasation of material into the spinal canal and/or disk space, which minimizes the risk of inadvertently injecting more material, causing further neural, vascular, and/or other injury.[49-52] A few studies have shown that intraoperative imaging with CT in vertebroplasty is a safe and effective method for the treatment of compression fractures.[49,51] With increased time and use, iCT will continue to allow for better technical and patient outcomes.

Spinal Trauma

The anatomy of the spine can be obscured in the setting of acute trauma to the spine. The assessment of the spine by the neurosurgical team can be enhanced with the use of iCT when there is a need for spinal stabilization. Studies utilizing iCT in the care of patients who have sustained spinal trauma have revealed improved outcomes for patients. iCT has resulted in decreased reoperative rates or no reoperation needed after intraoperative assessment of screw placement in addition to no noted neurological complications.[53,54] This has highlighted the need for further use and evaluation of iCT in cases of spinal trauma.[55]

SAFETY AND EFFICACY

There is limited data available on the safety and efficacy of the use of iCT in various neurosurgical procedures. However, a number of studies, as noted above, have shown improved technical outcomes of patients, such as better placement of hardware, improved tumor resection and repair of vascular pathology, with little to no adverse effects noted.[1-6] However, a recent study revealed that while iCT resulted in improved accuracy of screw placement in spinal instrumentation, the use of the intraoperative imaging resulted in a decreased threshold for screw revision compared to free-hand technique using anatomic landmarks when compared to patients who only received postoperative imaging.[9] Limited data exists that examines the consequence of possible increased radiation exposure to patients. However, the few limited studies that have been performed note no significantly increased radiation exposure compared to postoperative CT imaging.

COMPLICATIONS

Studies to date have reported little to no complications secondary to the use of iCT. There have been no increased risks of infection or neurologic deficits associated with the intraoperative imaging. There have likewise been no complications associated with contrast injection such as allergic or anaphylactic reactions or impairment in renal function.[1-6]

FUTURE DIRECTIONS

The implications of the use of iCT in patient care are particularly exciting. Further improvements in CT will potentially lead to even better imaging quality. Advances in the software will likewise allow for enhancement of the images as well as the improved ability to merge iCT with various imaging modalities, such as MRI to improve soft tissue assessment. These improved qualities will likewise make iCT an invaluable tool for neuronavigation for various neurosurgical procedures.

CONCLUSION

The use of intraoperative imaging has several applications for various neurosurgical procedures, from tumor resections, screw placement, vascular repair, or electrode placement. iCT provides excellent images for use in the operating room and allows for improved technical outcomes for patients. It appears clear that the advanced versatility of this modality in dealing with the widest spectrum of neurosurgical procedures holds the most convincing appeal for its expanded utilization. While more studies need to be performed to fully characterize long-term patient outcomes following the use of iCT in various neurosurgical procedures, there is hope that with increasing improvements in the technology, iCT will become even more valuable and increasingly integral to the neurosurgical team.

REFERENCES

1. Gasiński P, Zieliński P, Harat M, et al. Application of intraoperative computed tomography in a neurosurgical operating theatre. Neurol Neurochir Pol. 2012;46(6):536-41.
2. Costa F, Dorelli G, Ortolina A, et al. Computed tomography-based image-guided system in spinal surgery: state of the art through 10 years of experience. Neurosurgery. 2015;11(Suppl 2):59-67.
3. Schulz C, Waldeck S, Mauer UM. Intraoperative image guidance in neurosurgery: development, current indications, and future trends. Radiol Res Pract. 2012;2012:197364.
4. Rahmathulla G, Nottmeier EW, Pirris SM, et al. Intraoperative image-guided spinal navigation: technical pitfalls and their avoidance. Neurosurg Focus. 2014;36(3):E3
5. Uhl E, Zausinger S, Morhard D, et al. Intraoperative computed tomography with integrated navigation system in a multidisciplinary operating suite. Neurosurgery. 2009;64(5 Suppl 2):231-9.
6. Drazin D, Kim TT, Polly DW, et al. Introduction: Intraoperative spinal imaging and navigation. Neurosurg Focus. 2014;36(3):Introduction.
7. Albayrak B, Samdani AF, Black PM. Intraoperative magnetic resonance imaging in neurosurgery. Acta Neurochir (Wien). 2004;146(6):543-56.
8. Mason A, Paulsen R, Babuska JM, et al. The accuracy of pedicle screw placement using intraoperative image guidance systems. J Neurosurg Spine. 2014;20(2):196-203.
9. Bydon M, Xu R, Amin AG, et al. Safety and efficacy of pedicle screw placement using intraoperative computed tomography: consecutive series of 1148 pedicle screws. J Neurosurg Spine. 2014;21(3):320-8.
10. Tormenti MJ, Kostov DB, Gardner PA, et al. Intraoperative computed tomography image-guided navigation for posterior thoracolumbar spinal instrumentation in spinal deformity surgery. Neurosurg Focus. 2010;28(3):E11.
11. Goren O, Monteith SJ, Hadani M, et al. Modern intraoperative imaging modalities for the vascular neurosurgeon treating intracerebral hemorrhage. Neurosurg Focus. 2013;34(5):E2.
12. Tronnier VM, Bonsanto MM, Staubert A, et al. Comparison of intraoperative MR imaging and 3D-navigated ultrasonography in the detection and resection control of lesions. Neurosurg Focus. 2001;10(2):E3.
13. Hammoud MA, Ligon BL, elSouki R, et al. Use of intraoperative ultrasound for localizing tumors and determining the extent of resection: a comparative study with magnetic resonance imaging. J Neurosurg. 1996;84(5):737-41.
14. Fox WC, Wawrzyniak S, Chandler WF. Intraoperative acquisition of three-dimensional imaging for frameless stereotactic guidance during transsphenoidal pituitary surgery using the Arcadis Orbic System. J Neurosurg. 2008;108(4):746-50.
15. Maesawa S, Fujii M, Nakahara N, et al. Clinical indications for high-field 1.5 T intraoperative magnetic resonance imaging and neuro-navigation for neurosurgical procedures. Review of initial 100 cases. Neurol Med Chir (Tokyo). 2009;49(8):340-9.
16. Seifert V. Intraoperative MRI in neurosurgery: technical overkill or the future of brain surgery? Neurol India. 2003;51(3):329-32.
17. Wen DY, Hall WA, Miller DA, et al. Targeted brain biopsy: a comparison of freehand computed tomography-guided and stereotactic techniques. Neurosurgery. 1993;32(3):407-12.
18. Ranjan A, Rajshekhar V, Joseph T, et al. Nondiagnostic CT-guided stereotactic biopsies in a series of 407 cases: influence of CT morphology and operator experience. J Neurosurg. 1993;79(6):839-44.
19. Ferreira MP, Ferreira NP, Pereira Filho Ade A, et al. Stereotactic computed tomography-guided brain biopsy: diagnostic yield based on a series of 170 patients. Surg Neurol. 2006;65 Suppl 1:S1:27-1:32.
20. Chen CC, Hsu PW, Erich Wu TW, et al. Stereotactic brain biopsy: Single center retrospective analysis of complications. Clin Neurol Neurosurg. 2009;111(10):835-9.
21. Nishihara M, Sasayama T, Kudo H, et al. Morbidity of stereotactic biopsy for intracranial lesions. Kobe J Med Sci. 2011;56(4):E148-53.
22. Moran D, Kosztowski TA, Jusué-Torres I, et al. Does CT wand guidance improve shunt placement in patients with hydrocephalus? Clin Neurol Neurosurg. 2015;132:26-30.
23. Lee DJ, Zwienenberg-Lee M, Seyal M, et al. Intraoperative computed tomography for intracranial electrode implantation surgery in medically refractory epilepsy. J Neurosurg. 2015;122(3):526-31.
24. Barone DG, Lawrie TA, Hart MG. Image guided surgery for the resection of brain tumours. Cochrane Database Syst Rev. 2014;1:CD009685.

25. Li F, Lin J, Zhu G, et al. Neuroimaging and functional navigation as potential tools to reduce the incidence of surgical complications of lateral ventricular meningiomas. Clin Neurol Neurosurg. 2011;113(7):564-9.

26. Esposito F, Di Rocco F, Zada G, et al. Intraventricular and skull base neuroendoscopy in 2012: a global survey of usage patterns and the role of intraoperative neuronavigation. World Neurosurg. 2013;80(6):709-16.

27. Caversaccio M, Langlotz F, Nolte LP, et al. Impact of a self-developed planning and self-constructed navigation system on skull base surgery: 10 years experience. Acta Otolaryngol. 2007;127(4):403-7.

28. Anand VK, Kacker A. Value of radiologic imaging and computer assisted surgery in surgical decisions of the anterior skull base lesions. Rhinology. 2000;38(1):17-22.

29. Hamada H, Hayashi N, Asahi T, et al. Efficacy of a navigation system in neuro-endoscopic surgery. Minim Invasive Neurosurg. 2005;48(4):197-201.

30. Batra PS, Manes RP, Ryan MW, et al. Prospective evaluation of intraoperative computed tomography imaging for endoscopic sinonasal and skull-base surgery. Int Forum Allergy Rhinol. 2011;1(6):481-7.

31. Batra PS, Kanowitz SJ, Citardi MJ. Clinical utility of intraoperative volume computed tomography scanner for endoscopic sinonasal and skull base procedures. Am J Rhinol. 2008;22(5):511-5.

32. Solares CA, Ong YK, Carrau RL, et al. Prevention and management of vascular injuries in endoscopic surgery of the sinonasal tract and skull base. Otolaryngol Clin North Am. 2010;43(4):817-25.

33. Raza SM, Papadimitriou K, Gandhi D, et al. Intra-arterial intraoperative computed tomography angiography guided navigation: a new technique for localization of vascular pathology. Neurosurgery. 2012;71(2 Suppl Operative):ons240-52.

34. Schichor C, Rachinger W, Morhard D, et al. Intraoperative computed tomography angiography with computed tomography perfusion imaging in vascular neurosurgery: feasibility of a new concept. J Neurosurg. 2010;112(4):722-8.

35. Chauhan H, Rao SG, Chandramurti BA, et al. Neuro-navigation: An adjunct in craniofacial surgeries: Our experience. J Maxillofac Oral Surg. 2011;10(4):296-300.

36. Morrison CS, Taylor HO, Collins S, et al. Use of intraoperative computed tomography in complex craniofacial trauma: an example of on-table change in management. Craniomaxillofac Trauma Reconstr. 2014;7(4):298-301.

37. Rabie A, Ibrahim AM, Lee BT, et al. Use of intraoperative computed tomography in complex facial fracture reduction and fixation. J Craniofac Surg. 2011;22(4):1466-7.

38. Eggers G, Kress B, Rohde S, et al. Intraoperative computed tomography and automated registration for image-guided cranial surgery. Dentomaxillofac Radiol. 2009;38(1):28-33.

39. Crowley RW, Dumont AS, Asthagiri AR, et al. Intraoperative ultrasound guidance for the placement of permanent ventricular cerebrospinal fluid shunt catheters: a single-center historical cohort study. World Neurosurg. 2014;81(2):397-403.

40. Whitehead WE, Riva-Cambrin J, Wellons JC, et al. Factors associated with ventricular catheter movement and inaccurate catheter location: post hoc analysis of the hydrocephalus clinical research network ultrasound-guided shunt placement study. J Neurosurg Pediatr. 2014;14(2):173-8.

41. Janson CG, Romanova LG, Rudser KD, et al. Improvement in clinical outcomes following optimal targeting of brain ventricular catheters with intraoperative imaging. J Neurosurg. 2014;120(3):684-96.

42. Kim TT, Drazin D, Shweikeh F, et al. Clinical and radiographic outcomes of minimally invasive percutaneous pedicle screw placement with intraoperative CT (O-arm) image guidance navigation. Neurosurg Focus. 2014;36(3):E1.

43. Hecht AC, Koehler SM, Laudone JC, et al. Is intraoperative CT of posterior cervical spine instrumentation cost-effective and does it reduce complications? Clin Orthop Relat Res. 2011;469(4):1035-41.

44. Karandikar M, Mirza SK, Song K, et al. Complex pediatric cervical spine surgery using smaller nonspinal screws and plates and intraoperative computed tomography. J Neurosurg Pediatr. 2012;9(6):594-601.

45. Hum B, Feigenbaum F, Cleary K, et al. Intraoperative computed tomography for complex craniocervical operations and spinal tumor resections. Neurosurgery. 2000;47(2):374-80.

46. Freidberg SR, Pfeifer BA, Dempsey PK, et al. Intraoperative computerized tomography scanning to assess the adequacy of decompression in anterior cervical spine surgery. J Neurosurg. 2001;94(1 Suppl):8-11.

47. Costa F, Tomei M, Sassi M, et al. Evaluation of the rate of decompression in anterior cervical corpectomy using an intra-operative computerized tomography scan (O-Arm system). Eur Spine J. 2012;21(2):359-63.

48. Deinsberger R, Regatschnig R, Ungersböck K. Intraoperative evaluation of bone decompression in anterior cervical spine surgery by three-dimensional fluoroscopy. Eur Spine J. 2005;14(7):671-6.

49. Pitton MB, Herber S, Koch U, et al. CT-guided vertebroplasty: analysis of technical results, extraosseous cement leakages, and complications in 500 procedures. Eur Radiol. 2008;18(11):2568-78.

50. Ge JZ, Zhang HD, Jin WJ, et al. [Clinical analysis of CT guided unilateral PVP for the treatment of osteoporotic vertebral compression fracture in senile patients]. Zhongguo Gu Shang. 2011;24(10):824-7.

51. Seong JY, Kim JS, Jung B, et al. CT-Guided percutaneous vertebroplasty in the treatment of an upper thoracic compression fracture. Korean J Radiol. 2009;10(2):185-89.

52. Epstein NE. Computed tomography-guided vertebroplasty using a stereotactic guidance system (stereo-guide). Surg Neurol Int. 2010;1:10.

53. Patil AA. Computed tomography-guided vertebroplasty using a stereotactic guidance system (stereo-guide). Surg Neurol Int. 2010;1:17.

54. Costa F, Ortolina A, Attuati L, et al. Management of C1-2 traumatic fractures using an intraoperative 3D imaging-based navigation system. J Neurosurg Spine. 2015;22(2)128-33.

55. Schouten R, Lee R, Boyd M, et al. Intra-operative cone-beam CT (O-arm) and stereotactic navigation in acute spinal trauma surgery. J Clin Neurosci. 2012;19(8):1137-43.

9

CT-based Navigation in Brain and Spine Surgery

Ivan Ng Hua Bak

INTRODUCTION

In brain surgery, localization of intracranial surgical targets has been traditionally based on anatomical landmarks. Although landmarks are sufficient for skull base and posterior fossa surgery, the cerebral hemispheres contains relatively few consistent landmarks. The size, shape, and course of the cerebral convolutions differ between individuals and between hemispheres in the same individual. Furthermore, intra-axial surgical targets below the cortical surface are frequently hidden from view. Unlike surgery elsewhere in the body, exploration with surgical dissection will cause an unacceptable amount of morbidity. A high degree of accuracy is therefore paramount. The development of frame-based stereotaxy, and subsequently, frameless stereotaxy or neuronavigation has been instrumental in providing the modern neurosurgeon with the ability for precise localization of intracranial surgical lesions.

C-arm fluoroscopy has been the traditional work-horse in spinal surgery in providing definite localization of spinal levels and guidance for instrumentation. Nevertheless, C-arm fluoroscopy has a number of limitations. The images obtained are in the anteroposterior and lateral planes with the bony details superimposed. It is impossible to obtain images in the axial plane. In spinal regions of complex anatomy such as the craniocervical junction, the available views are inadequate. The upper thoracic spine is difficult to visualize in the lateral projection. Multiple repeated views in alternating planes are often needed, leading to frequent re-positioning of the C-arm. The risk of radiation exposure[1] requires the surgeon to wear leaded gowns, which are uncomfortable and fatigue-inducing. The development of virtual fluoroscopy,[2,3] by allowing the surgeon to navigate based on the anteroposterior and lateral fluoroscopic images, reduces radiation exposure and multiple C-arm repositioning but do not address the other limitations of conventional fluoroscopy. The principles of frameless stereotaxy were first applied to spinal surgery in the 1990s[4-8] and have matured significantly since.

NEURONAVIGATION

The specific technical details of each neuronavigation system vary but common elements exist. A reference array is fixed in relation to the patient's cranium or spine. A tracking system determines the spatial relationship between the reference array and the navigated instruments. A display monitor provides the surgeon with the position of the instruments and the patient's anatomical images in real time.

Optical Tracking Neuronavigation

Optical tracking neuronavigational systems, such as Brainlab's Vector Vision (Brainlab AG, Feldkirchen, Bavaria, Germany) and Medtronic's StealthStation (Medtronic, Minneapolis, Minnesota, USA) employ a pair of stereoscopic optical cameras, an infrared emitter, and reflective markers. Reflective markers on a reference array are fixed in relation to the patient's head or spine. Instruments usually have two or more markers. The optical cameras track the exact location and spatial relationship of these markers, allowing the neuronavigation system to identify the type, location and orientation of the instrument, and its relationship to the patient's position. This information is then displayed on a monitor, providing the surgeon with a real-time relationship between the tracked instruments and the anatomical images.

Electromagnetic Neuronavigation

AxiEM technology (Medtronic, Minneapolis, Minnesota, USA) utilizes a magnetic field generator placed near the surgical field. Using multiple transmitter coils, a hemisphere-shaped electromagnetic field of approximately 50 cm in diameter is created. The reference array is taped to the patient's head. By tracking the exact strength and direction of the magnetic field with an electromagnetic probe, the exact location and orientation of the probe in relation to the reference array is determined. Since the magnetic reference array may be taped to the patient's head, this system avoids the need for rigid head fixation. This is particularly advantageous in the pediatric population. Line-of-sight issues encountered with optical neuronavigation system are avoided.

Neuronavigation Registration for Brain Surgery

The accuracy of frameless neuronavigation relies heavily on the process of registration.[9] Put simply, registration is the process of aligning the patient's anatomy in radiological images to the anatomy in actual space.

The most common methods of registration in brain surgery involve the use of anatomical points (paired-point matching), facial anatomical features or the usage of fiducials. Anatomical points, whether it be fiducials, facial anatomy or anatomical points, on the patient are matched to the equivalent points on the patient's scan.

These methods suffer from a common methodological weakness in their reliance on the skin surface, which is not fixed in relation to the cranium and its contents. This introduces a degree of error into the registration process. Perioperative anesthetic preparation, including taping of the endotracheal tube and neuromuscular blockade, may render facial features dissimilar to their position in the preoperative radiological images. Scalp fiducials may move or become dislodged from their original position during positioning and head fixation. Comparing the location of skin fiducials on preoperative and intraoperative magnetic resonance imaging (MRI), Mitsui and colleagues[10] reported a mean extent of "skin shift" of 5.34 mm.

Intraoperative CT for Brain Surgery

The initial development of intraoperative CT (iCT) in brain surgery was for the purpose of tumor resection control.[11-13] This has been superseded by intraoperative MRI[14-16] with its superior visualization of the intracranial contents, particularly intracerebral tumors. iCT was subsequently applied to stereotactic neurosurgery[17,18] and frameless neuronavigation.[19] Although initial attempts to converge the technologies of iCT and frameless neuronavigation still relied on skin fiducials,[19] improved techniques of automatic registration has been developed.[20]

Automatic iCT registration for neuronavigation requires the placement of markers on the CT gantry. These markers are precalibrated to the position of the intraoperatively acquired CT images. During the scanning process, the positions of the iCT gantry and reference array are tracked by the neuronavigation system. Automatic registration between the scanned images and the patient's position is then performed by specialized neuronavigation software. Utilizing such a system in a phantom study, Eggers and colleagues[20] were able to achieve highly accurate registration, with an average target registration error of less than 1.2 mm. Image fusion with preoperative MRI may also be performed,[21] allowing the surgeon to navigate with superior, albeit preoperative, MRI images.

There are a number of additional benefits of iCT in neuronavigation beyond the benefits of highly accurate registration. Neuronavigation based on previously acquired neuroimaging (preoperative or intraoperative) becomes increasingly inaccurate due to the phenomenon of brain shift. The opening of the cranium and dura, release of cerebrospinal fluid, tumor resection and use of osmotic agents induce deformational changes in the cerebrum. In a study on intraoperative brain shift with serial intraoperative MRI scans, Nabavi and colleagues[22] concluded:

Brain shift is a continuous dynamic process that evolves differently in distinct brain regions. Therefore, only serial imaging or continuous data acquisition can provide consistently accurate image guidance.

With iCT based neuronavigation, the neuronavigation may be updated with the latest iCT images[23] as many times as deemed necessary in order to overcome the problem of brain shift.

Postintervention iCT may also be used to confirm the accuracy or completeness of the intervention.[19,24,25] In stereotactic procedures such as stereotactic thalamotomy, an iCT may be obtained after placement of the probe to confirm its appropriate position before ablation is carried out.[18] The use of iCT in this manner adds to the surgeon's confidence in the accuracy of the operation.

Neuronavigation Registration for Spine Surgery

A number of issues are encountered in the registration process in neuronavigation for spine surgery. The spine is a deep structure, with an overlying thick, mobile layer of soft tissue, and skin. Hence, registration based on skin-based landmarks or fiducials is frankly unreliable. The registration commonly utilizes exposed bony landmarks as anatomical points or surfaces. Unfused spinal segments are mobile in relation with one another. Registration of the spine may require separate registration of each spinal segment, which is time consuming. Preoperative spinal imaging is most commonly obtained with the patient supine, whereas surgery for spinal instrumentation is mostly performed with the patient prone in various degrees of spinal flexion and extension.

Intraoperative CT for Spine Surgery

In a study in 2000, Haberland and colleagues[26] attempted to improve the accuracy of neuronavigation registration in spine surgery by incorporating iCT into the process of registration. After surgical exposure of the spine, small titanium screws were implanted in the dorsal elements at every level involved in neuronavigation. This was followed by acquisition of an iCT scan. These screws serve as unambiguous landmarks for registration. With this method, a registration error of less than 1 mm was achieved.

Current techniques of iCT based spinal neuronavigation most commonly utilizes a reference array attached to bony structure, usually the spinous process. Automatic registration is performed after acquisition of an iCT scan. Non-CT based cross sectional imaging such as Iso-C C-arm (Siemens, Munich, Bavaria, Germany) and O-arm (Medtronic, Minneapolis, Minnesota, USA) provides adequate bony resolution for use in spine surgery.

Using iCT based spinal neuronavigation, CT images are acquired with the patient in the surgical position. In the event of shift occurring during the course of surgery or suspected neuronavigational inaccuracy, a repeat iCT scan may be obtained to update the neuronavigation system with the most up-to-date images. Operative time may be shorter using this method, as the time consuming processes of repeated repositioning of the C-arm in fluoroscopy and the steps of registration and verification in non-iCT neuronavigation are eliminated.[27]

The benefit of iCT in spine surgery also extends beyond neuronavigational accuracy. The immediate verification of appropriate implant position allows the surgeon to revise any misplaced screws to prevent subsequent return to the operating theatre for revision.[28-33]. With the availability of reliable intraoperative confirmation of implant position, a postoperative CT scan is no longer necessary. In decompressive surgery, the adequacy of bony decompression can be assessed and optimized if required.[30,31,34] Finally, as there is no need for significant bony exposure for registration, neuronavigation may be used in minimally invasive spinal surgery for the percutaneous placement of screws.

Options for Intraoperative CT

For iCT imaging, conventional CT technology is required for cranial surgery. However, for spinal surgery where bony anatomy is the critical component, a number of technologies, such as the O-arm (Medtronic, Minneapolis, Minnesota, USA), and Iso-C C-arm (Siemens, Munich, Bavaria, Germany) are able to produce cross-sectional imaging for multiplanar reconstruction with bone resolution similar to those obtained with CT scans.

Intraoperative CT Scanner

The setup at our iCT operating theatre (Brainsuite, Brainlab AG, Feldkirchen, Bavaria, Germany) consists of a 32-slice CT scanner (Siemens Somatom Sensation Open, Siemens, Munich, Bavaria, Germany) with a mobile gantry mounted

on rails. From the parked position at the side of the operating theater, the CT scanner is moved on rails to the operating table at the center of the operating theatre when a scan is needed. For intraoperative scans, the gantry is draped with transparent sterile drapes prior to entering the sterile field. Reflective markers on the CT gantry allow tracking during scan acquisition. The iCT scanner transfers the scan data to the integrated neuronavigation system (Brainlab Vectorvision, Brainlab, Feldkirchen, Bavaria, Germany). Automatic registration is performed with the surgical software (Brainlab iPlan, Brainlab, Feldkirchen, Bavaria, Germany) and transferred to the neuronavigation panel for intraoperative use.

Mobile CT Scanner

Mobile CT scanners are becoming increasing popular for intraoperative use. They may be used without the need for extensive installation of rails and operating theatre modification. The flexibility for use in the emergency department and intensive care unit are additional benefits.

O-arm

The O-arm (Medtronic, Minneapolis, Minnesota, USA) utilizes cone beam technology to produce 2D fluoroscopic images and 3-D multiplanar CT-quality images. Its footprint is slightly larger than a traditional C-arm. Initial positioning is similar to that of a C-arm, where the gantry is moved into the scanning position from the side of the operating table. Once the operating table is placed in the central bore, the telescoping door at the gantry opening is closed, forming a complete ring or "O" around the patient. A scanning volume, in cylindrical shape, of 15 cm length and 20 cm diameter is available. Seamless integration with the StealthStation neuronavigation system (Medtronic, Minneapolis, Minnesota, USA) reduces the hassle and time required for data transfer and registration.

Iso-C C-arm

Iso-C C-arm (Siemens, Munich, Bavaria, Germany) is a specially designed C-arm which maintains the area of interest in the center of the C-arm throughout the full 190° rotation of the C-arm. For 3D imaging, multiple 2D fluoroscopic images are acquired during a full automated, motorized "spin". Specialized software reconstructs the data into a cube-shaped 3D volumetric dataset, measuring 12 cm × 12 cm × 12 cm. Multiplanar reconstruction allows the visualization of the imaged anatomy in cross section in the axial, sagittal, and coronal planes. Integration with a neuronavigation system allows for neuronavigation with multiplanar CT-quality images.

Technical Issues

All current intraoperative imaging technology requires the scanner to be placed into the operative field. Physical attributes of the scanner and potential interactions with the components of the operating theatre are important considerations. The size of the central bore must be larger than the dimensions of the patient and operating table with its accessories. Intraoperative CT scanners, by virtue of the closed gantry, must approach the operating table from the end of the table. This precludes their use with the Jackson table in spine surgery. In contrast, C-arm and O-arm may be placed through the side of the operating table. The use of the sitting position for posterior fossa surgery is incompatible with current iCT technologies. The scanner and its movements are a potential source of contamination during surgery. Strict sterile draping and positioning protocols must be enforced.

Radiolucent operating table and accessories, including head holder, straps, arm-boards, should be radiolucent to prevent artifacts due to the differential penetration of X-rays. For the use of head holders in cranial surgery, pin artifact remains a significant problem. Use of specialized polymer pins should be used if available.

The addition of iCT for neuronavigation to the operating theater workflow introduces a layer of complexity. Unfamiliarity with the new technology may increase surgical time. The key to successful integration of iCT relies on proper planning, adequate staff training and the provision of technical support. Significant changes to the anesthetic workflow may also be required.[35]

The intraoperative acquisition of CT scan and update of the neuronavigation system do not greatly increase operative time. Duration of interruption of surgery of 9 minutes and 10–15 minutes have been reported in spine[33,36] and brain[36] surgery, respectively. This is offset by the elimination of the need for frequent C-arm repositioning or the time consuming process of non-iCT-based registration for neuronavigation.

Disadvantages of Intraoperative CT

The main barrier to the widespread adoption of iCT in neurosurgical units worldwide is the cost of acquisition and setup of an iCT operating theatre. A diagnostic CT scanner in most hospitals is used frequently on a daily basis and generates a steady and significant income, thus justifying the initial high costs. In contrast, the iCT scanner is used less frequently. In the initial 3-years after the installation of an iCT system in our operating theatre, the iCT scanner was utilized in 524 cases (429 brain operations and 95 spine operations) (unpublished data). A mathematical calculation gives an average of 3.4 cases per week. These usage rates may not provide sufficient economical justification for the acquisition of an iCT system at many hospitals. The costs of an Isi-C C-arm (Siemens, Munich, Bavaria, Germany) and O-arm (Medtronic, Minneapolis, Minnesota, USA) are lower than iCT and may be an option for spinal surgery as the soft tissue resolution is, at present, unsuitable for brain surgery.

The use of iCT scans exposes the patient to more ionizing radiation compared to the use of fluoroscopy, virtual fluoroscopy or non-iCT-based neuronavigation. The surgeon should ensure that all steps are taken to minimize the amount of intraoperative scans required.

BRAIN SURGERY: INDICATIONS

Although MRI-based neuronavigation is the imaging modality of choice for intracerebral pathology, there remains a role for CT-based neuronavigation in brain surgery.

Aspiration of Intracerebral Hematoma

Spontaneous intracerebral hematomas are a significant cause of morbidity and mortality in the elderly population worldwide. Frequently, concomitant comorbidities increase the risks of major surgical intervention. The advent of minimally invasive techniques for hematoma evacuation guided by CT-based neuronavigation is a major advancement for the treatment of this condition.

Barlas and colleagues[37] performed evacuation of spontaneous intracerebral hematomas through a 2.5 cm minicraniotomy in 20 elderly patients. CT-based neuronavigation facilitated the choosing of the optimal entry site and trajectory, avoiding eloquent cortex while providing the shortest route to the hematoma. 90% of these patients were independent at 6 months. The authors concluded that their minimally invasive technique allowed the prompt evacuation of intracerebral hematomas, resulting in a high rate of functional recovery with minimal surgical morbidity. In a similar cohort, Vespa and colleagues[38] performed neuronavigation-guided catheter placements into spontaneous intracerebral hematomas for clot aspiration and infusion of a thrombolytic agent. In 28 patients so treated, there was significant reduction in clot volume and improvement of their clinical status.

Catheter Placement

Ventricular puncture has traditionally been performed 'freehand', guided by anatomical landmarks. This suffices in straightforward cases. However, in cases of slit ventricles or altered anatomy, landmark-based ventricular catheter insertion may have a lower ventricular cannulation rate, requiring multiple passes or leading to abandonment of the procedure. Neuronavigation is beneficial in these cases.

Reig and colleagues[39] studied 26 patients requiring ventriculoperitoneal shunting but had ventricular configuration that was deemed challenging to cannulate. CT-based neuronavigation with facial surface mapping registration was utilized in the ventriculoperitoneal shunting procedure. The ventricle was cannulated successfully in every case.

Hermann and colleagues[40] utilized neuronavigation for ventricular catheter placement in 29 pediatric patients with difficult or abnormal ventricular anatomy undergoing shunting. Ventricular catheter placement was accurate in all cases, with no shunt revision for proximal blockage at a mean of 23.5 months follow-up.

In a nonrandomized study comparing ventriculoperitoneal shunting with and without navigation, Hayhurst and colleagues[41] found that a lower rate of poor ventricular catheter placement and early shunt revision rate in the navigated group. The shunt revision rate in the navigated group was 5.9%, compared to 22% in the non-navigated group.

When an intraventricular infusion of a chemotherapeutic agent through a ventricular catheter is planned, appropriate positioning of the tip of the ventricular catheter is essential. Malpositioning of the ventricular catheter may lead to disastrous consequences when the toxic agent is delivered. Takahashi and colleagues[42] utilized CT navigation for Ommaya reservoir placement in 85 cases, including 6 cases with slit ventricles. They achieved appropriate catheter positioning in all except one case.

Skull Base

In skull-base surgery, MRI provides superior visualization of cranial nerves, brainstem and basal cisterns, while CT has better resolution for bony and, with CT angiography for vascular structures. In the anatomically complex skull base, combining these complementary imaging methods for neuronavigation is beneficial.[43] The surgical approach may be tailored to the individual patient. Important neural and vascular structures could be identified early and protected during tumor resection.

Sure and colleagues[44] reported a series of 10 cases, in which CT-MRI played a crucial role in surgical planning. All patients had extra-axial tumors of the skull base. The authors could optimize the surgical approach and achieved complete resection in 80% of the cases.

Kurtsoy and colleagues[45] reported their results in 87 patients with skull base tumors. Depending on the location and extent of the tumor, four main surgical approaches were utilized in each: (1) extended frontobasal; (2) craniorbitozygomatic; (3) subtemporal and; (4) presigmoid transpetrosal. Gross total resection was achieved in 82 out of the 87 patients in their series. Fiducial-based registration required less than 10 minutes in each case, with a mean registration accuracy of 1.1 mm.

Nakamura and colleagues[46] applied CT-MRI based neuronavigation to the craniofacial resection of anterior skull base tumors. They found that image guidance allowed safe tumor resection and improved spatial orientation during surgery. The latter is particularly important in these cases where the anatomy is frequently distorted by tumor growth and invasion.

Vascular

In vascular neurosurgery, CT angiography provides superior visualization of intracranial vessels compared to MRI. This makes CT angiography an attractive solution for neuronavigation for neurovascular disorders. In addition, the MR angiographic "time of flight" sequence requires fusion with a volumetric T1 MRI sequence prior to usage in neuronavigation, hence, introducing a potential source of error.

Modern neuronavigation software offers the capability to reconstruct CT angiographic data into 3D rendered images for surgical planning and neuronavigation. This provides the surgeon with the opportunity to study the anatomical features of the aneurysm, plan the surgical approach, localize the aneurysm accurately with minimal unnecessary dissection and visualize hidden structures.[47]

Kim and colleagues[48] report a series of 12 patients who undergone surgical clipping of distal anterior cerebral artery aneurysms. These aneurysms may be difficult to localize during surgery, due to a lack of anatomical landmarks that guide the surgeon towards the aneurysm. Neuronavigation with CT angiography aided the localization of the aneurysm for clipping. In addition, a smaller craniotomy may be used with confidence in this setting.

Minimally Invasive Brain Surgery

Modern neuronavigation allows neurosurgeons to tailor the surgical approach to the patient's specific anatomical and pathological features. With the optimal skin incision, craniotomy and surgical trajectory, one may potentially reduce complications, lower transfusion rate and decrease the length of hospital stay.[49] Although larger openings are unavoidable in many cases, minimally invasive approaches guided by neuronavigation may be used in selected cases. The surgical approach may be tailored.

Coppens and colleagues[50] described their method of STA-MCA bypass through an enlarged burr hole. CT angiography is performed for preoperative planning and intraoperative neuronavigation. The donor and recipient vessels are selected preoperatively and localized intraoperatively with neuronavigation. This allows them to limit the size of the cranial opening to 2–2.5 cm.

In a study on unruptured intracranial aneurysms, Schmid-Elsaesser and colleagues[51] found that CT angiography based neuronavigation allowed the planning and execution of small, precisely-placed craniotomies for clipping of middle cerebral artery aneurysms. However, neuronavigation did not lead to small craniotomies for internal carotid artery or anterior communicating artery aneurysms.

Gharabaghi and colleagues[52] used CT navigation for avoidance of the frontal sinus during frontolateral craniotomies for approach to the skull base. Inadvertent entry into the frontal sinus may require obliteration of the frontal sinus to prevent mucocele formation or lead to infective complications such as meningitis. Avoidance of the frontal sinus may reduce the risk of these complications and potentially reduce operative time.

SPINE SURGERY: INDICATIONS

Pedicle Screw Insertion

Modern techniques of spinal stabilization and deformity correction rely heavily on the use of spinal instrumentation. In posterior spinal instrumentation, currently available pedicle screw based constructs are among the most robust and biomechanically strong instruments. Pedicle screws traverse all three columns of the spine. Stabilization with pedicle screws provides short and rigid segmental stabilization and may be used in the absence of intact posterior elements.[53] Breach of the spinal canal with wiring and laminar hook techniques is avoided.

However, pedicle screw insertion is technically challenging for a number of reasons. The size and angle of the vertebral pedicle varies between spinal regions. Malplacement of pedicle screws can potentially cause neurovascular injuries and dural tears. A high degree of accuracy is critical for safe pedicle screw instrumentation, especially the midcervical, midthoracic and thoracolumbar junction.[54]

The application of neuronavigation by Kalfas and colleagues[7] was a significant milestone in the history of pedicle screws. Neuronavigation in pedicle screw insertion has been demonstrated to be associated with a significantly lower risk of screw misplacements. In a meta-analysis by Shin and colleagues,[55] the risk of pedicle perforation is 6% with neuronavigation and 15% without neuronavigation, with no difference in operative time and blood loss. In a larger meta-analysis by Kosmopoulos and colleagues[56] which included 37,337 pedicle screws, accuracy of pedicle screw placement was higher with neuronavigation (95.2%) than without neuronavigation (90.3%). These results clearly favor the use of neuronavigation in pedicle screw insertion.

The subaxial cervical pedicle is in close proximity to the transverse foramen containing the vertebral artery. The potentially catastrophic consequences of vertebral artery injury dissuade most surgeons from inserting pedicle screws in this region. Although lateral mass instrumentation is safer than pedicle screw insertion, pedicle screw constructs are stronger and provides a more robust instrumentation.[57] This may be required in selected cases. The use of neuronavigation may enable surgeons to place pedicle screws in the subaxial cervical spine accurately and safely. Ito and colleagues[58] reported superior placement of cervical pedicle screws with CT-based neuronavigation than without neuronavigation.

At the thoracic spine, similarly good results of neuronavigation for pedicle screw insertion have been reported. Allam and colleagues[59] report a rate of accurate screw placement of 89.8% without neuronavigation and 98% with neuronavigation. Dinesh and colleagues[28] report 2.3% pedicle violations in thoracic pedicle screw placement with the use of iCT-based neuronavigation. In a randomized trial in thoracic pedicle screw insertion for deformity correction surgery, Rajasekaran and colleagues[60] report a pedicle breach rate of 2% with Iso-C 3-D neuronavigation and 23% without neuronavigation. In addition, the length of time required for navigated pedicle screw insertion was almost half of the time required for non-navigated pedicle screw insertion (2.37 minutes vs 4.61 minutes).

In a study on pedicle screw insertion in the lumbosacral spine utilizing O-arm neuronavigation, Silbermann and colleagues[61] report an extremely high accuracy, with only 2 (1%) of 197 screws causing cortical penetration. In comparison, 25(5.9%) of 152 non-navigated screws had evidence of cortical penetration, including four screws which required immediate intraoperative revision.

Tumor Resection

Thorat and colleagues[62] described their experience with iCT and neuronavigation in single stage, complete resection of thoracic dumbbell tumors. Intraoperative CT was employed for localization, determining the extent of the paraspinal tumor extension as well as neuronavigation for instrumentation.

For bony lesions such as osteomas, CT-based neuronavigation may be used for precise localization.[63] In addition, an iCT scan can confirm the adequacy of excision.[63]

Trauma

Significant spinal trauma with bony fractures and soft tissue injury may potentially distort the normal spinal anatomy, disrupting the relationships between spinal elements and between adjacent spinal segments. CT-based neuronavigation is useful in these circumstances to orientate the surgeon to the patient's anatomy and guide surgical treatment.

Schouten and colleagues[64] applied intraoperative O-arm technology with neuronavigation 27 cases of spinal trauma, concluding that this use of the technology allowed them to overcome the anatomical challenges and broaden the stabilization options in these cases.

Wang and colleagues[65] inserted 140 pedicle screws in 21 patients undergoing instrumentation for thoracolumbar spine fractures. All screws were inserted successfully, with a 0% of pedicle cortical perforation of more than 2 mm.

Utilizing Iso-C 3-D neuronavigation, Rajasekaran and colleagues[66] successfully placed pedicle screws for direct repair of hangman fractures for 20 patients with good clinical results. Direct screw fixation of these fractures is technically demanding but provide simple and biomechanically sound fixation.

Craniocervical Junction

Instrumentation of the craniocervical junction is indicated in cases with instability and deformity. Options for C1-2 stabilization include posterior wiring and screw-based techniques. Screw-based techniques are biomechanically stronger, may be used in the absence of C1 posterior arch or C2 lamina and do not require placement of wires into the spinal canal. However, screw insertion in this region is technically challenging due to the complexity of the anatomy of C1 and C2. A significant risk of vertebral artery injury is present during C2 pedicle screw insertion and C1-2 transarticular screw insertion.[67] This risk is increased in the presence of aberrant vertebral artery anatomy.

Numerous authors have reported their results in the insertion of C1-C2 transarticular screws using neuro-navigation.[68,69] Acosta and colleagues[68] placed 36 C1-C2 transarticular screws for atlantoaxial instability. 92% of these screws were deemed to be well-positioned. Uehara and colleauges[69] reported their results with CT-based neuronavigation in C1-2 transarticular screw placement in 20 patients. Only one screw (2.6%) had caused cortical perforation. There were no neurovascular injuries.

The mobility of atlanto-axial joint, particularly in the setting of instability, poses significant challenges for neuronavigation based on preoperative CT. Gluf and colleagues,[70] with their experience with 353 transarticular screws in 191 patients, reported frequent difficulty with neuronavigation. Inaccuracy arises from limitations of using tracking devices on C2 and difficulties in registration.

Given the limitations in the application preoperative CT-based neuronavigation to the craniocervical junction, it is natural that surgeons apply iCT neuronavigation for this purpose. Yang and colleagues[71] compared Iso-C 3-D neuronavigation with conventional fluoroscopy in C1 lateral mass and C2 pedicle screw insertion in a series of 24 patients. Screw accuracy was found to be significantly higher with the use of Iso-C 3-D neuronavigation.

In a non-randomized study of 51 patients undergoing odontoid screw insertion, Martirosyan and colleagues[72] found the use of Iso-C 3-D neuronavigation to be associated with superior screw positioning and higher fusion rates compared to conventional fluoroscopy.

Our results in this setting are similarly favorable. In 21 patients with C1/C2 subluxation treated with the aid of iCT neuronavigation, Ling and colleagues[73] achieved ideal positioning in 98% of screws (lateral mass, translaminar and pedicle screws) with a 0% incidence of neurological and vascular injury.

Basilar invagination requires, in selected cases, resection of the odontoid process through an anterior approach. Neuronavigation may be used for surgical guidance in place of traditional C-arm fluoroscopy. Gempt and colleagues[74] found CT-based neuronavigation to be an important adjunct in three cases of endoscopic transnasal approach for the resection of the odontoid process.

Minimally Invasive Spinal Instrumentation

Minimally invasive spinal instrumentation avoids a long surgical wound, extensive surgical dissection and excessive blood loss. The use of C-arm fluoroscopy in minimally invasive spinal instrumentation requires frequent repositioning of the C-arm and multiple fluoroscopic images, which increases radiation exposure to the patient and surgeon.

CT-based neuronavigation is an attractive alternative. The reference clamp may be placed percutaneously or through a small midline opening. As registration based on bony anatomy is impossible, iCT is a critical component in this setting. Percutaneous spinal instrumentation is carried out guided by neuronavigation. In the event of loss of neuronavigational accuracy, the iCT scan and registration process may be repeated. iCT can also confirm the appropriate placement of these implants and, generally, obviates the need for a postoperative CT.

Houten and colleagues[75] reported their results in percutaneous lumbar pedicle screw placement in 42 patients with fluoroscopic guidance and 52 patients with O-arm neuronavigation guidance. In addition to avoiding the use of fluoroscopy, there was a lower rate of pedicle cortical perforation and lower operative time with the use of O-arm neuronavigation. Likewise, Nakashima and colleagues[76] reported higher accuracy of percutaneous pedicle screw placement with CT-based neuronavigation compared to fluoroscopic guidance.

Vertebroplasty

Comparing CT-based neuronavigation and conventional fluoroscopic methods, Kaso and colleagues[77] achieved improved accuracy of needle placement with a reduction in the frequency of cement leakage with neuronavigation.

SUMMARY

CT-based neuronavigation is beneficial in brain and spine surgery. Although it does not obviate the need for a sound knowledge of anatomy and careful study of the specific case at hand, it complements the skills of the surgeon and improves the accuracy and safety of surgical procedures.

REFERENCES

1. Rampersaud YR, Foley KT, Shen AC, et al. Radiation exposure to the spine surgeon during fluoroscopically assisted pedicle screw insertion. Spine (Phila Pa 1976). 2000;25(20):2637-45.

2. Foley KT, Simon DA, Rampersaud YR, et al. Virtual fluoroscopy: computer-assisted fluoroscopic navigation. Spine (Phila Pa 1976). 2001;26(4):347-51.

3. Merloz P, Troccaz J, Vouaillat H, et al. Fluoroscopy-based navigation system in spine surgery. Proc Inst Mech Eng H. 2007;221(7):813-20.

4. Carl AL, Khanuja HS, Gatto CA, et al. In vivo pedicle screw placement: image-guided virtual vision. J Spinal Disord. 2000;13(3):225-9.

5. Carl AL, Khanuja HS, Sachs BL, et al. In vitro simulation. Early results of stereotaxy for pedicle screw placement. Spine (Phila Pa 1976). 1997;22(10):1160-4.

6. Glossop ND, Hu RW, Randle JA. Computer-aided pedicle screw placement using frameless stereotaxis. Spine (Phila Pa 1976). 1996;21(17):2026-34.

7. Kalfas IH, Kormos DW, Murphy MA, et al. Application of frameless stereotaxy to pedicle screw fixation of the spine. J Neurosurg. 1995;83(4):641-7.

8. Murphy MA, McKenzie RL, Kormos DW, et al. Frameless stereotaxis for the insertion of lumbar pedicle screws. J Clin Neurosci. 1994;1(4):257-60.

9. Steinmeier R, Rachinger J, Kaus M, et al. Factors influencing the application accuracy of neuronavigation systems. Stereotact Funct Neurosurg. 2000;75(4):188-202.

10. Mitsui T, Fujii M, Tsuzaka M, et al. Skin shift and its effect on navigation accuracy in image-guided neurosurgery. Radiol Phys Technol. 2011;4(1):37-42.

11. Lunsford LD, Parrish R, Albright L. Intraoperative imaging with a therapeutic computed tomographic scanner. Neurosurgery. 1984;15(4):559-61.

12. Shalit MN, Israeli Y, Matz S, et al. Intra-operative computerized axial tomography. Surg Neurol. 1979;11(5):382-4.

13. Shalit MN, Israeli Y, Matz S, et al. Experience with intraoperative CT scanning in brain tumors. Surg Neurol. 1982;17(5):376-82.

14. Black PM, Alexander E, Martin C, et al. Craniotomy for tumor treatment in an intraoperative magnetic resonance imaging unit. Neurosurgery. 1999;45(3):423-33.

15. Black PM, Moriarty T, Alexander E, et al. Development and implementation of intraoperative magnetic resonance imaging and its neurosurgical applications. Neurosurgery. 1997;41(4):831-45.

16. Knauth M, Wirtz CR, Tronnier VM, et al. Intraoperative MR imaging increases the extent of tumor resection in patients with high-grade gliomas. AJNR Am J Neuroradiol. 1999;20(9):1642-6.

17. Lunsford LD, Latchaw RE, Vries JK. Stereotactic implantation of deep brain electrodes using computed tomography. Neurosurgery. 1983;13(3):280-6.

18. Patil A, Kumar P, Leibrock L, et al. The value of intraoperative scans during CT-guided stereotactic procedures. Neuroradiology. 1992;34(5):453-6.

19. Grunert P, Müller-Forell W, Darabi K, et al. Basic principles and clinical applications of neuronavigation and intraoperative computed tomography. Comput Aided Surg. 1998;3(4):166-73.

20. Eggers G, Kress B, Mühling J. Automated registration of intraoperative CT image data for navigated skull base surgery. Minim Invasive Neurosurg. 2008;51(1):15-20.

21. Eboli P, Shafa B, Mayberg M. Intraoperative computed tomography registration and electromagnetic neuronavigation for transsphenoidal pituitary surgery: accuracy and time effectiveness. J Neurosurg. 2011;114(2):329-35.

22. Nabavi A, Black PM, Gering DT, et al. Serial intraoperative magnetic resonance imaging of brain shift. Neurosurgery. 2001;48(4):787-97.

23. Matula C, Rössler K, Reddy M, et al. Intraoperative computed tomography guided neuronavigation: concepts, efficiency, and work flow. Comput Aided Surg. 1998;3(4):174-82.

24. Broggi G, Ferroli P, Franzini A, et al. CT-guided neurosurgery: preliminary experience. Acta Neurochir Suppl. 2003;85:101-4.

25. Fiegele T, Feuchtner G, Sohm F, et al. Accuracy of stereotactic electrode placement in deep brain stimulation by intraoperative computed tomography. Parkinsonism Relat Disord. 2008;14(8):595-9.

26. Haberland N, Ebmeier K, Grunewald JP, et al. Incorporation of intraoperative computerized tomography in a newly developed spinal navigation technique. Comput Aided Surg. 2000;5(1):18-27.

27. Costa F, Cardia A, Ortolina A, et al. Spinal navigation: standard preoperative versus intraoperative computed tomography data set acquisition for computer-guidance system: radiological and clinical study in 100 consecutive patients. Spine (Phila Pa 1976). 2011;36(24):2094-8.

28. Dinesh SK, Tiruchelvarayan R, Ng I. A prospective study on the use of intraoperative computed tomography (iCT) for image-guided placement of thoracic pedicle screws. Br J Neurosurg. 2012;26(6):838-44.

29. Hecht AC, Koehler SM, Laudone JC, et al. Is Intraoperative CT of posterior cervical spine instrumentation cost-effective and does it reduce complications? Clin Orthop Relat Res. 2011;469(4):1035-41.

30. Hum B, Feigenbaum F, Cleary K, et al. Intraoperative computed tomography for complex craniocervical operations and spinal tumor resections. Neurosurgery. 2000;47(2):374-81.

31. Steudel WI, Nabhan A, Shariat K. Intraoperative CT in spine surgery. Acta Neurochir Suppl. 2011;109:169-74.

32. Tormenti MJ, Kostov DB, Gardner PA, et al. Intraoperative computed tomography image-guided navigation for posterior thoracolumbar spinal instrumentation in spinal deformity surgery. Neurosurg Focus. 2010;28(3):E11.

33. Zausinger S, Scheder B, Uhl E, et al. Intraoperative computed tomography with integrated navigation system in spinal stabilizations. Spine (Phila Pa 1976). 2009;34(26):2919-26.

34. Freidberg SR, Pfeifer BA, Dempsey PK, et al. Intraoperative computerized tomography scanning to assess the adequacy of decompression in anterior cervical spine surgery. J Neurosurg. 2001;94(1 Suppl):8-11.

35. Fritz HG, Kuehn D, Haberland N, et al. Anesthesia management for spine surgery using spinal navigation in combination with computed tomography. Anesth Analg. 2003;97(3):863-6.

36. Uhl E, Zausinger S, Morhard D, et al. Intraoperative computed tomography with integrated navigation system in a multidisciplinary operating suite. Neurosurgery. 2009;64(5 Suppl 2):231-9.

37. Barlas O, Karadereler S, Bahar S, et al. Image-guided keyhole evacuation of spontaneous supratentorial intracerebral hemorrhage. Minimally invasive neurosurgery. Minim Invasive Neurosurg. 2009;52(2):62-8.

38. Vespa P, McArthur D, Miller C, et al. Frameless stereotactic aspiration and thrombolysis of deep intracerebral hemorrhage is associated with reduction of hemorrhage volume and neurological improvement. Neurocrit care. 2005;2:274-281.

39. Reig AS, Stevenson CB, Tulipan NB. CT-based, fiducial-free frameless stereotaxy for difficult ventriculoperitoneal shunt insertion: experience in 26 consecutive patients. Stereotact Funct Neurosurg. 2010;88(2):75-80.

40. Hermann EJ, Capelle HH, Tschan CA, et al. Electromagnetic-guided neuronavigation for safe placement of intraventricular catheters in pediatric neurosurgery. J Neurosurg Pediatr. 2012;10(4):327-33.

41. Hayhurst C, Beems T, Jenkinson MD, et al. Effect of electromagnetic-navigated shunt placement on failure rates: a prospective multicenter study. J Neurosurg. 2010;113(6): 1273-8.

42. Takahashi M, Yamada R, Tabei Y, et al. Navigation-guided Ommaya reservoir placement: implications for the treatment of leptomeningeal metastases. Minim Invasive Neurosurg. 2007;50(6):340-5.

43. Nemec SF, Donat MA, Mehrain S, et al. CT-MR image data fusion for computer assisted navigated neurosurgery of temporal bone tumors. Eur J Radiol. 2007;62(2):192-8.

44. Sure U, Alberti O, Petermeyer M, et al. Advanced image-guided skull base surgery. Surg Neurol. 2000;53(6):563-72.

45. Kurtsoy A, Menku A, Tucer B, et al. Neuronavigation in skull base tumors. Minim Invasive Neurosurg. 2005;48(1):7-12.

46. Nakamura M, Stöver T, Rodt T, et al. Neuronavigational guidance in craniofacial approaches for large (para)nasal tumors involving the anterior skull base and upper clival lesions. Eur J Surg Oncol. 2009;35(6):666-72.

47. Rohde V, Hans FJ, Mayfrank L, et al. How useful is the 3-dimensional, surgeon's perspective-adjusted visualisation of the vessel anatomy during aneurysm surgery? A prospective clinical trial. Neurosurg Rev. 2007;30(3):209-16.

48. Kim TS, Joo SP, Lee JK, et al. Neuronavigation-assisted surgery for distal anterior cerebral artery aneurysm. Minim Invasive Neurosurg. 2007;50(3):140-4.

49. Paleologos TS, Wadley JP, Kitchen ND, et al. Clinical utility and cost-effectiveness of interactive image-guided craniotomy: clinical comparison between conventional and image-guided meningioma surgery. Neurosurgery. 2000;47(1):40-7; discussion 47-8.

50. Coppens JR, Cantando JD, Abdulrauf SI. Minimally invasive superficial temporal artery to middle cerebral artery bypass through an enlarged bur hole: the use of computed tomography angiography neuronavigation in surgical planning. J Neurosurg. 2008;109(3):553-8.

51. Schmid-Elsaesser R, Muacevic A, Holtmannspötter M, et al. Neuronavigation based on CT angiography for surgery of intracranial aneurysms: primary experience with unruptured aneurysms. Minim Invasive Neurosurg. 2003;46(5):269-77.

52. Gharabaghi A, Krischek B, Feigl GC, et al. Image-guided craniotomy for frontal sinus preservation during meningioma surgery. Eur J Surg Oncol. 2008;34(8):928-31.

53. Boos N, Webb JK. Pedicle screw fixation in spinal disorders: a European view. Eur Spine J. 1997;6(1):2-18.

54. Rampersaud YR, Simon DA, Foley KT. Accuracy requirements for image-guided spinal pedicle screw placement. Spine (Phila Pa 1976). 2001;26(4):352-9.

55. Shin BJ, James AR, Njoku IU, Härtl R.Pedicle screw navigation: a systematic review and meta-analysis of perforation risk for computer-navigated versus freehand insertion. J Neurosurg Spine. 2012;17(2):113-22.

56. Kosmopoulos V, Schizas C. Pedicle screw placement accuracy: a meta-analysis. Spine (Phila Pa 1976). 2007;32(3):E111-20.

57. Abumi K, Ito M, Sudo H. Reconstruction of the subaxial cervical spine using pedicle screw instrumentation. Spine (Phila Pa 1976). 2012;37(5): E349-56.

58. Ito H, Neo M, Yoshida M, et al. Efficacy of computer-assisted pedicle screw insertion for cervical instability in RA patients. Rheumatology International. 2007;27(6):567-74.

59. Allam Y, Silbermann J, Riese F, et al. Computer tomography assessment of pedicle screw placement in thoracic spine: comparison between free hand and a generic 3D-based navigation techniques. Eur Spine J. 2013;22(3):648-53.

60. Rajasekaran S, Vidyadhara S, Ramesh P, et al. Randomized clinical study to compare the accuracy of navigated and non-navigated thoracic pedicle screws in deformity correction surgeries. Spine (Phila Pa 1976). 2007;32(2):E56-64.

61. Silbermann J, Riese F, Allam Y, et al. Computer tomography assessment of pedicle screw placement in lumbar and sacral spine: comparison between free-hand and O-arm based navigation techniques. Eur Spine J. 2011;20(6):875-81.

62. Thorat JD, Rajendra T, Thirugnanam A, et al. Single-stage posterior midline approach for dumbbell tumors of the thoracic spine, with intraoperative CT guidance. Surg Neurol Int. 2011;2:31.

63. Rajasekaran S, Kamath V, Shetty AP. Intraoperative Iso-C three-dimensional navigation in excision of spinal osteoid osteomas. Spine (Phila Pa 1976). 2008;33(1):E25-9.

64. Schouten R, Lee R, Boyd M, et al. Intra-operative cone-beam CT (O-arm) and stereotactic navigation in acute spinal trauma surgery. J Clin Neurosci. 2012;19(8):1137-43.

65. Wang HC, Yang YL, Lin WC, et al. Computer-assisted pedicle screw placement for thoracolumbar spine fracture with separate spinal reference clamp placement and registration. Surgical Neurology. 2008;69(6):597-601.

66. Rajasekaran S, Tubaki VR, Shetty AP. Results of direct repair of type 2 hangman fracture using Iso-C3D navigation: 20 cases. J Spinal Disord Tech. 2012;25(5):E134-9.

67. Yoshida M, Neo M, Fujibayashi S, et al. Comparison of the anatomical risk for vertebral artery injury associated with the C2-pedicle screw and atlantoaxial transarticular screw. Spine (Phila Pa 1976). 2006;31(15):E513-7.

68. Acosta FL, Quinones-Hinojosa A, Gadkary CA, et al. Frameless stereotactic image-guided C1-C2 transarticular screw fixation for atlantoaxial instability: review of 20 patients. J spin disord tech. 2005;18(5):385-91.

69. Uehara M, Takahashi J, Hirabayashi H, et al. Computer-assisted C1-C2 Transarticular Screw Fixation "Magerl Technique" for Atlantoaxial Instability. Asian Spine J. 2012;6(3): 168-77.

70. Gluf WM, Schmidt MH, Apfelbaum RI. Atlantoaxial trans-articular screw fixation: a review of surgical indications, fusion rate, complications, and lessons learned in 191 adult patients. J Neurosurg Spine. 2005;2(2):155-63.

71. Yang YL, Liang Y, Sheng ZD, et al. Comparison of isocentric C-arm 3-dimensional navigation and conventional fluoroscopy for C1 lateral mass and C2 pedicle screw placement for atlantoaxial instability. J Spinal Disord Techs. 2013;26(3):127-34.

72. Martirosyan NL, Kalb S, Cavalcanti DD, et al. Comparative analysis of isocentric 3-dimensional C-arm fluoroscopy and biplanar fluoroscopy for anterior screw fixation in odontoid fractures. J Spinal Disord Tech. 2013;26(4):189-93.

73. Ling JM, Tiruchelvarayan R, Seow WT, et al. Surgical treatment of adult and pediatric C1/C2 subluxation with intraoperative computed tomography guidance. Surg Neurol Int. 2013;4(Suppl 2):S109-17.

74. Gempt J, Lehmberg J, Grams AE, et al. Endoscopic transnasal resection of the odontoid:case series and clinical course. Eur Spine J. 2011;20(4):661-6.

75. Houten JK, Nasser R, Baxi N. Clinical assessment of percutaneous lumbar pedicle screw placement using the O-arm multidimensional surgical imaging system. Neurosurg. 2012;70(4):990-5.

76. Nakashima H, Sato K, Ando T, et al. Comparison of the percutaneous screw placement precision of isocentric C-arm 3-dimensional fluoroscopy-navigated pedicle screw implantation and conventional fluoroscopy method with minimally invasive surgery. J Spinal Disord Tech. 2009;22(7):468-72.

77. Kasó G, Horváth Z, Szenohradszky K, et al. Comparison of CT characteristics of extravertebral cement leakages after vertebroplasty performed by different navigation and injection techniques. Acta Neurochir (Wien). 2008;150(7):677-83.

10

Intraoperative Ultrasound

Gavin Quigley

INTRODUCTION

Neurosurgery remains a highly technology-dependent specialty with numerous advances over the years. Imaging technology, in particular has dramatically changed since the pioneering days of the discipline. Yet, no one imaging modality is all encompassing enough to replace the others. Intraoperative ultrasound has remained a vital part of this multimodality approach to intraoperative imaging.

Whilst it is beyond the scope of this chapter to describe the physics of ultrasonography, the reader is directed any of the standard reference texts on the subject.[1] The basic premise is that a piezoelectric crystal converts electrical energy into high frequency sound waves (typically in the range of 2–20 MHz). The subsequent reflections are received by the crystal and converted back into a black and white display, so called B (Brightness) mode imaging. This is the most commonly used imaging mode. Doppler imaging is also used and provides information about blood flow. In simple terms, the Doppler mode examines the characteristics of direction and speed of tissue motion and blood flow, and presents it in audible or color displays. Color Doppler ultrasound is also known as color-flow ultrasound. It can show blood flow in a selected two-dimensional (2D) area. Direction and velocity of tissue motion and blood flow are color coded and superimposed on the corresponding B-mode image. Power Doppler does not demonstrate velocity or direction of flow but can show blood flow even in very low flow states.

Few neurosurgeons appreciate that ultrasound's first diagnostic use was in neurological disease.[2,3] Unfortunately Dussik's method was later shown to ineffective and the images were in fact due to a reflection artifact.[4] There was considerable initial interest in ultrasound of the brain and French et al. published a report demonstrating the safety and efficacy of A mode scanning.[5]

Despite these early reports few neurosurgeons persisted with ultrasound with the exception of a few centers. Professor Kenji Tanaka and colleagues published 5 papers in the 1950s describing their experience of diagnostic ultrasound use in brain disorders in Japan.[6] For those wishing to learn more about the history of ultrasound are directed to Dr Joseph Woo's excellent work at *www.ob-ultrasound.net*. Publications describing ultrasound use in the brain are few and far between from 1950 until the early 1980s. This contrasts sharply with obstetrics and gynecology, which experienced a massive rise in publications with widespread adoption of the technology. This limited uptake of ultrasound is perhaps unsurprisingly given the developments in computed tomography (CT) and the magnetic resonance (MR) scanning. The development of the microchip permitted these highly computer-dependent modalities to flourish.

However, this technological progress made real-time ultrasound imaging possible by the late 1970s. The machinery and probes remained large and cumbersome for practical intraoperative use. The first true intraoperative uses of ultrasound in neurosurgery are described in the early 1980s.[3,7-9] This resurgence of interest in intraoperative ultrasound was limited by poor signal to noise ratio and subsequent disappointing image quality. The last two decades have witnessed considerable improvements in ultrasound image quality and publication numbers have risen markedly.

The primary focus of intraoperative imaging in neurosurgery has been to guide and judge resection in tumor removal and this remains the case. Increasing scientific evidence has suggested gross total resection as the aim of surgery in low-grade, high-grade, and recurrent gliomas.[10-13] Numerous strategies have been recommended over the years to maximize resection including intraoperative CT or MR, awake surgery, neuronavigation, and 5-aminolevulinic acid. Intraoperative ultrasound must be considered as part of the surgeons' armamentarium to be used in combination with these existing modalities. Several studies have confirmed the utility of ultrasound in this regard and the authors conclude that the real-time nature of the imaging and the lack of ionizing radiation are major benefits.[14,15] Clearly, other procedures such as ventricular cannulation, syrinx drainage, and hematoma evacuation can be performed with ultrasound assistance.[3,7] Ultrasound remains a safe, portable, and low-cost addition to any neurosurgical operating theater. Practice, patience, and a standard procedure for use are crucial to obtaining maximal benefit from intraoperative ultrasound.

CLINICAL USE

The brain and spinal cord are ideal mediums for ultrasound examination since they are primarily water. However, basic ultrasound principles must be adhered to obtain good quality images.

The bone opening must be large enough to accommodate the array; the bone edges should be free of the probe otherwise poor acoustic contact will result in suboptimal images. If safe, consider enlarging burr holes with a punch to allow the array to sit comfortably within the bone opening.

Good acoustic contact requires the use of a sterile ultrasound gel or saline between the transducer and brain or dura. This can be achieved by a number of methods; the probe can be covered with a sterile sleeve and gel placed inside, gel or saline to fill burr holes and larger cavities should be filled with saline. Selbekk et al. describe a number of methods to improve image quality and the reader is encouraged to read this excellent article.[16]

If available, integration with a navigation system will allow faster and more intuitive orientation. When using ultrasound alone, it is useful to obtain two initial scans prior to dural opening, one coronally-orientated and the other at 90° in either the sagittal or axial plane depending in the position of the lesion (sagittal imaging is easier with lesions closer to the vertex). Ideally, these two images are saved to allow future comparison. The initial scans are used to orientate the operator in combination with the depth. The importance of the depth display cannot be over-emphasized, particularly, where the user is new to ultrasound.

A larger craniotomy probe is recommended, wherever, possible since it has a wider field of view and permits quicker recognition of structures. Smaller burr hole probes are very useful but require practice and experience to gain the most from them.

The display screen should be positioned in the surgeon's eyeline, and be clearly visible without the need to move away from the surgical field. Consider dimming ambient light when scanning.

Doppler is very helpful to identify vessels, particularly in intracerebral hemorrhage; biphasic flow in the center of a hematoma is suggestive of an arteriovenous malformation (AVM). Color Doppler can be combined with standard B mode imaging to outline vascularity around tumors or delineate larger intracranial vessels.

SUGGESTED STEPS PRIOR TO USE

Transducers

Usually, a choice between craniotomy and burr hole transducer **(Figures 10.1 and 10.2)** depends on access and aims of surgical procedure. Most craniotomy probes are of a curved array design. Consider the use of sterilizable probes to give improved image quality; otherwise a sterile cover is required.

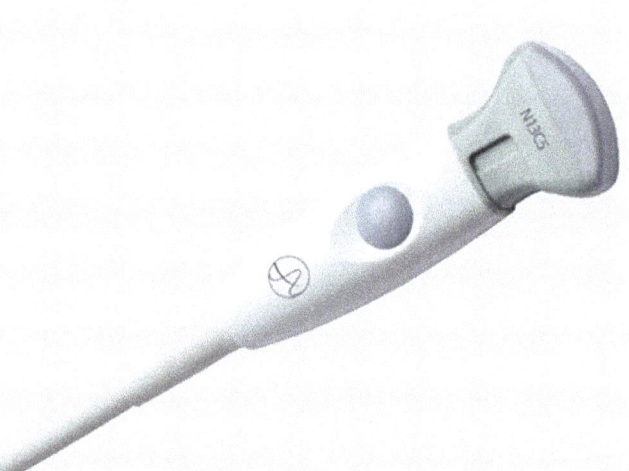

Figure 10.1 Craniotomy probe

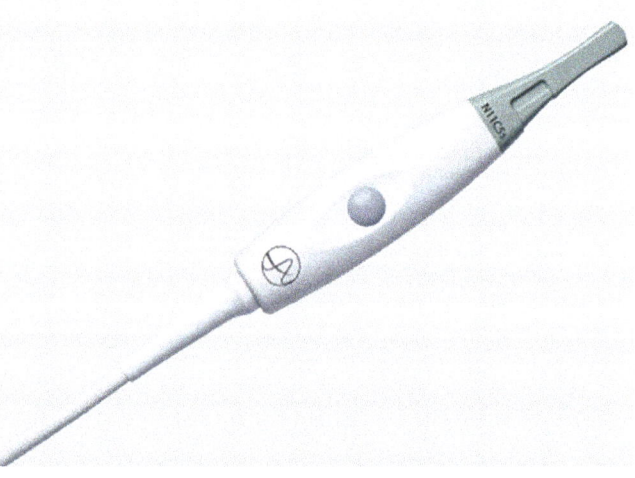

Figure 10.2 Burr hole transducer

Patient

- Patient ID entered so images can be saved allowing serial comparison.
- Position is vital for good acoustic contact.

Orientation

Identify left side of *probe*. If necessary, gently tap probe on one side to confirm.

Frequency

Check with manufacturer 5–8 MHz typically for most cranial lesions. Obviously, increasing frequency will reduce depth penetration. It might be appropriate to increase frequency, if trying to demonstrate a superficial lesion or pathology just the skin under skin, such as shunt tubing (consider linear probe).

Depth

- Depth is extremely important; the scale must be clearly displayed.
- The majority of cranial pathology is no deeper than 6 cm; in spinal cases this may be considerably less.

Gain

- Excessive gain will decrease resolution.
- Ideally, the gain should be increased to maximum, and then reduced to as low a level as possible.

Focus

Each transducer has a specific focal zone and this should be adjusted to correspond to pathology, seek manufacturer's advice.

Difficulties

Previous surgery and radiotherapy can cause difficulties using ultrasound in the brain or spine. It may not be possible to delineate lesions from the effects of previous surgery and or radiotherapy with ultrasound.[15]

Poor image quality is usually due to inadequate acoustic contact between transducer and neural tissue. Either because of patient position or bony opening that is too small to accommodate the transducer. Both scenarios result in air between the transducer and target tissue.

Loss of orientation occurs either because of poor image quality, transducer movement whilst scanning or oblique rather than standard plane imaging. Combined use with a neuronavigation system reduces these difficulties and helps to develop experience faster **(Figure 10.3)**.

IMAGE-GUIDANCE INTEGRATION

As ultrasound technology improved in the 1990s, neuronavigation systems become increasingly commonplace. These allowed the surgeon to navigate intraoperatively based on preoperative CT or MR scans without the need for a stereotactic frame. Early attempts at combining this technology with ultrasound, were still somewhat cumbersome.[17]

A group from Trondheim developed the first navigation system with an integrated ultrasound scanner.[18] The system appealed to many surgeons and soon had a number of centers using the technology. The SonoWand produced excellent ultrasound images and crucially seamlessly produced three-dimensional (3D) ultrasound volumes, which were used for intraoperative navigation. In particular, the brain shift was easily apparent and the team described several methods to improve image quality.[19,20] Sadly despite a number of centers worldwide investing in the SonoWand system the company ceased trading in 2015.

Navigation systems have continued to progress and optical tracking became the dominant technology. Most modern neuronavigation systems still use this method, manufactures such as Brainlab, Medtronic, and Stryker account for the majority of systems in use today. Brainlab and Medtronic systems both have the facility to connect real-time tracked ultrasound probes. Brainlab connects to a large number of vendors ultrasound systems. At present, the combination Brainlab navigation and BK Medical Flex Focus ultrasound represents the most advanced commercially

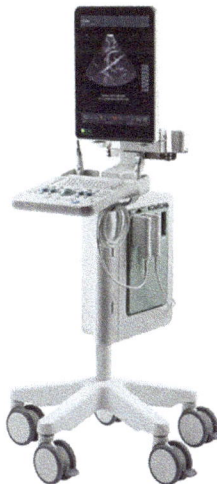

Figure 10.3 Modern portable intraoperative ultrasound system

available solution. This combination allows tracking of the ultrasound probe and automatic depth changes via a digital connection. Both 2D overlay ultrasound and 3D ultrasound volumes can be fused to preoperative CT or MR or diffusion tensor imaging (DTi) or functional MRI images. Automated object shift correction to compensate for brain shift is a particularly useful feature (**Figures 10.4 and 10.5**).

VENTRICULAR CANNULATION WITH BURR HOLE PROBE

Dependent on the size of the burr hole created, it may be useful to enlarge the opening as shown to accommodate the cannula and probe.

The depth scale is vital since the ventricular wall is most often seen 3–4.5 cm from the cortical surface, i.e. the probe tip. The angle of insonation should be 90° between probe and cortex or dura.

Occasionally, a reverberation artifact is seen caused by the highly reflective falx and the probe tip. This can give the appearance of second much deeper falx. Depth orientation will allow the user to identify this potential error (**Figure 10.6**).

ULTRASOUND FEATURES OF INTRACRANIAL STRUCTURES

The ultrasound features of intracranial structures have been described in **Table 10.1**.

High-grade Glioma

Ultrasound characteristics are of a *heterogeneous lesion with a hyperechoic* margin and hypoechoic portions (related to necrotic areas within the tumor). Surrounding edema is *hyperechoic*, clinical judgment is required to estimate its extent (**Figures 10.7 to 10.13**).

Meningioma

The meningioma has been shown in **Figure 10.14**.

Metastasis

Metastasis has been shown in **Figures 10.15 and 10.16**.

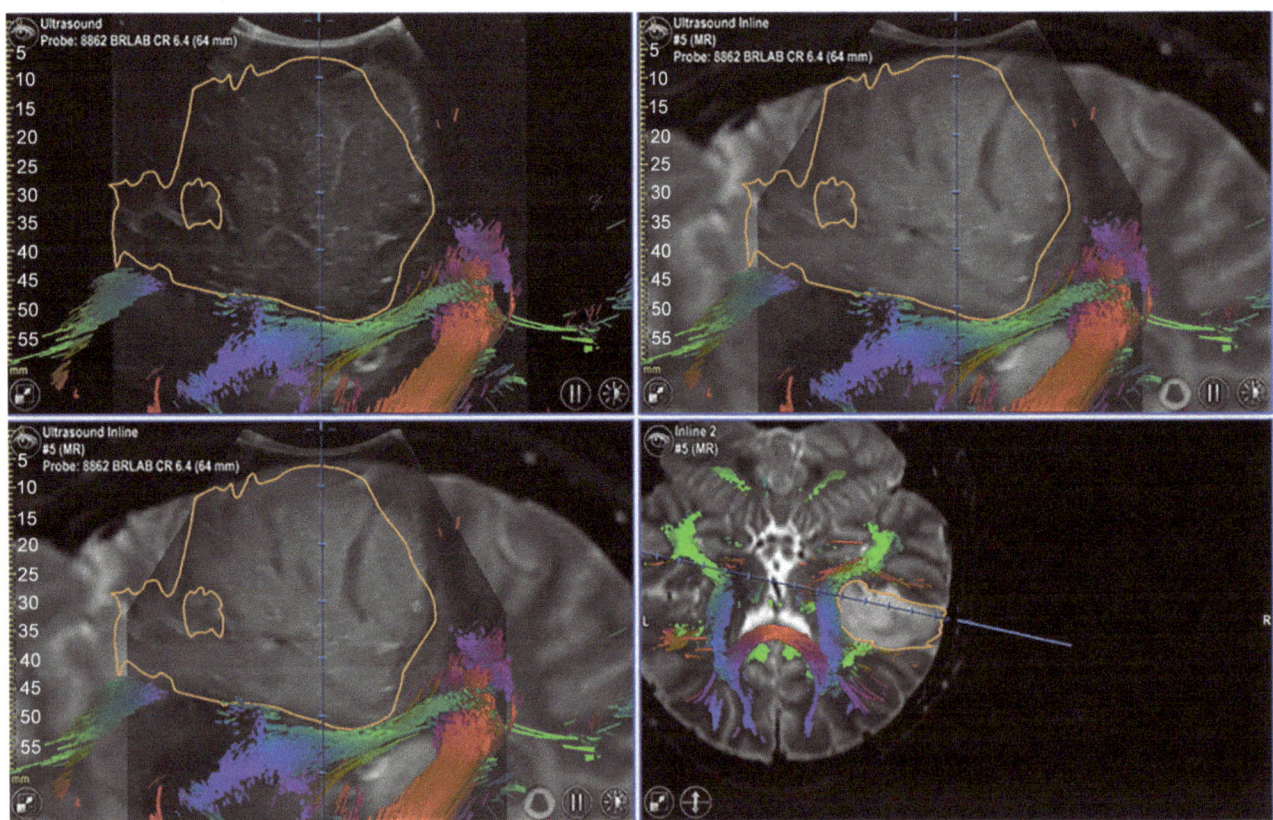

Figure 10.4 Two-dimensional ultrasound overlaid on preoperative magnetic resonance and diffusion tensor images. Minor brain shift is apparent early in the procedure

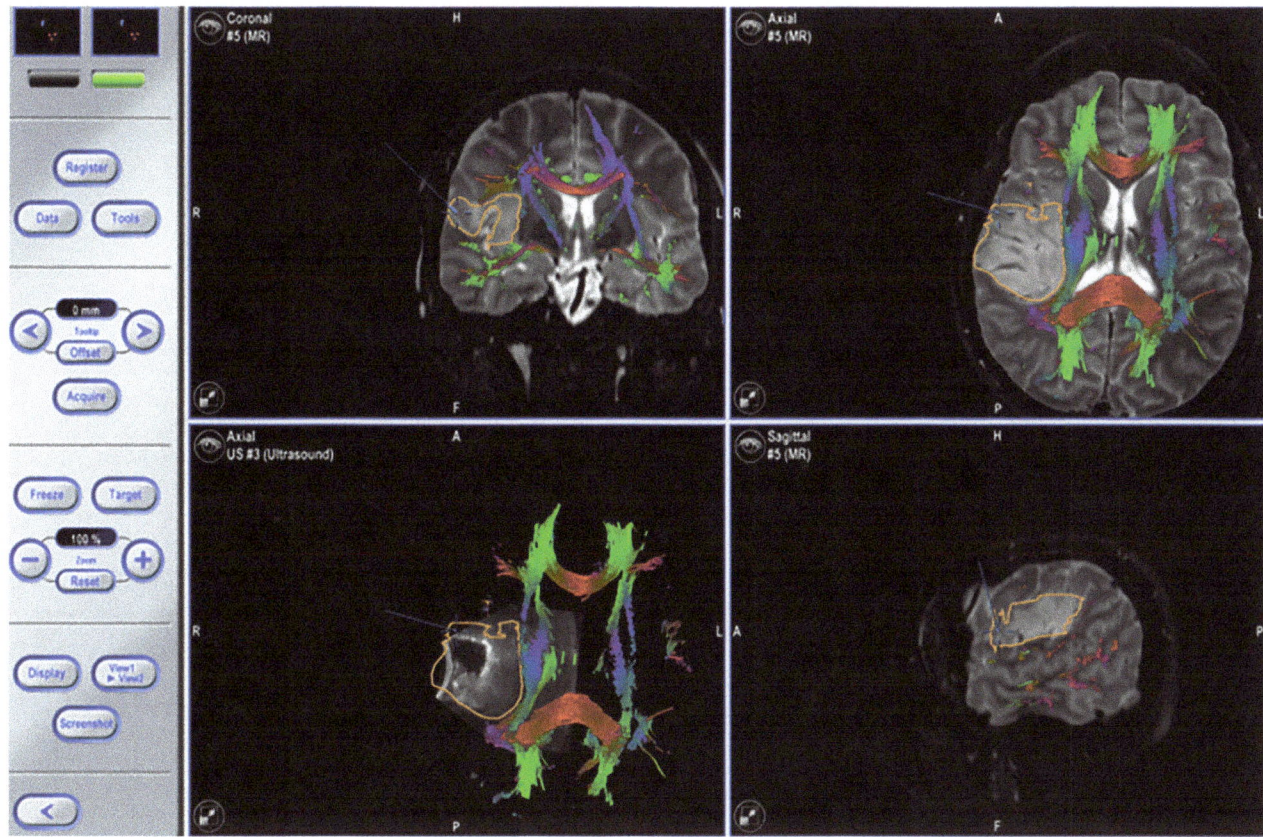

Figure 10.5 Images during resection shows a three-dimensional ultrasound volume being used for navigation

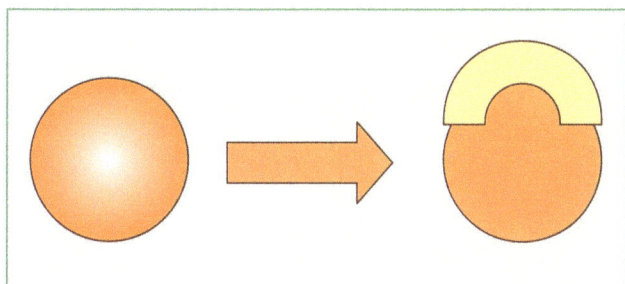

Figure 10.6 Often slight enlargement of the burr hole with a punch allows easier passage of cannulas or needles

Table 10.1 Ultrasound characteristics of intracranial structure

Structure	Ultrasound Characteristics
Gray mater	Isoechoic to hypoechoic, homogeneous
White mater	Isoechoic and homogeneous
Sulci	Hyperechoic and heterogeneous
Ventricle	Hypoechoic and homogeneous
Brainstem	Hypoechoic and homogeneous
Choroid plexus	Hyperechoic and heterogeneous

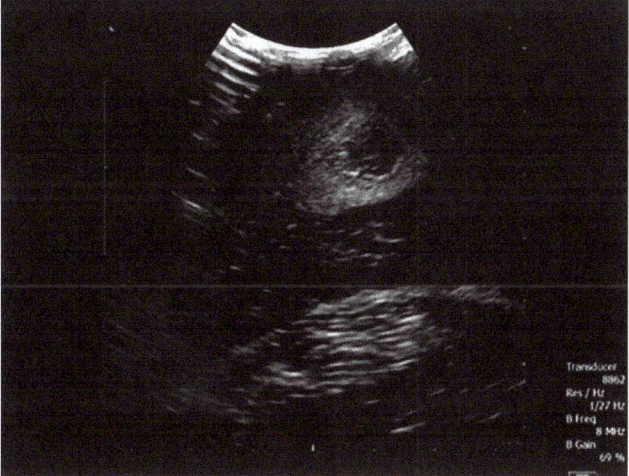

Figure 10.7 Typical appearance of a high-grade glioma with very cellular (hyperechoic) rim. The center is necrotic and hypoechoic

Patient Position is Crucial

For optimal imaging, the patient should be positioned as demonstrated in **Figures 10.17A and B.**

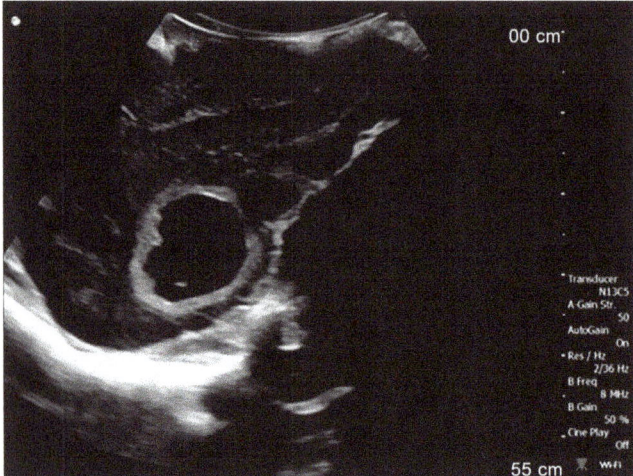

Figure 10.8 High-grade glioma

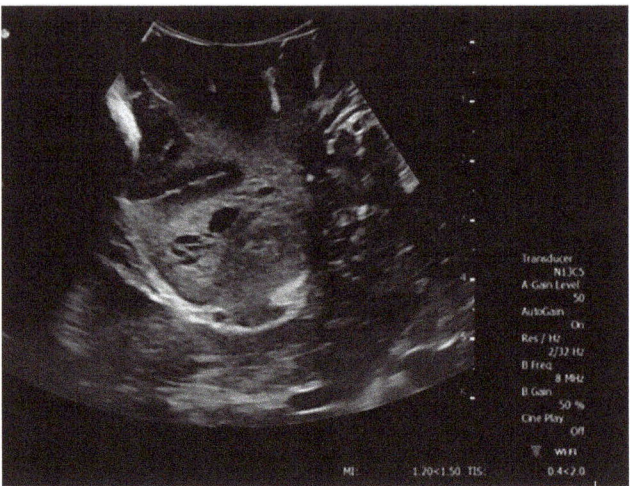

Figure 10.11 Low-grade glioma of temporal lobe, pathologically oligodendroglioma grade 2

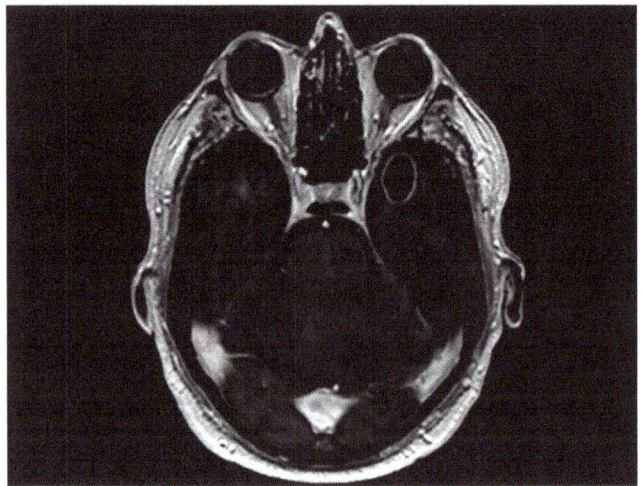

Figure 10.9 Magnetic resonance image of Figure 10.8 (High-grade glioma)

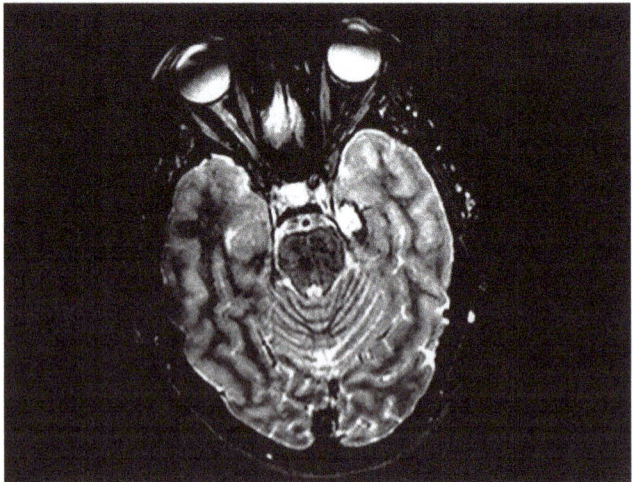

Figure 10.12 Magnetic resonance image of cavernous malformation

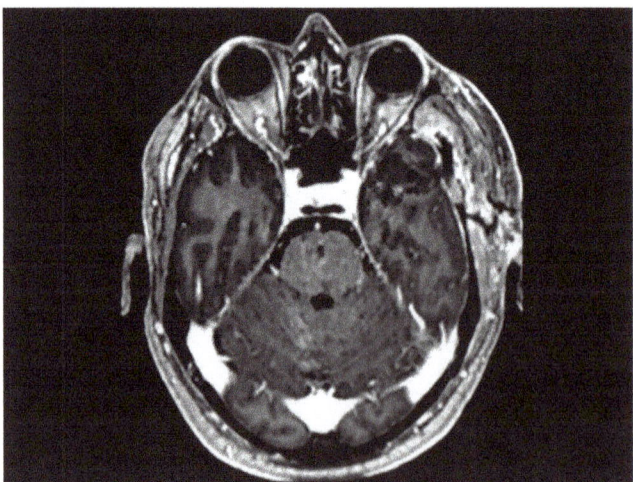

Figure 10.10 Postoperative magnetic resonance image of Figure 10.9 (High-grade glioma)

CONCLUSION

The author's own experience is typical of many neurosurgeons, starting with borrowed anesthetic machinery to assist in tumor resection. Interest in the technology grew until, we were fortunate enough to purchase a modern intraoperative ultrasound specifically for our operating department. The workflow varies from surgeon to surgeon but all follow the basic steps outlined previously.

The author encourages all interested readers to try to incorporate ultrasound into their operative practice. Portable ultrasound systems are now ubiquitous in many operating departments worldwide and can be used to gain experience before making the jump to a dedicated neurosurgical system.[21] Good practice is to carefully image before dural opening and save images for future comparison. As discussed previously, image guidance can speed the learning curve and reassure surgeons unfamiliar with ultrasound imaging.

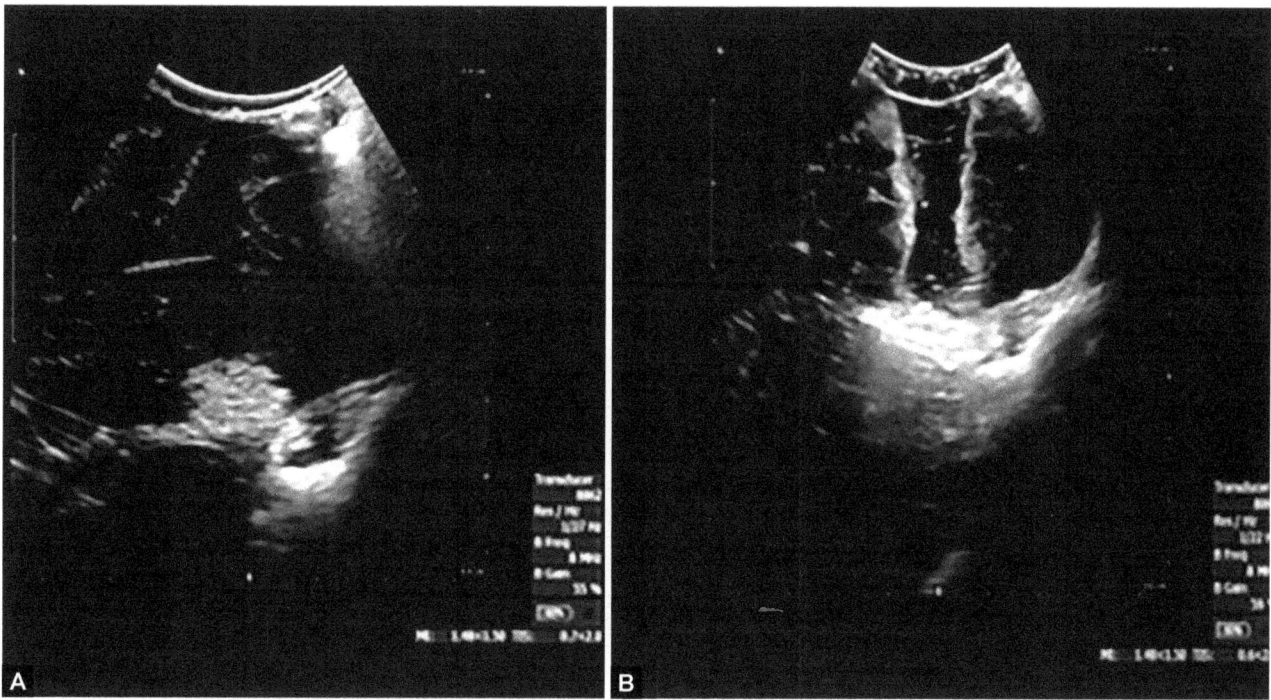

Figures 10.13A and B (A) Two-dimensional ultrasound image of the cavernoma shown in Figure 10.12; (B) Demonstrates the use of ultrasound to confirm approach to the lesion. Note the increased brightness at the base of the resection cavity due to changes in attenuation as a result of dissection

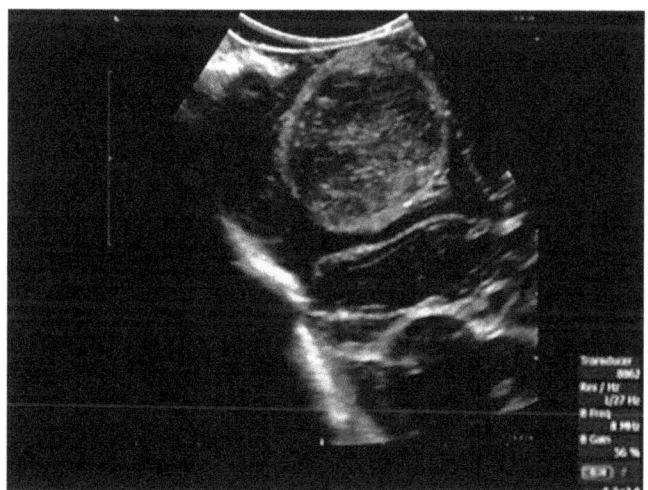

Figure 10.14 Usually well-defined with a homogeneous hyperechoic appearance. Often with a cleft of cerebrospinal fluid between mass and surrounding brain. Occasional flecks of calcification as in this example are seen. Some meningiomas are heavily calcified

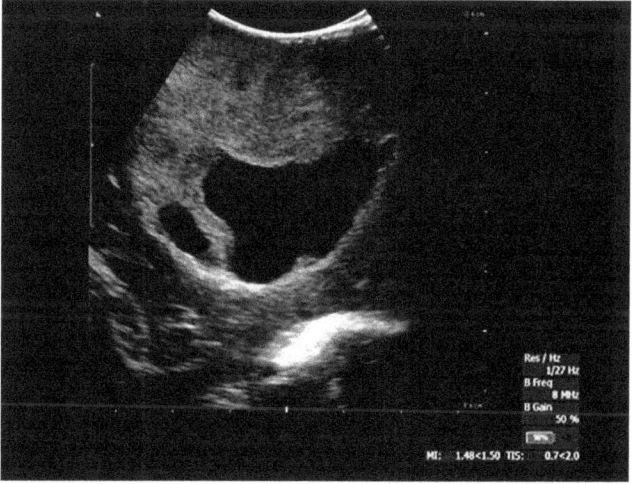

Figure 10.15 Variable appearances, usually hyperechoic with a heterogeneous appearance. This example of a lung cancer metastasis shows hyperechoic tissue with a large cyst. There is a well-defined edge to the lesion

Encouragingly many units are developing intraoperative ultrasound technology and research is ongoing. Intravenous contrast media is available and beginning to find its place in neurosurgery, further studies are clearly required.[22]

Intraoperative ultrasound deserves its place in the modern neurosurgical operating theater; recent years have seen improvements in image quality, probe design, portability, and display resolution. The major attractions of

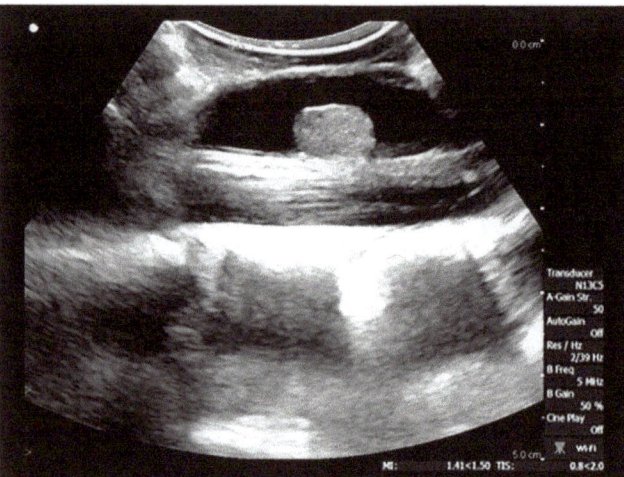

Figure 10.16 Sagittal image shows an intradural neurofibroma at the region of the conus

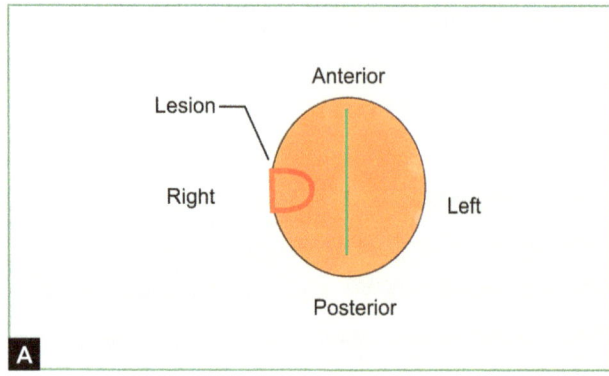

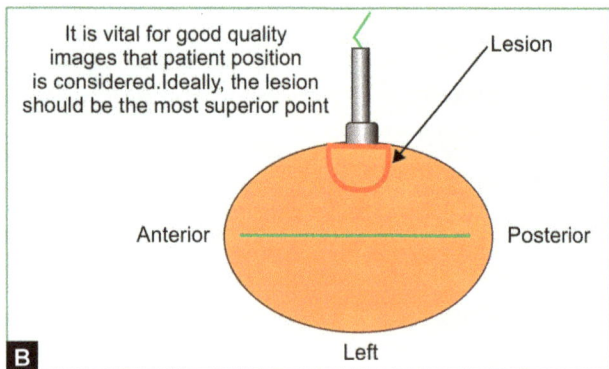

Figures 10.17A and B If possible the patient should be positioned as demonstrated for optimal imaging. This may not always be possible

ultrasound remain unchanged; real-time images, low cost, and ease of use. Challenges persist, particularly in relation to image interpretation during or after surgical procedures on neural tissue.

REFERENCES

1. McGahan JP, Goldberg BB. Diagnostic ultrasound: a logical approach. Philadelphia: Lippincott-Raven; 1998.
2. Dussik KT, Dussik F, Wyt L. Auf dem Wege zur Hyperphonographie des Gehirnes. Wien Med Wochenschr. 1947; 97:425-9.
3. Knake JE, Chandler WF, McGillicuddy JE, et al. Intraoperative sonography for brain tumor localization and ventricular shunt placement. Am J Roentgenol. 1982;139:733-8.
4. Guttner W, Fiedler G, Patzold J. Über Ultraschallabbildungen am menschlichen Schädel. Acta Acustica united with Acustica. 1952;2:148-56.
5. French L. The experimental application of ultrasonics to the localisation of brain tumours. J Neurosurg. 1951;8:1-6.
6. Tanaka K, Wagai T, Kikuchi Y, et al. Studies on detection of intracranial anatomical pathology by ultrasound. J Acoust Soc Jap. 1952;2.
7. Chandler WF, Knake JE, McGillicuddy JE, et al. Intraoperative use of real-time ultrasonography in neurosurgery. J Neurosurg. 1982;57:157-63.
8. Tsutsumi Y, Andoh Y, Inoue N. Ultrasound-guided biopsy for deep-seated brain tumors. J Neurosurg. 1982;57:164-7.
9. Sjölander U, Lindgren PG, Hugosson R. Ultrasound sector scanning for the localization and biopsy of intracerebral lesions. J Neurosurg. 1983;58:7-10.
10. Sanai N, Polley MY, McDermott MW, et al. An extent of resection threshold for newly diagnosed glioblastomas. J Neurosurg. 2011;115:3-8.
11. Sanai N, Berger MS. Glioma extent of resection and its impact on patient outcome. Neurosurgery. 2008;62:753-64.
12. Duffau H. Long-term outcomes after supratotal resection of diffuse low-grade gliomas: a consecutive series with 11-year follow-up. Acta Neurochir (Wien). 2016;158:51-8.
13. Bloch O, Han SJ, Cha S, et al. Impact of extent of resection for recurrent glioblastoma on overall survival: clinical article. J Neurosurg. 2012;117:1032-8.
14. LeRoux PD, Winter TC, Berger MS, et al. A comparison between preoperative magnetic resonance and intraoperative ultrasound tumor volumes and margins. J Clin Ultrasound. 1994;22:29-36.
15. Hammoud MA, Ligon BL, elSouki R, et al. Use of intraoperative ultrasound for localizing tumors and determining the extent of resection: a comparative study with magnetic resonance imaging. J Neurosurg. 1996;84:737-41.
16. Selbekk T, Jakola AS, Solheim O, et al. Ultrasound imaging in neurosurgery: approaches to minimize surgically induced image artefacts for improved resection control. Acta Neurochir (Wien). 2013;155:973-80.

17. Koivukangas J, Louhisalmi Y, Alakuijala J, et al. Ultrasound-controlled neuronavigator-guided brain surgery. J Neurosurg. 1993;79:36-42.
18. Gronningsaeter A, Kleven A, Ommedal S, et al. SonoWand, an ultrasound-based neuronavigation system. Neurosurgery. 2000;47:1373-9.
19. Unsgaard G, Ommedal S, Muller T, et al. Neuronavigation by intraoperative three-dimensional ultrasound: initial experience during brain tumor resection. Neurosurgery. 2002;50:804-12.
20. Unsgaard G, Gronningsaeter A, Ommedal S, et al. Brain operations guided by real-time two-dimensional ultrasound: new possibilities as a result of improved image quality. Neurosurgery. 2002;51:402-11.
21. Solanki SP, White BD. The anaesthetist's SonoSite Probe - Successful adjunct to complex intradural spinal surgery or poor man's intraoperative ultrasound? Br J Neurosurg. 2016;30:464-6.
22. Prada F, Perin A, Martegani A, et al. Intraoperative contrast-enhanced ultrasound for brain tumor surgery. Neurosurgery. 2014;74:542-52.

11

ALA Dye in High-grade Gliomas

Gord Von Campe

INTRODUCTION

Gliomas represent a heterogeneous group of malignant primary brain or spinal cord tumors of neuroepithelial origin arising from glial cells, mainly of astrocytic and oligodendrocytic lineage. They account for about 28% of all central nervous system (CNS) tumors and 80% of all malignant CNS neoplasms. High-grade gliomas, defined as World Health Organization (WHO) histological grades III and IV, have an average annual age-adjusted incidence for all ages of about 5.8/100,000 with a slight male predominance.[1] Due to their fast-growing rate, highly infiltrative nature and consequently ill-defined borders, the surgical treatment of these tumors represents a considerable challenge, especially when guided only by conventional white light microscope illumination (under 30% complete resections in several published series).[2-7] This is all the more relevant as there is growing evidence from the literature to support the positive impact of gross total resection (GTR), removal of more than 98% of the visible contrast enhancement on magnetic resonance imaging[8] on progression-free survival (PFS) and overall survival (OS) in malignant gliomas,[9,10] especially when followed by combined radiochemotherapy.[11] Also, recurrences of high-grade gliomas usually occur within approximately 2 cm of the resection margin.[12,13] Since infiltrative glioma tissue is often difficult to recognize, various intraoperative monitoring and visualization techniques, described elsewhere in this book, have been developed to help the neurosurgeon safely maximize the extent of resection of these tumors. The present discussion outlines the use of 5-aminolevulinic acid (5-ALA)-mediated protoporphyrin IX (PpIX) tumor fluorescence in the setting of high-grade glioma surgery.

PRINCIPLES OF FLUORESCENCE

Due to their high sensitivity and selectivity, fluorescent dyes are commonly used to visualize structures and processes in biological tissue. Fluorescence is the phenomenon of light emission after excitation of a molecule via absorption of light energy. Cyclic molecules that are capable of fluorescing are called fluorophores. In their ground state, these molecules are in a relatively low energy stable configuration and do not emit any light.

Fluorescence is a three stage process (Jablonski diagram): (1) excitation—light of sufficient energy is absorbed by the fluorophore which reaches a higher energy state called excited state; (2) non-radiative excited lifetime—the fluorophore is unstable at high energy configurations and therefore, adopts the lowest energy excited state which is semi-stable and lasts for a very short time (10^{-15}–10^{-9} seconds); and (3) emission— the fluorophore rearranges from the semi-stable excited state back to the ground state, releasing the excess energy as emitted light. In most cases, the emitted light is of lower energy and thus, longer wavelength than the absorbed light, meaning that the color of the emitted light is different from the color of the light that has been absorbed.

Although a fluorophore can repeatedly undergo the cyclical fluorescence process and thus, generate a signal multiple times, the structural instability during the excited lifetime makes it susceptible to degradation. High intensity illumination can cause the fluorophore to finally change its structure, preventing any further fluorescence, which is called photobleaching.

Fluorophores absorb and emits light over a range of wavelengths (characteristic fluorescence excitation and emission spectra) with a specific excitation and emission maximum. This "optical fingerprint" can be used to detect or identify specific molecules in biological tissue.

5-AMINOLEVULINIC ACID AND PROTOPORPHYRIN IX

Delta-aminolevulinic acid (δ-ALA or 5-aminolevulinic acid or 5-ALA, $C_5H_9NO_3$, molecular weight: 131.13 g/mol) is the first compound in the intracellular porphyrin biosynthetic pathway, leading to heme in mammals (and other nonphotosynthetic eukaryotes) and chlorophyll in plants. If given exogenously, δ-ALA can be referred to as a prodrug.

In humans, the enzyme ALA synthase catalyzes the mitochondrial synthesis of δ-ALA through the condensation of glycine and succinyl-CoA, also known as the Shemin pathway.[14] In the cell cytosol, two linear molecules of δ-ALA are then combined to give the cyclical compound porphobilinogen. Further intracytoplasmic modifications lead to uroporphyrinogen III and coproporphyrinogen III, which, transported back into the mitochondrion via the adenosine triphosphate (ATP)-binding cassette (ABC) transporter ABCB6, is finally transformed into the main end-product PpIX, among others through the enzyme coproporphyrinogen oxidase (CPOX). The further combination of divalent iron (Fe^{2+}) and PpIX, catalyzed by the enzyme ferrochelatase, leads to the formation of heme.[15]

This biosynthetic pathway is regulated by a negative feedback mechanism through the control of ALA synthase by the concentration of free mitochondrial heme **(Figure 11.1)**. The negative feedback mechanism can be overcome by providing the cells with an excess amount of exogenous 5-ALA (thus, effectively bypassing the ALA synthase step), resulting in intracellular accumulation of fluorescent porphyrins, mainly PpIX.

5-AMINOLEVULINIC ACID: GENERAL APPLICATIONS

Industrial uses of 5-ALA are mainly found in wool growers and land farming. A photodynamic follicle-ablating method with topical application of 5-ALA to permanently reduce or prevent wool growth at selected locations in sheep was filed in Australia (World International Property Organization Number WO 00/71089 A1). Since, 5-ALA is also a key precursor in the chlorophyll biosynthetic pathway, the Japanese company Cosmo Oil developed a process to produce a 5-ALA containing solid fertilizer (European Patent Application Number EP 2 623 486 A1); different preparations of this fertilizer are commercially available under the Pentakeep® and Pentagarden® line of products.

Medical applications are based on the observation that local or systemic application of exogenous 5-ALA induces a strong accumulation of PpIX in epithelial and glandular structures such as epidermis, mucosa, conjunctiva, endometrium, urothelium, liver, kidney, gallbladder, and mammary glands. On the other side, tissue of mesodermal origin (muscle, bone and connective tissue) exhibits only very limited and clinically irrelevant PpIX accumulation under the same conditions. This resulted in a number of publications describing novel methods for *in situ* visualization and/or photodynamic therapy of various skin,[16] oral,[17,18] bladder[19]

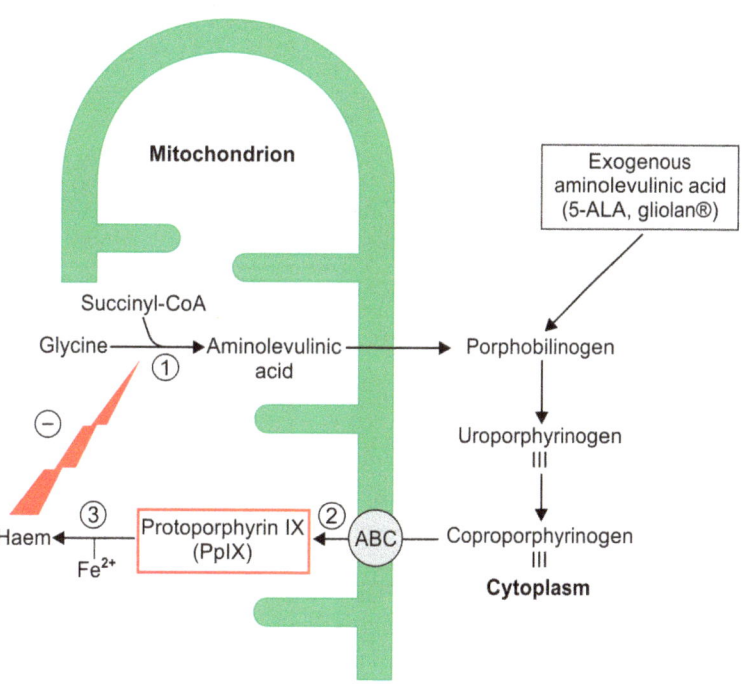

Figure 11.1 Schematic diagram of the haem biosynthetic pathway. Enzymes: (1) ALA synthase, (2) coproporphyrinogen III oxidase (CPOX); (3) ferrochelatase. ABC = ABCB6 transporter, CoA = coenzyme A. Haem concentration regulates the 5-ALA synthase activity through a negative loop-back mechanism. Exogenous 5-ALA can enter the cell by active transport and passive diffusion

and gastrointestinal[20,21] neoplasms. Several factors play a role in the accumulation of PpIX within these tumor cells, like cellular uptake of 5-ALA, increased PpIX synthesis, low availability of iron and/or reduced PpIX conversion into heme.

Glial cells are of neuroepithelial (neuroectodermal) origin and should, therefore, exhibit the same behavior as other epithelial tissue when placed in the presence of excess amounts of 5-ALA. This behavior was confirmed under experimental conditions, showing that neoplastic glial cells do indeed demonstrate a strong intracellular accumulation of fluorescent PpIX after exogenous administration of 5-ALA in C6 cell cultures,[22] C6 spheroids,[23] or 9L/C6 glioma animal models.[22,24,25] These encouraging findings opened the prospect of using 5-ALA-mediated PpIX fluorescence for the intraoperative detection and visualization of high-grade gliomas in humans. A detailed description of the technical principles and its prospective application in 52 glioblastoma patients was first published in 2000 by Stummer et al. effectively demonstrating the usefulness of the method in guiding tumor resection in high-grade gliomas.[10]

Cellular uptake of 5-ALA (via the oligopeptide transporters PEPT1 or PEPT2), increased PpIX synthesis, reduced PpIX conversion into heme and low availability of iron are probably the principal factors influencing the potential amount of PpIX accumulation within a cell. Although still little is known on the exact underlying molecular mechanisms specific to glioma cells, it is considered that one of the main reasons for the pathological intracellular accumulation of PpIX in these tumors is the reduced conversion of PpIX into heme due to a selective down-regulation of the ferrochelatase enzyme expression,[7,26] with consequent loss of the negative feedback mechanism. In addition, Takahashi et al. have shown a correlation between 5-ALA-mediated PpIX fluorescence intensity, up-regulation of the *CPOX* gene and decreased ABCG2 (a cell membrane PpIX transporter to maintain intracellular porphyrin homeostasis) messenger ribonucleic acid (mRNA) levels.[27] Furthermore, Zhao et al. could demonstrate an increase in ABCB6 expression levels in gliomas, proportionate to their histological grade.[28]

5-AMINOLEVULINIC ACID AND PHOTODYNAMIC DETECTION OF HIGH-GRADE GLIOMAS

A large controlled multicenter phase III trial undertaken in Germany demonstrated that 5-ALA-mediated PpIX fluorescence-guided microsurgery enabled more complete resection of the contrast-enhancing tumor and thus improved PFS in patients with high-grade gliomas, when compared to conventional white light microsurgery.[7] Based on these findings, the method was approved by the European Medicines Agency (EMA) in September 2007 for its limited application in neurosurgery, restricted to (radiological) suspected high-grade gliomas (WHO grades III and IV) in adult patients over 18 years of age.

The drug is available as 5-aminolevulinic acid hydrochloride (5-ALA HCl, molecular weight: 167.59 g/mol), which is marketed in Europe and other parts of the world under the brand name Gliolan® (Medac GmbH, Wedel, Germany). Lyophilized 5-ALA HCl presents as a white, odorless, readily water soluble powder, stable for 36 months when stored undissolved at +25°C and 60% relative humidity. 5-ALA HCl itself is a linear, not light-sensitive and nonfluorescent substance; only its biotransformation into PpIX will result in a fluorescence capable molecule. 5-ALA HCl is dissolved in water and given exclusively by oral route at a dosage of 20 mg/kg body weight. It is readily absorbed with an almost instant bioavailability lasting around 3–4 hours (Stummer W, personal communication). Despite its small molecular size, 5-ALA does not usually enter normal brain tissue, but in glioma tissue, the blood-brain barrier is disrupted, allowing the substrate to reach the target cells; steroid overtreatment or concurrent steroid and 5-ALA administration should therefore be avoided. Also, 5-ALA should be kept away from antacids, since it is easily decomposed at high pH values,[29] and phenytoin has been shown to reduce the accumulation of PpIX in malignant glioma cells.[30] The exogenously given 5-ALA acts as a prodrug, leading to a preferential transformation into PpIX within glioma cells due to the previously described mechanisms (mainly ferrochelatase down-regulation). The intracellular accumulation of PpIX results in a strong visible specific red-violet fluorescence (λpeak = 635 nm, secondary peak at 705 nm) under blue light illumination (λ = 400–440 nm, λpeak = 405 nm). Maximal PpIX fluorescence is reached 6–8 hours after 5-ALA administration and lasts for at least 12 hours. The resulting fluorescence is relatively resistant to photobleaching, as it takes 25.7 minutes under blue light (87.2 minutes under white light) for the initial fluorescent signal intensity to fall to 36%.[31] Due to the limited general tissue penetration of blue light, photobleaching is of no practical concern and does not require specific light protective measures of the brain or neoplastic tissue. Qualitative visual assessment of the fluorescence signal distinguishes between intense (vital solid tumor), vague (tumor infiltration zone) and no fluorescence (either tumor necrosis or tumor cells burden less than 10% or areas of lower malignancy) **(Figures 11.2A to C)**.[32] A tumor cell count below 10% cannot be reliably perceived as visible fluorescence by the human eye any more, but is still detectable using more sensitive spectrophotometric methods. More generally, these spectrophotometric methods can be used to detect and precisely quantify the amount of fluorescence present in the examined tissue.[33-35] Regardless whether using direct observation or spectrophotometric methods, increasing the 5-ALA dose above 20 mg/kg body weight does not result in a better fluorescence signal and may even induce unwanted adverse reactions.

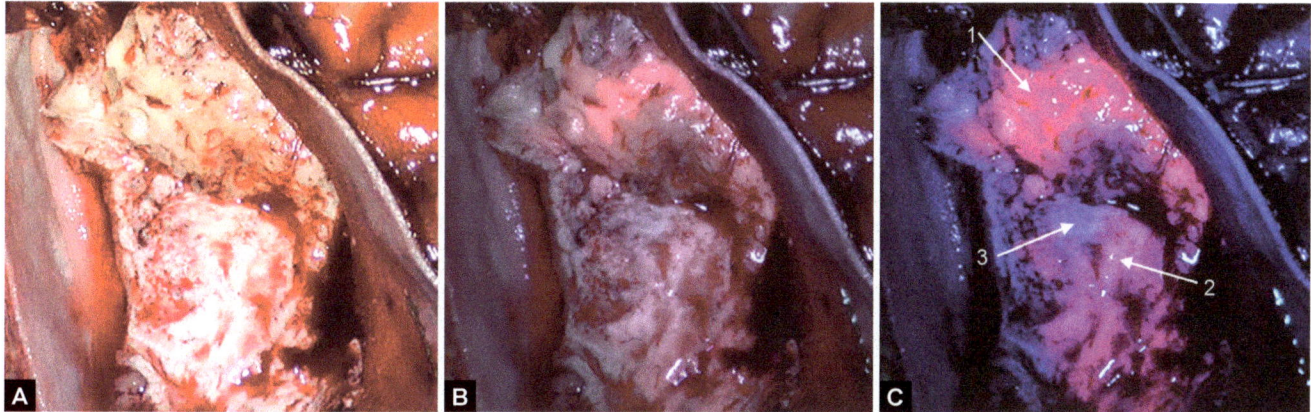

Figures 11.2A to C Intraoperative fluorescence. (A) Regular white light aspect. (B) Montage overlaying the blue light image (C, 50% transparency) on the white light image (A). C. Same area as in A, as seen intraoperatively under blue light illumination: (1) = Intense/strong fluorescence (solid tumor visible on gadolinium-enhanced magnetic resonance images, positive predictive value 100%), (2) = Vague/faint fluorescence (10–60% of infiltrating tumor cells, positive predictive value 92%), (3) = No fluorescence (necrotic tissue, if surrounded by positive fluorescence)

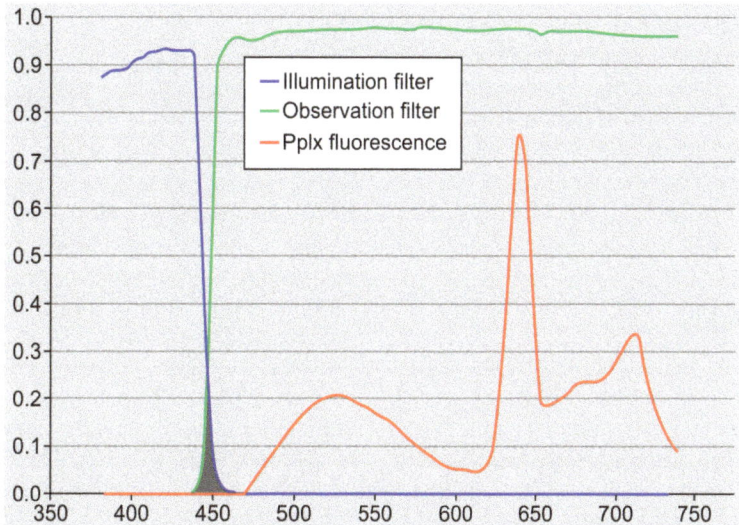

Figure 11.3 Filter properties and emission spectra. Red = protoporphyrin IX (PpIX) emission spectrum. Blue = low-pass excitation filter. Green = high-pass observation filter. Note greyed area representing the small amount of remitted excitation light. Units: x-axis = nm, y-axis = arbitrary units. Adapted from Stummer et al. 1988a and courtesy of Leica Microsystems/Mr Roger Spink

Many modern operating microscopes from leading manufacturers either already come with or can easily be retrofitted to enable the ability of intraoperative photodynamic tumor detection using 5-ALA-mediated PpIX fluorescence. In addition to a powerful Xenon light source, this encompasses special filters for excitation in the 400–440 nm wavelength range, as well as a special dichroic mirror or high-pass observation filter to visualize the resulting fluorescence while also allowing a small amount of excitation light pass through in order to illuminate the surrounding nonfluorescent anatomical brain structures (remitted excitation light) **(Figure 11.3)**.[31] Such a modified neurosurgical microscope

enables the surgeon to theoretically perform the entire tumor resection under blue light, only switching to white light for hemostasis (blood blocks the excitation light and covers the fluorescent tissue).

Although mainly used in the setting of elective surgery for intended GTR of newly diagnosed high-grade gliomas, the method is not necessarily restricted to these cases. Based on 354 biopsies in 36 patients, Nabavi et al. found that surgical guidance using 5-ALA-mediated PpIX fluorescence is an effective adjunct in the surgery of *recurrent* high-grade gliomas, with a high positive predictive value of 97.2%.[36] The method could also be a promising marker for intraoperative visualization of anaplastic foci in noncontrast-enhancing diffuse low-grade gliomas.[37] Furthermore, photodynamic detection can be used for accuracy verification in (stereotactic) brain biopsies. In order to avoid a sampling bias due to tissue heterogeneity, often multiple specimens are obtained in these procedures, which in turn increase their morbidity and mortality risk. Given the high positive predictive value of the 5-ALA method, the immediate and simple intraoperative demonstration of a positive fluorescence in the biopsy specimen would confirm the successful targeting of the lesion, thus obviating the need for further samples and reducing the overall duration of the procedure.[38,39]

Visible 5-ALA-mediated PpIX fluorescence extends beyond the magnetic resonance imaging (MRI) T1-enhancing tumor and closely matches the preoperative MRI fluid-attenuated inversion recovery (FLAIR) signal abnormalities or ^{18}F-fluoroethyl-L-tyrosine positron emission tomography (^{18}F-FET PET) positive areas.[40-42] Removing fluorescent tumor beyond the contrast-enhancing areas visible on preoperative MRI while maintaining functional boundaries has been shown to have a statistically relevant positive impact on surgical outcome, resulting in longer mean overall survival.[43] 5-ALA-mediated photodynamic detection of malignant tissue has been shown to have a sensitivity of 81–87% and specificity of 88.8–90%.[44-46] The positive predictive value of observable intraoperative PpIX fluorescence for pathological tissue is found to be as high as 98.9%.[10,40,47-49]

5-AMINOLEVULINIC ACID: ADVERSE REACTIONS

Given orally and being a naturally occurring endogenous amino acid, 5-ALA has no significant side effects at the recommended oral dose of 20 mg/kg body weight. 5-ALA uptake happens in all epithelial tissues, including the skin, causing a temporary increase in photosensitization of the latter for approximately 24 hours after administration (due to the phototoxicity of PpIX). Exposition to strong light sources (e.g. direct sunlight, brightly focused light, ultraviolet A) and coadministration with other potentially phototoxic substances (e.g. certain antibiotics and neuroleptic drugs)[50] should, therefore, be avoided during that time interval.

As a result of the preferential liver uptake, a transient increase in liver enzymes and blood bilirubin without clinical symptoms is expected and frequently observed. Approximately 30% of the orally administered dose of 5-ALA is excreted unchanged into the urine within 12 hours after administration.

Published dose-dependent side effects of 5-ALA include various degrees of increased skin phototoxicity, nausea or vomiting, hypotension and/or tachycardia.[21,51-54] Since exogenous administration of 5-ALA leads to an increase in porphyrin biosynthesis, its use is contraindicated in cases of porphyria.

5-AMINOLEVULINIC ACID AND PHOTODYNAMIC THERAPY

Photodynamic therapy (PDT) is a treatment modality consisting of the administration of a specific inactive light-absorbing photosensitizer which, in the presence of oxygen and (laser) light of appropriate wavelength, induces a photo-oxidative reaction generating highly reactive singlet oxygen.[55] PDT was primarily developed for the treatment of cancerous or precancerous lesions due to the propensity of several photosensitizers to be absorbed preferentially by hyperproliferative cells. Owing to the accessibility of the skin, its main applications are found in dermatology, but PDT has also been used for the management of certain bladder, lung, and esophageal cancers, and early preclinical studies on PDT in glioma cell cultures were published in 1972.[56] A well-known and approved first-generation photosensitizer is hematoporphyrin derivative (porfimer sodium, also known as Photofrin® or Photosan-3), which however needs to be given systemically and causes severe long-lasting (up to 2 months) skin photosensitivity. Therefore, several second-generation photosensitizers are currently being evaluated, and 5-ALA has been successfully used for the treatment of solar (or actinic) keratosis.[57] Most sensitizers already in clinical use or being evaluated for PDT are porphyrins or porphyrin-based molecules. As tissue light penetration increases with higher wavelengths, irradiation is performed at wavelengths greater than 630 nm, corresponding to the last porphyrin absorption bands. The biological mechanisms underlying the photodamage caused by PDT can be direct and indirect in nature, depending on the tissue oxygenation, photosensitizer involved, and light intensity or dose. Known direct cytotoxic effects include damage to various cell structures (subcellular damage) and cell membrane breakdown, ultimately leading to cell apoptosis. Indirect effects occur at the vascular level (collapse or leakage of the tumor vasculature), as well as involving inflammatory and immunological responses.[58]

In high-grade gliomas, the 5-ALA-mediated intracellular accumulation of PpIX does not only render the tumor cells fluorescent, but also makes them photosensitive and thus, potentially amenable to PDT. PpIX becomes a potent photosensitizer when illuminated with light at a wavelength of 635 nm and, in combination with oxygen, causes cell death by apoptosis and necrosis,[59-61] possibly through a mitochondrial pathway with release of cytochrome c and activation of caspase-3 and caspase-9.[62,63] In addition to this direct effect, initiation of an adaptive immunological response with activation of dendritic cells and modulation of migratory activity and invasiveness of PDT treated human glioblastoma spheroids could also be demonstrated.[64,65] The photodamaging effect appears limited and selective, causing cell death only in the affected neoplastic tissue, without damage to the surrounding normal tissue.[66] As suggested by early clinical reports, PDT could therefore be used to effectively destroy residual glioma cells that cannot be completely and safely removed by surgery alone.[61,67-69]

Currently, the major drawbacks of PDT are the limited depth of tissue penetration as well as the high costs of the optical systems (laser lights, high-power density optical fibers) and their maintenance. Also, optimizing the various PDT parameters is difficult, expensive and time-consuming. Therefore, as of 2015, PDT of high-grade gliomas using 5-ALA has not yet reached routine clinical application and still warrants further studies.

PERSPECTIVES

Due to its safety profile, ease of use, high sensitivity, and specificity, photodynamic tumor detection using 5-ALA-mediated PpIX fluorescence has now become an established and valuable adjunct in the routine surgical management of high-grade gliomas. On the other hand, 5-ALA-mediated PDT has emerged as a potential new adjuvant modality in high-grade gliomas by its ability to selectively photokill residual tumor cells infiltrating normal brain, e.g. when a radical surgical resection is not possible due to the close proximity to eloquent areas. Although not carrying the risk of secondary oncogenesis or therapy resistance, and despite encouraging preliminary reports, there still is a clear need for defined protocols before PDT of high-grade gliomas can be formally established in clinical practice.

Several efforts are being undertaken to broaden the use of photodynamic detection using 5-ALA-mediated PpIX fluorescence to other, especially malignant, CNS tumors, where the extent of resection has a clear impact on outcome as well. Positive fluorescence marked not only the main tumor, but also distant meningeal infiltrations and areas of bone invasion in meningiomas.[70,71] These findings might have some importance in histological benign looking, but genetically potentially malignant meningiomas,[72] especially since bone invasion can be present without prior radiological identification and directly affects outcome.[73,74]

As of 2015, photodynamic tumor detection using 5-ALA-mediated PpIX fluorescence in the CNS is restricted to be used in adults. A recently published survey, however, showed that the method might also be useful for contrast-enhancing supratentorial pediatric tumors, calling for appropriate controlled studies.[75]

REFERENCES

1. Ostrom QT, Gittleman H, Liao P, et al. CBTRUS statistical report: primary brain and central nervous system tumors diagnosed in the United States in 2007-2011. Neuro Oncol. 2014;16 Suppl 4:iv1-63.
2. Wood JR, Green SB, Shapiro WR. The prognostic importance of tumor size in malignant gliomas: a computed tomographic scan study by the Brain Tumor Cooperative Group. J Clin Oncol. 1988;6(2):338-43.
3. Vecht CJ, Avezaat CJ, van Putten WL, et al. The influence of the extent of surgery on the neurological function and survival in malignant glioma. A retrospective analysis in 243 patients. J Neurol Neurosurg Psychiatry. 1990;53(6):466-71.
4. Barker FG, Prados MD, Chang SM, et al. Radiation response and survival time in patients with glioblastoma multiforme. J Neurosurg. 1996;84(3):442-8.
5. Albert FK, Forsting M, Sartor K, et al. Early postoperative magnetic resonance imaging after resection of malignant glioma: objective evaluation of residual tumor and its influence on regrowth and prognosis. Neurosurgery. 1994;34(1):45-60.
6. Kowalczuk A, Macdonald RL, Amidei C, et al. Quantitative imaging study of extent of surgical resection and prognosis of malignant astrocytomas. Neurosurgery. 1997;41(5):1028-36.
7. Stummer W, Pichlmeier U, Meinel T, et al. Fluorescence-guided surgery with 5-aminolevulinic acid for resection of malignant glioma: a randomised controlled multicentre phase III trial. Lancet Oncol. 2006;7(5):392-401.
8. Lacroix M, Abi-Said D, Fourney DR, et al. A multivariate analysis of 416 patients with glioblastoma multiforme: prognosis, extent of resection, and survival. J Neurosurg. 2001;95(2):190-8.
9. McGirt MJ, Chaichana KL, Gathinji M, et al. Independent association of extent of resection with survival in patients with malignant brain astrocytoma. J Neurosurg. 2009;110(1):156-62.
10. Stummer W, Novotny A, Stepp H, et al. Fluorescence-guided resection of glioblastoma multiforme by using 5-aminolevulinic acid-induced porphyrins: a prospective study in 52 consecutive patients. J Neurosurg. 2000;93(6):1003-13.
11. Stupp R, Mason WP, van den Bent MJ, et al. Radiotherapy plus concomitant and adjuvant temozolomide for glioblastoma. N Engl J Med. 2005;352(10):987-96.
12. Wallner KE, Galicich JH, Krol G, et al. Patterns of failure following treatment for glioblastoma multiforme and anaplastic astrocytoma. Int J Radiat Oncol Biol Phys. 1989;16(6):1405-9.
13. Aydin H, Sillenberg I, von Lieven H. Patterns of failure following CT-based 3-D irradiation for malignant glioma. Strahlenther Onkol. 2001;177(8): 424-31.
14. Kreske N, Simoni RD, Hill RL. A pathway for heme biosynthesis: the work of David Shemin. J Biol Chem. 2006;281(34):e28.
15. Colditz MJ, Leyen KV, Jeffree RL. Aminolevulinic acid (ALA)-protoporphyrin IX fluorescence guided tumour resection. Part 2: theoretical, biochemical and practical aspects. J Clin Neurosci. 2012;19(12):1611-6.
16. Fritsch C, Verwohlt B, Bolsen K, et al. Influence of topical photodynamic therapy with 5-aminolevulinic acid on porphyrin metabolism. Arch Dermatol Res. 1996;288(9):517-21.
17. Grant WE, Hopper C, MacRobert AJ, et al. Photodynamic therapy of oral cancer: photosensitisation with systemic aminolaevulinic acid. Lancet. 1993;342(8864):147-8.
18. Loh CS, MacRobert AJ, Bedwell J, et al. Oral versus intravenous administration of 5-aminolaevulinic acid for photodynamic therapy. Br J Cancer. 1993;68(1):41-51.
19. Kriegmair M, Baumgartner R, Knüchel R, et al. Detection of early bladder cancer by 5-aminolevulinic acid induced porphyrin fluorescence. J Urol. 1996;155(1):105-9.
20. Loh CS, Vernon D, MacRobert AJ, et al. Endogenous porphyrin distribution induced by 5-aminolaevulinic acid in the tissue

layers of the gastrointestinal tract. J Photochem Photobiol B. 1993;20(1):47-54.

21. Regula J, MacRobert AJ, Gorchein A, et al. Photosensitisation and photodynamic therapy of oesophageal, duodenal, and colorectal tumours using 5 aminolaevulinic acid induced protoporphyrin IX: a pilot study. Gut. 1995;36(1):67-75.

22. Stummer W, Stocker S, Novotny A, et al. In vitro and in vivo porphyrin accumulation by C6 glioma cells after exposure to 5-aminolevulinic acid. J Photochem Photobiol B. 1998;45(2-3):160-9.

23. Zelenkov P, Baumgartner R, Bise K, et al. Acute morphological sequelae of photodynamic therapy with 5-aminolevulinic acid in the C6 spheroid model. J Neurooncol. 2007;82(1):49-60.

24. Sterenborg HJ, Hebeda KM, Saarnak AE, et al. ALA-induced endogenous porphyrins in brain tumours. Clin Neurol Neurosurg. 1997;99(1):S133.

25. Hebeda KM, Saarnak AE, Olivo M, et al. 5-Aminolevulinic acid induced endogenous porphyrin fluorescence in 9L and C6 brain tumours and in the normal rat brain. Acta Neurochir (Wien). 1998;140(5):503-12.

26. Teng L, Nakada M, Zhao SG, et al. Silencing of ferrochelatase enhances 5-aminolevulinic acid-based fluorescence and photodynamic therapy efficacy. Br J Cancer. 2011;104(5):798-807.

27. Takahashi K, Ikeda N, Nonoguchi N, et al. Enhanced expression of coproporphyrinogen oxidase in malignant brain tumors: CPOX expression and 5-ALA-induced fluorescence. Neuro Oncol. 2011;13(11):1234-43.

28. Zhao SG, Chen XF, Wang LG, et al. Increased expression of ABCB6 enhances protoporphyrin IX accumulation and photodynamic effect in human glioma. Ann Surg Oncol. 2013;20(13):4379-88.

29. Bunke A, Zerbe O, Schmid H, et al. Degradation mechanism and stability of 5-aminolevulinic acid. J Pharm Sci. 2000;89(10):1335-41.

30. Hefti M, Albert I, Luginbuehl V. Phenytoin reduces 5-amino-levulinic acid-induced protoporphyrin IX accumulation in malignant glioma cells. J Neurooncol. 2012;108(3):443-50.

31. Stummer W, Stepp H, Möller G, et al. Technical principles for protoporphyrin-IX-fluorescence guided microsurgical resection of malignant glioma tissue. Acta Neurochir (Wien). 1998;140(10):995-1000.

32. Hefti M, von Campe G, Moschopulos M, et al. 5-aminolevulinic acid induced protoporphyrin IX fluorescence in high-grade glioma surgery: a one-year experience at a single institution. Swiss Med Wkly. 2008;138(11-12):180-5.

33. Utsuki S, Oka H, Sato S, et al. Possibility of using laser spectroscopy for the intraoperative detection of nonfluorescing brain tumors and the boundaries of brain tumor infiltrates. Technical note. J Neurosurg. 2006;104(4):618-20.

34. Eljamel MS, Leese G, Moseley H. Intraoperative optical identification of pituitary adenomas. J Neurooncol. 2009; 92(3):417-21.

35. Valdés PA, Kim A, Leblond F, et al. Combined fluorescence and reflectance spectroscopy for in vivo quantification of cancer biomarkers in low- and high-grade glioma surgery. J Biomed Opt. 2011;16(11):116007.

36. Nabavi A, Thurm H, Zountsas B, et al. Five-aminolevulinic acid for fluorescence-guided resection of recurrent malignant gliomas: a phase ii study. Neurosurgery. 2009;65(6):1070-6.

37. Widhalm G, Wolfsberger S, Minchev G, et al. 5-Aminolevulinic acid is a promising marker for detection of anaplastic foci in diffusely infiltrating gliomas with nonsignificant contrast enhancement. Cancer. 2010;116(6):1545-52.

38. von Campe G, Moschopulos M, Hefti M. 5-Aminolevulinic acid-induced protoporphyrin IX fluorescence as immediate intraoperative indicator to improve the safety of malignant or high-grade brain tumor diagnosis in frameless stereotactic biopsies. Acta Neurochir (Wien). 2012;154(4):585-8.

39. Widhalm G, Minchev G, Woehrer A, et al. Strong 5-aminolevulinic acid-induced fluorescence is a novel intraoperative marker for representative tissue samples in stereotactic brain tumor biopsies. Neurosurg Rev. 2012;35(3):381-91.

40. Diez Valle R, Tejada Solis S, Idoate Gastearena MA, et al. Surgery guided by 5-aminolevulinic fluorescence in glioblastoma: volumetric analysis of extent of resection in single-center experience. J Neurooncol. 2011;102(1):105-13.

41. Roessler K, Becherer A, Donat M, et al. Intraoperative tissue fluorescence using 5-aminolevolinic acid (5-ALA) is more sensitive than contrast MRI or amino acid positron emission tomography ((18)F-FET PET) in glioblastoma surgery. Neurol Res. 2012;34(3):314-7.

42. Schucht P, Knittel S, Slotboom J, et al. 5-ALA complete resections go beyond MR contrast enhancement: shift corrected volumetric analysis of the extent of resection in surgery for glioblastoma. Acta Neurochir (Wien). 2014;156(2):305-12.

43. Aldave G, Tejada S, Pay E, et al. Prognostic value of residual fluorescent tissue in glioblastoma patients after gross total resection in 5-aminolevulinic Acid-guided surgery. Neurosurgery. 2013;72(6):915-20.

44. Friesen SA, Hjortland GO, Madsen SJ, et al. 5-Aminolevulinic acid-based photodynamic detection and therapy of brain tumors (review). Int J Oncol. 2002;21(3):577-82.

45. Eljamel S. 5-ALA fluorescence image guided resection of glioblastoma multiforme: a meta-analysis of the literature. Int J Mol Sci. 2015;16(5):10443-56.

46. Zhao S, Wu J, Wang C, et al. Intraoperative fluorescence-guided resection of high-grade malignant gliomas using 5-aminolevulinic acid-induced porphyrins: a systematic review and meta-analysis of prospective studies. PLoS One. 2013;8(5):e63682.

47. Roberts DW, Valdés PA, Harris BT, et al. Coregistered fluorescence-enhanced tumor resection of malignant glioma: relationships between delta-aminolevulinic acid-induced protoporphyrin IX fluorescence, magnetic resonance imaging enhancement, and neuropathological parameters. Clinical article. J Neurosurg. 2011;114(3):595-603.

48. Valdés PA, Leblond F, Kim A, et al. Quantitative fluorescence in intracranial tumor: implications for ALA-induced PpIX as an intraoperative biomarker. J Neurosurg. 2011;115(1):11-7.

49. Stummer W, Tonn JC, Goetz C, et al. 5-Aminolevulinic acid-derived tumor fluorescence: the diagnostic accuracy of visible fluorescence qualities as corroborated by spectrometry and histology and postoperative imaging. Neurosurgery. 2014;74(3):310-9.

50. Eberlein-König B, Bindl A, Przybilla B. Phototoxic properties of neuroleptic drugs. Dermatology. 1997;194(2):131-5.

51. Waidelich R, Hofstetter A, Stepp H, et al. Early clinical experience with 5-aminolevulinic acid for the photodynamic therapy of upper tract urothelial tumors. J Urol. 1998;159(2):401-4.

52. Herman MA, Webber J, Fromm D, et al. Hemodynamic effects of 5-aminolevulinic acid in humans. J Photochem Photobiol B. 1998;43(1):61-5.

53. Ackroyd R, Brown N, Vernon D, et al. 5-Aminolevulinic acid photosensitization of dysplastic Barrett's esophagus: a pharmacokinetic study. Photochem Photobiol. 1999;70(4):656-62.

54. Ladner DP, Steiner RA, Allemann J, et al. Photodynamic diagnosis of breast tumours after oral application of aminolevulinic acid. Br J Cancer. 2001;84(1):33-7.

55. Norum OJ, Selbo PK, Weyergang A, et al. Photochemical internalization (PCI) in cancer therapy: from bench towards bedside medicine. J Photochem Photobiol B. 2009;96(2):83-92.

56. Diamond I, Granelli SG, McDonagh AF, et al. Photodynamic therapy of malignant tumours. Lancet. 1972;2(7788):1175-7.

57. Fink-Puches R, Hofer A, Smolle J, et al. Primary clinical response and long-term follow-up of solar keratoses treated with topically applied 5-aminolevulinic acid and irradiation by different wave bands of light. J Photochem Photobiol B. 1997;41(1-2):145-51.

58. Castano AP, Mroz P, Hamblin MR. Photodynamic therapy and anti-tumour immunity. Nat Rev Cancer. 2006;6(7):535-45.

59. Olzowy B, Hundt CS, Stocker S, et al. Photoirradiation therapy of experimental malignant glioma with 5-aminolevulinic acid. J Neurosurg. 2002;97(4):970-6.

60. Krammer B. Plaetzer K. ALA and its clinical impact, from bench to bedside. Photochem Photobiol Sci. 2008;7(3):283-9.

61. Eljamel MS, Goodman C, Moseley H. ALA and Photofrin fluorescence-guided resection and repetitive PDT in glioblastoma multiforme: a single centre Phase III randomised controlled trial. Lasers Med Sci. 2008;23(4):361-7.

62. Inoue H, Kajimoto Y, Shibata MA, et al. Massive apoptotic cell death of human glioma cells via a mitochondrial pathway following 5-aminolevulinic acid-mediated photodynamic therapy. J Neurooncol. 2007;83(3):223-31.

63. Karmakar S, Banik NL, Patel SJ, et al. 5-Aminolevulinic acid-based photodynamic therapy suppressed survival factors and activated proteases for apoptosis in human glioblastoma U87MG cells. Neurosci Lett. 2007;415(3):242-7.

64. Etminan N, Peters C, Ficnar J, et al. Modulation of migratory activity and invasiveness of human glioma spheroids following 5-aminolevulinic acid-based photodynamic treatment. Laboratory investigation. J Neurosurg. 2011;115(2):281-8.

65. Etminan N, Peters C, Lakbir D, et al. Heat-shock protein 70-dependent dendritic cell activation by 5-aminolevulinic acid-mediated photodynamic treatment of human glioblastoma spheroids in vitro. Br J Cancer. 2011;105(7):961-9.

66. Dougherty TJ. Photodynamic therapy. Photochem Photobiol. 1993;58(6):895-900.

67. Beck TJ, Kreth FW, Beyer W, et al. Interstitial photodynamic therapy of nonresectable malignant glioma recurrences using 5-aminolevulinic acid induced protoporphyrin IX. Lasers Surg Med. 2007;39(5):386-93.

68. Stummer W, Beck T, Beyer W, et al. Long-sustaining response in a patient with non-resectable, distant recurrence of glioblastoma multiforme treated by interstitial photodynamic therapy using 5-ALA: case report. J Neurooncol. 2008;87(1):103-9.

69. Sherman JH, Hoes K, Marcus J, et al. Neurosurgery for brain tumors: update on recent technical advances. Curr Neurol Neurosci Rep. 2011;11(3):313-9.

70. Kajimoto Y, Kuroiwa T, Miyake S, et al. Use of 5-aminolevulinic acid in fluorescence-guided resection of meningioma with high risk of recurrence. Case report. J Neurosurg. 2007;106(6):1070-4.

71. Morofuji Y, Matsuo T, Hayashi Y, et al. Usefulness of intraoperative photodynamic diagnosis using 5-aminolevulinic acid for meningiomas with cranial invasion: technical case report. Neurosurgery. 2008;62(3 Suppl 1):102-3.

72. Al-Mefty O, Kadri PA, Pravdenkova S, et al. Malignant progression in meningioma: documentation of a series and analysis of cytogenetic findings. J Neurosurg. 2004;101(2):210-8.

73. Pieper DR, Al-Mefty O, Hanada Y, et al. Hyperostosis associated with meningioma of the cranial base: secondary changes or tumor invasion. Neurosurgery. 1999;44(4):742-6.

74. Gabeau-Lacet D, Aghi M, Betensky RA, et al. Bone involvement predicts poor outcome in atypical meningioma. J Neurosurg. 2009;111(3):464-71.

75. Stummer W, Rodrigues F, Schucht P, et al. Predicting the "usefulness" of 5-ALA-derived tumor fluorescence for fluorescence-guided resections in pediatric brain tumors: a European survey. Acta Neurochir (Wien). 2014;156(12):2315-24.

12

Intraoperative Imaging in Epilepsy Surgery

Aditya Gupta, Rishabh Kedia, Pawan Goyal

INTRODUCTION

Chronic neurodegenerative diseases are rarely treatable by surgery, epilepsy being one of the exceptions.

Medical management is effective in majority of patients, however, up to 40% epilepsy patients are resistant to any type of treatment with drugs.[1] These drug-resistant patients should be given a trial of surgical management for better control of seizures.

WHO NEEDS SURGERY?[1]

- The patient with intractable seizures, i.e. the one having persistent seizures even after proper treatment with two or major antiepileptic drugs under the supervision of a competent neurologist.
- Epilepsy is proving to be disabling for the patient.
- Surgery should offer patient a reasonable chance to improve without much risk.

Surgical treatments for many neurodegenerative disorders do exist, but they are merely palliative. On the other hand, epilepsy surgeries can be curative for a well-defined lesion in as many as 70–80% cases.[2]

Surgery for epilepsy is aimed towards identifying abnormal cortical area responsible for seizures and removing it safely without causing any damage to eloquent brain. More localized is the lesion, better are the chances of curing epilepsy. That is why it is very important to have accurate localization of lesion for successful outcome.

While operating on an epileptic brain, one may find himself to be operating on an absolutely normal structure unlike the case of a tumor or a vascular lesion. Even under microscopic magnification and illumination, it may not be possible to differentiate epileptic focus from normal anatomic structures. Intraoperative imaging helps us to identify abnormal areas of brain in real-time and thus aid in resection in operating room.

There are certain other uses of intraoperative imaging in epilepsy like navigation-guided placement of electrodes, identification of functional cortex by doing real-time functional magnetic resonance imaging (MRI) or to assess response of tissue to photoablative therapy. The main tool of intraoperative imaging is MRI besides ultrasound and computed tomography (CT).

INTRAOPERATIVE MAGNETIC RESONANCE IMAGING

Intraoperative magnetic resonance imaging (iMRI) along with frameless stereotaxy has brought a revolution in the field of neurosurgery. Black and colleagues[3] first introduced iMRI at the Brigham and Women's Hospital in Boston.

The basic idea is to get three-dimensional view of a point in the patient's head with the help of imaging modality to assist in the surgical procedure. It is particularly helpful in epilepsy surgery as (1) it helps to delineate anatomic boundaries which are not visible to naked eye, (2) to help locate and decide a trajectory for a focal lesion as pathology in a case of epilepsy is not visible to naked eye, (3) to help assess intraoperatively the extent of resection and residual pathological tissue left.

During surgery, due to opening of dura, resection of tissue, and cerebrospinal fluid (CSF) loss, there occurs a shift of 1–1.5 cm in brain structures.[4-8] This is the time where iMRI plays a very important role (**Figures 12.1 and 12.2**).

INTRAOPERATIVE ULTRASOUND

To compensate for CSF loss and brain shifts, real-time imaging is needed. Intraoperative ultrasound (IOUS) provides that imaging with high level of accuracy. IOUS not only provides continuous and real-time imaging but also has wider and easy availability and also is very cost-effective.

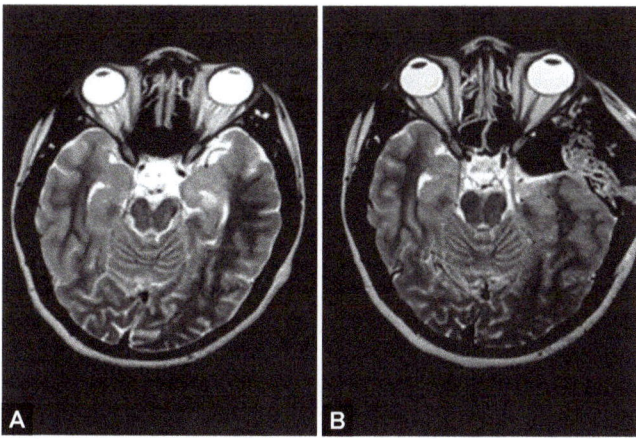

Figures 12.1A and B (A) A 20-year-old female with focal cortical dysplasia, Preoperative magnetic resonance imaging; (B) intraoperative magnetic resonance imaging (MRI) helped to assess the extent of resection and re-resection was done

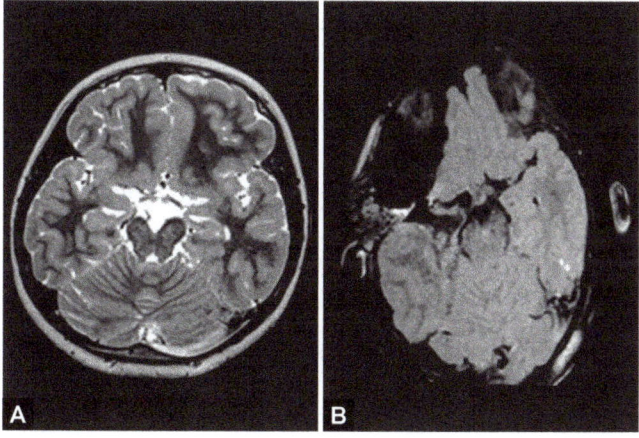

Figures 12.2A and B (A) An 11-year-old female with mesial temporal sclerosis, resection extended surgery done after (B) intraoperative magnetic resonance imaging (MRI)

Irrespective of brain shift, it provides information regarding extent of lesion. Cases of focal cortical dysplasia have been operated by Miller et al.[9] and Lee et al.[10] using IOUS.

Only disadvantage with IOUS is that imaging quality is not so good.[11]

INTRAOPERATIVE COMPUTED TOMOGRAPHY

Intraoperative CT is one more imaging for the purpose but disadvantage is poor image quality as compared to MRI and bone artifacts, especially in posterior fossa interfere with the accurate assessment.[12]

EXTRATEMPORAL EPILEPSY

Extratemporal epilepsy is a very challenging entity in the area of surgery for epilepsy.

Extratemporal lesionectomies only represent a small percentage of about 9–18% of all epilepsy surgeries.[13-15]

Extratemporal lobe lesions present with a variety of histopathological findings, which are unsteady and diffuse and not that well-defined as, e.g. hippocampal sclerosis.

The localization of extratemporal lesions in the vicinity of functional cortex or fiber tracts make them difficult to resect without harming susceptible brain tissue and causing severe permanent neurological deficits.

A good clinical outcome in the form of significant seizure reduction and improvement in overall life quality between 58% and greater than 80%,[14,16-18] is expected in a case of temporal epilepsy after surgery. On the other hand, extratemporal seizures are more difficult to treat surgically, with reported seizure freedom rates of only 10–54%.[19-23]

Awake craniotomy with intraoperative cortical brain mapping is considered to be the primary method to monitor eloquent brain areas during surgery.[24]

However, the superiority of this technique regarding efficiency and safety is still a matter of debate, lacking randomized controlled trials with larger patient cohorts.[25,26]

Inadequate pain control, airway obstruction leading to intubation, vomiting, brain swelling and intraoperative seizures are among the common objectionable events during awake surgery. The risk of new appearance or worsening of permanent neurological deficits using this technique has been reported to be between 0% and 29%, with surgical complication rates between 0% and 14.8%.[24-26]

Considering the aforementioned obstacles of awake craniotomy, a non-invasive preoperative targeting of eloquent structures of brain using functional MRI (fMRI) and diffusion tensor imaging (DTI) with general anesthesia seems to be a better option.

The advent of iMRI has made it possible to analyze the extent of lesion resection. Additionally, a dynamic adaptation to different perioperative phenomena such as brain shift and localization of a residual lesion by redoing navigation using fresh intraoperative images has become possible. Moreover, damage of eloquent brain areas, such as speech or sensorimotor areas can be avoided by integrating data from fMRI [blood oxygen level-dependent (BOLD) imaging]. Thus, resections adjacent to these important brain regions can be performed with more safety and efficiency.[27-29]

TEMPORAL EPILEPSY

The risk profile of epilepsy surgery in the dominant temporal lobe is generally serious.[30]Various eloquent structures are at risk: (1) sensory speech function within the dorsal superior temporal gyrus, (2) memory-related functions within the hippocampus and parahippocampal gyrus, and (3) Meyer's loop, part of the visual tract within the superior-lateral border of the temporal ventricular horn.[31-33]

In patients with hippocampal sclerosis (HS), resection of a significant amount of hippocampus, parahippocampal gyrus as well as amygdala and uncus is necessary to achieve at least a 60–70% success rate in Engel class I outcome.[18]

Use of depth electrodes aids in demonstrating ictal onsets from amygdala, hippocampal and parahippocampal regions.[34-37]Several studies have shown that a residual hippocampal and parahippocampal region has significant impact in the form of recurrent seizures.[38-41] There is a definitive higher seizure-free outcome after complete or near complete resection of hippocampus. That is why, in temporal lobe resections, aggressive amygdalohippocampectomy is considered an essential part nowadays.[42-45]

Operating surgeons generally tend to overestimate their extent of resection while on operating table, despite the availability of best of operating microscope. This is why intraoperative imaging is essential as it gives a real update of the situation on operating table and iMRI is most useful for all.[43,45-48]

iMRI especially helps to delineate the end of amygdala and start of basal ganglia and helps prevent disastrous outcome.

Bilateral Wada testing may help to define the dominant temporal lobe and investigate reorganization of speech and memory to ipsilateral distant areas or to the contralateral side, but it is not able to demonstrate the topographical localization of functional areas on the magnetic resonance (MR) scans used for navigated surgery.[49,50]

Employing fMRI, localization of eloquent brain areas involved in speech and memory processing can be fused with MR scans and thus guide surgical interventions by using neuronavigation.[51]

Furthermore, neuronavigation is able to co-localize fMRI functional areas to the intraoperatively exposed cortex.[29]

Additionally, DTI localizes subcortical tracts, which can also be integrated in the intraoperative neuronavigation to avoid damage.[52-54]

Moreover, issues like brain shift can be effectively dealt with using iMRI and may help to guide maximized resection and to avoid injury to adjacent eloquent cortical or white matter tract systems.[55]

Combining fMRI, neuronavigation and iMRI for surgery of lesional dominant temporal lobe epilepsy is promising and may lead to favorable postoperative results and enhance the percentage of seizure-free patients.

Deep Brain Stimulation

Deep brain stimulation (DBS) also has an important place in treating epilepsy cases.[56]

Preoperative MR has been already accepted as a modality to do target planning. But iMRI provides immediate information regarding lead location **(Figures 12.3A to C).**

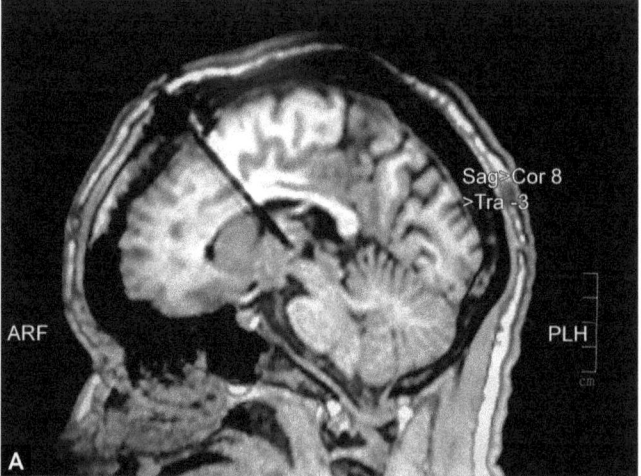
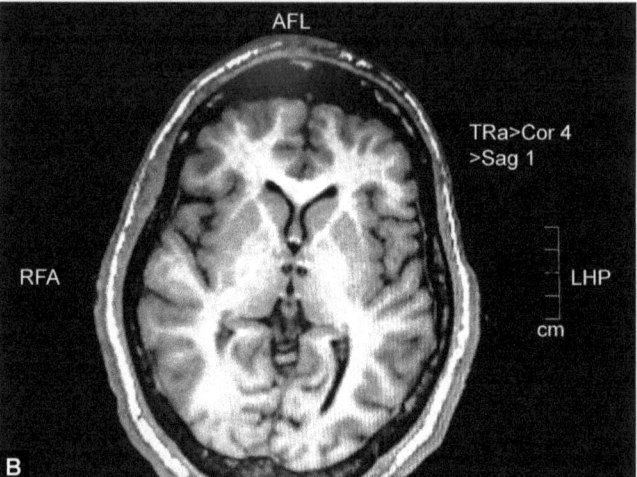
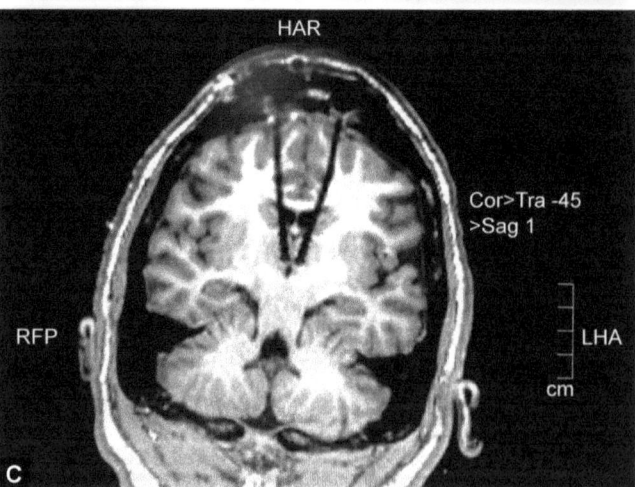

Figures 12.3A to C Intraoperative MRI for checking the placement of DBS electrodes before connecting and placing the battery

Also, it helps to screen for undesired complications. This information regarding lead location can further be helpful for rapid and accurate programming when patient returns back.

However, with DBS leads in situ, there is a risk of lesioning during MRI acquisition due to heat transmission to DBS leads.[57,58]

Hence, MRI should be done with caution. Ideally a transmit or receive head coil rather than a body coil should be used.

CONCLUSION

Advantages in Lesional Epilepsy

- Planning of location and extent of skin incision, craniotomy and dural opening
- Segmentation of lesion and surrounding epileptogenic tissue
- Planning of the trajectories for atraumatic targeting of deep-seated lesions
- Outlining of lesion borders (e.g. in ganglioglioma resection)
- Implementation of functional imaging (fMRI or DTI) data for sparing of eloquent tissue
- Intraoperative outlining of residual lesions and resection during the same operation.

Advantages in Non-lesional Epilepsy

- Implementation of preoperative positron emission tomography (PET) or magnetoencephalography (MEG) data into resection planning via image fusion
- Verification of resected PET or MEG foci w/ iMRI during operation [e.g. ganglioglioma, focal cortical dysplasia (FCD)]
- Verification of preplanned electrode position during electrode implantation and intraoperative correction of electrode malposition
- Implementation of electroencephalography (EEG) data from invasive monitoring into the resection approach; implementation of functional imaging (fMRI or DTI) data for sparing of eloquent tissue.

Use of iMRI is going to become a routine in near future in neurosurgical field. With technological advancement, the area of utility of this modality is widening. Quality of image is better with high-field magnets but it interferes with equipment due to high-field strength. This shortcoming can be overcome by using low-field magnets, but it has its own disadvantages like poor image quality and difficult surgical positioning.

With further advanced technology, if these issues can be overcome, then iMRI will definitely become a standard armamentarium in neurosurgery, especially epilepsy procedures.

REFERENCES

1. Michaelides C, Cosgrove GR, Cole AJ. Evaluation of patients for epilepsy surgery. In: Winn HR (Ed). Youmans Neurological Surgery, 6th edition. New York: Elsevier Saunders; 2011. pp. 714-20.
2. Doyle WK, Spencer DD. Anterior temporal resections. In: Engel JJ, Pedley TA (Ed). Epilepsy. A Comprehensive Textbook. Philadelphia: Lippincott-Raven Publishers; 1997. pp. 1807-17.
3. Black PM, Moriarty T, Alexander E, et al. Development and implementation of intraoperative magnetic resonance imaging and its neurosurgical applications. Neurosurgery. 1997;41(4):831-42.
4. Nimsky C, Ganslandt O, Cerny S, et al. Quantiication of, visualization of, and compensation for brain shift using intraoperative magnetic resonance imaging. Neurosurgery. 2000;47(5):1070-9.
5. Dorward NL, Alberti O, Velani B, et al. Postimaging brain distortion: magnitude, correlates, and impact on neuronavigation. J Neurosurg. 1998;88(4):656-62.
6. Hill DL, Maurer CR, Maciunas RJ, et al. Measurement of intraoperative brain surface deformation under a craniotomy. Neurosurgery. 1998;43(3):514-26.
7. Nabavi A, Black PM, Gering DT, et al. Serial intraoperative magnetic resonance imaging of brain shift. Neurosurgery. 2001;48(4):787-97.
8. Roberts DW, Hartov A, Kennedy FE, et al. Intraoperative brain shift and deformation: a quantitative analysis of cortical displacement in 28 cases. Neurosurgery. 1998;43(4):749-58.
9. Miller D, Knake S, Bauer S, et al. Intraoperative ultrasound to define focal cortical dysplasia in epilepsy surgery. Epilepsia. 2008;49(1):156-8.
10. Lee CC, Lin CF, Yu HY, et al. Applications of intraoperative ultrasound in epilepsy surgery for focal cortical dysplasia. J Med Ultrasound. 2014;22(1):43-6.
11. Chandler WF, Knake JE, McGillicudy JE, et al. Intraoperative use of real-time ultrasonography in neurosurgery. J Neurosurg. 1982;57(2):157-63.
12. Lunsford LD, Parrish R, Albight L. Intraoperative imaging with a therapeutic computed tomographic scanner. Neurosurgery. 1984;15(4):559-61.
13. Binder DK, Podlogar M, Clusmann H, et al. Surgical treatment of parietal lobe epilepsy. J Neurosurg. 2009;110(6):1170-8.
14. Chaudhry N, Radhakrishnan A, Abraham M, et al. Selection of ideal candidates for extratemporal resective epilepsy surgery in a country with limited resources. Epileptic Disord. 2010;12(1):38-47.
15. Frater JL, Prayson RA, Morris HH, et al. Surgical pathologic findings of extratemporal-based intractable epilepsy: a study of 133 consecutive resections. Arch Pathol Lab Med. 2000;124(4):545-9.
16. Engel J, Wiebe S, French J, et al. Practice parameter: temporal lobe and localized neocortical resections for epilepsy. Epilepsia. 2003;44(6):741-51.
17. Téllez-Zenteno JF, Dhar R, Wiebe S. Long-term seizure outcomes following epilepsy surgery: a systematic review and meta-analysis. Brain. 2005;128(5):1188-98.

18. Wiebe S, Blume WT, Girvin JP, et al. A randomized, controlled trial of surgery for temporal-lobe epilepsy. N Engl J Med. 2001;345(5):311-8.

19. Elsharkawy AE, Pannek H, Schulz R, et al. Outcome of extratemporal epilepsy surgery experience of a single center. Neurosurgery. 2008;63(3):516-25.

20. Haglund MM, Ojemann GA. Extratemporal resective surgery for epilepsy. Neurosurg Clin N Am. 1993;4:283-92.

21. Kutsy RL. Focal extratemporal epilepsy: clinical features, EEG patterns, and surgical approach. J Neurol Sci. 1999;166(1):1-15.

22. McIntosh AM, Averill CA, Kalnins RM, Mitchell LA, Fabinyi GC, Jackson GD, et al. Long-term seizure outcome and risk factors for recurrence after extratemporal epilepsy surgery. Epilepsia. 2012;53(6):970-8.

23. Zentner J, Hufnagel A, Ostertun B, et al. Surgical treatment of extratemporal epilepsy: clinical, radiologic, and histopathologic findings in 60 patients. Epilepsia. 1996;37(11):1072-80.

24. Serletis D, Bernstein M. Prospective study of awake craniotomy used routinely and nonselectively for supratentorial tumors. J Neurosurg. 2007;107(1):1-6.

25. Gupta DK, Chandra PS, Ojha BK, et al. Awake craniotomy versus surgery under general anesthesia for resection of intrinsic lesions of eloquent cortex--a prospective randomised study. Clin Neurol Neurosurg. 2007;109(4):335-43.

26. Pereira LC, Oliveira KM, L'Abbate GL, et al. Outcome of fully awake craniotomy for lesions near the eloquent cortex: analysis of a prospective surgical series of 79 supratentorial primary brain tumors with long follow-up. Acta Neurochir (Wien). 2009;151(10):1215-30.

27. Gasser T, Szelenyi A, Senft C, et al. Intraoperative MRI and functional mapping. Acta Neurochir Suppl. 2011;109:61-5.

28. Hall WA, Kim P, Truwit CL. Functional magnetic resonance imaging-guided brain tumor resection. Top Magn Reson Imaging. 2009;19(4):205-12.

29. Roessler K, Donat M, Lanzenberger R, et al. Evaluation of preoperative high magnetic field motor functional MRI (3 Tesla) in glioma patients by navigated electrocortical stimulation and postoperative outcome. J Neurol Neurosurg Psychiatry. 2005;76(8):1152-7.

30. Hader WJ, Tellez-Zenteno J, Metcalfe A, et al. Complications of epilepsy surgery: a systematic review of focal surgical resections and invasive EEG monitoring. Epilepsia. 2013;54(5):840-7.

31. Baxendale S, Thompson PJ, Sander JW. Neuropsychological outcomes in epilepsy surgery patients with unilateral hippocampal sclerosis and good preoperative memory function. Epilepsia. 2013;54(9):e131-4.

32. Davies KG, Bell BD, Bush AJ, et al. Naming decline after left anterior temporal lobectomy correlates with pathological status of resected hippocampus. Epilepsia. 1998;39(4):407-19.

33. Winston GP. Epilepsy surgery, vision, and driving: what has surgery taught us and could modern imaging reduce the risk of visual deficits? Epilepsia. 2013;54(11):1877-88.

34. Spencer DD, Spencer SS, Mattson RH, et al. Access to the posterior medial temporal lobe structures in the surgical treatment of temporal lobe epilepsy. Neurosurgery. 1984; 15(5):667-71.

35. Jooma R, Yeh HS, Privitera MD, et al. Seizure control and extent of mesial temporal resection. Acta Neurochir (Wien). 1995;133(1-2):44-9.

36. Hudson LP, Munoz DG, Miller L, et al. Amygdaloid sclerosis in temporal lobe epilepsy. Ann Neurol. 1993;33(6):622-31.

37. Weiser HG. Electroclinical Features of Psychomotor Seizures. London: Butterworths; 1983.

38. Holmes MD, Wilensky AJ, Ojemann LM, et al. Predicting outcome following reoperation for medically intractable epilepsy. Seizure. 1999;8(2):103-6.

39. Germano IM, Poulin N, Olivier A. Reoperation for recurrent temporal lobe epilepsy. J Neurosurg. 1994;81(1):31-6.

40. Awad IA, Nayel MH, Lüders H. Second operation after the failure of previous resection for epilepsy. Neurosurgery. 1991;28(4):510-8.

41. Wyler AR, Hermann BP, Richey ET. Results of reoperation for failed epilepsy surgery. J Neurosurg. 1989;71(6):815-9.

42. Wyler AR, Hermann BP, Somes G. Extent of medial temporal resection on outcome from anterior temporal lobectomy: a randomized prospective study. Neurosurgery. 1995;37(5):982-90; discussion, 990-1.

43. Awad IA, Katz A, Hahn JF, et al. Extent of resection in temporal lobectomy for epilepsy. I. Interobserver analysis and correlation with seizure outcome. Epilepsia. 1989;30(6):756-62.

44. Bengzon AR, Rasmussen T, Gloor P, et al. Prognostic factors in the surgical treatment of temporal lobe epileptics. Neurology. 1968;18:717-31.

45. Nayel MH, Awad IA, Luders H. Extent of mesiobasal resection determines outcome after temporal lobectomy for intractable complex partial seizures. Neurosurgery. 1991;29:55-61.

46. Van Roost D, Schaller C, Meyer B, et al. Can neuronavigation contribute to standardization of selective amygdalohippocampectomy. Stereotact Funct Neurosurg. 1997;69(1-4):239-42.

47. Jack CR, Sharbrough FW, Marsh WR. Use of MR imaging for quantitive evaluation of resection for temporal lobe epilepsy. Radiology. 1988;169:463-8.

48. Siegel AM, Wieser HG, Wichmann W, et al. Relationship between MR-imaged total amount of tissue removed, resection scores of specific mediobasal limbic subcompartments and clinical outcome following selective amygdalohippocampectomy. Epilepsy Res. 1990;6(1):56-65.

49. Uijl SG, Leijten FS, Arends JB, et al. The intracarotid amobarbital or Wada test: unilateral or bilateral? Acta Neurol Scand. 2009;119(3):199-206.

50. Schulze-Bonhage A, Quiske A, Loddenkemper T, et al. Validity of language lateralisation by unilateral intracarotid Wada test. J Neurol Neurosurg Psychiatry. 2004;75(9):1367-68.

51. Grummich P, Nimsky C, Pauli E, et al. Combining fMRI and MEG increases the reliability of presurgical language localization: a clinical study on the difference between and congruence of both modalities. Neuroimage. 2006;32(4):1793-803.

52. Zhang J, Mei S, Liu Q, et al. fMRI and DTI assessment of patients undergoing radical epilepsy surgery. Epilepsy Res. 2013;104(3):253-63.

53. Winston GP, Yogarajah M, Symms MR, et al. Diffusion tensor imaging tractography to visualize the relationship of the optic radiation to epileptogenic lesions prior to neurosurgery. Epilepsia. 2011;52(8):1430-8.

54. Nimsky C, Ganslandt O, Hastreiter P, et al. Preoperative and intraoperative diffusion tensor imaging-based fiber tracking in glioma surgery. Neurosurgery. 2005;56(1):130-7.

55. Nimsky C, Ganslandt O, Hastreiter P, et al. Intraoperative diffusion-tensor MR imaging: shifting of white matter tracts during neurosurgical procedures – initial experience. Radiology. 2005;234:218-25.

56. Fisher R, Salanova V, Witt T, et al. Electrical stimulation of the anterior nucleus of thalamus for treatment of refractory epilepsy. Epilepsia. 2010;51(5):899-908.

57. Henderson JM, Tkach J, Phillips M, et al. Permanent neurological deficit related to magnetic resonance imaging in a patient with implanted deep brain stimulation electrodes for Parkinson's disease: case report. Neurosurgery. 2005;57(5):E1063.

58. Spiegel J, Fuss G, Backens M, et al. Transient dystonia following magnetic resonance imaging in a patient with deep brain stimulation electrodes for the treatment of Parkinson disease. Case report. J Neurosurg. 2003;99(4):772-4.

13

Impact of Intraoperative Magnetic Resonance Imaging on Extent of Resection

Moritz Scherer

BACKGROUND

Intraoperative magnetic resonance imaging (iMRI) has been introduced into neurosurgical operating rooms (ORs) almost 20 years ago to provide accurate image-based resection guidance and compensation for brain shift in neuronavigation. From the initial description of iMRI implementation and workflows from Brigham and Women's Hospital in Boston and Heidelberg University Hospital[1-3] until today, various studies have been published analyzing the benefit of iMRI guidance in neurosurgical procedures and evaluating the impact of iMRI on patient outcome. Today, resection guidance is still the main indication for its use during surgery in high- and low-grade gliomas, pituitary tumors, and other skull base lesions. However, it also provides an image framework for stereotactic procedures, biopsies, deep brain stimulation and can assist in resections of vascular brain pathology and epilepsy surgery.[4-9]

This article aims at summarizing the evolution of iMRI in modern neurosurgery with a special focus on glioma surgery. An overview of different aspects of resection guidance and the impact on surgical results are presented.

IMPACT OF INTRAOPERATIVE MAGNETIC RESONANCE IMAGING IN GLIOMA SURGERY

Extent of Resection is a Key Outcome Parameter

Diagnosed with an intracranial mass lesion, patients need confirmation of histological diagnosis in order to receive adequate and specific therapy. Beyond delivering a histologic diagnosis, however, a radical preferably complete resection of the tumor has been identified as a key outcome parameter in glioma patients in recent years. Routine acquisition of early postresection MRI scans within 48–72 hours after surgery allowed for a correlation of the extent of resection (EOR) and different outcome measures in high- and low-grade gliomas.

Up-to-date, no large randomized study has explicitly evaluated outcome after gross total resections (GTR) versus partial resections (PR) in intracranial gliomas and from the current point of view, ethical considerations will prohibit such studies in the future. Existing studies therefore have to be interpreted in the light of known limitations of retrospective studies or subgroup evaluations. Nevertheless, a solid body of evidence has evolved in the past to conclude that a radical tumor resection harbors survival benefits, which lead to the establishment of EOR as a key outcome parameter in glioma treatment lately.

Extent of Resection in High-grade Gliomas

In high-grade gliomas (HGG), surgery has been shown to impact on survival but is also performed to relief symptoms caused by the rapidly growing tumor mass and brain edema. Due to the infiltrative growth behavior of HGG, a complete resection of the tumor is never feasible but a GTR of solid tumor is usually defined by the removal of the contrast-enhancing portion of the tumor apparent on preoperative MRI.

Highest available evidence was derived from a German multicenter randomized controlled trial by Stummer et al., comparing 5-aminolevulinic acid (5-ALA) fluorescence-guided with conventional white-light HGG resections. In a balanced restratification for resection extent, all patients that with GTR had significantly longer overall survival compared to incompletely resected patients (16.7 vs 11.8 months, respectively, p < 0.0001). Regarding the role of a tumor resection compared to mere tumor biopsy, Kreth et al. have prospectively shown that survival after incomplete or subtotal resection is clearly inferior to patients with GTR and is comparable to patients that only received tumor biopsy.

The value of incomplete resections is hence questioned in this context, since this would suggest the limitation of surgical treatment to sole tumor biopsy in cases where GTR is not feasible because of impending neurologic deficits. Sanai et al. present a review of literature with a focus on precise calculation of EOR and clear statistical measures. They report a statistically significant beneficial effect from maximized EOR in 16/28 HGG studies. Moreover, another series by the same author including 500 primary glioblastomas (GBM) could also illustrate EOR thresholds for improved survival and demonstrated pronounced survival effects even in the 95–100% EOR range. Besides primary GBM, which were primarily evaluated for their outcome after surgery, also recurrent GBM were susceptible to surgical treatment with significant effect on survival.[10-17]

Extent of Resection in Low-grade Gliomas

Low-grade gliomas (LGG) patients often show no to mild clinical symptoms but eventual malignant tumor progression will aggravate symptoms and reduce life expectancy. The infiltrative growth behavior of low-grade tumors and their eventual tendency to infiltrate, progress and dedifferentiate pose a tremendous therapeutic challenge. Surgery used to be the only promising treatment option for LGG, since results from radiotherapy or chemotherapy were limited. However, recent randomized studies also suggest benefits from radiation therapy, which might affect treatment regimen in the future.

Due to their slow growth, mild symptoms, and a younger age of the patients at first diagnosis watch and wait regimen are still applied in LGG until a definite therapy is initiated later on. Based on current evidence, this approach should be questioned, however, when surgery alternately can safely remove the tumor, diminishing the risk of malignant transformation or appearance of neurologic symptoms or seizures. Literature provides support for radical surgery in supratentorial LGG that are amenable for a safe resection as the treatment of choice. Jakola et al. present a cohort study based on a national registry clearly favoring an early radical resection of LGG over an initial watch and wait regimen. Smith et al. present the largest series of World Health Organization (WHO) grade II LGG and illustrate a significant and independent benefit of higher EOR for progression-free and overall survival in their cohort. In the systematic review of Sanai et al., 9/10 selected LGG-studies were in favor of extensive resection of LGG lesions. EOR was an independent positive prognosticator in seven of these studies. Even in case of tumor recurrence, Ahmadi et al. could show a beneficial effect of repeat surgery in terms of time to malignant progression an overall survival.[13,18-23]

In summary, GTR in contrast to a subtotal resection (STR) or PR of the tumor has been identified as an independent prognostic factor for survival in HGG. A radical surgical approach has significant survival benefits also in LGG and recent results should call the utility of watch-and-wait regimen into question.

IMPACT OF INTRAOPERATIVE MAGNETIC RESONANCE IMAGING GUIDANCE ON EXTENT OF RESECTION

With the identification of EOR as a key outcome parameter in glioma patients, this clearly defines the target in contemporary glioma surgery being a GTR of the tumor while warranting neurologic integrity and function after surgery. Accurate delineation of tumor and normal brain parenchyma remains one of the major challenges in glioma surgery, however, in recent years many technical advancements have been developed to assist the surgeon in locating and precisely confining brain tumors. Alongside with multimodal neuronavigation, intraoperative ultrasound and 5-ALA in GBM, iMRI is used in a growing number of centers for tumor resection control. Reports of increased EOR and improved patient prognosis have accumulated over recent years and other advantages such as compensation for brain shift through intraoperative update of neuronavigation have been pointed out. At the Department of Neurosurgery at Heidelberg University Hospital, iMRI guidance is implemented into daily routine in the resection process of intracranial gliomas since 2010. Nowadays, up to 180 iMRI-guided tumor resections are performed per year. iMRI is additionally used for resection control in pituitary surgery and for planning in stereotactic biopsies and deep brain stimulations as illustrated in **Figure 13.1**.

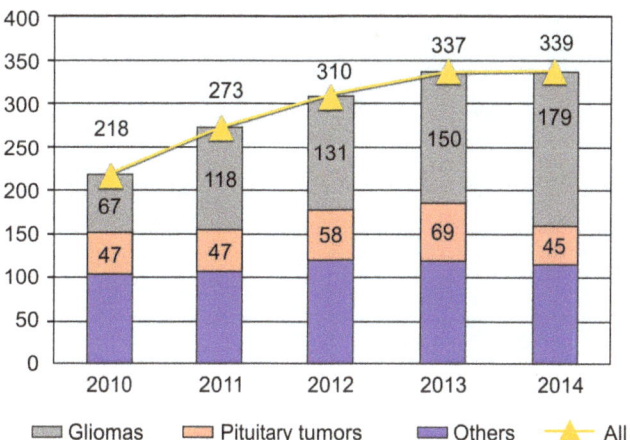

Figure 13.1 Cases of intraoperative magnetic resonance imaging-guided surgery at Heidelberg University Hospital from 2010–2014

Intraoperative MRI in High-grade Gliomas

To corroborate the contribution of iMRI to higher EOR and better rates of GTR, a bundle of retrospective studies and cohort analyses have been published including analysis of patient survival. Among them, Senft et al. conducted the only randomized controlled trial concerning the benefit of iMRI for resection results and survival. In their cohort of 49 HGG cases scheduled for a total resection of the tumor, randomization assigned patients either to receive iMRI-guided (0.15 Tesla), or conventional microneurosurgical extirpation of the tumor. In the iMRI resection group, rate of GTR at 96% was significantly larger compared to 68% of cases in the conventional surgery group (p = 0.023). This randomized study successfully showed an improvement of the primary outcome measure which was the rate of GTR but lacked power and cohort size to also underscore survival benefits directly associated with iMRI surgery. Another criticism arouse about the comparably small median tumor size of 20 cm included in this randomized study. Even though this selection is a limitation, which was most likely the trade-off for its randomization, potential benefits of iMRI guidance would be expected to be even larger in bigger tumors. In other words, the failure-to-achieve GTR under white-light conventional surgery in 32% of cases particularly underscores the need for resection guidance even in comparably small tumors and advocates the use of iMRI in this regard.[8] An illustrative case for iMRI guidance in GBM surgery is given in **Figures 13.2A to C**. In similar fashion, multiple clinical studies conducted volumetric analysis of tumor size throughout the resection process to illustrate the volumetric contribution of iMRI guidance to tumor resections. Results concordantly show an increase in EOR on postoperative imaging compared to iMRI values and yield final EOR values of 85–96%.[24-27] Oftentimes,

iMRI is challenged by 5-ALA fluorescence particularly as a more time and cost-effective and as a real-time tissue staining for intraoperative resection guidance in high-grade gliomas. However, both methods should be regarded as two alternate guidance tools with specific advantages as well as drawbacks that justify its use in certain cases. This will be discussed on later in this chapter. So far, the advantage of iMRI is depiction of EOR during surgery and delineation of residual tumor independently from tumor location, extension, craniotomy size, and visual angles compared to 5-ALA procedures. Moreover, by showing residual contrast enhancing tumor and also EOR, iMRI *directly* depicts the primary outcome parameter in glioma surgery to the surgeon during resection and gives the possibility to immediately impact on this outcome parameter.

The impact on survival was also evaluated in some iMRI series. However, a direct effect of use of iMRI and improved survival could not be found in any iMRI series up-to-date. Instead, an indirect effect was observed since GTR has repeatedly been shown to positively correlate with improved survival, which was in turn significantly more frequently achieved when iMRI was employed for resection guidance. In that manner, Wirtz et al. reported improved survival in GTR patients compared to PR after iMRI surgery back in the year 2000.[28] More recent results suggest a significant increase in progression-free survival (PFS) and overall survival (OS) after GTR achieved by iMRI surgery.[26,29-31]

Above all, iMRI series unequivocally emphasize the safety aspect of this method. Patient transport or intraoperative scanning in the OR environment did not cause any significant morbidity during or related to the procedure itself. Moreover, literature does not suggest any correlation for continued resections after iMRI and appearance of new postoperative neurologic deficits. Permanent new neurologic deficits are

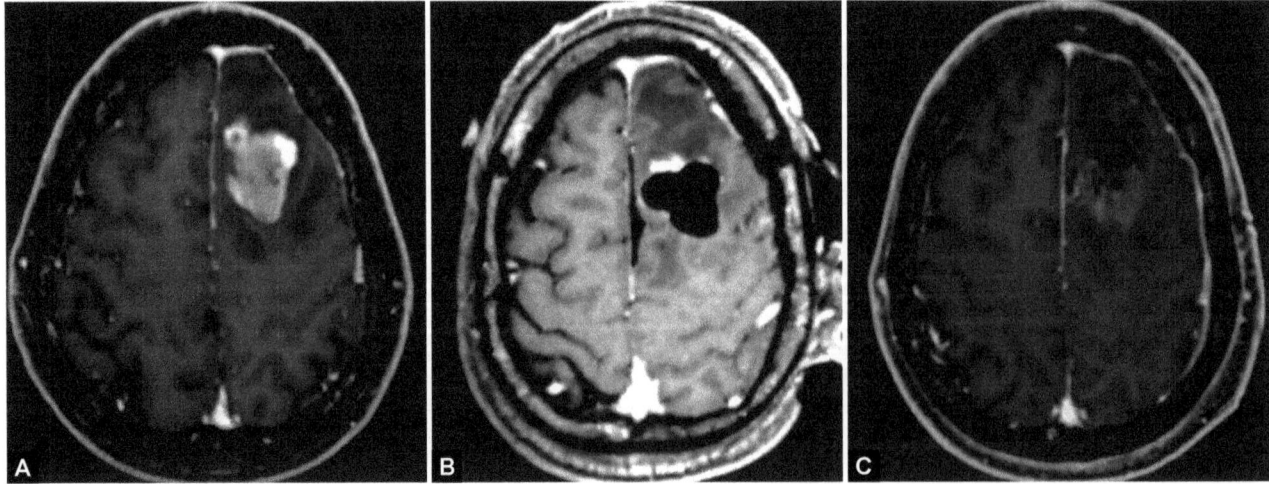

Figures 13.2A to C Intraoperative magnetic resonance imaging-guided resection of a glioblastoma: (A) Preoperative MRI; (B) Intraoperative MRI with residual tumor at the ventral aspect of the resection cavity; (C) Early postoperative MRI showing complete resection of contrast-enhancing tumor

reported in 5–13% of cases after iMRI-guided surgery which is in good concordance to other series from 5-ALA-guided or conventional resection series.[8,11,15,24,26] Concluding from the impact of iMRI on EOR, survival analysis and safety evaluation, iMRI has the potential to assist the surgeon in achieving the seemingly contradictory goal of a safe and radical tumor resection.

Intraoperative MRI in Low-grade Gliomas

Especially in LGG cases, high-field iMRI scanners harbor a great potential benefit for resection guidance providing imaging at full diagnostic quality to delineate nonenhancing tumor. Up-to-date, there are only few retrospective studies available evaluating LGG outcomes after iMRI-guided resection. In 2005, a group from Brigham and Women's Hospital in Boston compared long-term survival from 156 iMRI-guided LGG resections to a matched cohort from a national registry. Their central finding was a significant reduction of 1-, 2- and 5-years age and histology-adjusted death rates compared to the national registry when iMRI was used for resection guidance. Stratifying for total and subtotal LGG tumor removal, a 1.4 times higher risk of recurrence [95% confidence interval (CI), 0.7–3.1] and a 4.9 times higher risk of death (95% CI, 0.61–40.0) was apparent when lesions were only removed subtotally.[32] A retrospective multicenter analysis of benefits of iMRI guidance in WHO grade II gliomas confirmed these previous results. In this analysis, 288 cases were included from six German iMRI centers and analyzed for the effect of GTR or PR on tumor progression and survival. As a central finding in this series, GTR significantly increased PFS [hazard ratio (HR) 0.44, p < 0.01] compared to a partial resection of the tumor. Moreover, survival was significantly

inferior in patients where GTR was intended but not achieved despite use of iMRI. These cases of "failed" GTR after iMRI surgery had PFS comparable to intended PR. This suggests a strong correlation of residual tumor volume and tendency to progression in WHO grade II tumors and puts radical surgery in favor for first-line therapy of resectable tumors.[23] Additionally, the effect of low-field (<0.5 Tesla) and high-field (1.5 Tesla) iMRI upon resection guidance was evaluated in this series. GTR of a tumor was significantly more likely when a high-field iMRI machine was used compared to a low-field machine in this multicenter analysis (OR 0.51, p < 0.01). This points at better tissue discrimination and image resolution on fluid-attenuated inversion recovery (FLAIR) imaging, which is facilitated by higher-field-strength magnets.[7] Not to mention, neurologic morbidity was comparable to other surgical LGG series and no association of iMRI guidance and neurologic deficits after surgery could be found in these series. An example for iMRI-guided resection of a LGG is given in **Figures 13.3A to C**. Evidence is in favor for use of iMRI as a valuable and safe tool for resection guidance in LGG comparable to benefits observed in HGG. Moreover, tumor resections in LGG offer the potential to significantly postpone progression and malignization, which makes the pursuit of even minimal tumor remnants worth the effort.[23]

IMPACT OF INTRAOPERATIVE MAGNETIC RESONANCE IMAGING UPON THE RESECTION PROCESS

Few studies have evaluated the impact of iMRI guidance upon the course of surgery and upon surgical decision making during surgery. Knowledge about factors that influence

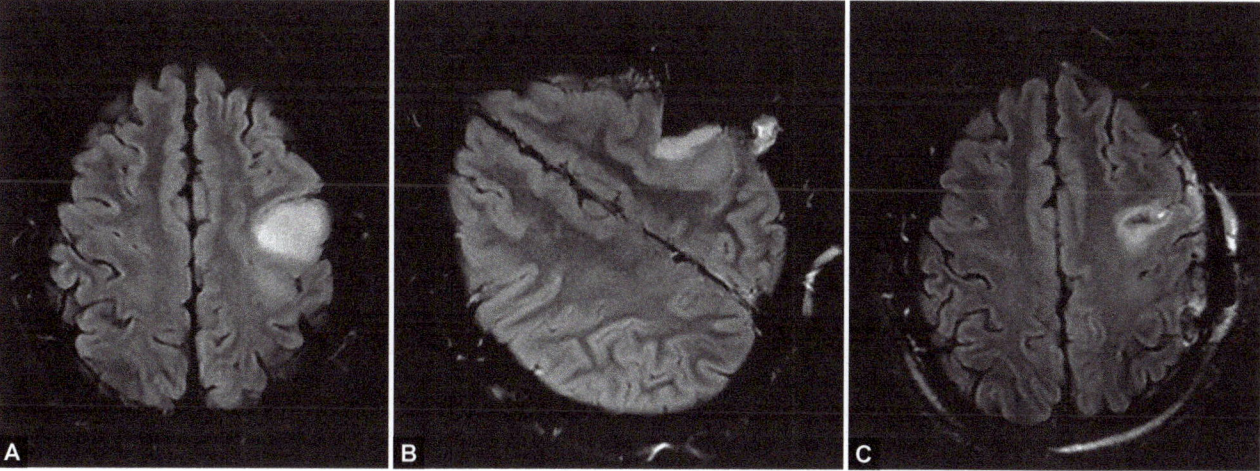

Figures 13.3A to C Intraoperative magnetic resonance imaging-guided resection of a low-grade astrocytoma: (A) Preoperative MRI; (B) Intraoperative MRI showing residual tumor at the dorsal aspect of the resection cavity; (C) Early postoperative MRI showing complete resection of FLAIR hyperintensity despite signs of postresection injury around the resection cavity
Abbreviation: FLAIR, fluid-attenuated inversion recovery.

the frequency of additional resections after iMRI and the surgeon's intraoperative impression of EOR can be of interest for preoperative planning and identification of ideal cases to book for iMRI surgery.

Additional Resections after Intraoperative MRI

Depending upon the iMRI set-up (one-room versus two-room, magnet-to-patient versus patient-to-magnet) and upon the individual workflows at iMRI centers throughout the world, the rate of additional resections after iMRI to remove residual tumor can be affected. Repeat intraoperative scanning can assist in safe approximation of tumor boundaries but is achieved at the expense of prolonged duration of the procedure and also accumulation of contrast media within the parenchyma. This can cause fainted tissue contrasts in repeat scanning and also systemic, dose-dependent side effects.[33,34]

In literature, continued resections after iMRI are reported in 25–70% of cases throughout all types of gliomas WHO grade I–IV with a peak for additional resections in WHO grade II tumors with up to 80%.[7,8,24,26,35] This suggests a benefit of iMRI guidance in a majority of cases assuming that resections would have been terminated unless an iMRI would have been available. However, the surgeon could rely on the intraoperative scan in most of the studies reporting their additional resection rates, which could have lead to premature interruption of surgery and premature scanning. Consequently, the amount of tumor removed after iMRI does not represent the true benefit of iMRI guidance due to this limitation. To answer the question in how many cases an iMRI really is needed and provides additional information about residual tumor to the surgeon at a point where he would otherwise terminate surgery can be expected by a randomized, triple-blind study by Wu et al. In this study design, the surgeon is blinded to whether iMRI is used or not during surgery until the surgeon terminates his resection based on personal criterions. After that, he is unblinded and resection can be continued after iMRI was performed according to randomization[36] (clinicaltrails.gov: NCT01479686).

Concerning variables that trigger additional resections after iMRI, we could identify initial tumor volume (p < 0.01) and WHO grade (p < 0.05) as significant variables in a prospective series of 224 cases of mixed glioma entities. Interestingly, tumor location, proximity to eloquent regions and the goal of surgery being GTR or PR did not affect the rate of additional resections in this series. Moreover, a mutual benefit of iMRI guidance for junior as well as senior neurosurgeons has been suggested, since surgical experience did not correlate with observed rates of additional resections after iMRI in this series.[35]

Under the condition that iMRI guidance is implemented routinely in all glioma resections at a certain center, it has to be assumed that the rate of additional resections after iMRI will swing into a certain level over time. Depending upon application of additional surgical guidance tools and different iMRI set-ups, rates are expected to be rather high and could affect up to two-thirds of resections.

INTRAOPERATIVE IMPRESSION OF EXTENT OF RESECTION

The infiltrative nature of gliomas complicate the delineation of tumor tissue from normal brain during surgery and thus, require additional guidance tools to improve surgical results. The surgeon's intraoperative impression of EOR is known to be commonly incorrect in this regard. Surgeons have been shown to regularly overestimate EOR judged from their intraoperative perception. As discussed earlier, iMRI is an established guidance tool to improve results after glioma surgery and to reduce undesired incomplete resections.

Another aspect in some iMRI studies was to evaluate the discrepancy between the surgeons intraoperative perception of EOR and the objective depiction of intraoperative EOR delivered by iMRI. Moreover, the value of iMRI guidance for surgeons of different experience levels was analyzed.

From previous series, it has been reported that GTR is successfully achieved in only 36–68% of cases with conventional white-light surgery. Hence, residual tumor is unintentionally overlooked in a significant number of cases without additional guidance tools. A series by Orringer et al. evaluated the surgeons impression of EOR during conventional surgery. When a GTR was perceived by the surgeon according to his intraoperative impression, residual tumor was still delineated on postoperative MRI in 70% of these cases. However, when the surgeon expected an incomplete resection, this was true in 96% of cases according to postoperative imaging. In other words, when it comes to rule out residual tumor there is frequent dissonance of subjective impression and objective evaluation of EOR provided by postoperative MRI.

In a before mentioned prospective series of 224 iMRI-guided resections, the ability of the surgeon to predict the likelihood of an additional resection after iMRI was analyzed by inquiring the intraoperative impression prior to the acquisition of an iMRI.

Results were similar to conventional surgical techniques. When the surgeon expected residual tumor on iMRI and also expected an additional resection accordingly, additional resections were frequently performed. The positive predictive value (PPV) of the intraoperative impression was 93.1% (95% CI, 77.2–99.15%) in this study. When it came to rule out residual tumor and to exclude an additional resection however, these evaluations were correct in only 44% (95% CI, 34.2–53.4%) of cases and additional resections were performed in 56% of cases against the surgeon's initial expectation. This study indicates how iMRI can compensate for the imprecise intraoperative impression of EOR and also illustrates how often surgical results and intraoperative decision-making is influenced by results from iMRI.

A pronounced benefit of iMRI guidance could moreover be expected in junior surgeons that lack surgical experience to delineate residual tumor by conventional visual and haptic techniques. However, the earlier mentioned study found no significant correlation for surgical experience with either residual intraoperative tumor volume or rate of additional resections after iMRI in uni- and multiple regression analysis. Junior, intermediate experienced and senior neurosurgeons with more than 10 years of surgical experience had comparable rates of additional resections in this series suggesting a comparable amount of uncertainty regarding the EOR achieved under conventional surgical techniques. As mentioned before, the ability to rule out residual tumor from visual perception was poor but interestingly improved with increasing surgical experience. In the earlier mentioned study, residual tumor was correctly ruled out in 26.7% (95% CI, 7.8–55.1%) by junior surgeons. Intermediate experienced surgeons evaluated EOR correctly in 38.2% (95% CI, 22.2–56.4%) of cases and senior colleagues reached 50.0% (95% CI, 36.6–63.4%) of correct estimations.

Nevertheless, overall accuracy remained poor and did not exceed 50% even in senior surgeons with experience more than 10 years in glioma surgery. This discrepancy justifies the implementation of surgical guidance tools in general and iMRI in particular in order to improve resection results in the light of survival benefits conveyed by a radical resection. Another aspect of this analysis was, that omission of iMRI guidance in experienced surgeons or presumed straightforward tumor resections cannot be supported after interpretation of data. The mutual value of iMRI guidance for surgeons of various experience levels recommends iMRI as a surgical learning tool and also as a measure of quality control. Immediate feedback about intraoperative EOR, iMRI can promote an optimized learning progress in junior surgeons, while warranting uncompromised resection results comparable to senior colleagues.[15,24,35,37,38]

LIMITATIONS OF INTRAOPERATIVE MAGNETIC RESONANCE IMAGING RESEARCH AND FUTURE CONSIDERATIONS

Limitation of Intraoperative MRI Surgery

Besides iMRI surgery being a costly procedure by financial and timely means, some limitations lie in the method itself that can only be overcome by addition of other resection tools. The interaction between iMRI and neuronavigation solved problems with brain shift to some extent. However, iMRI surgery still suffers from limitations of image-guided surgery and does not provide real-time guidance compared to 5-ALA or intraoperative ultrasound guidance. Another

aspect that is not sufficiently covered by iMRI resection guidance is monitoring of neurologic function during surgery. Various attempts have been made to integrate functional data into multimodal neuronavigation and also to acquire updated functional imaging during surgery. These surrogate parameters for functionality help to define safety margins and have been shown to increase safety during resections of eloquent tumors. However, only in combination with awake craniotomy and electrophysiological monitoring and mapping, functional boundaries can really be safely approached during a tumor resection.[39-42]

DEFINITION OF TUMOR DIMENSION AND TARGET RESECTION VOLUME

The accurate definition of tumor dimension and the target resection volume accordingly is still an unsolved issue up to day. Regarding the significance for patient outcome that is ascribed to EOR nowadays, recommendations how to handle and define tumor dimensions are very limited. Usually high-grade tumors are defined according to contrast enhancement on preoperative T1-weighted imaging, while low-grade, nonenhancing tumors are delineated on T2 based FLAIR sequences. In HGG, one has to keep in mind that contrast enhancement is only an indirectly enhancement of pathology since enhancement is based upon extravasation of contrast media into the parenchyma instead of directly staining pathologic tissue. The value of other imaging sequences like FLAIR or magnetic resonance (MR) perfusion and diffusion imaging in the evaluation and prognosis of high-grade tumors have been evolving lately and might impact the way, we appraise the extension of brain tumors into the parenchyma in the future.[43-45] Alongside with better understanding of tumor imaging on preoperative MRI, also the definition of resection targets might change based on these new criterions. The role of iMRI will be to pursuit this development and to provide the surgeon with all imaging information needed also intraoperatively in order to achieve a best possible resection for the patient. However, the boundaries to every tumor resection in the brain are always set by functionality which always have to be respected regardless of the imaging sequences used for definition of tumor dimension.

DELINEATION OF RESIDUAL TUMOR ON INTRAOPERATIVE MAGNETIC RESONANCE IMAGING

Delineation of residual tumor on iMRI appears trivial to persons that are not involved in the method. In fact, iMRI data needs careful interpretation of trained radiologists and the surgeon in charge in order to tap the full potential of intraoperative imaging. Intraoperative artifacts at liquid or tissue or air borders, blood clots or hemostatic agents complicate image evaluation intraoperatively. Especially, the temporary disruption of the blood-brain barrier and subsequent leakage of contrast media due to surgical trauma can cause contrast enhancement in otherwise healthy brain parenchyma. This challenge has been addressed by different methods of contrast media appliance. Dynamic susceptibility contrast enhancement (DSC) and also intraoperative MR perfusion imaging helps to increase the diagnostic yield in iMRI and to provide accurate delineation of residual tumor.[46,47] Both dynamic imaging methods have been shown to improve anatomic resolution and show better delineation of neoplastic tissue compared to standard contrast-enhanced anatomic T1 sequences and should be routinely available in iMRI protocols to clear equivocal intraoperative imaging.

UNINTENDED INCOMPLETE RESECTIONS

Despite the use of iMRI guidance in glioma surgery, some patients experience unwanted incomplete resections although a complete, i.e. GTR, was planned. This does not include cases where tumor was deliberately left behind for reasons of safety and preservation of functionality but unintended incomplete resections. This is observed in roughly 18% of GBM resections (personal observation) and in 24% of LGG resections in a multicenter series.[7,48] There are some possible explanations to the failure to achieve GTR, which should thoroughly be addressed since the affected patients suffer from a significantly reduced survival prognosis compared to patients were an intended GTR was also achieved.

Firstly, different field strength and imaging protocols in intraoperative and postoperative MRI could result in inferior tissue contrast intraoperatively. When postoperative imaging is performed at 3 Tesla, this could delineate small contrast enhancing remnants that were invisible on intraoperative 1.5 Tesla imaging. Secondly, the time from appliance of contrast media to imaging acquisition should be comparable on intraoperative and postoperative imaging. If the time is insufficient for contrast media saturation intraoperatively, this can result in inadequate tissue contrast or absence of enhancement in some regions of interest and prevents accurate resection of residual tumor after iMRI.

After ruling out technical explanations for unwanted residual tumor postoperatively, a ceiling effect for iMRI resection guidance should be discussed. Hypothetically, a 100% GTR is not always feasible with iMRI guidance alone but requires multimodal resection guidance. A study by Coburger et al. suggests an additional benefit of combined iMRI and 5-ALA guidance in GBM surgery compared to iMRI-guided surgery alone in a matched-pair analysis of primary GBM.[48] The benefits of combined resection guidance and also the interaction of iMRI with electrophysiological mapping and monitoring and awake craniotomies will have to be evaluated in the future in order to minimize unwanted incomplete resections in glioma surgery.

PATIENT SELECTION AND NEED FOR RANDOMIZATION IN OUTCOME STUDIES

One flaw in studies evaluating the impact on iMRI on patient outcome is the lack of randomization. Absence of adequate control groups and random allocation to either iMRI or non-iMRI surgery limit conclusions in many series in literature. Moreover, many published case series reporting on the effect of iMRI-guided surgery often have significant selection bias as to the allocation of their patients to iMRI surgery. This was rarely performed according to clear criterions. But instead patients with suspected intracranial gliomas were scheduled to iMRI surgery according to the surgeon's preference or simple availability of the magnet. To our knowledge, there are only two studies evaluating the impact of iMRI on resection results in a randomized setting. Senft et al. first published their results from an ultra-low-field scanner (0.15 Tesla) and randomized their eligible patients to either iMRI or conventional white-light microneurosurgery. The second study was conducted by Wu et al. and an interims analysis was published in 2014. Both series suggest a benefit of iMRI guidance for both safety of a resection and outcome of the patients and therefore confirm results from other, non-randomized studies.[8,36]

With a growing body of evidence supporting a radical surgical approach, ethical considerations defeat the conduction of a randomized study today regarding a comparison against conventional white-light surgery. Moreover, high drop-out rates or patient crossover would have to be expected in a randomization to white-light surgery nowadays. After potentially unsuccessful white-light surgery, patients could seek a second resection of tumor remnants at a different center or would be lost in follow-up. Also, surgeons could be urged to perform an iMRI-guided, second resection after an unsuccessful first white-light attempt based on the results and recommendations in literature.

A potential aspect of future randomized research might be a comparison of different methods of resection guidance given that both methods have comparable impact and benefits on its own. From an ethical point of view, a comparison of 5-ALA guidance and iMRI guidance or a combination of both methods in high-grade gliomas might be approachable in a randomized setting since both methods have been shown to improve resection results and survival to a comparable extent.

Another approach was chosen by a German multicenter iMRI study group to evaluate benefits of intraoperative guidance tools in GBM surgery in a large, multicenter setting. To compare results after iMRI and 5-ALA-guided surgery, a parallel-group clinical trial is under way since 2015 comparing centers exclusively using iMRI with other centers which use

5-ALA fluorescence for resection guidance (clinicaltrials.gov: NCT02379572). Like in all other parallel group trials, strict inclusion criteria have to warrant comparability of patient cohorts. Results from this series are expected during the next years.

In LGG, iMRI has unparalleled ability for image-guided surgery and until today there is no comparable guidance tool available. Intraoperative ultrasound has been shown to help in tumor delineation, but accuracy and predictive value is known to be very user-dependent which limit its comparability within clinical studies.[20,49] Additionally, extensive follow-up periods necessary in the evaluation of surgical results and outcome in LGG is a major drawback for the conduction of prospective studies, also from a financial point of view.

SUMMARY AND OUTLOOK

In summary, a considerable amount of literature has evaluated the contribution and value of iMRI guidance and supports this concept for glioma surgery. Different aspects have been studied so far suggesting improved surgical results in low- and high-grade glioma surgery, which also translates into beneficial outcome and survival of the patients. Also, analysis of technical aspects of iMRI-guided resections are in favor for this method as the influence of tumor- and surgeon-related factors upon the resection result can be significantly reduced through image guidance. Since, the conduction randomized controlled trials evaluating the impact of iMRI guidance on the EOR and survival are ethically debatable from current state of knowledge, well-designed prospective observational studies might be the only way to underscore the importance and benefit of a more radical surgery for the treatment of intracranial gliomas in the future. A parallel-group clinical trial is under way to compare effects of iMRI versus 5-ALA-guided surgery for GBM. Beyond that, accurate volumetric definition of resection targets and postoperative EOR should create a common ground for future data collections and facilitate meta-analyses.

Another future challenge will be to redefine surgical outcome in the light of the revised WHO classification of gliomas. Evaluation of EOR in histology-adjusted cohorts with stratification for molecular characteristics will be required to provide sustainable estimates of survival in surgical outcome studies in the future. Beyond technical aspects, future studies also have to focus on clinical performance and quality of life after surgery in order to work out well-grounded treatment concepts also in borderline cases of elderly patients or recurrent malignant tumors.

REFERENCES

1. Black PM, Alexander E, Martin C, et al. Craniotomy for tumor treatment in an intraoperative magnetic resonance imaging unit. Neurosurgery. 1999;45(3):423-31.

2. Moriarty TM, Kikinis R, Jolesz FA, et al. Magnetic resonance imaging therapy. Intraoperative MR imaging. Neurosurg Clin N Am. 1996;7(2):323-31.

3. Wirtz CR, Bonsanto MM, Knauth M, et al. Intraoperative magnetic resonance imaging to update interactive navigation in neurosurgery: method and preliminary experience. Comput Aided Surg. 1997;2(3-4):172-9.

4. Bekelis K, Missios S, Desai A, et al. Magnetic resonance imaging/magnetic resonance angiography fusion technique for intraoperative navigation during microsurgical resection of cerebral arteriovenous malformations. Neurosurg Focus. 2012;32:E7.

5. Buchfelder M, Fahlbusch R, Ganslandt O, et al. Use of intraoperative magnetic resonance imaging in tailored temporal lobe surgeries for epilepsy. Epilepsia. 2002;43(8): 864-73.

6. Coburger J, König R, Seitz K, et al. Determining the utility of intraoperative magnetic resonance imaging for transsphenoidal surgery: a retrospective study. J Neurosurg. 2014;120(2):346-56.

7. Coburger J, Merkel A, Scherer M, et al. Low-grade glioma surgery in intraoperative magnetic resonance imaging: results of a multicenter retrospective assessment of the German Study Group for intraoperative magnetic resonance imaging. Neurosurgery. 2016;78(6):775-86.

8. Senft C, Bink A, Franz K, et al. Intraoperative MRI guidance and extent of resection in glioma surgery: a randomised, controlled trial. Lancet Oncol. 2011;12(11):997-1003.

9. Sillay KA, Rusy D, Buyan-Dent L, et al. Wide-bore 1.5 T MRI-guided deep brain stimulation surgery: initial experience and technique comparison. Clin Neurol Neurosurg. 2014;127:79-85.

10. Gorlia T, van den Bent MJ, Hegi ME, et al. Nomograms for predicting survival of patients with newly diagnosed glioblastoma: prognostic factor analysis of EORTC and NCIC trial 26981-22981/CE.3. Lancet Oncol. 2008;9(1):29-38.

11. Kreth FW, Thon N, Simon M, et al. Gross total but not incomplete resection of glioblastoma prolongs survival in the era of radiochemotherapy. Ann Oncol. 2013;24(12):3117-23.

12. Oppenlander ME, Wolf AB, Snyder LA, et al. An extent of resection threshold for recurrent glioblastoma and its risk for neurological morbidity. J Neurosurg. 2014;120(4):846-53.

13. Sanai N, Berger MS. Glioma extent of resection and its impact on patient outcome. Neurosurgery. 2008;62(4):753-64.

14. Sanai N, Polley MY, McDermott MW, et al. An extent of resection threshold for newly diagnosed glioblastomas. J Neurosurg. 2011;115(1):3-8.

15. Stummer W, Pichlmeier U, Meinel T, et al. Fluorescence-guided surgery with 5-aminolevulinic acid for resection of malignant glioma: a randomised controlled multicentre phase III trial. Lancet Oncol. 2006;7(5):392-401.

16. Stummer W, Tonn JC, Mehdorn HM, et al. Counterbalancing risks and gains from extended resections in malignant glioma surgery: a supplemental analysis from the randomized 5-aminolevulinic acid glioma resection study. Clinical article. J Neurosurg. 2011;114(3):613-23.

17. Stummer W, van den Bent MJ, Westphal M. Cytoreductive surgery of glioblastoma as the key to successful adjuvant therapies: new arguments in an old discussion. Acta Neurochir (Wien). 2011;153(6):1211-8.

18. Ahmadi R, Dictus C, Hartmann C, et al. Long-term outcome and survival of surgically treated supratentorial low-grade

glioma in adult patients. Acta Neurochir (Wien). 2009;151(11): 1359-65.

19. Jakola AS, Myrmel KS, Kloster R, et al. Comparison of a strategy favoring early surgical resection vs a strategy favoring watchful waiting in low-grade gliomas. JAMA. 2012;308(18):1881-8.

20. Jakola AS, Unsgård G, Myrmel KS, et al. Surgical strategy in grade II astrocytoma: a population-based analysis of survival and morbidity with a strategy of early resection as compared to watchful waiting. Acta Neurochir (Wien). 2013;155(12): 2227-35.

21. Potts MB, Smith JS, Molinaro AM, et al. Natural history and surgical management of incidentally discovered low-grade gliomas. J Neurosurg. 2012;116(2):365-72.

22. Sanai N, Chang S, Berger MS. Low-grade gliomas in adults. J Neurosurg. 2011;115(5):948-65.

23. Smith JS, Chang EF, Lamborn KR, et al. Role of extent of resection in the long-term outcome of low-grade hemispheric gliomas. J Clin Oncol. 2008;26(8):1338-45.

24. Hatiboglu MA, Weinberg JS, Suki D, et al. Impact of intraoperative high-field magnetic resonance imaging guidance on glioma surgery: a prospective volumetric analysis. Neurosurgery. 2009;64(6):1073-81.

25. Kubben PL, ter Meulen KJ, Schijns OE, et al. Intraoperative MRI-guided resection of glioblastoma multiforme: a systematic review. Lancet Oncol. 2011;12(11):1062-70.

26. Kuhnt D, Ganslandt O, Schlaffer SM, et al. Quantification of glioma removal by intraoperative high-field magnetic resonance imaging: an update. Neurosurgery. 2011;69(4): 852-62.

27. Schneider JP, Trantakis C, Rubach M, et al. Intraoperative MRI to guide the resection of primary supratentorial glioblastoma multiforme: a quantitative radiological analysis. Neuroradiology. 2005;47(7):489-500.

28. Wirtz CR, Knauth M, Staubert A, et al. Clinical evaluation and follow-up results for intraoperative magnetic resonance imaging in neurosurgery. Neurosurgery. 2000;46(5):1112-20.

29. Coburger J, Wirtz CR, König RW. Impact of extent of resection and recurrent surgery on clinical outcome and overall survival in a consecutive series of 170 patients for glioblastoma in intraoperative high field iMRI. J Neurosurg Sci. 2015. [Epub ahead of print].

30. Kuhnt D, Becker A, Ganslandt O, et al. Correlation of the extent of tumor volume resection and patient survival in surgery of glioblastoma multiforme with high-field intraoperative MRI guidance. Neuro Oncol. 2011;13(12):1339-48.

31. Roder C, Bisdas S, Ebner FH, et al. Maximizing the extent of resection and survival benefit of patients in glioblastoma surgery: high-field iMRI versus conventional and 5-ALA-assisted surgery. Eur J Surg Oncol. 2014;40(3):297-304.

32. Claus EB, Horlacher A, Hsu L, et al. Survival rates in patients with low-grade glioma after intraoperative magnetic resonance image guidance. Cancer. 2005;103(6):1227-33.

33. Knauth M, Aras N, Wirtz CR, et al. Surgically induced intracranial contrast enhancement: potential source of diagnostic error in intraoperative MR imaging. Am J Neuroradiol. 1999;20(8):1547-53.

34. Knauth M, Wirtz CR, Tronnier VM, et al. Intraoperative MR imaging increases the extent of tumor resection in patients with high-grade gliomas. Am J Neuroradiol. 1999;20(9): 1642-6.

35. Scherer M, Jungk C, Younsi A, et al. Factors triggering an additional resection and determining residual tumor volume on intraoperative MRI: analysis from a prospective single-center registry of supratentorial gliomas. Neurosurg Focus. 2016;40(3):E4.

36. Wu JS, Gong X, Song YY, et al. 3.0-T intraoperative magnetic resonance imaging-guided resection in cerebral glioma surgery: interim analysis of a prospective, randomized, triple-blind, parallel-controlled trial. Clin Neurosurg. 2014;61(1): 145-54.

37. Albert FK, Forsting M, Sartor K, et al. Early postoperative magnetic resonance imaging after resection of malignant glioma: objective evaluation of residual tumor and its influence on regrowth and prognosis. Neurosurgery. 1994;34(1):45-60.

38. Orringer D, Lau D, Khatri S, et al. Extent of resection in patients with glioblastoma: limiting factors, perception of resectability, and effect on survival. J Neurosurg. 2012;117(5):851-9.

39. Duffau H. The conceptual limitation to relying on intraoperative magnetic resonance imaging in glioma surgery. World Neurosurg. 2014;82(5):601-3.

40. Kuhnt D, Bauer MH, Becker A, et al. Intraoperative visualization of fiber tracking based reconstruction of language pathways in glioma surgery. Neurosurgery. 2012;70(4):911-9.

41. Nimsky C, Ganslandt O, Buchfelder M, et al. Intraoperative visualization for resection of gliomas: the role of functional neuronavigation and intraoperative 1.5 T MRI. Neurol Res. 2006;28(5):482-7.

42. Nimsky C, Ganslandt O, von Keller B, et al. Intraoperative high-field MRI: anatomical and functional imaging. Acta Neurochir Suppl. 2006;98:87-95.

43. Elson A, Bovi J, Siker M, et al. Evaluation of absolute and normalized apparent diffusion coefficient (ADC) values within the post-operative T2/FLAIR volume as adverse prognostic indicators in glioblastoma. J Neurooncol. 2015;122(3):549-58.

44. Grabowski MM, Recinos PF, Nowacki AS, et al. Residual tumor volume versus extent of resection: predictors of survival after surgery for glioblastoma. J Neurosurg. 2014;121(5):1115-23.

45. Li YM, Suki D, Hess K, et al. The influence of maximum safe resection of glioblastoma on survival in 1229 patients: Can we do better than gross-total resection? J Neurosurg. 2016;124(4):977-88.

46. Roder C, Bender B, Ritz R, et al. Intraoperative visualization of residual tumor: the role of perfusion-weighted imaging in a high-field intraoperative magnetic resonance scanner. Neurosurgery. 2013;72(2):ons151-8.

47. Ulmer S, Helle M, Jansen O, et al. Intraoperative dynamic susceptibility contrast weighted magnetic resonance imaging (iDSC-MRI)—Technical considerations and feasibility. Neuroimage. 2009;45(1):38-43.

48. Coburger J, Hagel V, Wirtz CR, et al. Surgery for glioblastoma: impact of the combined use of 5-aminolevulinic acid and intraoperative MRI on extent of resection and survival. PLoS One. 2015;10(6):e0131872.

49. Majchrzak K, Kaspera W, Bobek-Billewicz B, et al. The assessment of prognostic factors in surgical treatment of low-grade gliomas: a prospective study. Clin Neurol Neurosurg. 2012;114(8):1135-44.

14

Intraoperative Imaging in Pituitary Surgeries

Sudhir Dubey, Deepak Bhangale

INTRODUCTION

Pituitary adenomas are among the most frequent primary intracranial neoplasms and account for 10–15% of all intracranial tumors. Annual incidence is of 0.4–8.2/100,000 population. The overall estimated prevalence as assessed by imaging and autopsy studies is 16.7%. Symptomatic pituitary adenomas may occur in up to 1 in 1,064 patients, with overall prevalence of 80–90 per 100,000 patients. They account for 25% of surgical resections for brain tumors.[1]

Pathophysiologically, they result from the monoclonal expansion of genetically altered adenohypophyseal cells. Mutations along the traditional oncological pathways and epigenetic changes lead to tumor formation.[1] Pathologically, they are mostly benign. In only 0.1–0.2% cases, they are pituitary carcinomas.

Benign tumors present anywhere in the body can normally be cured if they can be excised totally. But, pituitary adenomas are a challenge. They straddle both extra- and intra-axially, especially when they invade through the boundaries of sella. They are in relation to the cavernous sinus on either sides (containing one pair of internal carotid arteries and three pair of nerves) and the suprasellar, interpeduncular, and interoptic cisterns with their constituent structures (internal carotid artery and basilar artery with their branches, optic apparatus, pituitary stalk, floor of III ventricle, hypothalamus, thalamus, medial frontal, and temporal lobe). Thus they have been described to occupy the most precious real estate of the body.[2]

The goals of pituitary surgery are:
- Total excision is the primary goal which leads to cure from the disease
- Decompression of the optic apparatus (four pair of cranial nerves)
- Preservation and restoration of pituitary functions.

The surgery for lesions of pituitary gland has been evolving since 1889 when Sir Victor Horsley attempted transcranial pituitary excision. Discovery of X-rays by Roentgen in 1895 leads to its rapid use in diagnosis and management of pituitary disorders. Italian physician, David Giordano, developed the transsphenoidal approach. In 1907, the first transsphenoidal surgery was performed by Schloffer. Hirsch performed the first endonasal, transseptal transsphenoid approach in 1910. Halstead contributed to sublabial approach. Cushing embraced transnasal submucosal approach but transitioned to transcranial approach, though his patients who underwent transphenoid approach were discharged in better state without any increase in mortality.[1] Norman Dott and Guiot persisted with transnasal approach and introduction of intraoperative fluoroscopy by Guiot led to wider acceptance of transsphenoidal approach. Hardy used fluoroscopy with microscopy and this approach is in vogue till the present day.[1] Fluroscope assisted microsurgery became the "gold standard" for excision of pituitary adenomas. Endoscopy was pursued by Guiot and Janikowski. But, it was the work of Jho and Carrau was seminal in establishing endoscopy for resection of pituitary adenomas. Intraoperative magnetic resonance imaging (iMRI) was first used in 1994 by Black for intracranial pathologies including for pituitary adenomas.[3]

Despite such advancement, complete resection and cure remains elusive in a significant percentage of patients. Recurrence and residual tumor is attributed to:
- Cavernous sinus invasion
- Encasement of carotid artery
- Frond-like extension to temporal or frontal lobes
- Multicompartment disease
- Incomplete visualization.

The removal of tumor adjacent to vital structures (as earlier) may lead to catastrophe which leads to morbidity and mortality. On the other hand, incomplete visualization may lead to postoperative residual tumor that could have been safely removed during initial operation. Residual tumor requires treatment with radiation therapy, repeat operation or pharmacotherapy, all of which could have been avoided had the residual tumor been appreciated during the operation.

INTRAOPERATIVE MAGNETIC RESONANCE IMAGING

The field of neurosurgery has always been the one in which the accuracy of its procedures is very important. It is closely linked to the innovations in neuroimaging that accompany it. The surgical microscope was introduced by Carl-Olof Siggesson Nylén, a Swedish otolaryngologist in 1921. This was a very important milestone in the development of neurosurgical techniques. It increased the precision of interventions beyond the limitations of the naked eye.[4] Its use started in the late 1950s when William House developed new techniques for temporal bone surgery. However, Gazi Yasargil in 1953 was the first neurosurgeon to make use of the surgical microscope when he was working with Professor Hugo Krayenbühl in Switzerland.[5]

Later on, frame-based and frameless stereotactic systems were developed. They used preoperative computed tomography (CT) and MRI and offered three-dimensional maps for neuronavigation. These aided immensely in the exploration of the brain.[6] MRI in particular was appealing because it provided unique soft tissue resolution and multiple contrast mechanisms. Furthermore, the ability to acquire tomographic images in multiple planes greatly helped.[7,8] Despite these benefits, the use of preoperatively obtained images to guide stereotactic navigation results in inconsistencies between the virtually mapped space and the actual anatomy in real time.

These discrepancies in neuronavigation are a result of "brain shift", secondary to loss of cerebrospinal fluid (CSF), patient position, tissue resection, edema, and other factors that change the brain environment intraoperatively from its previous state during preoperative scanning.[8-12] Although these changes are minimal from the time of opening of dura but they slowly progress with time, leading to increased stereotactic errors as the operation continues.[9] To keep pace with these dynamic shifts throughout surgery, a high-resolution, intraoperative imaging solution which could appreciate these changes and redirect the neuronavigation was required. iMRI was developed for this purpose in mind. iMRI was first developed for neurosurgical operations in the mid 1990s at Brigham and Women's Hospital of the Harvard Medical School in Boston, USA with a 0.5 Tesla (T) open MRI system. Interest and acceptance of the use of iMRI technology in neurosurgical procedures grew after the work done by Black and Jolesz in 1997.[3,13]

The initial years of iMRI consisted of estimating the setup and protocols to perform procedures within the operating theater with MRI guidance.[3,14] In their beginning, iMRI systems helped to improve the efficacy of surgical resection and monitoring intraoperative complications such as acute hemorrhage, ischemia and diffuse brain edema. They were becoming increasingly present in the neurosurgical operating room, and therefore it was essential to ask if these results

extrapolated into better patient outcomes. Furthermore, it was also necessary to know, for which procedures was this benefit significant.[15] The transition from low-field iMRI systems with basic acquisition techniques and poorer imaging quality to systems with high-field magnets, the degree of precision has increased along with better image quality. The indications therefore may also continue to increase for which iMRI appears to be useful. The iMRI systems have continued to improve in their ease of use and resolution.

Intraoperative MRI systems consist of magnets ranging in field strength from 0.12–3.0T. They are subdivided accordingly into low-field (0.12–0.5T) and high-field (1.5–3.0T) systems. Although, the high-field systems enjoy advanced imaging capabilities and superior image quality such as functional MRI (fMRI) and diffusion tensor imaging (DTI), they sometimes sacrifice surgical access to the patient or time by requiring patient to be transported (within the operation room or to an adjacent but separate MRI suite).[16] Alternatively, low-field systems emphasize patient access and real-time imaging in the truest sense because many of these configurations do not require patient movement; however, their imaging resolution and capabilities are somewhat limited.[3]

Other factors that differentiate the currently available iMRI systems include the need for magnetic resonance-compatible surgical equipment and the methodology through which the patient or magnet is mobilized during imaging. These practical and potentially financial differences have led to the evolution of various iMRI systems for most effective intraoperative imaging.

TRANSSPHENOIDAL RESECTION OF PITUITARY ADENOMAS

Transsphenoidal resection quite recently has become the method of choice in the resection of pituitary tumors.[17] Innovations such as intraoperative fluoroscopy, the operating microscope, frameless stereotaxy, and the neuroendoscope have helped in improving navigation to the tumor bed and tumor visualization to maximize resection.[2,17,18] But these advances were not without their limitations. Fluoroscopy allows for a rapid real-time imaging, but visualization is limited to the sellar bony structures only. It does not aid in tumor detection.[19] The operating microscope enhances visibility of the surgical field, but is limited by angles of viewing. The appreciation of the entire sella and its surroundings is not possible by microscopic visualization alone.[17] The brain shift phenomenon interferes with the accuracy of neuronavigation in frameless stereotactic systems. Further, these systems cannot be intraoperatively updated to identify residual tumor, thereby decreasing their utility. The improvement that endoscopy has provided relative to the surgical microscope alone in direct visualization of the tumor, is limited by the fact that it does not allow one to see beyond the surface anatomy.[17]

This is particularly troublesome in tumors with suprasellar and parasellar extension. In these cases, appreciation of structures beneath and around the surgical field is required for complete removal. Because of these limitations, complete removal of pituitary adenomas was achieved in only about 65% of macroadenoma cases.[20]

Intraoperative MRI is a distinctly advantageous tool for transsphenoidal navigation and neuroimaging. The iMRI provides intraoperative images of tissue that enables assessment of residual tumor. These updates allow the neurosurgeon to localize remnant tumor while considering brain shift intraoperatively. It aids in the direct resection with preservation of critical native structures (the optic chiasm and cavernous sinuses) in the vicinity. Further, dynamic image sequences help to distinguish between normal pituitary tissue (fast contrast enhancement), adenoma (slow contrast enhancement) and hemorrhage (heme-sensitive gradient echo).[18,19]

With low-field iMRI systems, some investigators have reported residual tumor in 20–66% of patients after initial resection using the transsphenoidal approach. They achieved complete removal in 75–100% of cases with the use of iMRI.[18] Several other groups have also reported similarly superior rates of complete tumor resection while using iMRI with transsphenoidal resection.[2,8,17-19,21] However, these studies varied greatly in their inclusion criteria, with some choosing nonfunctioning macroadenomas with suprasellar extension, whereas others did not specify the hormonal status or amount of tumor extension into neighbouring brain regions **(Table 14.1)**. Therefore, objective comparison of surgical outcomes is difficult to assess.

ROLE OF NAVIGATION

In endoscopic pituitary surgery, indications for neuro-navigation are obtaining additional anatomical information for complex dissections. It includes not only presurgical planning and surgical approach but also tumor resection and skull-base reconstruction. It allows the surgical team to understand the anatomical relationships preoperatively in a more precisely. The trajectory and area of interest can be planned.[29]

It may also be used for exploration of the tumor cavity including confirmation of the cavernous portion of the internal carotid arteries. However, the accuracy of image guidance is dependent upon dynamic "brain shift". Further, the bony margins of the sellar defect can be planned for surgical reconstruction.[30]

Endoscope offers panoramic view of the operative field. But its major limitation is its inability to see through bones or tissues. What lies beyond has special significance in structures of the sella as it is surrounded by lot of vital structures. For pituitary surgery, the crux of operation is to define the boundaries of the sella. There have been many studies which qualitatively describe the positive role played by navigation in endoscopic pituitary surgery.[31] The role of navigation becomes very critical in cases of anatomical variations, poor pneumatization of sphenoid sinus including conchal variant, dehiscence of carotid arteries or optic nerves, kissing carotids, Onodi cells, pediatric patients, chronic sinonasal disease, recurrent surgery, and complex pathology. In addition to safety, it has been found that the size of sphenoid and sellar opening has a bearing on extent of resection. Making the exposure of sphenoid sinus and sella, the widest helps in increasing the extent of resection.[32] Wang tried to qualitatively compare the accuracy of surgeons's impression of sellar margins with that of navigation. He found that there is 14% fiducial localization error.[31] The cause of this was investigated and thought to be due to movement of reference frame. In cases if it is needed, registration had to be done again. This also made us change our practice. Each time we use navigation, we check our accuracy again. In Wang's study, the mean error in surgeon's localization was 4.5 mm and it was more for medial border of carotids compared to

Table 14.1 Summary of the earlier studies on iMRI

Author	N = Sample size	Macroadenomas	Microadenomas	Complete resection (through iMRI)	Complications		
					VF	CSF	INF
Paternó[22]	72	All	NA	23 reoperated	–	–	–
Vitaz[23]	100	81	9	76%	1%	6%	5%
Corburger[24]	143	–	–	91%		NA	NA
Szerlip[25]	59	55	4	67%	NA	–	
Tabakow[26]	18	67%	–	65%	–	–	–
Berkmann[27]	60	–	–	85%	–	–	–
Bellut[28]	48	–	–	29% increase	–	–	–
Kuge[29]	35	–	–	30% increase	–	–	–

Abbreviations: iMRI, intraoperative magnetic resonance imaging; VF, visual field; CSF, cerebrospinal fluid; INF, infections.

superior or inferior borders. In our surgery, in 38% of our cases, we increased our exposure for mean of 4 mm on both sides. This, we believe, contributed to increase in volume of tumor resected. In our study, the image guidance facilitated endoscopy in defining sphenoid position of internal carotid arteries and cavernous sinus [medial opticocarotid recess (MOCR) and lateral opticocarotid recess (LOCR)] in majority of cases and widened the sellar opening in nearly third of our cases.

OPERATIVE TECHNIQUE

Preoperative Work-up and Planning

All patients undergo sophisticated preoperative and post-operative endocrinological and ophthalmological evaluation. Complete ophthalmological work-up which includes visual acuity, visual fields and fundus examination is done by an ophthalmologist. An endocrinological work-up including preoperative hormonal assessment [prolactin, serum cortisol (morning sample), thyroid function tests, growth hormone with insulin-like growth factor I (IGF-I), luteinizing hormone and follicle-stimulating hormone levels] is done preoperatively. Informed consent for the procedure and iMRI is taken. Patients receive dose of steroid (hydrocortisone) on the morning of surgery which is also given in the perioperative period. They also undergo a navigation protocol (Brain Suite)

MRI brain with contrast and neuronavigation. Registration is established after collimating the preoperative images with the position on Brain Suite table under anesthesia **(Figure 14.1)**. The accuracy of the neuronavigation system is doubly checked by the Brain Suite technician and also by the members of the operating team **(Figures 14.2 and 14.3)**. The endoscopic transnasal transsphenoidal approach is used and after achieving a reasonable resection (after demonstration of fall of arachnoid) and securing hemostasis, the tumor cavity is packed with fat and fascia (see operative details) and vascularized mucosal flap-Hadad flap is put over it and nasal cavity is packed.

Steps of Surgery

Positioning

Typically, the approach is begun with the patient supine and his head in an iMRI frame and pin head-holder. The neck is slightly extended and the head is gently turned to the right to face the surgeon, to permit a good view through the nares. Brain Suite neuronavigation system is used to register the current position of the patient and the images are collimated with a previously done MRI (navigation protocol) in the same Brain Suite. Once registered and confirmed that the images are properly matched with real-time position, the operation is begun with patient being draped in intraoperative drapes.

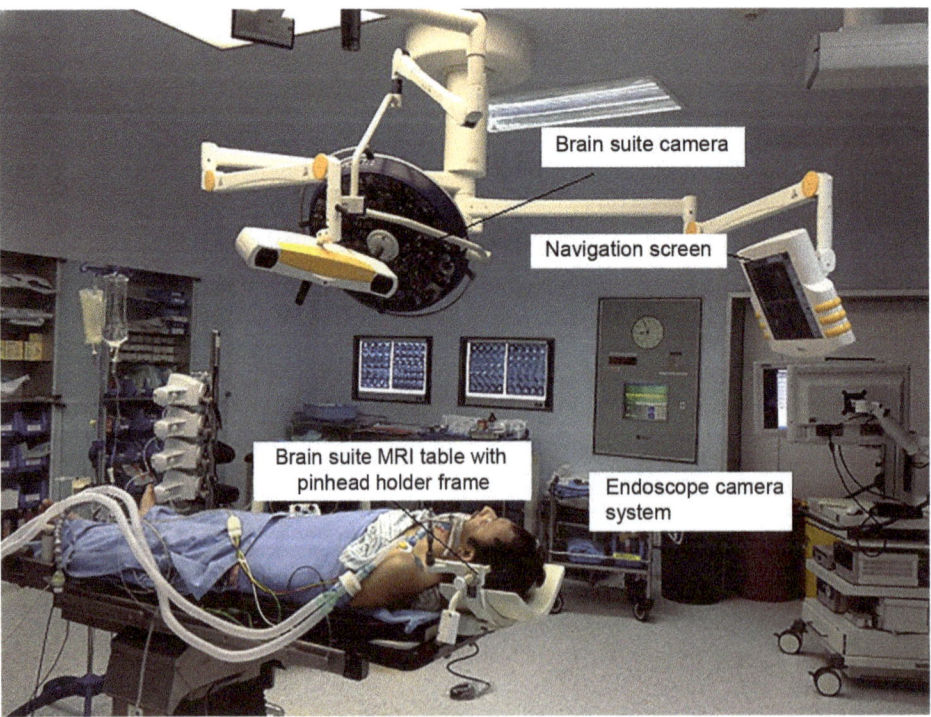

Figure 14.1 Setup for endoscopic surgery and neuronavigation

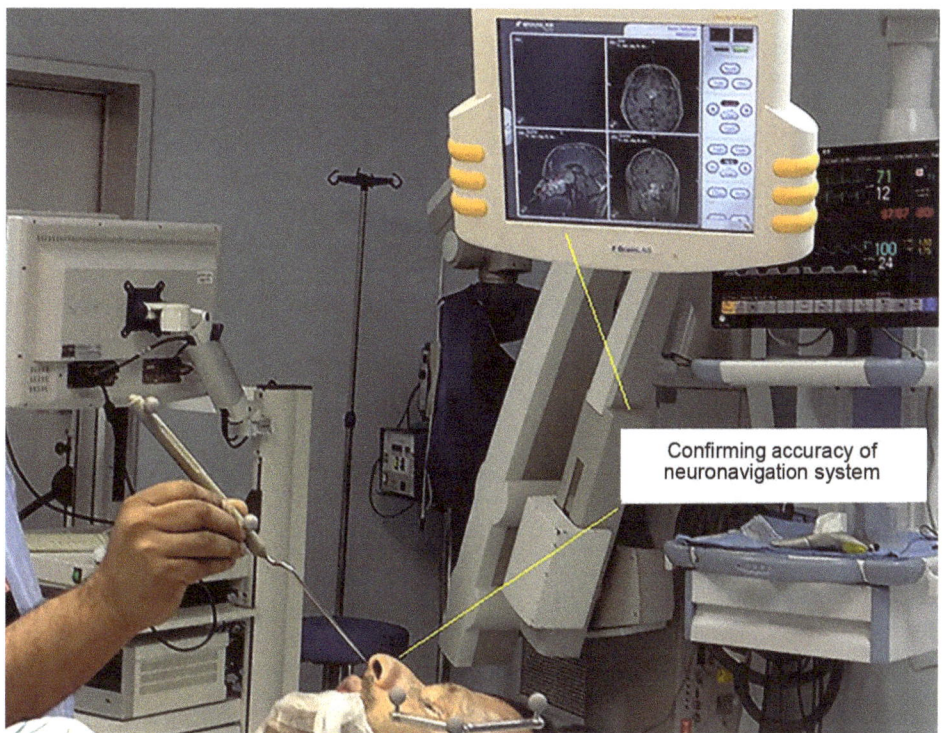

Figure 14.2 Checking accuracy of neuronavigation

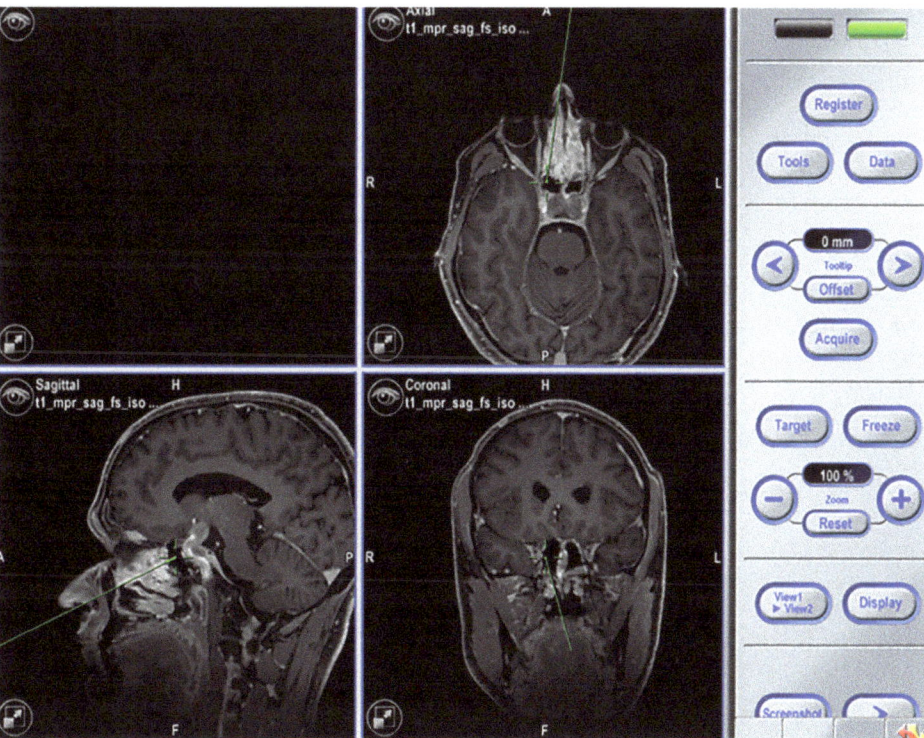

Figure 14.3 Accuracy of neuronavigation

The head is slightly elevated to reduce mucosal congestion and bleeding during the approach.

We routinely prepare the skin of the face or nasal cavity with antiseptic solution, and also graft sites such as the lateral thigh for fascia lata or adipose tissue should be prepared in a sterile standard fashion.

The nurse with the instrument trolley stands to the patient's left near the head end of the patient. The monitor with the camera and light source (on the trolley) is on the left side near the patient's head, opposite to the surgeon. The assistant stands opposite to the surgeon.

Nasal Stage

We use a unilateral, uninostril transnasal approach. We routinely use a 0 degree, 4 mm rigid endoscope (Karl Storz®) for visualizing the surgical site. The endoscope can be introduced via either nostril, although the right side is used more frequently. On introduction of the endoscope, the landmarks that should be initially identified in the nasal cavity are the inferior turbinate (laterally), the nasal septum (medially) and the choana (posteriorly). The choana is identified, maneuvering the endoscope superiorly allows identification of the middle turbinate, which arises from the region of the ethmoid sinuses superiorly. A Freer instrument is used to gently displace the middle turbinate laterally, attempting to preserve the integrity of the overlying mucosa and minimize bleeding at all times. Intermittent packing with lidocaine and/or epinephrine pledgets placed between the middle turbinate, and nasal septum helps to maintain the developed working space between the middle turbinate and nasal septum and achieve hemostasis. Following sufficient lateral displacement of the middle turbinate, the endoscope is advanced and angled slightly superiorly, to identify the superior turbinate posteriorly. In rare cases, resection of the middle turbinate will be required to widen the surgical corridor, and is typically reserved for extended skull base operations or hypertrophied turbinates. A small incision was made in the septal mucosa and a vascularized hadad flap. It is pedicled on the posterior nasoseptal artery, a branch of the posterior nasal artery.[33]

Localizing Sphenoid Sinus Ostium

Once the anterior wall of the sphenoid sinus has been exposed, the sphenoid sinus ostium may be seen about 1-1.5 cm above the nasopharynx. Often however, it is not seen, and one needs to lateralize the superior turbinate to see it. The superior turbinate is a very reliable landmark to localize the ostium, as it lies just behind the inferior aspect of the superior turbinate. If there is mucosal edema obscuring the ostium, then gentle probing should be done in the region of the ostium. Use of neuronavigation is also helpful in confirming the trajectory into the sphenoid sinus, after which a small dissector instrument, such as a Freer or a fine suction cannula, can be used to probe gently for the ostium and enter the sinus.[33,34]

Vomer Stage

Entire bony sphenoid rostrum is exposed by stripping the nasal mucosa along a subperiosteal plane on both sides of the vomer. Superior-most and inferior-most aspects of the bony keel of the vomer serve as useful midline markers during the remainder of the operation. It is also cross-checked by neuronavigation. It is advisable not to resect tissue in the inferolateral aspect of the exposure where the sphenopalatine artery enters the nasal cavity. Arterial bleeding encountered from the sphenopalatine artery at this point requires cauterization or even clipping of the artery and increases the risk for delayed arterial epistaxis despite initial hemostasis. The vomer is drilled and sphenoid sinus is exposed. The lateral and superior soft tissue and bony overhang of the sphenoid rostrum and sinus are resected using a Kerrison rongeur or a microdebrider, to provide adequate room. The sphenoid mucosa is gently stripped off.[33,34]

Sphenoidal Stage

Key anatomic landmarks are identified and correlated with the neuroimaging findings. It includes the curvature of the sellar floor, the location and course of the carotid arteries, and the configuration of any sphenoid septations that may be present. MOCR and LOCR are identified along with clival recess. Frequently, the entirety of these landmarks may not be plainly apparent and careful attention to the preoperative imaging combined with judicious use of neuronavigation will prevent inadvertent complications.[34] The floor of the sella is prominent and easily recognizable in most patients with neuronavigation.

Sellar Stage

The sellar position is confirmed using the neuronavigation. The sella can be opened in many different ways. If the tumor has eroded part of the bone, then it is quite easy to use the smallest Kerrison punch to remove loose bone to expose the dura. Another option is to use a drill to thin the bone prior to opening it. The limits of exposure are decided by neuronavigation guidance. The opening should be made as wide as possible being careful of the cavernous sinuses laterally. The superior limit is the tuberculum sella and inferiorly the floor is removed if required.

Incising the Dura: The dura is incised using endoscopic dural knife and enlarged using endoscissors **(Figure 14.4)**. A rectangular dural "window" can be resected. Horizontal cuts should be made in a lateral-to-medial direction to avoid

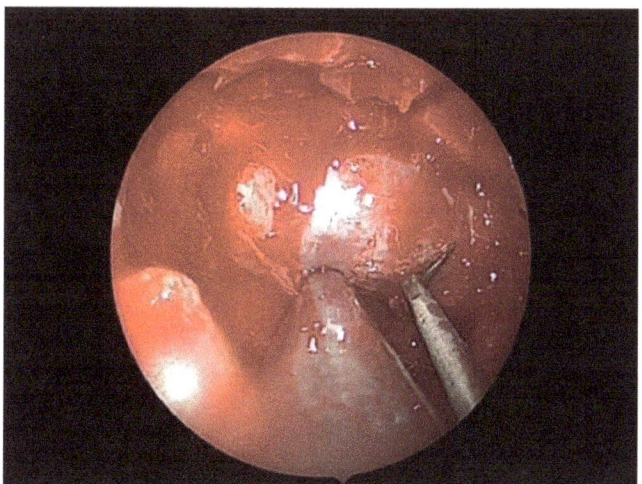

Figure 14.4 Dural opening with endoscissors

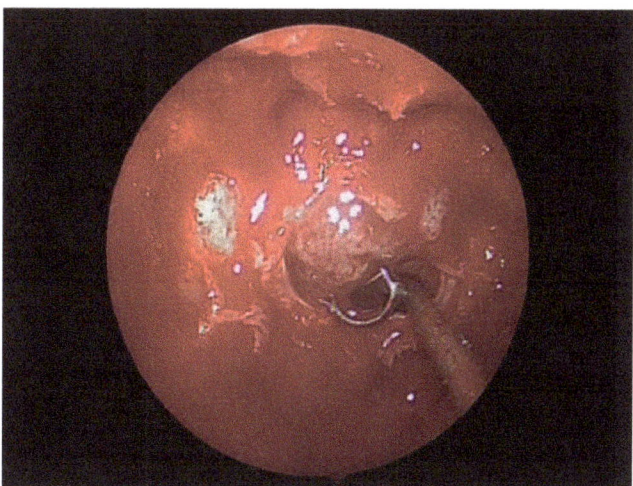

Figure 14.5 Removal of adenomatous tissue

carotid injury, while the vertical incision should be made in a superior-to-inferior direction to avoid inadvertent entry into the anterior arachnoid cistern with resultant CSF leakage.

Tumor removal: After dural opening, a blunt hockey dissector is used to develop a subdural, extraglandular, or extracapsular plane around the circumference of the dural opening. Usually soft tumor pops out and an anterior forceps, curettes, pituitary grasping forceps, gentle suction and irrigation may be used to extract the tumor piecemeal. The tissue is sent for histopathology. Further, tumor removal is done using ring curettes. Tumor is removed in the inferior and lateral aspects first and then superiorly **(Figure 14.5)**.[32] Our endpoint is redundant prolapse of the diaphragma sella and arachnoid into the surgical field. Direct suctioning on the arachnoid is avoided using cottonoids to prevent arachnoid breach.

The cavernous sinuses and suprasellar area are the most frequent areas of residual tumor. The sellar cavity is inspected directly once tumor resection is believed to be completed. Careful attention to these areas for detection of tumor remnants adherent to the normal pituitary gland is done. Symmetric descent of the diaphragm into the sella usually indicates optic chiasm decompression and failure of the diaphragm to descend, or asymmetric descent, should prompt further search for residual tumor. After final confirmation of complete tumor resection, meticulous hemostasis is achieved.

Closure and reconstruction of sella: Once the tumor is resected, complete hemostasis achieved with help of Surgicel®. The sellar floor was repaired with fat and fascia (harvested from patient's thigh). It is reinforced with fibrin glue. The sphenoid sinus is obliterated with a piece of fat harvested. The mucosal septal flap (Hadad flap) is used to further support the sella **(Figure 14.6)**.[33,34]

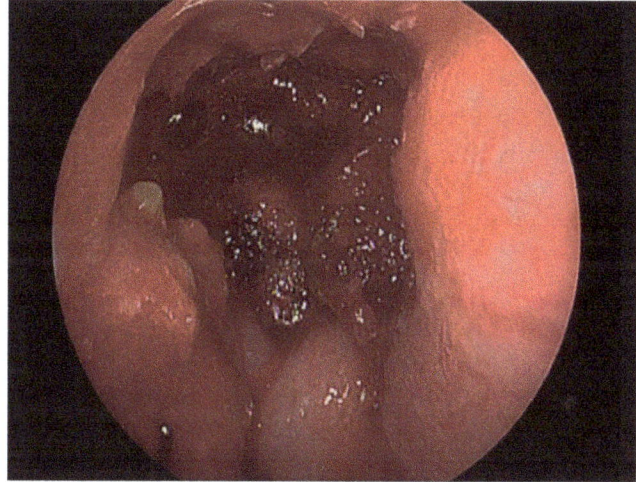

Figure 14.6 Hadad flap reinforcement of sellar floor

Intraoperative magnetic resonance imaging: The patient is immediately then shifted to the iMRI (1.5T-SIEMENS®) room, adjacent to the operating room, on a special Brain Suite transfer trolley. Under the same anesthesia, iMRI is performed with gadolinium contrast and the enhancing tissue is noted. Its amount and location is re-evaluated both by the operating team members and a neuroradiologist. Contrasts enhancing residual lesions in the sella are divided into three categories: (1) ring enhancement, (2) nodular and (3) mixed variety. In cases of mixed and nodular enhancement is seen, decision to operate was taken. Residual tissue of above variety in close proximity to carotids, cavernous sinus or optic chiasm and technical difficulty of approach are other hindrances to "relook". After the surgery is considered to be complete, the patient is reverted and extubated.

Technique of Intraoperative Magnetic Resonance Imaging and Volumetric Assessment

Intraoperative MRI was performed with a SIEMENS® 1.5T machine **(Figure 14.7)**. The imaging starts with localizer sequence [field of view (FOV): 280 mm; repetition time (TR): 20 ms; time (TE): 50 ms; scan time: 9 seconds]. T2-weighted (T2W) half-fourier single-shot turbo spin-echo sequences (slice thickness: 5 mm; FOV: 230 mm; TR: 1,000 ms; TE: 89 ms; scan time: 25 seconds at 5 acquisitions) in axial, coronal and sagittal orientation were measured next to give a quick overview. Afterward, T1-weighted (T1W) coronal and sagittal spin-echo sequences were applied (slice thickness: 3 mm; FOV: 270 mm; TR: 450 ms; TE: 12 ms; scan time: 4 minute 57 seconds at 4 acquisitions). In addition, high-resolution T2W turbo spin-echo sequence with an in-plane resolution of 0.6 × 0.4 mm were measured applied (slice thickness: 3 mm; FOV: 230 mm; TR: 4000 ms; TE: 97 ms; scan time: 6 minute 6 seconds at 3 acquisitions). This was followed by a T1W contrast (gadolinium) sequences. Same sequence methodology was used in the postoperative and follow-up scans.

For radiological collaboration, we define the resection rates in two ways:

Qualitative assessment: Gross total resection (GTR) is called when on a postoperative contrast MRI, the pituitary stalk, gland and surrounding granulation was seen. Three patterns of residual tissue are noted: (1) ring enhancement, (2) nodular and (3) mixed variety and were classified accordingly.

Quantitative assessment: To quantitatively define the resection status, the volume of residual tumor tissue is assessed and calculated in the pre-, intra- and postoperative 1.5T magnetic resonance (MR) images, respectively. Normally, a postoperative MRI shows a normal pituitary gland and granulation tissue after a resection. To establish

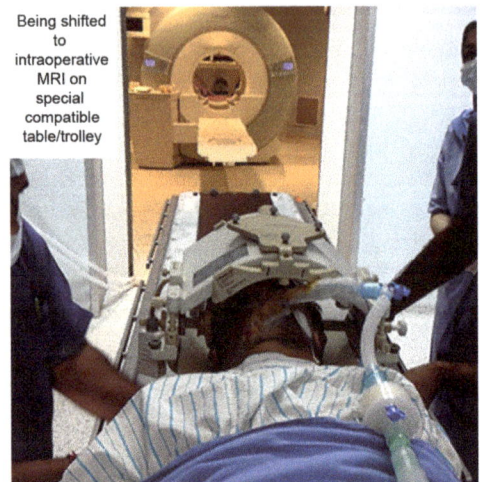

Being shifted to intraoperative MRI on special compatible table/trolley

Figure 14.7 *Intraoperative MRI:* Setup and transfer system

and standardize, the average volume of pituitary gland and granulation tissue was taken as 0.30 cubic centimeter (0.30 mL). This was calculated from 12 GTR patients who were followed long-term after pituitary surgery.[35] The images are transferred from syngo plaza interface (PACS) and Monaco contouring workstation version 5.00.04 is used for volumetric analysis utilizing 1 mm slices **(Figures 14.8 to 14.12)**.

POSTOPERATIVE PLAN

Postoperatively, patients are closely monitored and managed in a dedicated neurosciences intensive care unit. Perioperative monitoring for diabetes insipidus and hypo/hypernatremia is continued in the postoperative period and appropriate measures are taken to maintain homeostasis. Complications with regards to visual acuity, field defects, extraocular movements of eyes, CSF leak and infection (meningitis) are recorded when they occur. The histopathology of the specimen of tumor sent intraoperatively is followed up and the report along with immunohistochemistry is duly recorded. After reasonable recovery, the patients are discharged with detailed instructions on electrolyte monitoring, hormonal supplementation and follow-up.

OUR EXPERIENCE

We were able to perform GTR in 87.3% cases with percentage of resection above 80% which is better than most published series. This can be attributed to the fact that this prospective study was not at start of surgical experience but after more than 250 cases were performed.

Ammirati et al. in their meta-analysis did not find any difference in endoscopic and microsurgical approaches but, there were increased vascular complications with endoscopy.[36]

While retrospective cohort studies and meta-analysis generally favor endoscopy, but conflicting data and limited population make it difficult to assess the difference. Our study adds to benefit of endoscopes in extent of resection and lesser complications.

Table 14.2 shows the comparison of our study with other series using endoscope with iMRI.[37]

In our series, the average blood loss was 275 mL. Blood transfusion was required only in one patient and CSF leak rates were 5.4%. Time from induction to extubation was 240.8 minutes with the use of iMRI.

Goudakos et al. in their meta-analysis included 11 studies for comparison of endoscopy and microscopy. They found no statistical significant difference in remission rates of functional adenomas, complete tumor removal and CSF leak. They found more diabetes insipidus (p = 0.003) and intracranial complications (p = 0.05) in microsurgery group. The hospital stay was less in endoscopy group (p = 0.00001).[38] In our series, there were no diabetes insipidus at discharge.

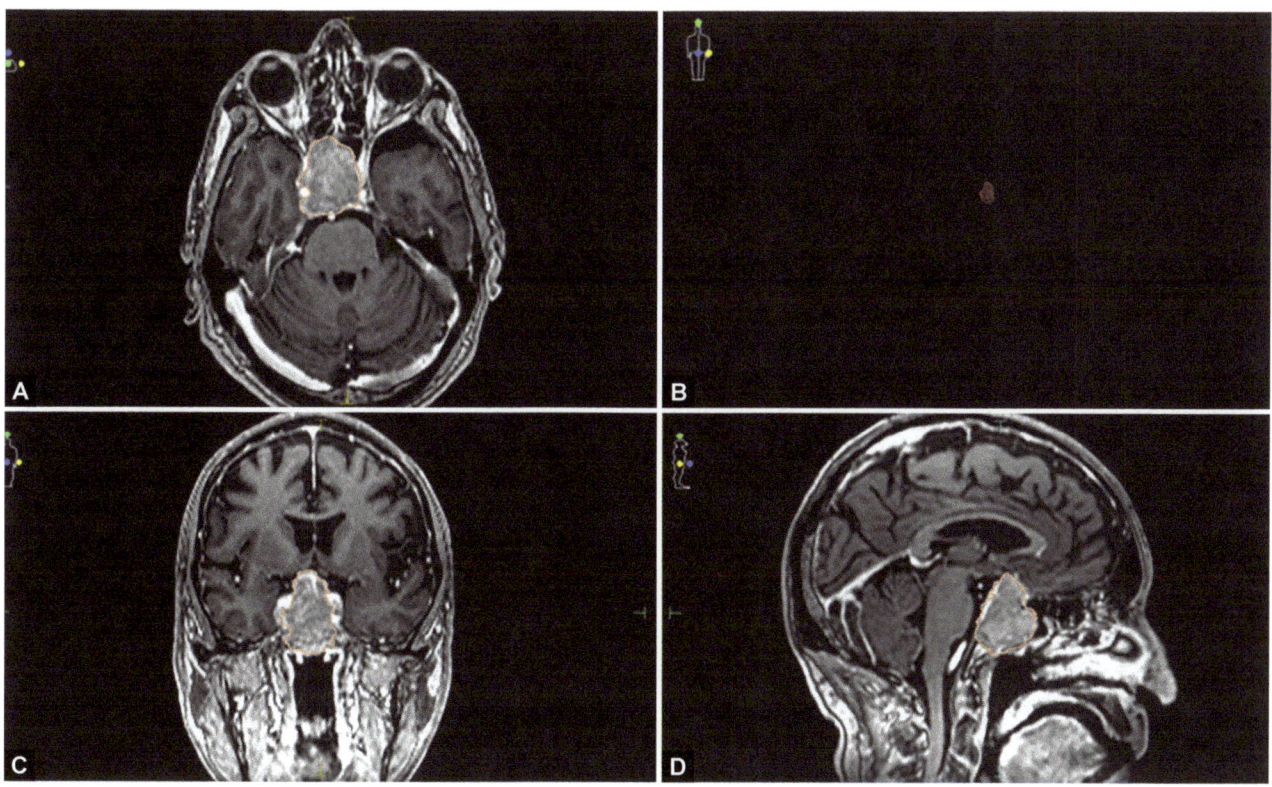

Figures 14.8A to D Preoperative images contouring for volumetric analysis

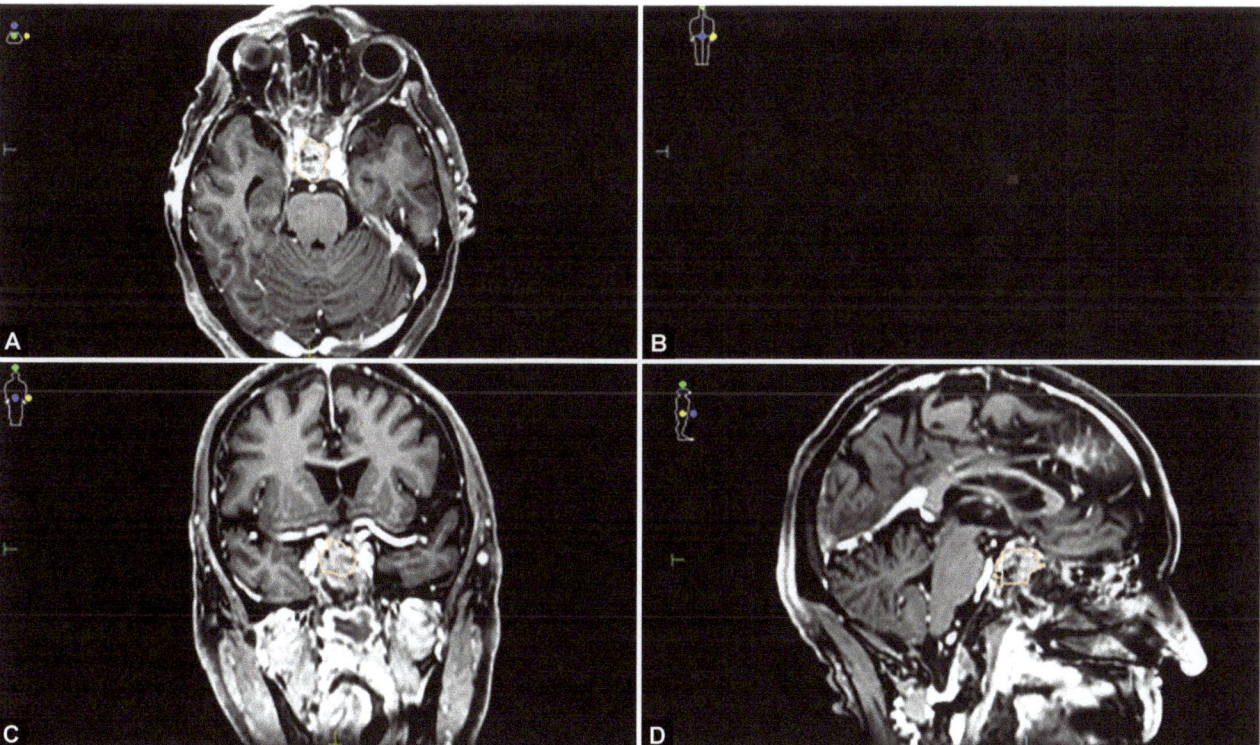

Figures 14.9A to D Intraoperative images contouring for volumetric analysis

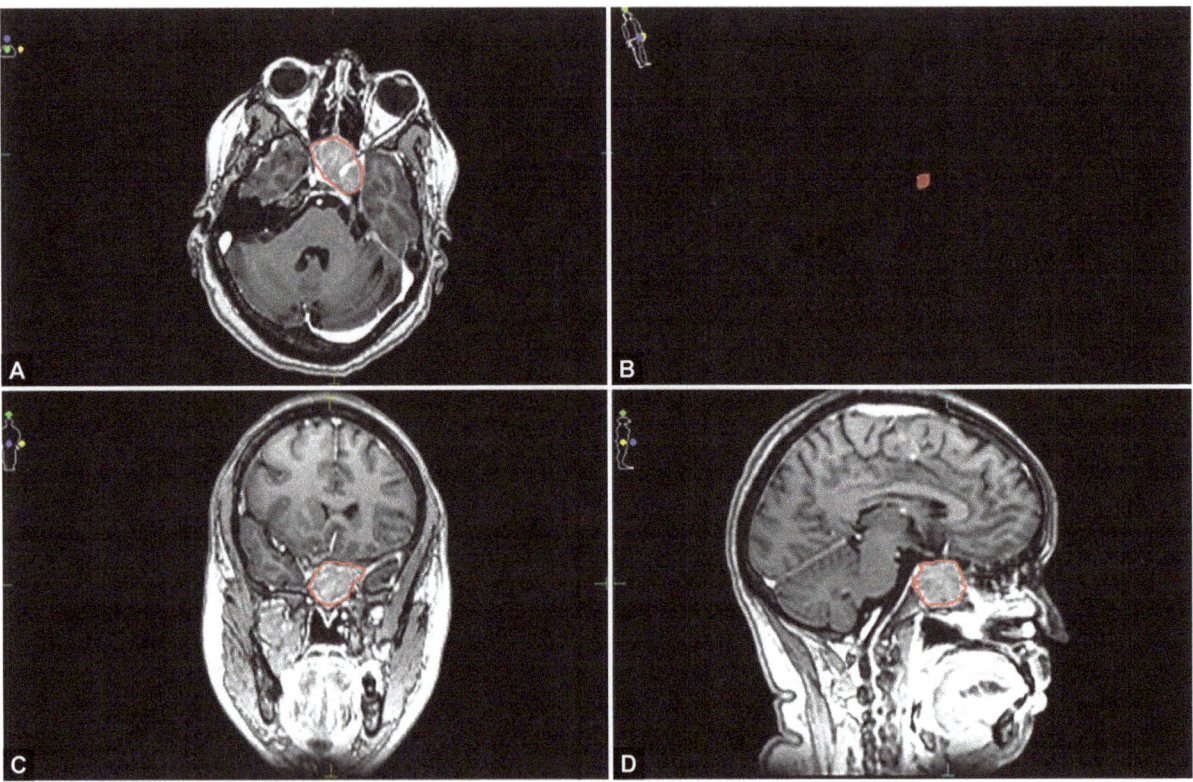

Figures 14.10A to D Preoperative images contouring for volumetric analysis.

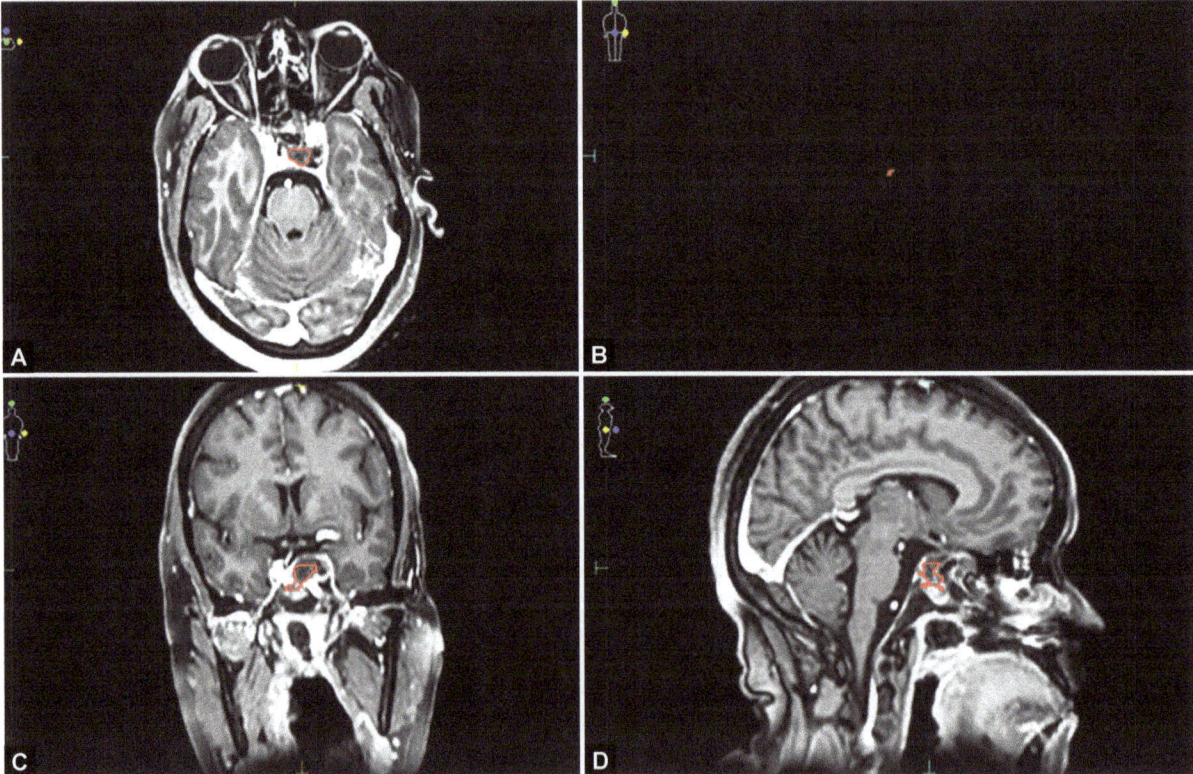

Figures 14.11A to D Intraoperative images contouring for volumetric analysis

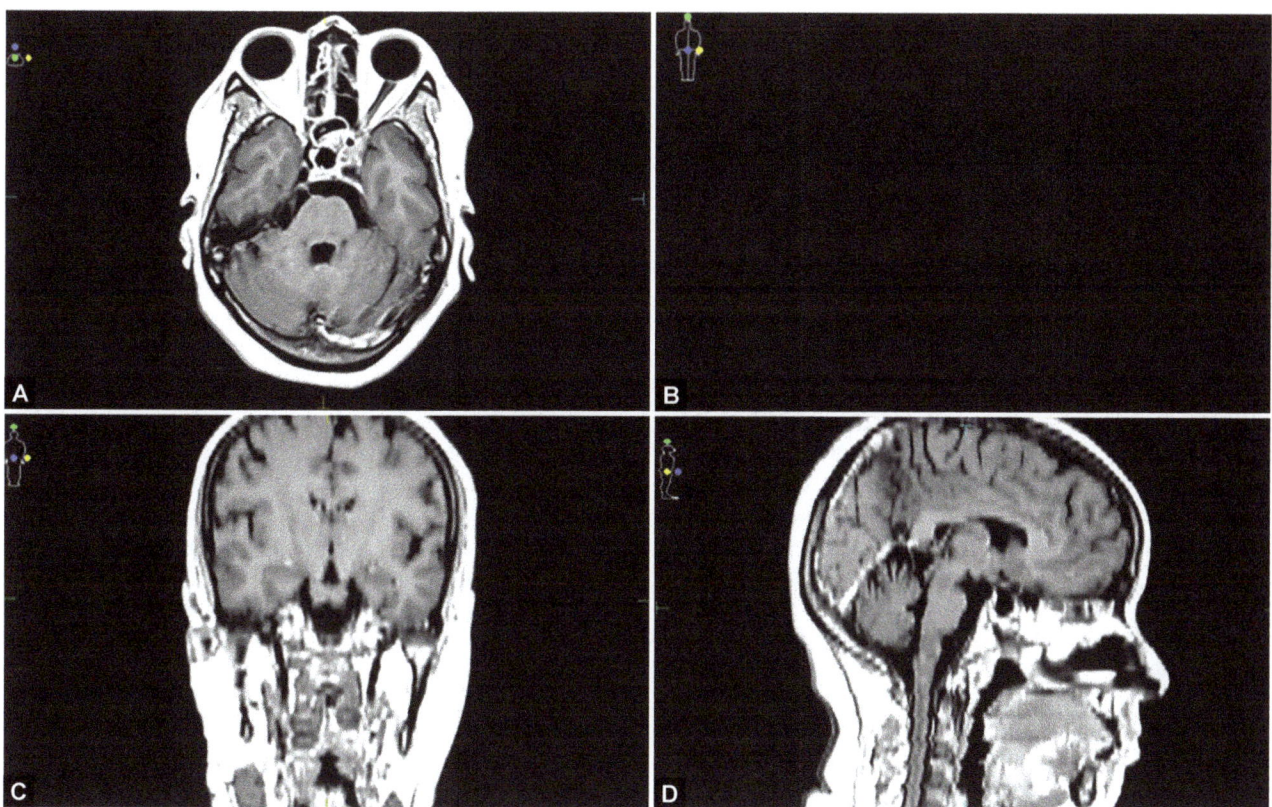

Figures 14.12A to D Postoperative images

Table 14.2 Comparison of resection in endoscopic and iMRI series

Authors and year	MRI	Number of patient and adenoma type	Unexpected residual tumor found on iMRI	Eligible for further resection	Pre-iMRI GTR → Post-iMRI GTR	iMRI let to further resection
Netuka et al. 2011	3.0T	86 (76 macro and 10 micro), intended GTR: 49, intended NTR or STR: 37	15.1% (13/86)	33.7% (29/86)	69.4–91.8%	33.70%
Theodosopoulos et al. 2010	0.3T	27 macro	14.8% (4/27)	12.6% (3/27)	62.9–70%	11%
Schwartz et al. 2006	0.12T	15 macro	20% (3/15)	20% (3/15)	80–100%	20%
Hasan et al. 2016	3.0T	20 macro intended GTR: 14, intended NTR or STR: 6	30% (6/20)	30% (6/20), 28.6% (4/14) and 33.3% (2/6)	60–80%	30%
Our experience	1.5T	385 macro	12.72% (49/385)	12.72% (49/385)	51.3–85.6%	34.30%

Abbreviations: GTR, gross total resection; iMRI, intraoperative magnetic resonance imaging; NTR, near total resection; STR, subtotal resection.

Zhu analyzed short- and long-term complications in both endoscopy and microscopy group and found statistically significant shorter follow-up (p = 0.02), lesser of diabetes insipidus (p = 0.0001), fewer complications (p = 0.0008), less blood loss (p = 0.03), higher rates of complete resections (p = 0.03) and shorter hospitalization (p = 0.0001) in endoscopic cases.[39] Contrast-enhanced iMRI theoretically holds lot of promise in resection of pituitary adenomas since its first use in 1994 by Black et al.[3] It has increasingly been used to attempt GTR and also maximal resection in those patients whom the GTR cannot be achieved. Most reports are based on claims of qualitative analysis and there are very few reports on quantitative analysis.[40] Also, most reports are on low-field scanners (less than 1.5T) which affect the technical resolution of images. We designed our present study to address these concerns.

One of the confounding errors in using the iMRI is the initial resection rates being lower before performing the MRI than groups who do not use any intraoperative imaging. Reported rates of endoscopic GTR in pituitary adenomas range from 44% to 88%. Endoscopic GTR after first resections before performing the iMRI ranged from 34% to 62%. The average GTR rates over lot of series without iMRI for endoscopy and microscopy are 79% and 65%. Volumetric resections up to 88% are achieved with endoscopy and iMRI. In our study too, the rate of resection increased from 51.3% (in initial resection) to 85.6% (in final resection).

In our study, the resection was measured in two ways: First, qualitative assessment was done by assessment of contrast enhancement. Ring enhancement was considered as granulation tissue. Small enhancement in continuation of pituitary stalk was considered as normal pituitary and any nodule was considered as residue. GTR was considered when no gross mass lesion was seen although there was residual gland and capsule enhancement. These patients did not undergo second surgery. Second, was quantitative measurement of volume of contrast enhancement on postoperative MRI scans. Out of 385 patients, GTR was planned in 287 (74.5%) cases and subtotal resection (Wilson-Hardy Grade III D and above) in 98 (25.5%) cases. Reoperation was done in 12.7% cases out of which 7.3% were from the subtotal resection group and rest 5.4% from the GTR planned group. Reoperation was more required in higher Hardy's Grades.

Our series that showed the amount of resection according to Hardy's Grade were described in **Table 14.3**.

Residual adenoma is a risk factor for regrowth in several series. In a retrospective study in 2008 on nonfunctioning adenomas, Chang et al. found a recurrence rate of 10% in a cohort of 663 patients with median follow-up of 8.4 years.[41] The predictive factors for recurrence were cavernous sinus invasion and subtotal resection without radiotherapy. No volumetric threshold was reported. According to Taneka et al.[42] and Honegger et al.,[43] MIB index varies conversely with tumor volume doubling time and is variable but can predict recurrence. The risk of recurrence is more in younger patients. The role of volumetric extent of resection in predicting recurrence still requires large studies with long-term follow-up.

The volumetric extent of resection is measured in the preoperative contrast enhancement, intraoperative contrast enhancement and postoperative contrast enhancement. The postoperative enhancement also occurs in normal pituitary and granulation tissue.

Initial resection rate as evident by the iMRI across the series was 71.44% (and was 80.32% at 3 months follow-up final resection rate). The range was 27.6–92.7%. As noted, 12.7% patients were reoperated. The mean initial resection in these cases was 51.33% which significantly increased to 85.59%. Due to intraoperative help of iMRI, the mean resection in reoperated cases was more than the mean resection across the series (85.59% and 80.32% respectively at final resections). This was statistically significant (p = 0.03).

In addition, we did a postoperative contrast-enhanced MRI at 3 months follow-up. In their study of 240 patients, Berkman and coworkers have shown about 20% reduction in enhancing tumor follow-up till 3 months.[44]

In our series also, there was volumetric reduction of enhancement which further increased the extent of resection from 75.24% to 80.77%.

In our study, there was no increase in morbidity due to iMRI. The mean duration of surgery was 240.8 minutes and

Table 14.3 Amount of tumor volume resection according to Hardy's grade

Hardy's grade	Mean preoperative volume (mL)	Mean intraoperative volume (mL)	Percentage resection (initial)	Mean postoperative volume (mL)	Percentage resection (final)
II-A	4.08	1.04	74.51%	0.79	80.64%
II-B	3.91	0.78	80.05%	0.65	83.38%
II-C	4.32	0.72	83.33%	0.72	83.33%
III-A	6.15	1.25	79.67%	0.91	85.20%
III-B	10.33	3.51	66.02%	2.19	78.80%
III-C	15.06	3.61	76.03%	2.62	82.60%
III-D	12.74	2.84	77.71%	1.94	84.77%
III-E	12.2	3.97	67.46%	3.82	68.69%
IV-C	17.51	4.93	71.84%	2.96	83.10%
IV-D	22.1	8.62	61.00%	7.46	66.24%
IV-E	27.55	13.29	51.76%	8.02	70.89%

there was no respiratory failure or deep vein thrombosis (DVT) due to prolonged surgery. This is across all series described in literature.

PATIENT-RELATED CHARACTERISTICS

Demographic studies show that pituitary adenoma is more common in females and occurs between 3rd decades and 6th decades of life. Demographics of our patients have showed a male preponderance, the reason for which may be heterogeneous nature of patient referral and a small study group. Mean age of 45.3 years corroborated well with the other series as evident by the study by Debede Theodros in 2015 which estimated the incidence of pituitary tumors only 3.5–8.5% prior to age of 20 years.[1] This was also consistent with the European and US pituitary tumor registries.[45,46]

The three major clinical presentations in our study were: (1) Headache 36.3%; (2) Visual disturbances 27.2%; and (3) Acromegaly 18.1%. Both in the Italian database,[45] as well as in the US registry,[46] have found half of the patients in their series presented with mass-related symptoms, such as visual defects, headache and hypogonadism symptoms. Recurrent pituitary adenoma was present in 5.4% of cases in our series and it was also incidentally discovered in 3.6% cases.

Visual examination was performed both clinically and also by ophthalmologist in our study. Defects in visual fields were observed in 47.2% cases in our study. Classical bitemporal hemianopia was as common as unilateral temporal hemianopia 20% each. Thomas et al. in 2002 reported atypical visual field pattern of 20%.[47] Another study from Brazil by Maria Licia et al. showed visual field defects to be present in 74% of patients in their series.[48]

The mean duration of the surgical procedure (induction to extubation) including the iMRI time was 240.8 minutes (around 4 hours). This was much higher than the study by Hlavica et al.[49] in 2013 who reported their procedure time to be 92.6 minutes and average 30 minutes of iMRI time (total 122.6 minutes) depending on the sequences obtained. But in their study, they used the microsurgical technique and also a 0.15T Polestar N20 MRI scanner was used, so their results are not comparable. Further, we kept our endpoints as induction to extubation, but the above study does not define the endpoints.

LIMITATIONS

The limitations associated with neuronavigation include those related to accuracy, anatomical disorientation, radiographic information, cost and outcomes literature. Accuracy in image guidance refers to the difference between the true positions of a point in space compared with its predicted radiographic position. The various methods of measuring accuracy differ based on the position of a fiducial marker, rather than an anatomical point. Fiducial registration error is the difference between the position of a fiducial point and its predicted radiographic location following registration, which in turn is calculated by image guidance software in terms of a root-mean-square value. Modern generations of image guidance systems have improved the fidelity and reproducibility related to accuracy by incorporating improved imaging data sets, increased fiducial points, improved three-dimensionality of fiducial points and automation of the registration process.[25] Although multiple studies have confirmed a reproducible accuracy of image guidance systems to within 2 mm, this is balanced against the anatomical precision necessary for skull base surgery where millimetric distances may be critical.

The expenses involved in purchasing and installing an iMRI unit as well as the ancillary support staff can be prohibitive. Many small academic medical centers as well as community hospitals may not have the necessary financial leverage. We have found that interpretation of images can be an important limiting factor, and it necessitates a multidisciplinary approach with a comprehensive discussion between the neurosurgeon and neuroradiologist. Finally, delays in surgery using iMRI initially posed a problem in over-extending the amount of time that the patient was in a state of general anesthesia.

SUMMARY

To summarize, the study had the following benefits and pitfalls.

Benefits

- Intraoperative MRI can be performed safely and effectively in all patients during the same anesthesia in the integrated operating room and MRI room setup.
- It gives the operating surgeon the ability to make real-time assessments to evaluate extent of adenoma resection.
- It further helps the surgeon to decide about dealing with the remnant tumor tissue and if any further resection is feasible safely.
- The technique helps in ascertaining the approach and technical difficulties and also offers alternatives of approach to deal with remnant disease.
- It can also give evidence of complications such as hemorrhage in the operative cavity and sellar area, which may be removed immediately, under the same anesthesia.
- Since it is all real-time assessment, many patients are saved of a re-do surgery later as all significant tissue can be reasonably removed in primary surgical procedure itself.
- This reduces the cost of overall management of the adenoma as well as the duration of treatment if significant tumor tissue was removed at the primary surgery with the help of iMRI.

- This all translates into a safe and effective technique of dealing with surgical management of pituitary macroadenomas.
- It ensures to a greater extent the remission of hormonally active tumors and decreased recurrences over a long-term follow-up.

Pitfalls

- Intraoperative MRI is state-of-the-art technology which involves setting up of the unit inside the operating room or in the adjacent room. This is expensive and all neurosurgical units cannot afford it, especially in a developing nation like India.
- It requires a dedicated and trained team of neurosurgeons, neuroanesthesiologists, technicians and scrub nurses who help in managing the whole setup.
- Special equipment such as compatible MRI frame and table, patient transfer system and a compatible neuronavigation system is required.
- The average duration of surgery (induction to extubation) is increased as compared to a standard endoscopic transsphenoidal procedure, as it includes the time to perform the intraoperative MRI.
- It needs a help of an experienced neuroradiologist to further endorse the results of iMRI scans as it is difficult to differentiate between enhancing residual tumor tissue, normal pituitary and postoperative edema.

CONCLUSION

Intraoperative MRI-guided resection is an evidence-based advancement in the surgical management of pituitary macroadenomas. This allows the operating neurosurgeon to accurately distinguish residual tumor tissue intraoperatively, and increases the incidence of complete resection of all enhancing tumor.

Complete resection results in improved patient outcome, greater response to adjuvant therapies and a decreased number of reoperations. It also reduces mortality in functional pituitary adenomas because of greater remission of hormone hyperproduction and its effects. In nonfunctional adenomas, it reduces the number of interventions required for disease control and hence, decreases mortality.

Image guidance with high-resolution MRI imaging increases the boundaries of gross total resection with safety and accuracy.

Endoscopes have emerged as standard of care in management of pituitary adenomas. They offer better visualization and increased completeness of resections. Though no study conclusively proves that endoscopic surgery is better than microscopic surgery but there has been acceptance of its use. Numbers of centers doing endoscopic surgeries have mushroomed over the years. The safety in the form of lesser complication rates and lesser hospital stay with similar or increased resection rates has been proven for endoscopic surgeries.

Volumetric extent of resection is going to play a major role in predicting recurrence and the need of adjuvant therapy. But, larger studies with longer follow-up are required to prove its role.

Immunostaining and genetic analysis are work in progress. Better definition of the "Hit" in tumor suppressor genes offers hope for genetic therapies in future.

PEARLS

- More radicality of surgery can be reached.
- Training for the effective and sensible use of intraoperative MRI is necessary and helpful.
- Interpretation of intraoperative images is difficult and requires the help of a neuroradiologist.
- Remnant tumor location, extrasellar extension or cavernous sinus invasion should be carefully recognized and decision to relook should be taken judiciously after the proper interpretation of intraoperative images.
- Not every residual tumor can be operated although the risk-benefits of reoperating should be assessed and maximal safe tumor resection should be advocated.

Basic problems to acknowledge, discuss and experience during such a course are:

- The pitfalls of intraoperative interpretation of MRI scans.
- Logistics involved and time required for performing the iMRI.
- Availability of trained technical and nursing staff.
- Intraoperative MRI-compatible equipment and settings inside the operating room and MRI room.
- Interpretation of normal versus abnormal and evident residual tumor tissue.

REFERENCES

1. Theodros D, Patel M, Ruzevick J, et al. Pituitary adenomas: historical perspective, surgical management and future directions. CNS Oncol. 2015;4(6):411-29.
2. Schwartz TH, Stieg PE, Anand VK. Endoscopic transsphenoidal pituitary surgery with intraoperative magnetic resonance imaging. Neurosurgery. 2006;58(1 Suppl):ONS44-51.
3. Black PM, Moriarty T, Alexander E, et al. Development and implementation of intraoperative magnetic resonance imaging and its neurosurgical applications. Neurosurgery. 1997;41(4):831-42.
4. Albayrak B, Samdani AF, Black PM. Intra-operative magnetic resonance imaging in neurosurgery. Acta Neurochir (Wien). 2004;146(6):543-57.
5. Tew JM. Yaşargil MG. Neurosurgery's man of the century. Neurosurgery. 1999;45(5):1010-4.

6. Willems PW, van der Sprenkel JW, Tulleken CA, et al. Neuronavigation and surgery of intracerebral tumours. J Neurol. 2006;253(9):1123-36.

7. Hushek SG, Martin AJ, Steckner M, et al. MR systems for MRI-guided interventions. J Magn Reson Imaging. 2008;27(2):253-66.

8. Nimsky C, Ganslandt O, Tomandl B, et al. Low-field magnetic resonance imaging for intraoperative use in neurosurgery: a 5-year experience. Eur Radiol. 2002;12(11):2690-703.

9. Nimsky C, Ganslandt O, Cerny S, et al. Quantification of, visualization of, and compensation for brain shift using intraoperative magnetic resonance imaging. Neurosurgery. 2000;47(5):1070-9.

10. Black PM, Alexander E, Martin C, et al. Craniotomy for tumour treatment in an intraoperative magnetic resonance imaging unit. Neurosurgery. 1999;45(3):423-31.

11. Nabavi A, Black PM, Gering DT, et al. Serial intraoperative magnetic resonance imaging of brain shift. Neurosurgery. 2001;48(4):787-97.

12. Nimsky C, Ganslandt O, Hastreiter P, et al. Intraoperative compensation for brain shift. Surg Neurol. 2001;56(6):357-65.

13. Seifert V. Intraoperative MRI in neurosurgery: technical overkill or the future of brain surgery? Neurol India. 2003;51(3):329-32.

14. Tronnier VM, Wirtz CR, Knauth M, et al. Intraoperative diagnostic and interventional magnetic resonance imaging in neurosurgery. Neurosurgery. 1997;40(5):891-900.

15. Bergsneider M, Sehati N, Villablanca P, et al. Mahaley Clinical Research Award: extent of glioma resection using low-field (0.2 T) versus high-field (1.5 T) intraoperative MRI and image-guided frameless neuronavigation. Clin Neurosurg. 2005;52:389-99.

16. Bergsneider M, Liau LM. Intraoperative magnetic resonance imaging. In: Badie B (Ed). Neurosurgical Operative Atlas. New York: Thieme; 2007. pp. 104-13.

17. Bohinski RJ, Warnick RE, Gaskill-Shipley MF, et al. Intraoperative magnetic resonance imaging to determine the extent of resection of pituitary macroadenomas during transsphenoidal microsurgery. Neurosurgery. 2001;49(5):1133-43.

18. Pergolizzi RS, Nabavi A, Schwartz RB, et al. Intra-operative MR guidance during trans-sphenoidal pituitary resection: preliminary results. J Magn Reson Imaging. 2001;13(1):136-41.

19. Martin CH, Schwartz R, Jolesz F, et al. Transsphenoidal resection of pituitary adenomas in an intraoperative MRI unit. Pituitary. 1999;2(2):155-62.

20. Mortini P, Losa M, Barzaghi R, et al. Results of transsphenoidal surgery in a large series of patients with pituitary adenoma. Neurosurgery. 2005;56(6):1222-33.

21. Fahlbusch R, Keller BV, Ganslandt O, et al. Transsphenoidal surgery in acromegaly investigated by intraoperative high-field magnetic resonance imaging. Eur J Endocrinol. 2005;153(2):239-48.

22. Paterno' V, Fahlbusch R. High-Field iMRI in transsphenoidal pituitary adenoma surgery with special respect to typical localization of residual tumor. Acta Neurochir (Wien). 2014;156 (3):463-74.

23. Vitaz TW, Inkabi KE, Carrubba CJ. Intraoperative MRI for transphenoidal procedures: short-term outcome for 100 consecutive cases. Clin Neurol Neurosurg. 2011;113(9):731-5.

24. Coburger J, König R, Seitz K, et al. Determining the utility of intraoperative magnetic resonance imaging for transsphenoidal surgery: a retrospective study. J Neurosurg. 2014;120(2):346-56.

25. Szerlip NJ, Zhang YC, Placantonakis DG, et al. Transsphenoidal resection of sellar tumours using high-field intraoperative magnetic resonance imaging. Skull Base. 2011;21(4):223-32.

26. Tabakow P, Czyz M, Jarmundowicz W, et al. Surgical treatment of pituitary adenomas using low-field intraoperative magnetic resonance imaging. Adv Clin Exp Med. 2012;21(4):495-503.

27. Berkmann S, Fandino J, Müller B, et al. Intraoperative MRI and endocrinological outcome of transsphenoidal surgery for non-functioning pituitary adenoma. Acta Neurochir (Wien). 2012;154(4):639-47.

28. Bellut D, Hlavica M, Muroi C, et al. Impact of intraoperative MRI-guided transsphenoidal surgery on endocrine function and hormone substitution therapy in patients with pituitary adenoma. Swiss Med Wkly. 2012;142:w13699.

29. Kuge A, Kikuchi Z, Sato S, et al. Practical use of a simple technique, insertion of wet cotton pledgets into the tumor resection cavity in transsphenoidal surgery of pituitary tumors, for a better comparison between pre- and intraoperative high-field magnetic resonance images. J Neurol Surg A Cent Eur Neurosurg. 2013;74(6):366-72.

30. Tabaee A, Anand VK, Schwartz TH. The Role of Stereotactic Navigation in Endoscopic Pituitary Surgery. In: Endoscopic Pituitary Surgery. Thieme; 2012 pp. 305-12.

31. Wang YY, Thiryayi WA, Ramaswamy R, et al. Accuracy of Surgeon's Estimation of Sella Margins during Endoscopic Surgery for Pituitary Adenomas: Verification Using Neuronavigation. Skull Base. 2011;21(3):193-200.

32. Lasio G, Ferroli P, Felisati G, et al. Image-guided endoscopic transnasal removal of recurrent pituitary adenomas. Neurosurgery. 2002;51(1):132-6.

33. Shah NJ, Navnit M, Deopujari CE, et al. Endoscopic pituitary surgery: a beginner's guide. Indian J Otolaryngol Head Neck Surg. 2004;56(1):71-8.

34. Lucas JW, Zada G. Endoscopic surgery for pituitary tumors. Neurosurg Clin N Am. 2012;23(4):555-69.

35. Lee CC, Lee ST, Chang CN, et al. Volumetric measurement for comparison of the accuracy between intraoperative CT and posoperative MR imaging in pituitary adenoma surgery. Am J Neuroradiol. 2011;32(8):1539-44.

36. Ammirati M, Wei L, Ciric I. Short-term outcome of endoscopic versus microscopic pituitary adenoma surgery: a systematic review and meta-analysis. J Neurol Neurosurg Psychiatry. 2013;84(8):843-9.

37. Zaidi HA, De Los Reyes K, Barkhoudarian G, et al. The utility of high-resolution intraoperative MRI in endoscopic transsphenoidal surgery for pituitary macroadenomas: early experience in the Advanced Multimodality Image Guided Operating suite. Neurosurg Focus. 2016;40(3):E18.

38. Goudakos JK, Markou KD, Georgalas C. Endoscopic versus microscopic trans-sphenoidal pituitary surgery: a systematic review and meta-analysis. Clin Otolaryngol. 2011;36(3):212-20.

39. Zhu M, Yang J, Wang Y, et al. Endoscopic transsphenoid surgery versus microsurgery for resection of pituitary adenomas: a systemic review. Zhonghua Er Bi Yan Hou Tou Jing Wai Ke Za Zhi. 2014;49(3):236-9.

40. Serra C, Burkhardt JK, Esposito G, et al. Pituitary surgery and volumetric assessment of extent of resection: a paradigm shift in the use of intraoperative magnetic resonance imaging. Neurosurg Focus. 2016;40(3):E17.

41. Chang EF, Zada G, Kim S, et al. Long-term recurrence and mortality after surgery and adjuvant radiotherapy for nonfunctional pituitary adenomas. J Neurosurg. 2008; 108(4):736-45.

42. Taneka Y, Hongo K, Tada T, et al. Growth pattern and rate in residual nonfunctioning pituitary adenomas: correlations among tumor volume doubling time, patient age, and MIB-1 index. J Neurosurg. 2003;98(2):359-65.

43. Honegger J, Zimmermann S, Psaras T, et al. Growth modelling of non-functioning pituitary adenomas in patients referred for surgery. Eur J Endocrinol. 2008;158(3):287-94.

44. Berkmann S, Schlaffer S, Buchfelder M. Tumor shrinkage after transsphenoidal surgery for nonfunctioning pituitary adenoma. J Neurosurg. 2013;119(6):1447-52.

45. Ferrante E, Ferraroni M, Castrignanò T, et al. Non-functioning pituitary adenoma database: a useful resource to improve the clinical management of pituitary tumors. Eur J Endocrinol. 2006;155(6):823-9.

46. Drange MR, Fram NR, Herman-Bonert V, et al. Pituitary tumor registry: a novel clinical resource. J Clin Endocrinol Metab. 2000;85(1):168-74.

47. Thomas R, Shenoy K, Seshadri MS, et al. Visual field defects in non-functioning pituitary adenomas. Indian J Ophthalmol. 2002;50(2):127-30.

48. Cury ML, Fernandes JC, Machado HR, et al. Non-functioning pituitary adenomas: clinical feature, laboratorial and imaging assessment, therapeutic management and outcome. Arq Bras Endocrinol Metab. 2009;53(1):31-39.

49. Hlavica M, Bellut D, Lemm D, et al. Impact of ultra-low-field intraoperative magnetic resonance imaging on extent of resection and frequency of tumor recurrence in 104 surgically treated nonfunctioning pituitary adenomas. World Neurosurg. 2013;79(1):99-109.

15

Intraoperative Imaging in Skull Base Surgeries

Michael R Chicoine

INTRODUCTION

The category of skull base tumors comprises a broad variety of benign and malignant lesions. The incidence of each skull base tumor type is difficult to quantify, since many are clinically silent. Meningioma, pituitary adenoma, and vestibular schwannomas (VS) are the most common benign skull base tumors, but paragangliomas, craniopharyngiomas, Rathke's cleft cysts, epidermoid cysts, dermoid cysts, teratomas, fibro-osseous processes such as fibrous dysplasia and other benign conditions can also involve the skull base. Chordomas and chondrosarcomas are more aggressive, but intermediate grade malignant tumors of the skull base. A variety of more malignant tumors including squamous cell carcinoma, adenoid cystic carcinoma, metastases from systemic cancers, and other carcinomas and sarcomas can also grow in and around the skull base. In this chapter, we will focus on the application of intraoperative imaging for these more common skull base tumors, with brief mention of specific applications for less common tumors that we have encountered or that have been presented in the literature. Pituitary adenoma and sellar tumors are covered elsewhere; however, we have added our recent experience with these tumors for completion as these represent, in a sense, the most common skull base tumor.

Skull base tumors, as a general category, are often difficult to surgically remove due to depth of resection required, narrow operative corridor for visualization, and/or proximity to eloquent structures. Tumor characteristics such as brain infiltration, neurovascular involvement, gross tumor size, and tumor consistency also impact ease of resection. Often times, the surgeon must judge whether to aggressively pursue gross total resection, or if a more conservative approach is warranted, leaving known or suspected residual tumor in the resection bed. This decision making process occurs preoperatively and dynamically during the surgery, with consideration of tumor type, cranial location, consistency and proximity to eloquent structures, as well as an understanding of possible postoperative adjunctive therapies that may have benefit.

The principle treatment for many of these tumors is microscopic surgical resection; however, other management options may be more appropriate in many cases. Radiotherapy can be used as a postoperative adjuvant or as a substitute for surgery in certain cases. Observation may also be a valid approach for a subset of these tumors with a demonstrated slow growth rate and benign clinical course. In more recent years, minimally invasive and endoscopic techniques have been proposed for many skull base tumors, replacing traditional complex and site-specific open cranial approaches in some instances. Studies have suggested that these advanced approaches may reduce surgical morbidity and improve extent of resection (EOR) for certain skull base tumors; however, the potential for unintended residual tumor remains.

Technologies such as intraoperative ultrasound (iUS), intraoperative computed tomography (iCT), and intraoperative magnetic resonance imaging (iMRI) have been introduced to identify residual disease during surgery and allow for additional resection efforts to improve EOR. Intraoperative bone scanning (iOBS) has been reported on a limited basis to assess EOR for osteoid osteomas. In addition to radiographic intraoperative imaging modalities, intraoperative fluorescent techniques have also begun to be used for skull base tumor resection. Photodynamic diagnostics using 5-aminolevulinic acid (5-ALA) has allowed for increased discrimination of tumor from normal structures and improved identification of residual tumor remnants. Similar to iCT and iMRI, 5-ALA has been most extensively studied for intra-axial brain tumors, particularly malignant gliomas. Fluorescent angiography using indocyanine green videoangiography (ICGV) has also been used to appreciate the relationship between tumor and adjacent vascular structures. Intraoperative neuromonitoring (iONM) is another method used for real-time surgical assessment, with the primary role of preventing iatrogenic injury. It could be argued that iONM also works towards improving EOR, since it allows accurate discrimination between functional and pathological tissue. Despite differences in mode and function, all of these intraoperative imaging and monitoring technologies have the same primary goal—maximize safe surgical resection.

The impact of EOR on postoperative outcome for skull base tumors is often difficult to determine due to patient individual presentation variations, tumor heterogeneity, proximity to normal brain, and the potential effectiveness of adjuvant therapies. Therefore, resection aggressiveness must always be balanced against potential surgical morbidity, keeping first in mind the patient's postoperative quality of life. This dichotomy of balancing between aggressiveness of resection and preservation of function impacts decision making regarding the clinical significance of intraoperative imaging for skull base tumors.

In this chapter, we will summarize the relevant surgical and clinical characteristics of skull base tumors. With pre-, peri-, and postoperative management in mind, we will evaluate the published experience with intraoperative imaging techniques. We will also describe our experience and offer a summary of a detailed analysis of high-field iMRI for pituitary adenomas at Washington University or Barnes-Jewish Hospital.

INTRAOPERATIVE IMAGING TECHNIQUES

Radiographic Modalities

- *Intraoperative magnetic resonance imaging*: It is a powerful, versatile tool for assessing EOR during the resection of intracranial tumors. The majority of studies evaluating iMRI use during low- or high-grade glioma[1-7] and pituitary adenoma[8-25] resection. Low-field iMRI devices tend to be less costly and easier to implement into an existing operating room, but the small field-of-view and lower resolution may limit the usefulness of this technology for many intracranial applications. For example, imaging the complex anatomy of the sellar region can be challenging even with the highest resolution scanners available. This situation is complicated by the intraoperative environment in which blood, air tissue interfaces and other artifacts of the surgical field may impair the sensitivity of the imaging. Low-field scanners have limited capability for identifying subtle, small foci of residual tumor given these constraints.[23] Nevertheless, a number of centers have reported increased EOR for pituitary adenomas using low-field iMRI techniques.

Studies evaluating the use of iMRI for skull base tumors other than pituitary adenomas are limited.[26,27]

- *Intraoperative computed tomography*: It is another modality that offers promise for assessing EOR during skull base resection. High-resolution iCT can provide high quality imaging for certain applications and has considerable advantage over iMRI for osseous anatomy and bone pathologies. Additional operational advantages of iCT include faster image acquisition, lower acquisition and maintenance cost, simpler operating room arrangement and no challenges of operating in or near a strong magnetic field. Compared to high-field iMRI, the principle limitations of iCT for skull base tumor evaluation are the poor soft tissue resolution and multichannel analysis. Also, similar to conventional CT scanning, iCT exposes the patient to limited doses of ionizing radiation.[28] The two principles of iCT modalities are conventional multidetector CT (MDCT) and cone-beam CT (CBCT).[29-31] The MDCT provides greater soft tissue resolution than CBCT, while CBCT can be purchased at a lower cost, with less radiation exposure and less artifact from metallic objects than MDCT.[32] The increased resolution may make MDCT more useful for skull base resection; however, Chan et al.[30] performed intraoperative CBCT on phantom models of anterior skull base tumors, and found that intraoperative CBCT improved accuracy and surgeon confidence for these lesions.

- *Intraoperative ultrasound*: It is perhaps the most efficient intraoperative imaging modalities for skull base tumor assessment. This modality is less costly and time consuming than either iCT or iMRI, but does not have the high degree of resolution or versatility. Comparative poor resolution makes this modality suboptimal for identifying small areas of residual tumor. In consideration of this limitation, some have advocated combining iMRI and iUS. Using this approach, the surgeon can use iUS frequently and repeatedly during resection, and then later perform iMRI for more definitive assessment of EOR.[33]

- *Intraoperative bone scan:* It is used in conjunction with nuclear medicine also has the potential to visualize residual tumor in the skull base. Limited literature is currently available regarding iOBS for osteoid osteomas,[34] but it is possible that this modality could be of particular use for other tumors with extensive bony involvement.

Non-radiographic Modalities

Two principle intraoperative fluorescent techniques used in neurosurgery are photodynamic diagnostics using *5-ALA* and fluorescent angiography using *ICGV*. Use of 5-ALA has been reported most frequently and with great clinical significance for malignant gliomas;[35-37] however, there are limited reports describing its use in tumors such as meningiomas and pituitary adenomas.[38-44] ICGV is a simple, cost-effective technique that is commonly used for intraoperative assessment of patency of native vessels and lesion obliteration during surgery for aneurysms, arteriovenous malformations and other cerebrovascular conditions, but has the potential to benefit patients with pituitary adenomas and other skull base tumors in close proximity to arterial or venous structures.[45] Several investigators have proposed that this technology could be used transdurally for surgical approach planning, which may have some application for more superficially located skull base tumors.[46,47]

Intraoperative neuromonitoring can help to confirm the location and function of neurological structures. In particular, we find motor electromyography (EMG) monitoring and direct stimulation of cranial nerves VII, XI and XII often quite helpful during skull base surgery. Monitoring of cranial nerves II, III, IV, VI, IX and X is also feasible, but a technique that we use less frequently during skull base procedures. Intraoperative recording of the brainstem auditory evoked response (BAER) can be useful for hearing preservation, and motor evoked potentials (MEPs) and somatosensory evoked potentials (SSEPs) are helpful to monitor brainstem function. This physiological data is an excellent complement to the anatomical data of the surgical navigation and intraoperative imaging modalities, and can help to avoid inadvertent damage to the brain stem, cranial nerves and other vital structures.

INTRAOPERATIVE IMAGING FOR SKULL BASE TUMORS

The majority of current reports regarding intraoperative imaging for skull base tumors have studied iMRI use during pituitary adenoma resection, which has been covered in a separate chapter. These studies largely support the use of iMRI for these tumors, reporting improvements in EOR directly attributable to iMRI. At Washington University and Barnes-Jewish Hospital, we have made efforts to relate EOR improvement to more patient-centered outcomes, which will be covered briefly in this chapter.

Intraoperative imaging modalities may improve EOR for skull base tumors other than pituitary adenomas, but the data thus far are limited. It is also not clear how well EOR improvement translates to clinical outcomes such as recurrence rate, long-term cost and quality of life for these tumors. There may be other roles for intraoperative imaging than EOR improvement, but these are also not well-reported. As suggested by the current literature, these techniques may be best suited to endonasal endoscopic procedures, where tumor visualization may be obstructed by the narrow field-of-view or the complex anatomy of the suprasellar region and/or cavernous sinus. We will cover the existing data regarding intraoperative imaging for nonpituitary adenoma skull base tumors in this chapter.

Pituitary Adenoma

Pituitary adenomas are benign tumors that account for 10–15% of intracranial neoplasms.[48] These tumors can cause significant morbidity through excess hormones production or mass effect on the optic chiasm or other adjacent structures. Surgery via the transsphenoidal route remains the primary treatment, with craniotomy approaches reserved for extensive tumors.[49] Endoscopic and microscopic approaches have been described, and controversy exists regarding the best technique. The use of radiographic intraoperative imaging for pituitary adenoma resection has been the most extensively studied of all skull base lesions, including many studies reporting the EOR benefits of both low-field[8,9,14,19-22] and high-field iMRI.[13,15-18,25,50] Groups have also begun to evaluate iCT for identification of residual pituitary adenoma.[51]

The role of iMRI in pituitary adenoma resection has been well studied, with many groups showing a clear EOR benefit. There are, however, a number of limitations to many of these studies including the potential for selection and treatment bias due to nonrandomization and use of surrogate markers of patient benefit as primary endpoints. The use of EOR as a surrogate marker for patient benefit during pituitary adenoma resection may also be particularly problematic for a number of reasons. First, these are slow-growing, benign neoplasms that often do not progress or recur after resection. Second, there are several postoperative adjuvant therapies (e.g. radiation, hormone suppressive medication) that are both safe and effective for controlling residual and recurrent disease in certain situations. Third, several additional surgical tools (i.e. operative endoscope, stereotactic neuronavigation) have been incorporated into the operating room in recent years with EOR benefit that potentially overlaps with iMRI.

At *Washington University and Barnes-Jewish Hospital in St Louis*, a movable high-field 1.5 Tesla iMRI device (IMRIS, Inc., Winnipeg, Manitoba, CA) has been used in nearly 1,000 neurosurgical procedures including over 200 endonasal, endoscopic approaches for pituitary adenomas and a variety of benign and malignant skull base tumor resections.[11,52-55] The MRI device is situated between two operating rooms **(Figures 15.1A to C)** and can be transported to the patient by a ceiling mounted rail system.

Prior publications by Theodosopoulos et al.[19], Anand et al.[9] and Schwartz et al.[20] have demonstrated *complementary efficacy of endoscopy and iMRI*, which has been our experience as well. Analysis of pituitary adenoma cases from our institution revealed that iMRI prompted further resection in approximately 35–40% of cases, with approximately 10% of patients receiving an increased EOR status (from subtotal to near or gross total, or near total to gross total). Multivariate analysis revealed that that the combination of iMRI and endoscopy increased EOR status compared to conventional microsurgery without iMRI. Unpublished data from our center also suggests that increased EOR lengthens progression-free survival when controlling for prognostic baseline factors such

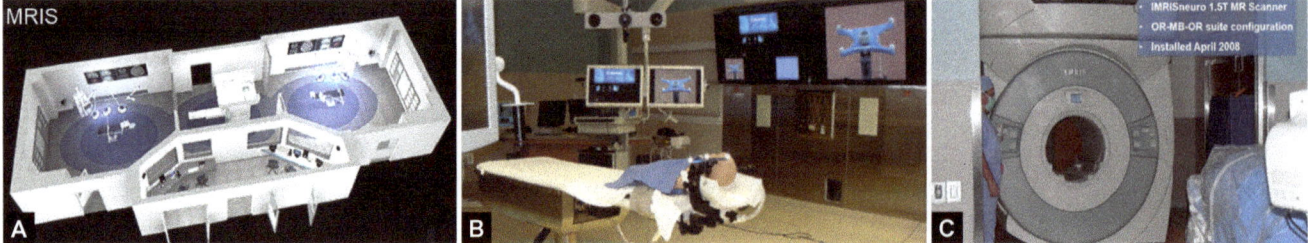

Figures 15.1A to C (A) Two operating room arrangement for the IMRIS 1.5 Tesla intraoperative magnetic resonance imaging (iMRI) suite installed in April 2008 at Barnes-Jewish Hospital; (B) The iMRI scanner is transfer to each operating room, and (C) On ceiling mounted rails by operating room technical staff

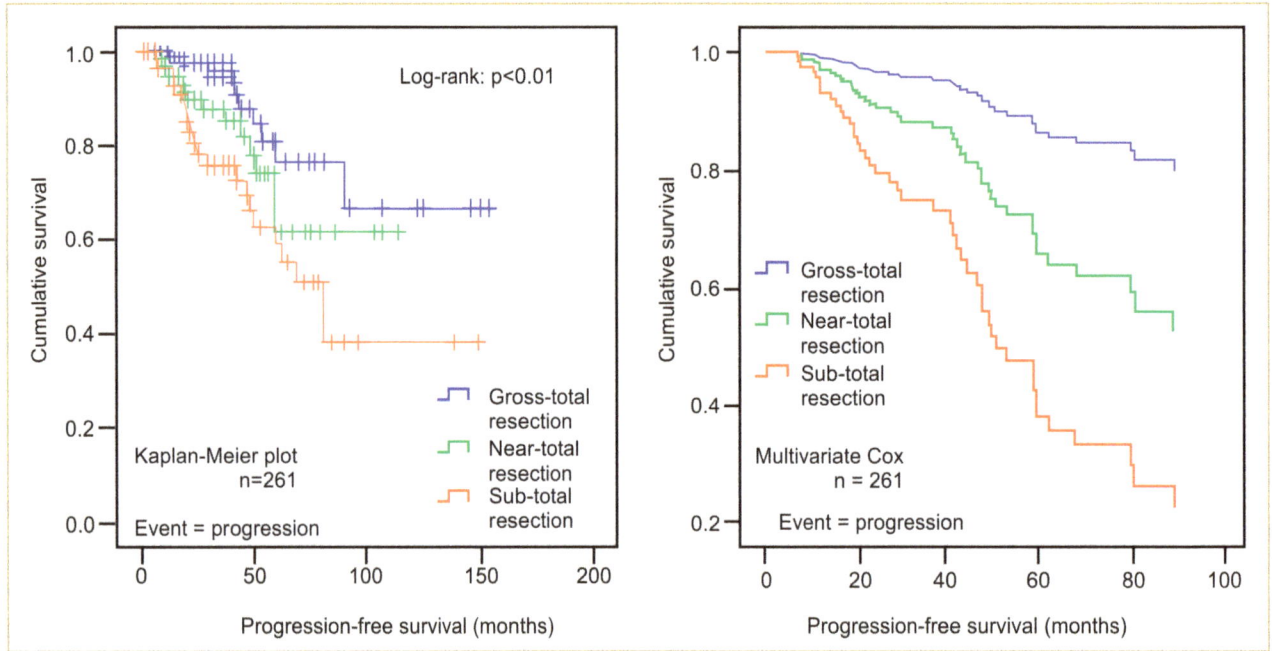

Figure 15.2 Survival analyses depicting progression-free survival for different extent of resection statuses. Kaplan-Meier plot (left) and multivariate Cox regression (right) of cases followed expectantly after surgery (i.e. no additional surgery, radiation, or hormone suppressive medication) showed a significantly longer progression-free survival for greater extent of resection status

as recurrent tumor, cavernous sinus invasion and tumor size **(Figure 15.2)**.

Some investigators have argued that iCT could be an adequate alternative to iMRI for a number of centers. A prospective study by Lee et al.[51] compared residual tumor volume determined from iCT (MDCT) to postoperative 1.5 Tesla MRI for 33 patients that received endoscopic resection of pituitary macroadenomas. They found a strong correlation in tumor volumes between modalities for gross total ($R^2 = 0.971$) and subtotal resected tumors ($R^2 = 0.957$), and concluded that iCT could be used effectively for pituitary adenoma resection with similar efficacy to iMRI. These results seem to support that iCT might be a suitable alternative iMRI for pituitary adenoma resection; however, further assessment is warranted.

The technique of iUS has been proven to be feasible and reasonably sensitive for pituitary adenomas resection,[56,57] and may be a useful adjunct. Combination with other intraoperative imaging modalities takes advantage of the ability to frequently recheck resection status with iUS and then perform a final check with the more sensitive iCT or iMRI,[33] which may be particularly useful during endoscopic or microscopic pituitary adenoma resection due to limits in direct tumor visualization.

Use of non-radiographic intraoperative imaging modalities such as fluorescence-guided resection with 5-ALA or ICGV has not been frequently reported. However, preliminary reports have suggested efficacy of ICGV for pituitary adenoma resection.[38,45]

Meningioma

Skull base meningiomas are benign tumors that represent approximately 25% of all intracranial meningiomas.[58] Resection of these tumors can be much more challenging than non-skull base counterparts, with a wide range of reported gross total resection rates from 14.5% to 76% depending on tumor site.[59-62] Lower EOR rates for these tumors suggests a potential usefulness for intraoperative imaging; however, determining the clinical effectiveness of these technologies is complicated by numerous factors including unclear potential for improvement, conflicting literature regarding the prognostic significance of EOR, as well as confounding effectiveness of other intraoperative modalities, preoperative endovascular embolization and radiotherapy. In addition, several studies have shown that skull base meningiomas may be slower growing than non-skull base counterparts, with lower World Health Organization (WHO) grade, slower growth and less recurrence,[63-66] but the proximity to the brain stem, cranial nerves, and vasculature of these skull base meningiomas can lead to unique challenges for surgery and preservation of function.

In 1957, Donald Simpson published a paper that showed compelling evidence that increased meningioma resection improved postoperative outcomes. A grading system was reported in this study including grade I (total resection of tumor and involved dura and bone), grade II (total resection with cauterization of involved dura), grade III (total tumor removal only), grade IV (subtotal resection), and grade V (decompression with or without biopsy). Patients with increasing Simpson grade had successively higher rates of recurrence or progression.[67] This paper was the first to show a correlation between EOR and long-term outcomes for patients with meningiomas; however, there are limitations to this study that reduce translation of this grading scheme to current skull base practices. First, EOR and recurrence in Simpson's were based on clinical judgment, rather than postoperative imaging. Second, tools for tumor visualization and removal have improved dramatically since 1957, allowing perhaps greater EOR of tumors that had previously not been possible. Examples include introduction of the operative microscope and endoscope, stereotactic neuronavigation, and advanced debridement and electrocautery devices. Third, advanced skull base surgical approaches were essentially nonexistent in the 1950s.

Several modern studies have supported the results presented by Simpson,[68-70] including a report by Kallio et al. who found a 4.2 higher relative risk of mortality over 15 years after surgery for cases receiving only subtotal resection.[71] A study by Ichinose et al.[72] also supported this theme, but suggested further that recurrence rate correlated best with postoperative tumor residual volume and EOR, even in the setting of postoperative radiosurgery.

Other recent studies have re-evaluated the current relevance of Simpson grade on postoperative outcomes given the availability of modern surgical equipment and skull base surgical techniques. Sughrue et al. retrospectively evaluated 373 WHO grade I meningiomas with no prior meningioma surgery, with the principle endpoints being recurrence or progression-free survival evaluated actuarially 5 years postoperatively and using Kaplan-Meier analysis.[61] The results showed no difference in recurrence or progression-free survival at 5 years for Simpson grade I, II, III, or IV resections (95%, 85%, 88%, 81%, respectively; chi-squared p = non-significant, value not reported) and no difference in recurrence or progression-free survival between Simpson grades on Kaplan-Meier analysis (log-rank p = non-significant, value not reported). Subgroup Kaplan-Meier analysis also revealed no significant difference in recurrence or progression-free survival between Simpson grades for skull base meningioma (log-rank p = non-significant, value not reported). Based on these results, the authors concluded that the importance of Simpson grade in preoperative planning should be strongly questioned, particularly for skull base meningioma since these cases were underrepresented in Simpson's study. Nonetheless, this and other studies have limited follow-up for a tumor that can recur 10–20 years or more after surgery, and most would agree that maximal resection, including complete resection if feasible, is advisable when it can be accomplished safely. This study from Sughrue and colleagues applied only to WHO grade I meningiomas, and typically at the time of surgery, one cannot be certain of the WHO grade of the tumor. Newer studies suggest that 30% or more of meningiomas are WHO II based on the current criteria.

In addition to the uncertainty regarding the clinical importance of EOR, and balancing the EOR with preservation of function, the value of intraoperative imaging may have been further marginalized by *other treatment options* that have emerged to assist in the management of skull base meningioma since Simpson's landmark paper.

Even though the primary treatment for most meningioma remains surgical resection, fractionated *radiotherapy and radiosurgery* have gained increased use in both as a postoperative adjuvant and replacement therapies. Pollock et al.[73] retrospectively compared outcomes in 528 meningioma resections to 170 meningioma radiosurgeries including small to medium size tumors without symptomatic mass effect. 7-year progression-free survival was similar between Simpson grade I resections and radiosurgery (96% vs 95%, respectively), but Simpson grade II and III–IV had lower 7-year progression-free survival than radiosurgery (82% and 34%, respectively), suggesting that radiosurgery may be indicated in cases where low EOR is expected. Subsequently, several groups have evaluated long-term results following the use of radiosurgery for skull base meningioma,[74-78] supporting radiation as an effective alternative to microsurgery. Ultimately, the decision to use radiation therapy as primary treatment involves careful assessment of the patient's individual presentation and surgical risks including tumor size, location and proximity to eloquent structures.

Preoperative *endovascular embolization* has also been introduced to potentially improve the safety of meningioma resection. Early postoperative comparison performed by Dean et al.[79] and Macpherson[80] retrospectively compared meningioma cases that did not receive preoperative embolization, and found that the embolization group had less blood loss and fewer surgical complications. Subjectively, some reports have suggested that embolization improved the ease of resection. To date, no randomized trials have been completed to assess outcomes following preoperative meningioma embolization, and the benefits and indications for this procedure are not well-characterized. In addition, endovascular embolization is not without risk. A review of 36 studies (459 cases) by Shah et al.[81] identified 21 complications directly resulting from embolization. Most complications were minor or temporary (18 cases), but one case received a major complication (permanent blindness) and two cases resulted in fatality. At our center, endovascular embolization is used selectively in a small subset of meningiomas prior to resection when the tumor is particularly large and highly vascular. Endovascular embolization is used more consistently for glomus jugulare tumors or other highly vascular lesions.

Radiographic intraoperative imaging techniques have been used on a limited basis in an attempt to improve the safety and efficacy of meningioma resection. To date, only a single study, performed by Soleman et al.[26], reported results of iMRI use for meningioma resection. Included cases were difficult to remove skull base lesions or tumors compressing eloquent areas where radical resection was termed difficult by the authors. A 0.15T low-field scanner was utilized for 27 cases. Based on the iMRI scan, residual tumor was identified in 13/27 cases. Only one patient (3.4%) received additional resection after iMRI (sphenoid ridge anaplastic meningioma, previous surgery, previous stereotactic radiosurgery), and this did not improve from Simpson grade IV. Based on these results, the authors did not support general the use of iMRI for complex meningioma resection; however, they did suggest iMRI may have a role in select applications. High-field iMRI may better define residual tumor, but the differentiation of meningioma from adjacent structures is typically not the limiting factor in meningioma surgery. The EOR during meningioma surgery is typically more limited by proximity and adherence to critical structures such as cranial nerves, vessels and brain.

At our institution, high-field iMRI has been used on a limited basis in a small subset of complex skull base meningioma cases. **Figures 15.3A to C** show the pre-, intra-, and postoperative imaging of a patient with a recurrent anterior fossa skull base meningioma (Case 1) 10 years after a prior resection via a bilateral frontal craniotomy. Residual tumor from this prior resection had progressed gradually over the years, with preoperative MRI showing a large lesion in the anterior cranial fossa **(Figure 15.3A)**. Pathologic evaluation of the tumor specimen from her initial resection revealed a WHO grade II meningioma with brain invasion. Repeat resection was performed via an endonasal, endoscopic midline basal frontal craniotomy. After generous, but subtotal resection, an iMRI scan was performed, which revealed residual tumor in the anterior most aspect of the anterior fossa and right orbit **(Figure 15.3B)**. Additional tumor was removed from the right orbit, which was confirmed by pathology to be meningioma. The patient was returned to the operating room a few days later for repair of a skull base defect causing pneumocephalus, as well as removal of the known residual tumor focus in the anterior cranial fossa via a combined endoscopic and traditional bifrontal craniotomy approach. Postoperative MRI 4 months after surgery revealed no residual tumor **(Figure 15.3C)**. Final available radiographic follow-up 23 months after surgery revealed no recurrence. In this case, iMRI improved the EOR during the initial surgery; however, gross total resection was only achieved after a later surgical resection. The quantifiable utility of iMRI for this case is difficult to discern, but it may have helped with intraoperative decision making as to the appropriate safe limit of resection.

Solheim et al. described the methods for using iUS during intracranial meningioma resection.[82] In this study, 15 cases with giant meningioma (>5 cm in largest diameter) were retrospectively evaluated, revealing gross total resection in all cases (12/15 cases were Simpson grade I or II). Three-dimensional ultrasound angiography was able to identify important feeder vessels in 14/15 cases. The authors state that iUS may improve the safety and efficacy of resection for giant meningiomas due to the frequent involvement of normal vessels, encroachment on eloquent brain structures, and the large amount of intraoperative brain shift resulting from intracapsular dissection. In an earlier study from the same institution, the authors judged that 5/9 skull base meningioma received benefit from iUS (the remaining 4/9 cases "probably" received some benefit) in terms of greater extent of intracapsular resection before starting capsule removal, and probable reduction in trauma to normal brain structures.[83]

Preliminary findings regarding the use of *non-radiographic intraoperative imaging* techniques have also been reported. Case reports and series have described methods and suggested the efficacy of *5-ALA* for certain meningioma resections, with visible fluorescence present in 80–94% of cases.[39-42] Valdes et al.[43] reported the use of an intraoperative probe capable of detecting nanogram levels of protoporphyrin IX (PpIX) to quantify fluorescence levels in 10 patients, which revealed a strongly significant difference in PpIX levels between tumor and normal dura. Hefti et al.[44] reported results of an *in vitro* study of two meningioma cell line, suggesting that the heterogeneity in PpIX is mainly due to differences in ferrochelatase levels, but the clinical

Preoperative   Intraoperative   Postoperative

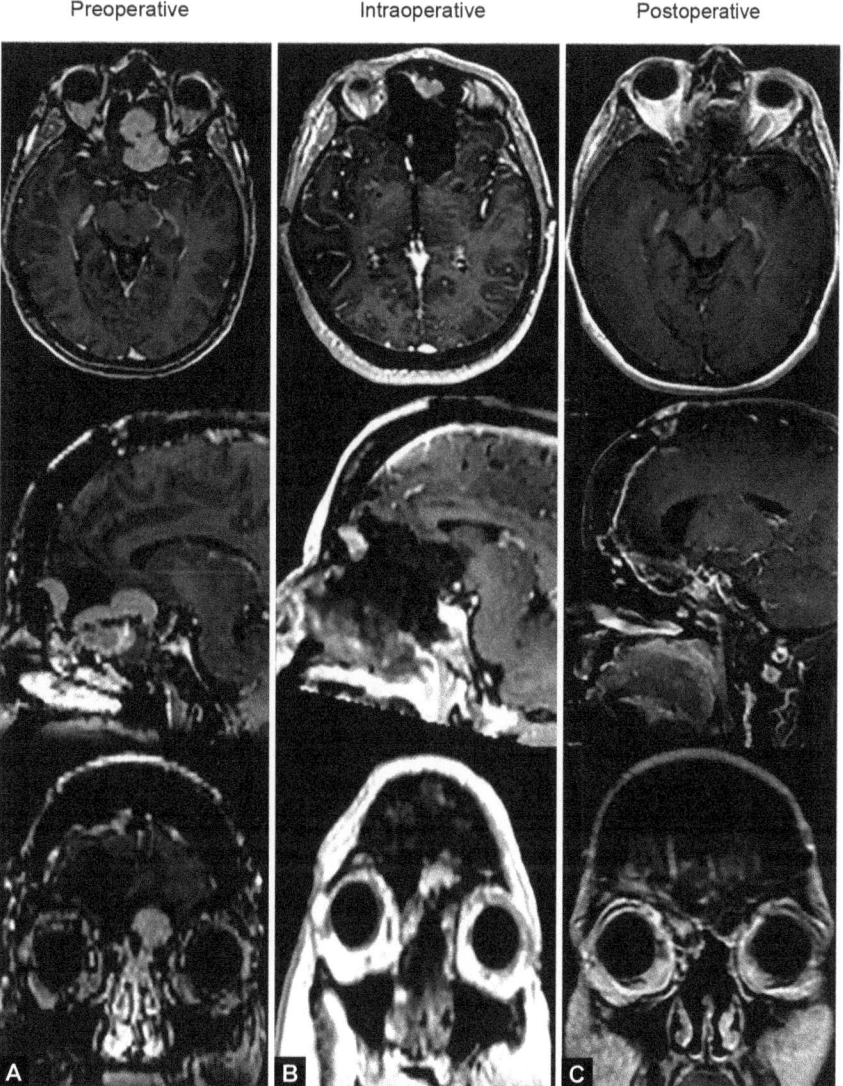

Figures 15.3A to C *Case 1:* Patient with recurrent World Health Organization (WHO) Grade II meningioma in the anterior cranial fossa skull base. Initial resection was 10 years prior. (A) Preoperative magnetic resonance imaging (MRI) demonstrated an enhancing lesion. Resection was performed by a combined endonasal, endoscopic and craniotomy approach; (B) On intraoperative MRI (iMRI), residual tumor was noted in the anterior resection cavity near the left orbit. Additional resection removed additional tumor, confirmed by pathology to be meningioma; and (C) Postoperatively, the patient developed pneumocephalus, and returned to the operating room for repair and additional tumor debulking via a combined endonasal, endoscopic and craniotomy approach. Postoperative MRI revealed gross total resection

relevance of this finding is not yet appreciated. Recent studies have also reported the use of transdural *ICGV* for the removal of meningioma, particularly for appropriate and safe dural opening. This strategy is perhaps most useful for convexity and parasagittal meningioma occluding the superior sagittal sinus;[46,47] however, foramen magnum meningioma may receive some benefit from ICGV.[47]

The idea of maximum tumor removal without damage to normal tissue has become increasingly accepted among skull base surgeons for certain lesions. Retrospective analysis

of 205 meningioma resection cases by Alkemade et al.[84] revealed a significant decrease in long-term survival for meningioma patients receiving surgery after age 45 due to tumor recurrence and stroke, and noted that 67% of patient had at least one neurological symptom postoperatively. These results highlight the vital importance of choosing appropriate patients for surgery and taking care to preserve normal structures.

In summary, intraoperative imaging modalities, particularly iMRI, have the potential to improve EOR for skull base meningiomas, but reports thus far have not favored routine use. It is difficult to assign specific prognostic significance to increased EOR, given conflicting results in recent literature regarding Simpson grade. The potential therapeutic benefit of radiation as adjuvant or replacement therapy in some cases might diminish the importance of iMRI for improving EOR. The use of iUS may have potential in reducing risk to vascular structures in giant skull base meningioma, but the currently available literature regarding this modality is also limited. A potential subgroup of meningioma that may receive the particular benefit from intraoperative imaging is the infiltrative type of meningioma; however, few studies have evaluated the prognostic influence and EOR capabilities associated with this factor.

Vestibular Schwannoma

Vestibular schwannomas (also known as acoustic neuromas) are benign skull base lesions that grow in the cerebellopontine angle (CPA) and internal auditory meatus. Based on registry data, VS, and nerve sheath tumors represent about 9% of primary brain tumors. Three main surgical approaches: (1) middle fossa, (2) translabyrinthine, and (3) retrosigmoid or suboccipital or combinations thereof are used to remove these tumors, often performed jointly between neurosurgery and otolaryngology.[85] Gross total resection rates from a large modern series are near 75%.[86] In addition, this same study found no difference in progression or recurrence free survival on Kaplan-Meier and multivariate Cox Proportional Hazards analysis between patients receiving gross versus subtotal resection. Like skull base meningiomas, it is typically not a difficulty with determination of the extent of the lesion that limits the resection of these tumors, but rather the intimate relationship to the cranial nerves, brainstem and other critical structures that leads the surgeon to perform a subtotal resection. Complete removal of VS, particularly for larger tumors carries distinct risk of injury to cranial nerves. To protect normal structures and mitigate nerve damage, iONM has been implemented during these surgeries and has become considered the standard of care.[87] Due to the CPA location of these tumors, the cranial nerves most at risk for a majority of these surgeries are the facial nerve [cranial nerve (CN) VII] and the vestibulocochlear nerve (CN VIII), but for larger tumors, CNs IV-VI, IX-XII can also be at risk. Other tumors of the CPA such as meningioma and epidermoid cysts also can benefit from iONM of the facial and vestibulocochlear nerve. As surgery for VS is largely based upon anatomy and iONM, intraoperative imaging such as iCT or iMRI in general probably has little utility.

Historically, surgical resection was the primary treatment for these tumors. Modern prospective studies have demonstrated excellent patient outcomes using stereotactic radiosurgery for many of these tumors. Observation, surgical resection (via middle fossa, translabyrinthine, or retrosigmoid

suboccipital approaches), or stereotactic radiosurgery are all viable treatment options. Subtotal resection followed by observation or radiosurgery are increasingly recognized as viable options for many patients that do require surgery, in an effort to preserve facial nerve and other neurological functions, particularly in patients with larger tumors, and in patients of older age. The choice of treatment should be tailored to address many factors including the patient's age and medical comorbidities, the size of the tumor, the status of the hearing, and other neurological parameters and patient preference.

Damage to the facial nerve during VS surgery can cause considerable morbidity to the patient due to the nerves innervation of muscles of facial expression. Damage to this nerve can cause facial drooping, loss of blinking, and impairments in speech, chewing and swallowing. In 1985, the House-Brackmann Grade was developed,[88] which classified the extent of facial nerve injury sustained during CPA surgery. This facial function grading system ranges from normal grade I function to profoundly impaired grade VI with no functional movement. In 2009, Vrabec et al.[89] proposed a new system term the Facial Nerve Grading System 2.0 (FNGS 2.0), which included primary movements from the brow, eye, mouth, and nasolabial fold, as well as synkinesis measured across the entire face. The number of grades was unchanged between House-Brackmann grading and the FNGS 2.0 (Grade I-VI); however, the authors of the FNGS 2.0 suggest better discrimination of mid-grade lesions using the new system.

The most common iONM techniques used during VS surgery for protecting the facial nerve is *EMG*. Using this technique, the surgeon can use a probe in regions proximal to the tumor site to stimulate a facial motor response, with the intention of localizing the facial nerve. Facial sensors can also detect irritation of the facial nerve in real-time, allowing the surgeon to avoid nerve damage during tumor manipulation and resection. A study by Sughrue et al.[90] showed that facial nerve stimulation detected by EMG is highly specific for nerve damage (90%), but has poor sensitivity (29%). *Intraoperative video monitoring (iOVM)* of facial movement has also be performed for facial nerve protection during VS surgery, but this technique is not as sensitive for nerve stimulation as EMG.[91] Studies have shown that patients with large tumors are particularly susceptible to facial nerve damage during VS surgery,[92] and may also receive the most benefit from iONM.

Hearing preservation during VS surgery is another crucially important quality of life concern for patients, but can be much more challenging than facial nerve preservation. Many of these patients have significant hearing impairment at the time of the initial diagnosis of the tumor. The severity of the hearing loss in addition to other anatomical features such as tumor size factor in the surgical planning decision making process. For example, a small intracanalicular tumor in an individual with good hearing might prompt resection via a middle fossa approach, whereas severe hearing loss in a patient with a tumor 2.5 cm in diameter in the CPA might prompt a translabyrinthine approach. The Gardner or Robertson grading system allows for quantitative comparisons of postoperative hearing outcomes.[93] Fischer et al.[94] reported preoperative predictive factors for hearing preservation included good low frequency hearing and small tumor size. Techniques for vestibulocochlear nerve iONM are commonly used for VS surgery employing either far-or near-field techniques. *Far-field techniques* such as brainstem auditory evoked potentials (BAER) measure electrical activity from the scalp surface. The large distance between source and electrode produce a small signal-to-noise ratio, which necessitates extensive signal averaging to produce meaningful information and slows response to the surgeon by as long as minutes. A series of 1000 VS cases using BAER, Samii et al.[95] reported anatomical cochlear nerve preservation in 682/1000, but good functional nerve preservation in only 289/732 cases (39.5%) with some preoperative hearing. Tonn et al. reported similar good functional hearing preservation rates (39.8%).[96] A separate study by Samii et al.[97] reported relatively increased good hearing preservation using the retrosigmoid approach (51%).

Near-field techniques such as electrocochleography and direct compound nerve action potential (CNAP) measurement have a significant advantage over far-field techniques in terms of signal-to-noise ratio, which alleviates the need for multiple signal averaging and long delays in iONM. Mechanistically, near-field techniques have greater efficacy for intraoperative monitoring than far-field counterparts, and work by Yamakami et al.[98] demonstrated the relative superiority of direct CNAP measurement in terms of sensitivity and specificity. The principle disadvantage of near-field techniques is the potential for not recording responses from the entire nerve, which could lead to iatrogenic injury. This may be particularly challenging with large tumors, where operative visibility is limited.

In summary, VS are benign, slow growing tumors that may be managed with observation, surgery or radiosurgery. Radiographic intraoperative imaging has little role for these extra-axial tumors, given the good operative visibility using modern skull base approaches and the frequent presence of a tumor capsule. Studies have also demonstrated a high rate of gross total resection. In some circumstances, subtotal resection may be advisable in order to preserve facial nerve or other neurological functions. After subtotal resection, observation or radiosurgery may be advisable. iONM of the facial nerve has been shown to improve postoperative outcomes following VS surgery using a validated grading system. iONM of the vestibulocochlear nerve may have utility in the patients with small tumors or excellent preoperative hearing, but for many patients, the size of the tumor and the severity of preoperative hearing loss limit the ability to preserve useful hearing. Similar strategies often also apply for other less common intracranial schwannomas such as

those of the trigeminal and vagal nerves, as well as other tumor types such as glomus jugulare tumors and epidermoid cysts. The primary outcome for these tumors should remain preservation of postoperative cranial nerve function, since residual tumor has not been shown to affect postoperative outcomes and can often be effectively treated with adjuvant radiosurgery, if needed.

Other Skull Base Tumors

Aside from pituitary adenoma resection, reports on the use of radiographic or non-radiographic intraoperative imaging for skull base tumors are relatively few. This is likely due to a combination of the rarity of these tumor types, as well as the limited access to and uncertain indication for intraoperative imaging. One suggested use for intraoperative imaging is for osteoid osteomas, an uncommon tumor that may be seen in the skull, which may receive some benefit from nuclear medicine iOBSs due to highly sensitive for lesion localization and verification of complete surgical extirpation.[34] These tumors are highly likely to recur if not completely resected, but will often be cured if completely removed. iOBS is a unique application for an uncommon condition, but may be very useful for this particular disease.

Our experience using iMRI for other skull base tumors is also limited due to lower surgeon interest and/or lower cases counts compared to pituitary adenoma. However, we have observed cases where iMRI has led to increased EOR during both traditional microsurgical and endonasal, endoscopic techniques **(Figures 15.4 to 15.7)**, so the opportunity exists for intraoperative imaging of these tumor resections even though at present the benefit is not well-defined. Here, we briefly present four cases, each an endoscopic resection for a large anterior or middle skull base lesion, which were selected to receive iMRI due to the expected complexity of resection.

Two cases were performed at our institution for patients with adenoid cystic carcinomas (Case 2 and Case 3) with similar pre- and postoperative courses. Preoperative MRI scans demonstrated large, enhancing base masses of the anterior skull base and sinonasal regions **(Figures 15.4A and 15.5A)**. Both cases received extensive, but subtotal resection via an endonasal, endoscopic approach prior to iMRI scanning **(Figures 15.4B and 15.5B)**. Continued soft tissue resection was performed, which was confirmed to be carcinoma, and postoperative MRI scanning revealed a reduction in residual tumor volume **(Figures 15.4C and 15.5C)**. Both patients received adjuvant fractionated radiotherapy to the residual tumor region, and available follow-up (16 months and 31 months, respectively) revealed no progression. Neither patient developed a neurologic deficit postoperatively.

A young patient received two operations at our institution using iMRI for surgical guidance during a *juvenile nasopharyngeal angiofibroma* resection (Case 4). The vascularity of this tumor was identified using catheter angiography **(Figure 15.6A)** and embolization was performed. Preoperative MRI demonstrated a sinonasal, skull base mass **(Figure 15.6B)**. Maximal resection was achieved via a combined endoscopic, endonasal and sublabial approach prior to iMRI, which demonstrated residual tumor involving the right petrous carotid and cavernous sinus. No further resection was attempted, and an early postoperative MRI was stable after surgery **(Figure 15.6C)**. Tumor progression was identified on a subsequent MRI, and a second combined endoscopic, endonasal and sublabial operation was attempted, with removal of additional tumor. The iMRI scan revealed persistent residual tumor surrounding the right

petrous carotid artery **(Figure 15.6D)**, which was further resected and confirmed to be angiofibroma. Postoperative MRI revealed a slight decrease in size from the prior iMRI scan **(Figure 15.6E)**. Final follow-up scan available 25 months later revealed stable residual tumor.

Another patient underwent endonasal, endoscopic resection of a recurrent middle fossa low-grade *chondrosarcoma* following prior craniotomy and subtotal resection (Case 5). Preoperative MRI demonstrated progression of a T2-enhancing mass **(Figure 15.7A)**. Resection was performed via an endoscopic, endonasal transsphenoidal approach. An iMRI scan performed after safe maximal resection revealed

| Preoperative | Intraoperative | Postoperative |

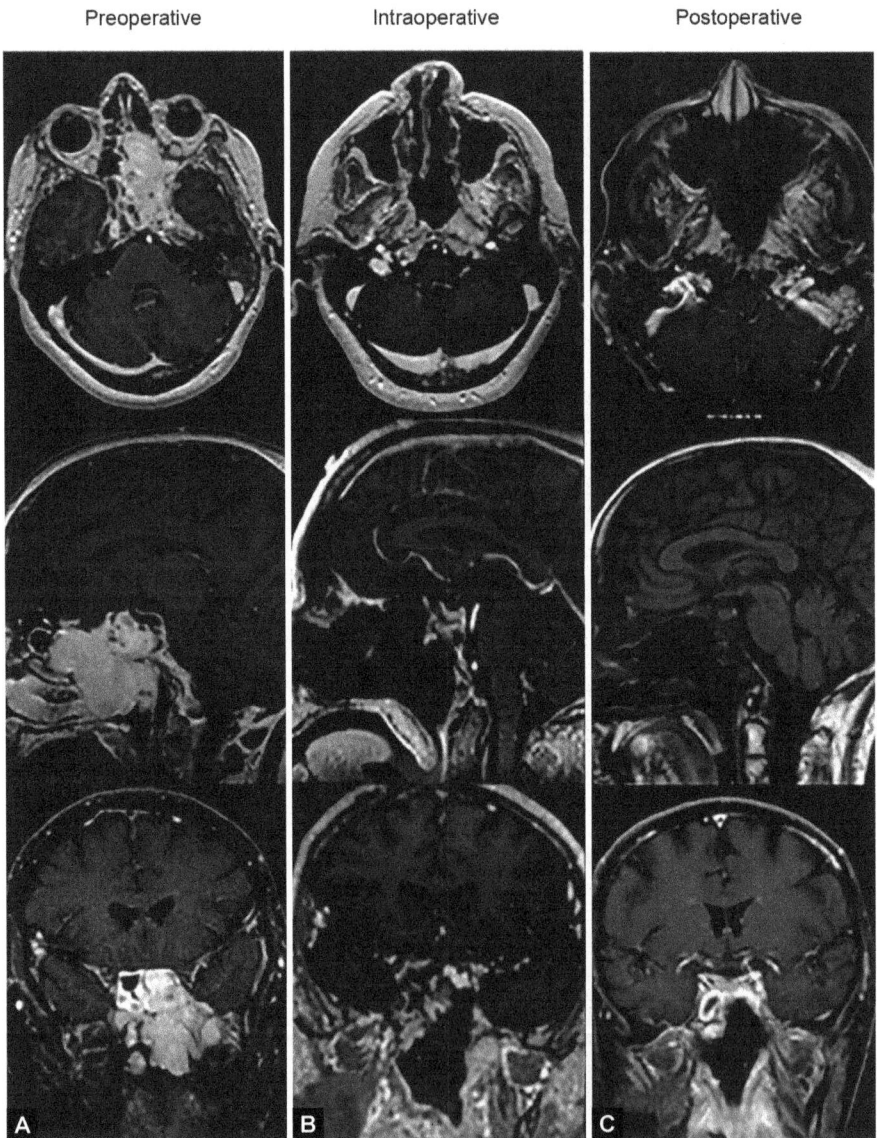

Figures 15.4A to C *Case 2:* (A) Patient with preoperative magnetic resonance imaging (MRI) demonstrating a large sinonasal mass. Endonasal, endoscopic resection was performed and pathology confirmed adenoid cystic carcinoma; (B) Intraoperative MRI revealed residual tumor in the inferior aspect of the resection bed. Resection was continued, and (C) Postoperative MRI revealed reduced residual tumor volume

| Preoperative | Intraoperative | Postoperative |

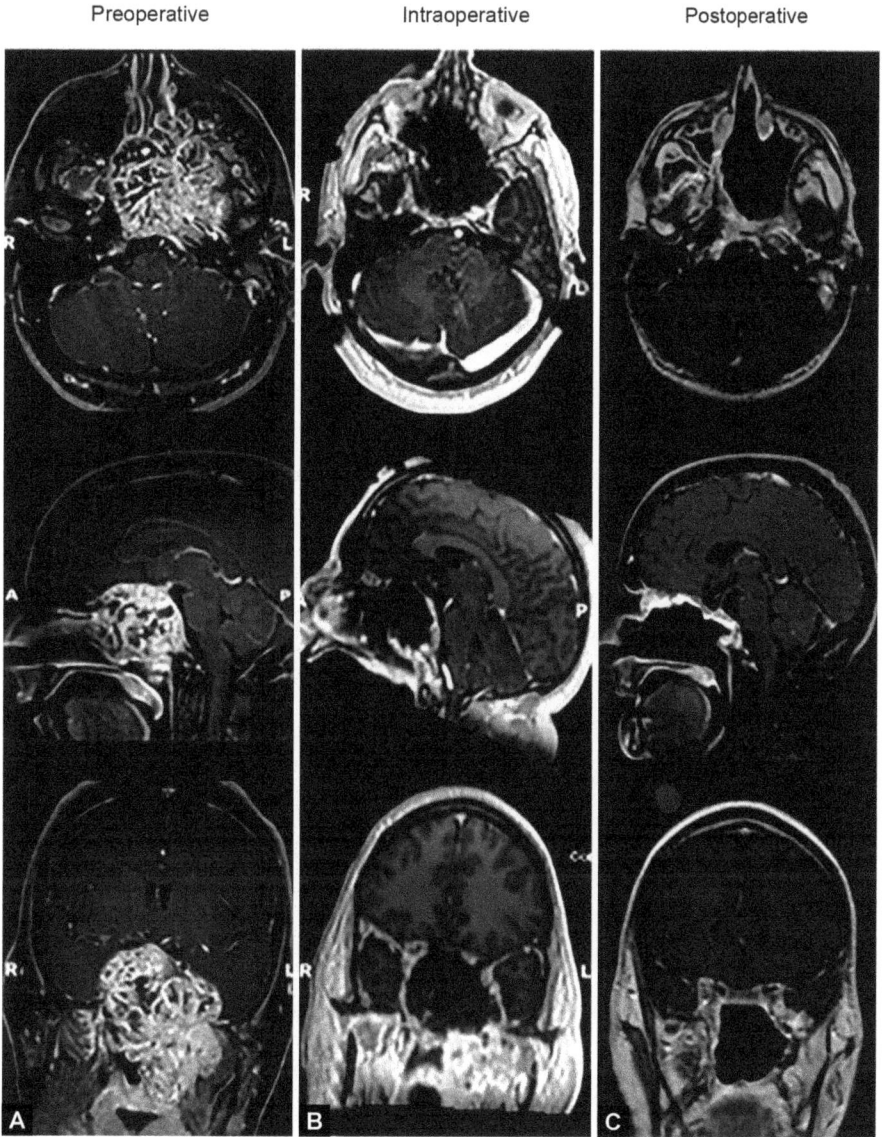

Figures 15.5A to C (A) *Case 3:* Patient with preoperative magnetic resonance imaging (MRI) demonstrating a large sinonasal mass. Endonasal, endoscopic resection was performed and pathology confirmed adenoid cystic carcinoma; (B) An intraoperative MRI scan revealed residual tumor in the inferior aspect of the resection bed near the soft palate; additional tumor was removed; and (C) Postoperative MRI revealed reduced residual tumor volume

residual enhancement on T2 sequence **(Figure 15.7B)**, which was further resected and confirmed to be chondrosarcoma. Postoperative MRI revealed potential areas of residual tumor **(Figure 15.7C)**, with radiographic progression identified 24 months after surgery that was subsequently treated with stereotactic radiosurgery. Final available imaging follow-up 46 months after surgery revealed continued slow growth of the residual lesion **(Figure 15.7D)**, but no clinical progression; therefore, continued observation was recommended.

Traditionally, malignant skull base tumor resections have been performed with the intention of gross and microscopic total resection, with frequent intraoperative biopsies taken to ensure clear margins. If resection to microscopically negative margins was deemed impossible preoperatively, these cases were often treated with fractionated radiotherapy alone or in combination with chemotherapy. In the four cases of rarer skull base tumors presented here, additional endoscopic resection guided by iMRI resulted in additional tumor removal. It is conceivable that additional debulking of these

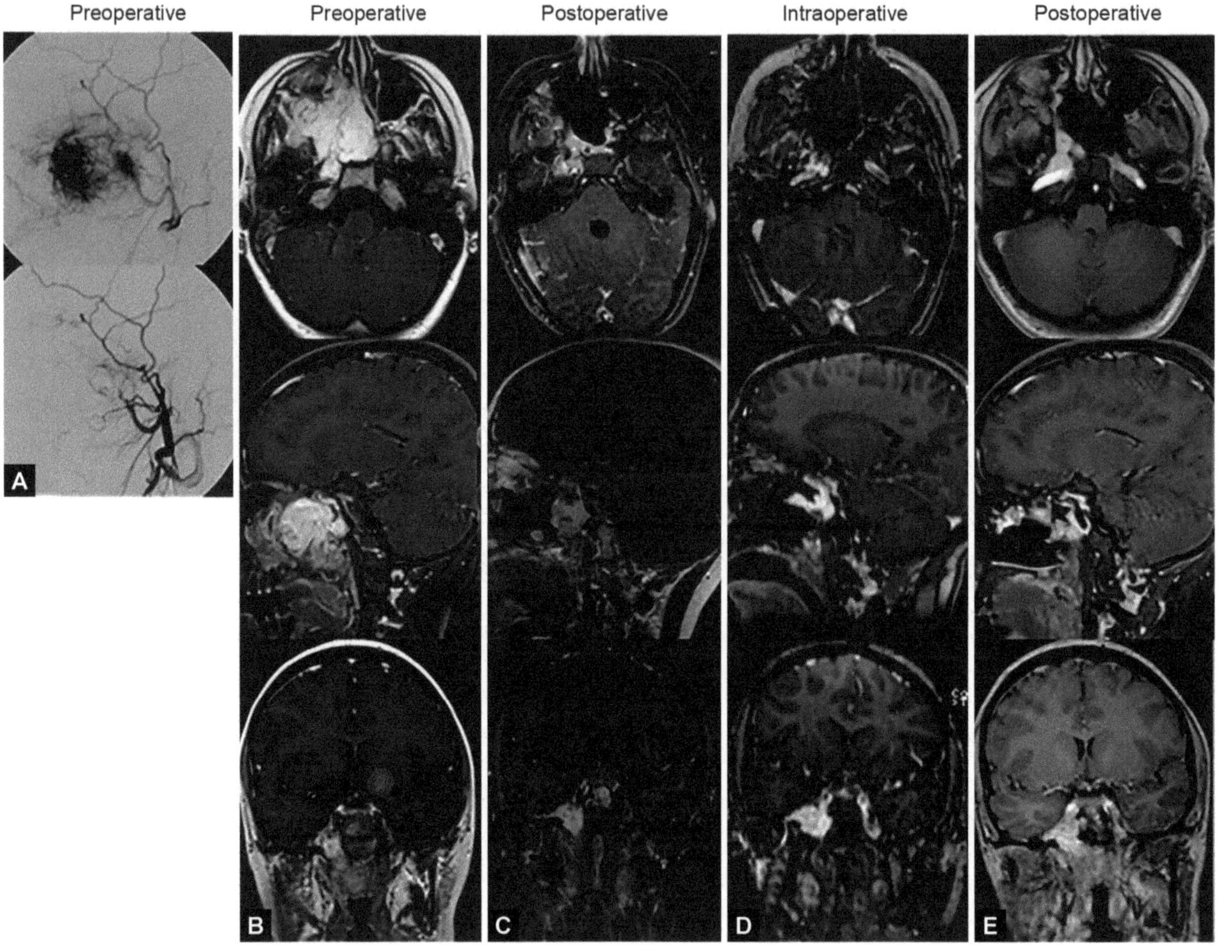

Preoperative	Preoperative	Postoperative	Intraoperative	Postoperative

Figures 15.6A to E *Case 4:* (A) Young patient with preoperative angiography demonstrating a vascular lesion; (B) Preoperative magnetic resonance imaging (MRI) revealed a large sinonasal mass. Endonasal, endoscopic resection was performed and pathology confirmed juvenile nasopharyngeal angiofibroma. Intraoperative MRI (iMRI) revealed residual tumor in the region of the right petrous carotid artery, which was not removed due to high vascular risk; (C) Postoperative MRI was unchanged from iMRI; (D) MRI 10 months after surgery revealed tumor progression, which prompted a second resection. After maximum safe resection was deemed complete and iMRI scan was performed that revealed residual tumor. Additional exposure was achieved, and resection was continued, and (E) Postoperative MRI revealed decreased tumor size

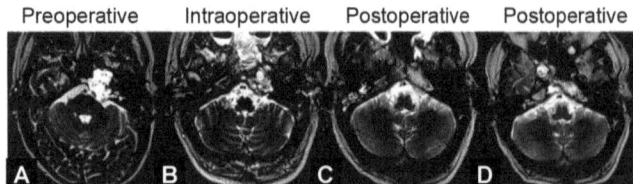

Preoperative	Intraoperative	Postoperative	Postoperative

Figures 15.7A to D *Case 5:* Patient presented with prior subtemporal craniotomy for resection of a low-grade chondrosarcoma. (A) Preoperative T2-weighted magnetic resonance imaging (MRI) showed a multinodular mass in the left petrous apex region. The patient underwent endonasal, endoscopic resection, which revealed recurrent low-grade chondrosarcoma; (B) Intraoperative MRI identified a focus of residual tumor that was further resected; (C) Postoperative MRI showed near total resection of the lesion; and (D) Final follow-up imaging 46 months after surgery revealed a small region of tumor progression

tumors improved postoperative patient outcomes, but the amount of benefit is difficult to quantify. It is also possible that iMRI did not improve postoperative outcomes for some or all of these cases, since iMRI led to only a small improvement in debulking, no gross total resection, and 3/4 cases were controlled postoperatively with adjuvant radiotherapy (two residual adenoid cystic carcinoma cases received fractionated radiotherapy, one low-grade chondrosarcoma case received stereotactic radiosurgery). These cases highlight the potential benefit of the combined strategy of endonasal, endoscopic skull base resection with iMRI for these complex tumors, but as mentioned, caution should be taken in interpretation of surrogate markers (i.e. EOR) for patient-oriented clinical outcomes. The good postoperative outcomes noted in this small number of patients suggest that less invasive palliative resection with endoscopy and intraoperative imaging may offer a suitable management option for cases that cannot achieve gross total resection, with the intention of performing postoperative adjuvant fractionated radiotherapy to control residual tumor. This technique of major, but subtotal tumor resection, might lessen the volume and intensity of the radiation required, reduce the immediate neurological impacts of tumor mass, and reduce some of the potential morbidity of radiotherapy. In addition, this strategy might offer some potential for better tumor control than palliative radiation alone for these tumors that traditionally have been deemed as unresectable. If there is a role for such a strategy, it likely has greater application for tumors such as some adenoid cystic carcinomas that have a somewhat less aggressive behavior in comparison to squamous cell carcinomas which are on average more notoriously aggressive.

AUTHOR COMMENTARY

Radiographic intraoperative imaging such as iCT or iMRI likely offers less benefit for skull base resection of extra-axial tumors such as meningiomas and VS than for transsphenoidal pituitary adenoma resection. Meningiomas and VS typically have relatively well-defined surgical margins, in contrast to intra-axial tumors such as gliomas, where the plane between tumor and adjacent normal brain tissue may be difficult to distinguish. However, the utility of these modalities for other less common skull base tumors may change over time. As technology improves and intraoperative imaging becomes more available in operating rooms, less time-consuming and less costly, one can imagine that skull base might be more inclined to integrate these technologies into these procedures, and appropriate indications will become more defined.

Healthcare technology and resources are by nature scarce; therefore, it is essential that the cost of intraoperative technologies be strongly considered when determining their suitability for a clinical practice. This decision making process will differ greatly for different practice environments, and large academic medical centers with strong research interests will continue to lead the way with these technologies. Radiographic intraoperative imaging techniques, particularly iMRI, have the highest upfront, maintenance, and operation cost and therefore, should probably be studied the most carefully.

Determining the cost-effectiveness of an iMRI scanner purchase is a complicated problem. Ideally, these analyses should be considered from a societal perspective, but hospitals and providers may measure the effectiveness of iMRI in part by patient recruitment and center reputation. Essentially, the effectiveness of iMRI is derived from translation of increased EOR to better quality of life, longer disease-specific progression or recurrence-free survival, or longer overall survival. The use of iMRI may lead to increased EOR and improved patient outcomes, which has reported to lead to decreased disease-related long-term costs in an early study,[99] but more current and large studies are needed.

A related, but different application of cost-effectiveness research would be determining the appropriate indications for iMRI use for centers that already have access to a scanner. Currently, studies have hinted at which disease would achieve the most benefit from iMRI, but none have analyzed this thoroughly. For malignant glioblastomas, increased EOR has been shown to lengthen overall survival,[100,101] and a randomized controlled trial by Senft et al.[1] demonstrated that low-field iMRI use resulted in a lower rate of subtotal resection compared to conventional surgery. These studies answer the question of effectiveness, but do not compare the cost of iMRI use to payer's willingness to pay for that benefit. For benign tumors like pituitary adenoma, work at our institution and prior studies have shown that increased EOR lengthens progression or recurrence-free survival for nonfunctional adenomas,[102] and it is self-evident that functional tumors require gross or near total resection to cure endocrinopathy. Determining the cost effectiveness specific to pituitary adenomas is perhaps more difficult than glioblastomas, due to high disease heterogeneity, confounding from effectiveness of adjuvant technologies, and a generally benign disease course. A cost-utility decision analysis model was developed at our institution using retrospective cohort of pituitary adenoma cases that either received or did not receive iMRI. Using this model, we assessed the 10-year disease-related healthcare cost differences (accounting for postoperative treatment with surgery, radiation, and/or hormone suppressive medication) associated with iMRI, and found that functional, recurrent and cavernous sinus invading tumors were most likely to benefit from iMRI in terms of cost and utility (unpublished data).

In addition to the direct financial cost, intraoperative imaging techniques cost the surgical team, time and effort, which are vitally precious resources. Particularly for skull base surgery, where resections tend to be by nature complicated and time-consuming, the surgeon must weigh carefully whether the benefit of intraoperative imaging outweighs real and theoretical risks including increased cost, operating time and operative complexity. A balance needs to be found to maximize the gains achievable with these technologies while controlling costs and improving efficiency. More aggressive resection encouraged by iMRI findings (or other modalities) can potentially increase complications related to resection technique [e.g. arterial injury and cerebrospinal fluid (CSF) leak]; therefore, more aggressive resection must be pursued only to the extent that it can be accomplished safely.

Currently, iMRI and iCT are mainly limited to major centers with large case volume and financial resources. The complexity and rarity of many complex skull base tumors also diverts these cases to surgeons either affiliated with an academic center or with a large surgical group. In the absence of iMRI or iCT, most surgical centers with high skull base volume have ready access to diagnostic high-resolution imaging modalities including MRI, CT, and catheter cerebral angiography. The availability of these diagnostic modalities, and increased pressures from budget constraints and healthcare financial oversight, will likely spur innovation to blur the lines between diagnostic and intraoperative imaging, with the creation of multipurpose surgical and diagnostic suites. Therefore, it is important to carefully evaluate these modalities specifically for each disease with changes in system integration.

In some instances, residual tumor identified on intraoperative imaging may not be accessible or safe for further resection. As an example, **Figures 15.8A to C** show the pre-, intra-, and postoperative imaging from a patient with a pituitary adenoma invading the cavernous sinus (Case 6). Advancement of tumor to such close proximity to the cavernous segment of the internal carotid artery precludes gross total resection in many cases due to unacceptable risk of intraoperative complication such as vascular injury. Cavernous sinus invasion occurs relatively frequently in pituitary adenoma cases, and is often defined radiographically when the tumor is noted on MRI to extend past the lateral aspect of the internal carotid artery on coronal magnetic resonance (MR) imaging (Knosp grade 3 or 4).[103] Other sellar and suprasellar lesions have the potential to invade the cavernous sinus, which limits the surgeon's ability to perform a gross total resection. These patients are often good candidates for postoperative radiotherapy such as stereotactic radiosurgery, as long as adequate decompression of the optic nerve is obtained.

For many endonasal, endoscopic procedures, the added complexity of techniques such as iMRI may be justified by the potential for increased EOR. In contrast, traditional microsurgical skull base approaches for tumors such as meningiomas and schwannomas, the added complexity of a technique such as iMRI may not be warranted. These tumors types may benefit most from simpler techniques such as iUS, iONM, and stereotactic neuronavigation, which add little complexity to the surgical environment, while offering the potential for more safe and accurate procedures.

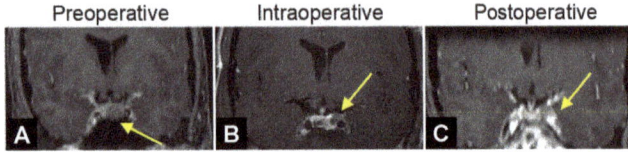

Figures 15.8A to C *Case 6:* (A) Preoperative magnetic resonance imaging (MRI) of a patient with acromegaly demonstrated a hypoenhancing focus in the sellar region (yellow arrow). Transsphenoidal resection was performed; (B) Subsequent intraoperative MRI (iMRI) identified a small residual focus of likely tumor encroaching into the left cavernous sinus, which was deemed inaccessible due to proximity to the left internal carotid artery, and (C) Postoperative MRI revealed no change in the residual tumor, which was then treated with adjuvant stereotactic radiotherapy

CONCLUSION

Intraoperative imaging offers great potential to improve the EOR for many intracranial tumors; however, the benefit for many skull base tumors is either small or not well-defined. Thus far, the majority of research has focused on the use of iMRI for pituitary adenoma resection, and the benefits of this modality have been reported extensively. Continued clinical investigation is needed to more carefully delineate the potential costs and benefits of each intraoperative imaging modality for all plausible skull base tumor types. Future technological advancement and system integration will likely increase the efficiency and accessible of intraoperative imaging techniques to the surgeon; therefore, the value of each modality for each indication should be monitored carefully over time.

ACKNOWLEDGMENTS

We would like to thank Feng Gao, PhD from the Department of Biostatistics at Washington University in St Louis for his advice regarding the statistical methods performed in this study. Furthermore, we would like to thank Bridget McCullough and Stan Goddard our MRI technologists, and Kathy Draege our neurosurgical operating room charge nurse and our entire operating room staff. These individuals enable the safe completion of these surgical procedures in the complex iMRI environment.

REFERENCES

1. Senft C, Bink A, Franz K, et al. Intraoperative MRI guidance and extent of resection in glioma surgery: a randomised, controlled trial. Lancet Oncol. 2011;12(11):997-1003.
2. Nimsky C, Fujita A, Ganslandt O, et al. Volumetric assessment of glioma removal by intraoperative high-field magnetic resonance imaging. Neurosurgery. 2004;55(2):358-70.
3. Özduman K, Yıldız E, Dinçer A, et al. Using intraoperative dynamic contrast-enhanced T1-weighted MRI to identify residual tumor in glioblastoma surgery. J Neurosurg. 2014;120(1):60-6.
4. Senft C, Seifert V, Hermann E, et al. Usefulness of intraoperative ultra low-field magnetic resonance imaging in glioma surgery. Neurosurgery. 2008;63(4 Suppl 2):257-66.
5. Schneider JP, Trantakis C, Rubach M, et al. Intraoperative MRI to guide the resection of primary supratentorial glioblastoma multiforme: a quantitative radiological analysis. Neuroradiology. 2005;47(7):489-500.
6. Hatiboglu MA, Weinberg JS, Suki D, et al. Impact of intraoperative high-field magnetic resonance imaging guidance on glioma surgery: a prospective volumetric analysis. Neurosurgery. 2009;64(6):1073-81.
7. Kuhnt D, Becker A, Ganslandt O, et al. Correlation of the extent of tumor volume resection and patient survival in surgery of glioblastoma multiforme with high-field intraoperative MRI guidance. Neuro Oncol. 2011;13(12):1339-48.

8. Ahn JY, Jung JY, Kim J, et al. How to overcome the limitations to determine the resection margin of pituitary tumours with low-field intra-operative MRI during trans-sphenoidal surgery: usefulness of Gadolinium-soaked cotton pledgets. Acta Neurochir (Wien). 2008;150(8):763-71.

9. Anand VK, Schwartz TH, Hiltzik DH, et al. Endoscopic transphenoidal pituitary surgery with real-time intraoperative magnetic resonance imaging. Am J Rhinol. 2006;20(4):401-5.

10. Berkmann S, Fandino J, Zosso S, et al. Intraoperative magnetic resonance imaging and early prognosis for vision after transsphenoidal surgery for sellar lesions. J Neurosurg. 2011;115(3):518-27.

11. Chicoine MR, Lim CC, Evans JA, et al. Implementation and preliminary clinical experience with the use of ceiling mounted mobile high field intraoperative magnetic resonance imaging between two operating rooms. Acta Neurochir Suppl. 2011;109:97-102.

12. Fahlbusch R, Ganslandt O, Buchfelder M, et al. Intraoperative magnetic resonance imaging during transsphenoidal surgery. J Neurosurg. 2001;95(3):381-90.

13. Fahlbusch R, Keller BV, Ganslandt O, et al. Transsphenoidal surgery in acromegaly investigated by intraoperative high-field magnetic resonance imaging. Eur J Endocrinol. 2005;153(2):239-48.

14. Gerlach R, du Mesnil de Rochemont R, Gasser T, et al. Feasibility of Polestar N20, an ultra-low-field intraoperative magnetic resonance imaging system in resection control of pituitary macroadenomas: lessons learned from the first 40 cases. Neurosurgery. 2008;63(2):272-84.

15. Lang MJ, Kelly JJ, Sutherland GR. A moveable 3-Tesla intraoperative magnetic resonance imaging system. Neurosurgery. 2011;68(1 Suppl Operative):168-79.

16. Netuka D, Masopust V, Belšán T, et al. One year experience with 3.0 T intraoperative MRI in pituitary surgery. Acta Neurochir Suppl. 2011;109:157-9.

17. Nimsky C, von Keller B, Ganslandt O, et al. Intraoperative high-field magnetic resonance imaging in transsphenoidal surgery of hormonally inactive pituitary macroadenomas. Neurosurgery. 2006;59(1):105-14.

18. Szerlip NJ, Zhang YC, Placantonakis DG, et al. Transsphenoidal resection of sellar tumors using high-field intraoperative magnetic resonance imaging. Skull Base. 2011;21(4):223-32.

19. Theodosopoulos PV, Leach J, Kerr RG, et al. Maximizing the extent of tumor resection during transsphenoidal surgery for pituitary macroadenomas: can endoscopy replace intraoperative magnetic resonance imaging? J Neurosurg. 2010;112(4):736-43.

20. Schwartz TH, Stieg PE, Anand VK. Endoscopic transsphenoidal pituitary surgery with intraoperative magnetic resonance imaging. Neurosurgery. 2006;58(1 Suppl):ONS44-51.

21. Wu JS, Shou XF, Yao CJ, et al. Transsphenoidal pituitary macroadenomas resection guided by PoleStar N20 low-field intraoperative magnetic resonance imaging: comparison with early postoperative high-field magnetic resonance imaging. Neurosurgery. 2009;65(1):63-70.

22. Vitaz TW, Inkabi KE, Carrubba CJ. Intraoperative MRI for transphenoidal procedures: short-term outcome for 100 consecutive cases. Clin Neurol Neurosurg. 2011;113(9):731-5.

23. Nimsky C, Ganslandt O, Fahlbusch R. Comparing 0.2 Tesla with 1.5 tesla intraoperative magnetic resonance imaging analysis of setup, workflow, and efficiency. Acad Radiol. 2005;12(9):1065-79.

24. Nimsky C, Ganslandt O, Von Keller B, et al. Intraoperative high-field-strength MR imaging: implementation and experience in 200 patients. Radiology. 2004;233(1):67-78.

25. Pamir MN, Peker S, Ozek MM, et al. Intraoperative MR imaging: preliminary results with 3 Tesla MR system. Acta Neurochir Suppl. 2006;98:97-100.

26. Soleman J, Fathi AR, Marbacher S, et al. The role of intraoperative magnetic resonance imaging in complex meningioma surgery. Magn Reson Imaging. 2013;31(6):923-9.

27. Zhou T, Meng XH, Xu BN, et al. Implementation and preliminary experience of high-field intraoperative magnetic resonance imaging in the endoscopic chordoma operation with transsphenoidal or transoral approach. Zhonghua Wai Ke Za Zhi. 2011;49(8):699-702.

28. Uhl E, Zausinger S, Morhard D, et al. Intraoperative computed tomography with integrated navigation system in a multidisciplinary operating suite. Neurosurgery. 2009;64(5 Suppl 2):231-9.

29. Rafferty MA, Siewerdsen JH, Chan Y, et al. Intraoperative cone-beam CT for guidance of temporal bone surgery. Otolaryngol Head Neck Surg. 2006;134(5):801-8.

30. Chan Y, Siewerdsen JH, Rafferty MA, et al. Cone-beam computed tomography on a mobile C-Arm: novel intraoperative imaging technology for guidance of head and neck surgery. J Otolaryngol Head Neck Surg. 2008;37(1):81-90.

31. Rafferty MA, Siewerdsen JH, Chan Y, et al. Investigation of C-arm cone-beam CT-guided surgery of the frontal recess. Laryngoscope. 2005;115(12):2138-43.

32. Conley DB, Tan B, Bendok BR, et al. Comparison of intraoperative portable CT Scanners in skull base and endoscopic sinus surgery: single center case series. Skull Base. 2011;21(4):261-70.

33. Pamir MN, Ozduman K, Dinçer A, et al. First intraoperative, shared-resource, ultrahigh-field 3-Tesla magnetic resonance imaging system and its application in low-grade glioma resection. J Neurosurg. 2010;112(1):57-69.

34. Blaskiewicz DJ, Sure DR, Hedequist DJ, et al. Osteoid osteomas: intraoperative bone scan-assisted resection: Clinical article. J Neurosurg Pediatr. 2009;4(3):237-44.

35. Stummer W, Stocker S, Wagner S, et al. Intraoperative detection of malignant gliomas by 5-aminolevulinic acid-induced porphyrin fluorescence. Neurosurgery. 1998;42(3):518-25.

36. Stummer W, Novotny A, Stepp H, et al. Fluorescence-guided resection of glioblastoma multiforme by using 5-aminolevulinic acid-induced porphyrins: a prospective study in 52 consecutive patients. J Neurosurg. 2000;93(6):1003-13.

37. Stummer W, Meinel T, Ewelt C, et al. Prospective cohort study of radiotherapy with concomitant and adjuvant temozolomide chemotherapy for glioblastoma patients with no or minimal residual enhancing tumor load after surgery. J Neurooncol. 2012;108(1):89-97.

38. Eljamel MS, Leese G, Moseley H. Intraoperative optical identification of pituitary adenomas. J Neurooncol. 2009;92(3):417-21.

39. Kajimoto Y, Kuroiwa T, Miyatake S, et al. Use of 5-aminolevulinic acid in fluorescence-guided resection of meningioma with high risk of recurrence. Case report. J Neurosurg. 2007;106(6):1070-4.

40. Morofuji Y, Matsuo T, Hayashi Y, et al. Usefulness of intraoperative photodynamic diagnosis using 5-aminolevulinic acid for meningiomas with cranial invasion: technical case report. Neurosurgery. 2008;62(3 Suppl 1):102-3.

41. Coluccia D, Fandino J, Fujioka M, et al. Intraoperative 5-aminolevulinic-acid-induced fluorescence in meningiomas. Acta Neurochir (Wien). 2010;152(10):1711-9.

42. Bekelis K, Valdés P, Erkmen K, et al. Quantitative and qualitative 5-aminolevulinic acid-induced protoporphyrin IX fluorescence in skull base meningiomas. Neurosurg Focus. 2011;30(5):E8.

43. Valdes PA, Bekelis K, Harris BT, et al. 5-Aminolevulinic-acid-induced protoporphyrin IX fluorescence in meningioma: qualitative and quantitative measurements in vivo. Neurosurgery. 2014;10 Suppl 1:74-82.

44. Hefti M, Holenstein F, Albert I, et al. Susceptibility to 5-aminolevulinic acid based photodynamic therapy in WHO I meningioma cells corresponds to ferrochelatase activity. Photochem Photobiol. 2011;87(1):235-41.

45. Litvack ZN, Zada G, Laws ER. Indocyanine green fluorescence endoscopy for visual differentiation of pituitary tumor from surrounding structures. J Neurosurg. 2012;116(5):935-41.

46. d'Avella E, Volpin F, Manara R, et al. Indocyanine green videoangiography (ICGV)-guided surgery of parasagittal meningiomas occluding the superior sagittal sinus (SSS). Acta Neurochir (Wien). 2013;155(3):415-20.

47. Ueba T, Okawa M, Abe H, et al. Identification of venous sinus, tumor location, and pial supply during meningioma surgery by transdural indocyanine green videography. J Neurosurg. 2013;118(3):632-6.

48. Ezzat S, Asa SL, Couldwell WT, et al. The prevalence of pituitary adenomas: a systematic review. Cancer. 2004;101(3):613-9.

49. Jane JA, Laws ER. The surgical management of pituitary adenomas in a series of 3,093 patients. J Am Coll Surg. 2001;193(6):651-9.

50. Coburger J, König R, Seitz K, et al. Determining the utility of intraoperative magnetic resonance imaging for transsphenoidal surgery: a retrospective study. J Neurosurg. 2014;120(2):346-56.

51. Lee CC, Lee ST, Chang CN, et al. Volumetric measurement for comparison of the accuracy between intraoperative CT and postoperative MR imaging in pituitary adenoma surgery. Am J Neuroradiol. 2011;32(8):1539-44.

52. Leuthardt EC, Lim CC, Shah MN, et al. Use of movable high-field-strength intraoperative magnetic resonance imaging with awake craniotomies for resection of gliomas: preliminary experience. Neurosurgery. 2011;69(1):194-205.

53. Shah MN, Leonard JR, Inder G, et al. Intraoperative magnetic resonance imaging to reduce the rate of early reoperation for lesion resection in pediatric neurosurgery. J Neurosurg Pediatr. 2012;9(3):259-64.

54. Haydon DH, Chicoine MR, Dacey RG. The impact of high-field-strength intraoperative magnetic resonance imaging on brain tumor management. Neurosurgery. 2013;60(Suppl 1):92-7.

55. Chicoine MR, Evans JA, Wippold FJ, et al. Comparison of intraoperative and postoperative MRI for endoscopic transsphenoidal resection of pituitary macroadenomas. Skull Base. 2011;21:A064.

56. Ram Z, Shawker TH, Bradford MH, et al. Intraoperative ultrasound-directed resection of pituitary tumors. J Neurosurg. 1995;83(2):225-30.

57. Doppman JL, Ram Z, Shawker TH, et al. Intraoperative US of the pituitary gland. Work in progress. Radiology. 1994;192(1):111-5.

58. Bondy M, Ligon BL. Epidemiology and etiology of intracranial meningiomas: a review. J Neurooncol. 1996;29(3):197-205.

59. Nakamura M, Roser F, Jacobs C, et al. Medial sphenoid wing meningiomas: clinical outcome and recurrence rate. Neurosurgery. 2006;58(4):626-39.

60. Ohba S, Kobayashi M, Horiguchi T, et al. Long-term surgical outcome and biological prognostic factors in patients with skull base meningiomas. J Neurosurg. 2011;114(5):1278-87.

61. Sughrue ME, Kane AJ, Shangari G, et al. The relevance of Simpson Grade I and II resection in modern neurosurgical treatment of World Health Organization Grade I meningiomas. J Neurosurg. 2010;113(5):1029-35.

62. Almefty R, Dunn IF, Pravdenkova S, et al. True petroclival meningiomas: results of surgical management. J Neurosurg. 2014;120(1):40-51.

63. Kane AJ, Sughrue ME, Rutkowski MJ, et al. Anatomic location is a risk factor for atypical and malignant meningiomas. Cancer. 2011;117(6):1272-8.

64. Sade B, Chahlavi A, Krishnaney A, et al. World Health Organization Grades II and III meningioma are rare in the cranial base and spine. Neurosurgery. 2007;61(6):1194-8.

65. McGovern SL, Aldape KD, Munsell MF, et al. A comparison of World Health Organization tumor grades at recurrence in patients with non-skull base and skull base meningiomas. J Neurosurg. 2010;112(5):925-33.

66. Hashimoto N, Rabo CS, Okita Y, et al. Slower growth of skull base meningiomas compared with non-skull base meningiomas based on volumetric and biological studies. J Neurosurg. 2012;116(3):574-80.

67. Simpson D. The recurrence of intracranial meningiomas after surgical treatment. J Neurol Neurosurg Psychiatry. 1957;20(1):22-39.

68. Bassiouni H, Ntoukas V, Asgari S, et al. Foramen magnum meningiomas: clinical outcome after microsurgical resection via a posterolateral suboccipital retrocondylar approach. Neurosurgery. 2006;59(6):1177-85.

69. Mathiesen T, Lindquist C, Kihlström L, et al. Recurrence of cranial base meningiomas. Neurosurgery. 1996;39(1):2-7.

70. Condra KS, Buatti JM, Mendenhall WM, et al. Benign meningiomas: Primary treatment selection affects survival. Int J Radiat Oncol Biol Phys. 1997;39(2):427-36.

71. Kallio M, Sankila R, Hakulinen T, et al. Factors affecting operative and excess long-term mortality in 935 patients with intracranial meningioma. Neurosurgery. 1992;31(1):2-12.

72. Ichinose T, Goto T, Ishibashi K, et al. The role of radical microsurgical resection in multimodal treatment for skull base meningioma. J Neurosurg. 2010;113(5):1072-8.

73. Pollock BE, Stafford SL, Utter A, et al. Stereotactic radiosurgery provides equivalent tumor control to Simpson Grade 1 resection for patients with small- to medium-size meningiomas. Int J Radiat Oncol Biol Phys. 2003;55(4):1000-5.

74. Kreil W, Luggin J, Fuchs I, et al. Long term experience of gamma knife radiosurgery for benign skull base meningiomas. J Neurol Neurosurg Psychiatry. 2005;76(10):1425-30.

75. Iwai Y, Yamanaka K, Ikeda H. Gamma Knife radiosurgery for skull base meningioma: long-term results of low-dose treatment. J Neurosurg. 2008;109(5):804-10.

76. Milker-Zabel S, Zabel-du Bois A, Huber P, et al. Fractionated stereotactic radiation therapy in the management of benign cavernous sinus meningiomas: long-term experience and review of the literature. Strahlenther Onkol. 2006;182(11): 635-40.

77. Vernimmen FJ, Harris JK, Wilson JA, et al Stereotactic proton beam therapy of skull base meningiomas. Int J Radiat Oncol Biol Phys. 2001;49(1):99-105.

78. Deinsberger R, Tidstrand J, Sabitzer H, et al. LINAC radiosurgery in skull base meningiomas. Minim Invasive Neurosurg. 2004;47(6):333-8.

79. Dean BL, Flom RA, Wallace RC, et al. Efficacy of endovascular treatment of meningiomas: evaluation with matched samples. AJNR Am J Neuroradiol. 1994;15(9):1675-80.

80. Macpherson P. The value of pre-operative embolisation of meningioma estimated subjectively and objectively. Neuroradiology. 1991;33(4):334-7.

81. Shah AH, Patel N, Raper DM, et al. The role of preoperative embolization for intracranial meningiomas. J Neurosurg. 2013;119(2):364-72.

82. Solheim O, Selbekk T, Lindseth F, et al. Navigated resection of giant intracranial meningiomas based on intraoperative 3D ultrasound. Acta Neurochir (Wien). 2009;151(9):1143-51.

83. Rygh OM, Nagelhus HT, Lindseth F, et al. Intraoperative navigated 3-dimensional ultrasound angiography in tumor surgery. Surg Neurol. 2006;66(6):581-92.

84. van Alkemade H, de Leau M, Dieleman EM, et al. Impaired survival and long-term neurological problems in benign meningioma. Neuro Oncol. 2012;14(5):658-66.

85. Theodosopoulos PV, Pensak ML. Contemporary management of acoustic neuromas. Laryngoscope. 2011;121(6):1133-7.

86. Sughrue ME, Kaur R, Rutkowski MJ, et al. Extent of resection and the long-term durability of vestibular schwannoma surgery. J Neurosurg. 2011;114(5):1218-23.

87. Acoustic neuroma. Consens Statement. 1991;9(4):1-24.

88. House JW, Brackmann DE. Facial nerve grading system. Otolaryngol Head Neck Surg. 1985;93(2):146-7.

89. Vrabec JT, Backous DD, Djalilian HR, et al. Facial nerve grading system 2.0. Otolaryngol Head Neck Surg. 2009;140(4): 445-50.

90. Sughrue ME, Kaur R, Kane AJ, et al. The value of intraoperative facial nerve electromyography in predicting facial nerve function after vestibular schwannoma surgery. J Clin Neurosci. 2010;17(7):849-52.

91. De Seta E, Bertoli G, De Seta D, et al. New development in intraoperative video monitoring of facial nerve: a pilot study. Otol Neurotol. 2010;31(9):1498-502.

92. Bernat I, Grayeli AB, Esquia G, et al. Intraoperative electromyography and surgical observations as predictive factors of facial nerve outcome in vestibular schwannoma surgery. Otol Neurotol. 2010;31(2):306-12.

93. Gardner G, Robertson JH. Hearing preservation in unilateral acoustic neuroma surgery. Ann Otol Rhino Laryngol. 1988;97(1):55-66.

94. Fischer G, Fischer C, Remond J. Hearing preservation in acoustic neuroma surgery. J Neurosurg. 1992;76:910-17.

95. Samii M, Matthies C. Management of 1000 vestibular schwannomas (acoustic neuromas): hearing function in 1000 tumor resections. Neurosurgery. 1997;40(2):248-60.

96. Tonn JC, Schlake HP, Goldbrunner R, et al. Acoustic neuroma surgery as an interdisciplinary approach: a neurosurgical series of 508 patients. J Neurol Neurosurg Psychiatry. 2000;69(2):161-6.

97. Samii M, Gerganov V, Samii A. Improved preservation of hearing and facial nerve function in vestibular schwannoma surgery via the retrosigmoid approach in a series of 200 patients. J Neurosurg. 2006;105(4):527-35.

98. Yamakami I, Yoshinori H, Saeki N, et al. Hearing preservation and intraoperative auditory brainstem response and cochlear nerve compound action potential monitoring in the removal of small acoustic neurinoma via the retrosigmoid approach. J Neurol Neurosurg Psychiatry. 2009;80(2):218-27.

99. Hall WA, Kowalik K, Liu H, et al. Costs and benefits of intraoperative MR-guided brain tumor resection. Acta Neurochir Suppl. 2003;85:137-42.

100. Stark AM, van de Bergh J, Hedderich J, et al. Glioblastoma: clinical characteristics, prognostic factors and survival in 492 patients. Clin Neurol Neurosurg. 2012;114(7):840-5.

101. Filippini G, Falcone C, Boiardi A, et al. Prognostic factors for survival in 676 consecutive patients with newly diagnosed primary glioblastoma. Neuro Oncol. 2008;10(1):79-87.

102. Chang EF, Zada G, Kim S, et al. Long-term recurrence and mortality after surgery and adjuvant radiotherapy for nonfunctional pituitary adenomas. J Neurosurg. 2008;108(4):736-45.

103. Knosp E, Steiner E, Kitz K, et al. Pituitary adenomas with invasion of the cavernous sinus space: a magnetic resonance imaging classification compared with surgical findings. Neurosurgery. 1993;33(4):610-7.

16

Role of Intraoperative Imaging in Cerebrovascular Surgeries

Peter Nakaji

INTRODUCTION

Intraoperative image guidance has come to play a central role in most cranial neurosurgery procedures. Its ability to provide accurate and precise localization of lesions in and around the brain has proven invaluable for surgeons. For cerebrovascular surgery, the relatively constant position of the vascular tree with respect to intracranial landmarks has made the use of neuronavigation less common in most practices. However, image guidance can in fact play an important role in managing cerebrovascular pathologies. Advances in technology continually increase the availability and utility of information acquired both preoperatively and intraoperatively for this purpose.

While many imaging modalities are used to preoperatively evaluate cerebrovascular lesions, such as digital subtraction angiography (DSA), rotational three-dimensional (3D) angiography, magnetic resonance angiography (MRA), and computed tomography angiography (CTA), the gold standard remains DSA, which provides excellent resolution for minor vascular structures. Nevertheless, DSA is an invasive procedure that is not always easily available, and on rare occasions, neurological or non-neurological complications occur. Furthermore, while DSA provides superior anatomical definition for cerebrovascular surgery, integration of DSA into intraoperative image guidance has proved challenging.

In this chapter, we present the current principles and modalities guiding intraoperative neuronavigation and intraoperative image acquisition in cerebrovascular surgery.

BASIC PRINCIPLES OF NEURONAVIGATION AND INTRAOPERATIVE IMAGING IN CEREBROVASCULAR SURGERY

Imaging studies obtained preoperatively are essential for planning cerebrovascular surgery. They can be used to provide preoperative definition of anatomy and to choose a treatment modality, including the alternative of endovascular treatments. Additionally, newer imaging platforms allow the opportunity for sophisticated preoperative surgical planning and simulation or rehearsal. These images can be carried into surgery for use on the intraoperative navigation platform.

During surgery, intraoperative image guidance allows intraoperative trajectory planning and navigation, albeit based on preoperative anatomy. Brain shift from lesion resection, or simply "brain sag" from cerebrospinal fluid removal, can negatively affect the accuracy of neuronavigation based on preoperative imaging. Acquisition of new images intraoperatively allows near real-time assessment of surgical results, so that interventions can still be carried out to alter the surgical plan and outcome. Intraoperative magnetic resonance (MR) image acquisition has become a powerful tool for selected neurosurgical lesions.[1,2] Intraoperative magnetic resonance imaging (MRI) provides a radiation-free environment for the surgeon and patient, and the multiplanar image quality provides superior brain parenchyma resolution compared with other forms of imaging. It also provides crucial capabilities for identifying the extent of many lesions and defining the relationship between the lesion and cerebral structures. Different groups have successfully used intraoperative MRI to provide updated neuronavigation data to the image guidance platform, mostly in neuro-oncology. This intraoperative imaging is used to continue surgery with an updated neuronavigational framework, and can just as easily be applied to cerebrovascular surgery when appropriate.[2-4]

PREOPERATIVE CEREBROVASCULAR IMAGING EVALUATION

Optimal surgical outcomes are bolstered via accurate preoperative surgical planning, especially for patients with lesions in eloquent areas of the brain.[5] These eloquent areas can be beyond the surgeon's perception for several reasons, which may include tissue edema, mass effect, and the shift of normal brain anatomy.[6] Therefore, preoperative evaluation using MRI, MRA, and/or CTA can be significantly useful for surgeons to determine the optimal surgical trajectory to a given vascular lesion, as well as elucidate the location of nearby eloquent cortex and white matter fiber tracts. For example, careful inspection of preoperative DSA or CTA may reveal that a posterior-pointing posterior communicating aneurysm should be approached from a lateral trajectory with splitting of the Sylvian fissure, while a laterally pointing one could be approached from a more anterior subfrontal approach. In this example, the former situation might call for a pterional approach, while the latter might be better served by an eyebrow minicraniotomy. Similarly, for an arteriovenous malformation (AVM), the positioning of the patient and the size and location of the craniotomy can best be served by a combination of preoperative inspection of the imaging and preincisional image guidance.

DynaCT and Flat-Panel Systems

Currently, frameless stereotactic navigation is based on preoperative computed tomography (CT) or MR images. For cerebrovascular lesions, CTA and MRA provide further visualization and better delineation. However, these procedures may still be inadequate for visualizing small lesions, such as small AVMs or small aneurysms, or for understanding other more complex cerebrovascular lesions. DSA remains the "gold standard" for cerebrovascular imaging and may be the only means to visualize and understand such lesions. However, catheter angiography data has not historically been easily integrated into the frameless stereotaxy protocol with the fidelity to support routine use.

As an alternative, DynaCT data obtained in the angiographic suite can now be fused with CT or MR stereotactic sequences for preoperative planning and intraoperative navigation. This technique enables more precise navigation during cerebrovascular surgery in lesions that are inadequately imaged or invisible to conventional CT or MR techniques. Tee et al. have found the DynaCT technique far superior to CTA or MRA datasets in the surgical resection of micro-AVMs, dural arteriovenous fistulas (AVFs) and small aneurysms.[7]

Schaller et al. in Geneva reported their experience with 99 patients with cerebrovascular lesions treated surgically. They used a flat-panel system that integrated intraoperative 2D and 3D DSA for automated segmentation of vascular structures and performance of an intraoperative CT. This system was connected with a surgical microscope and neuronavigation. All patients had intraoperative imaging for angiographic control or anatomical location. They concluded that this hybrid neurointerventional suite provides high-resolution angiographic or CT images that can be co-registered with a navigation system.[8]

Leng et al. introduced a technique that uses intraoperative flat-panel detector CT and 3D rotational angiography, which provides full neuronavigation capabilities during cerebrovascular surgery without the use of preoperative imaging studies. This technology allows accurate visualization of the vascular anatomy and localization of pathology. It requires a very short period of time (usually less than 15 minutes) to acquire the images and uses DSA images that are superior to conventional CT or MRI for the imaging of cerebrovascular pathology.[9]

PREOPERATIVE SURGICAL REHEARSAL

Increasingly, sophisticated imaging manipulation platforms are being used to provide preoperative rehearsal of surgery, both to improve surgical outcomes and deepen teaching. The concept of surgical rehearsal has intrinsic appeal for surgery. Surgery is not static, but rather is a narrative whose course is an amalgamation of the preoperative conceptualization of the neurosurgeon and the changing realities that the surgeon encounters in attempting to reach the surgical goal. Through rehearsal, the complexities of individual patient vascular anatomy and the relationship of the lesion to bony and neural structures can be virtually experienced before they are encountered, so that at each step the surgeon can anticipate problems and formulate strategies to avoid them, or devise optimal solutions for those that cannot be avoided. In other fields, such as laparoscopy, rehearsal has been shown to improve speed and accuracy and reduce the complication rate of surgery. Here, we discuss some of the platforms that support surgical rehearsal via image guidance.

Virtual Reality

The practice of surgical treatment of cerebral aneurysms has dramatically changed due to endovascular techniques. The volume of neurosurgery for these lesions has been reduced, but, at the same time, the complexity of aneurysms being treated with microsurgery has increased. Therefore, tools to improve surgeon experience are highly desirable. Simulation of cerebrovascular surgical approaches has been made possible by the introduction of high-resolution 3D-imaging techniques, such as 3D-CTA and 3D-DSA, enabling reproduction of a craniotomy and rotation of a vascular tree according to the orientation of the operative microscope. The Dextroscope® (Bracco Advanced Medical Technologies, Princeton, New Jersey, USA) is a virtual simulator that is available for these purposes.[10-12] This technology allows simulation of final clipping, enabling anticipation of aneurysm deformation during clip application and selection of the appropriate clip and its orientation.[13]

Specific cerebrovascular neuronavigation procedures have been developed based on 3D-CTA and 3D-DSA, which have helped to make the operation more secure by predicting the location and orientation of the aneurysm within the parenchyma.

Augmented Reality

Augmented reality (semi-immersive environment) is the integration of computer-generated images with the real-world field.[14] In neurosurgery, it implies the projection of segments and structures of interest from CT or MRI onto the real surgical field. These images can be projected using various technologies, such as heads-up displays, head-mounted displays and image injection into the operating microscope. Augmented reality represents a form of interactive image-guided neurosurgery that aids the surgeon with intraoperative orientation by showing what cannot be seen directly and by allowing the surgeon to integrate multimodal information without having to direct his or her attention away from the operating field.[15] Cabrilo et al. applied this technology to the surgical treatment of cerebral aneurysms. They used preoperative 3D-image datasets from 3D-DSA, CTA, or MRA to create virtual segmentation of patient's vessels, aneurysms, aneurysm necks, skulls and heads. These images were transferred into the operating microscope to allow a tailored minimally invasive approach and optimal clipping of aneurysms.[15] While segmentation of the vascular tree from the rest of the image guidance dataset can be cumbersome, once in place, it can be useful for roles such as finding a ruptured aneurysm within a clot or identifying vessel branches for proximal and distal control.

ANEURYSM MICROSURGERY

Intraoperative Neuronavigation

Traditional stereotactic image guidance is not often used for aneurysm microsurgery. This is predominantly because most aneurysms arise from the circle of Willis where the anatomy is generally fixed and can be easily located by following landmarks. In addition, the extra-axial subfrontal and pterional approaches most commonly used for aneurysm clipping rely on displacement of the brain, which tends to disturb the anatomy enough that its accuracy may be limited. Despite these caveats, there are some applications in which intraoperative neuronavigation using either preoperative CT or CTA or MR or MRA imaging can be useful for aneurysm microsurgery. These applications include surgery for aneurysms with very complex anatomy where finding all of the branches can be otherwise laborious, and for aneurysms in non-standard locations, for example, those that are very distal on the vascular tree.

Largely due to technical advances that have increased the precision, speed of image acquisition and capabilities for 3D reconstruction, CTA has become a primary imaging modality, providing initial diagnostic information for the care of patients with either ruptured or unruptured aneurysms. CTA images obtained by multislice scanners with very thin image thicknesses can provide exquisite rendering of vascular anatomy. Its convenience and flexibility often makes it useful in initial decisions about which treatment modality to use for aneurysms, e.g. microsurgical clipping versus endovascular coiling. If the decision is made to pursue a clipping strategy, a volumetric CTA, which has a large field of view (typically in the order of 25 cm), will also have sufficient rendering of external craniofacial landmarks to support image guidance registration.

Computed tomography angiography-based image guidance can be particularly useful for aneurysms in more distal or unusual locations in the vascular tree, such as the distal middle cerebral artery, pericallosal and callosomarginal arteries, posterior cerebral artery, distal superior cerebellar artery, posterior-inferior cerebellar artery, or locations where the anatomy is significantly distorted by unusual variants **(Figures 16.1A to G)**. For example, in the case of a distal middle cerebral artery aneurysm, a more highly focused dissection of the Sylvian fissure to obtain proximal and distal control may be made easier with the benefit of image guidance than without it. Very distal aneurysms can be difficult to locate without image guidance, which therefore, puts more brain at risk in dissection. The use of image guidance in this setting is no more cumbersome than that for any other type of case (e.g. tumor), and as noted above, systems can use the same CTA images that are used for diagnosis, if they are captured and stored in the proper format. At the Barrow Neurological Institute, it is our practice to always obtain CTA images in a format compatible with image guidance to leave this option open.

In addition to its usefulness for navigating to the aneurysm, the bone windows provide valuable information about the location of the air sinuses in the forehead and anterior skull base, which can be important in planning the type and extent of craniotomies in this region. While creating the desired exposure is essential, there are advantages in terms of operative risk and reconstruction to avoiding entering the air sinuses when possible, and we find stereotactic image guidance useful in this regard.

Intraoperative MRI or MRA-based image guidance can also be used in aneurysmal clipping. By providing "look-through" visualization of the vascular tree, it may assist the surgeon in applying a less invasive approach for access to the lesion by limiting how much proximal and distal exposure of the main vascular trunk or collateral vessels is needed.[16] Much as discussed with CTA earlier, this technique can also be useful for selected patients with distally located aneurysms

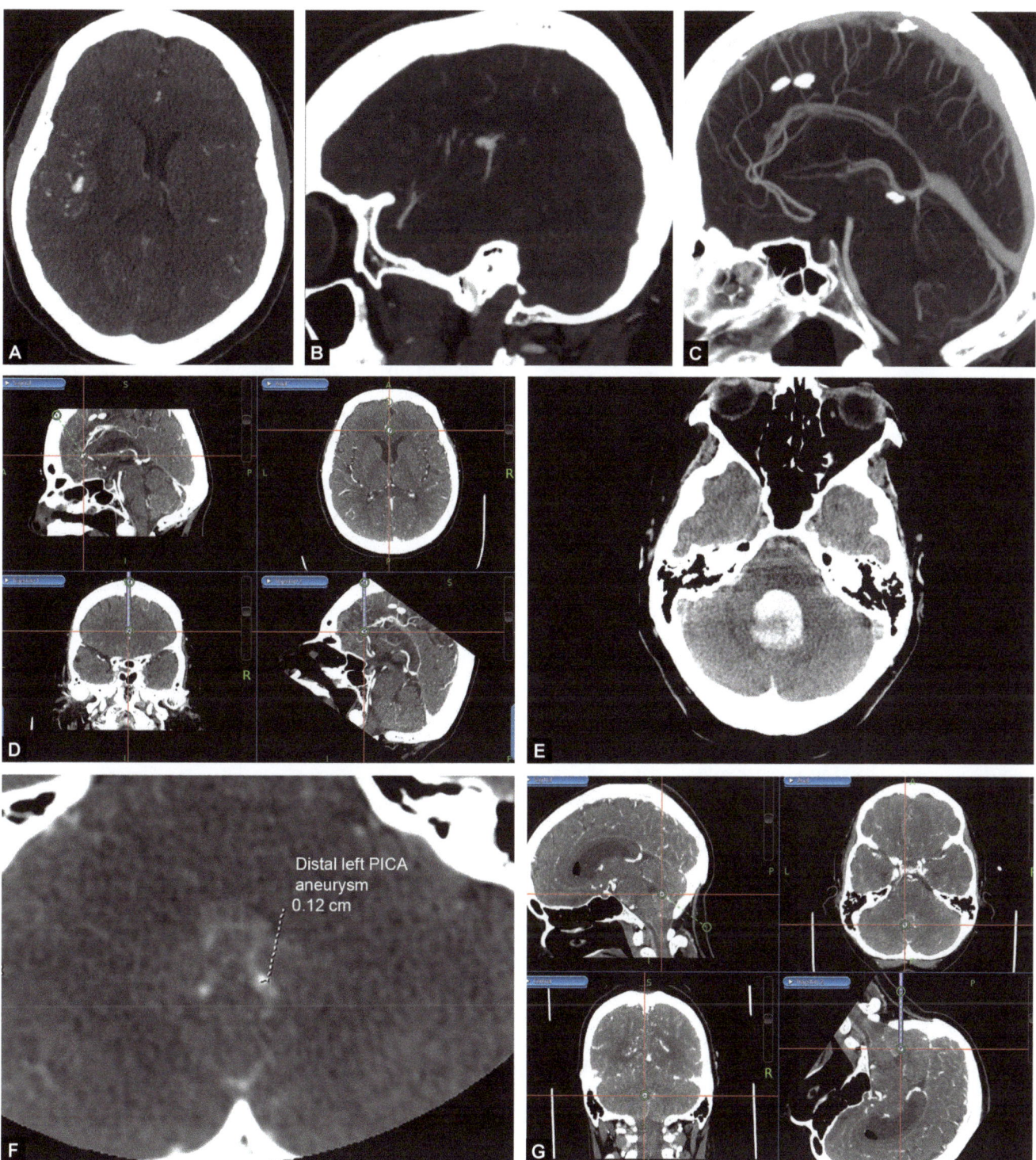

Figures 16.1A to G Image guidance may be helpful in localizing a variety of aneurysms, especially those in more unusual locations, as in these examples. A distal middle right cerebral artery is seen on (A) axial and (B) sagittal CT angiograms (CTAs); (C) Image guidance may be used to define the trajectory to a pericallosal artery aneurysm as shown in sagittal CTA views and (D) image guidance views; (E) A distal posterior-inferior cerebellar artery aneurysm in an unusually distal location within a fourth ventricular hematoma is visualized on (F) axial CTA and (G) image guidance views. *Source*: Used with permission from Barrow Neurological Institute, USA.

outside the basal cisterns, such as those of the pericallosal artery bifurcation or the far insular segment of the middle cerebral artery. Examples of these are very distal aneurysms of a mycotic nature that may be far out in the insula, for which otherwise very proximal and extensive dissection might be required.

Intraoperative Imaging Acquisition

Although we do not regularly use stereotactic neuro-navigation for aneurysm surgery, other than in the examples listed above, our institution has established routine intraoperative imaging to assess aneurysm obliteration and parent vessel patency. Multiple modalities can be used to intraoperatively assess the cranial vasculature, depending on the resources available to the surgeon, such as CTA, MRA, DSA, and indocyanine green videoangiography (ICGA).

Newer, faster, multislice portable or gantry-mounted CT scanners have begun to allow high-resolution intra-operative CTA. Modern CTA, with the ability to perform 3D reconstructions, is becoming an increasingly appealing substitute to intraoperative DSA at some institutions, with results comparable to other established techniques.[17]

Intraoperative MRI or MRA is useful for evaluating the brain parenchyma, but is less useful for evaluating the actual clipping, because the clip artifact often obscures the visualization of the neck of the aneurysm and the origin of the parent and distal arteries. Therefore, we consider intraoperative MRI or MRA the least useful of the intraoperative imaging modalities for aneurysm clipping.

The use of ICGA has become more popular in neurosurgery, since its introduction by Raabe and colleagues in 2003.[18] The advantages of ICGA in aneurysm surgery include that it can be performed at any time during surgery, there is no need to move the microscope or interrupt the operation, the results are available immediately within the surgical field, and the procedure can be repeated as needed without the use of iodinated contrast or radiation. Compared with DSA, another advantage of ICGA is that the surgeon can observe the patency of all vessels including small perforators and cortical arteries of sub-millimeter diameter that are not visualized even on high-quality DSA imaging. The disadvantages of ICGA include that the views are limited to the field of the microscope, so vessels covered by brain parenchyma, aneurysm clips, or blood clots cannot be viewed. Furthermore, its sensitivity for relative overclipping of the aneurysm neck causing mild to moderate parent vessel stenosis without complete vessel occlusion may be less than the sensitivity of a formal intraoperative DSA. Nonetheless, ICGA remains an extremely useful tool in aneurysm surgery and has supplanted about 88% of intraoperative catheter angiograms at our institution.[19]

ARTERIOVENOUS MALFORMATION MICROSURGERY

Intraoperative Neuronavigation

Surgical resection remains the most effective treatment for the majority of arteriovenous malformation microsurgery (AVM). At times, AVMs may be difficult to localize intra-operatively and to resect with minimal morbidity. Stereotactic neuronavigation in AVM surgery using CT-, MR- or DSA-based image guidance helps to define nidal margins, locate arterial feeders and identify draining veins (Figures 16.2A to C). This is especially useful during the final stages of resection along the deep periventricular margins, where vision is limited by the AVM nidus. In cases of preoperative embolization, image guidance also displays the extent and location of the embolization material. Other important components, such as small arterial feeders (down to at least 1.2 mm in diameter) and the presence of draining vein thrombosis, can also be identified using image guidance.[20]

Neuronavigation, usually with preoperatively obtained MRI, is most useful for planning a small, efficient and noneloquent cortical or sulcal incision when operating upon a deep-seated AVM with no cortical representation.[20] Well-planned cortical incisions and trajectories can decrease operative morbidity rates and minimize unnecessary parenchymal exploration. Image guidance can also be useful for localizing deep perinidal hematomas, allowing drainage of the hematoma and surgical excision of the AVM at the same time. Neuronavigation can also allow for safer placement of an external ventricular drain in the setting of an AVM with a periventricular location (Figures 16.3A and B). For small AVMs, intraoperative CTA acquisition linked with a neuronavigation platform enhances the safety of surgical treatment.[21] The incorporation of DSA to image guidance systems was introduced in 2010 by Gonzalez et al.[22], allowing the integration of catheter angiography images (acquired during preoperative embolization) to other neuronavigation imaging modalities during image-guided AVM resection. This technique reduces artifact from embolization materials, allowing for more precise neuronavigation. Overall, frameless stereotaxy may improve surgical outcomes for cerebral AVMs by allowing more precise localization, potentially decreasing operative times and minimizing blood loss.

Neuronavigation-Integrated Diffusion Tensor Imaging and Functional Imaging

For AVM surgery, the incorporation of diffusion tensor imaging (DTI) and preoperative functional data with standard image guidance allows more careful selection of the proper route to an AVM. Adding advanced image guidance to

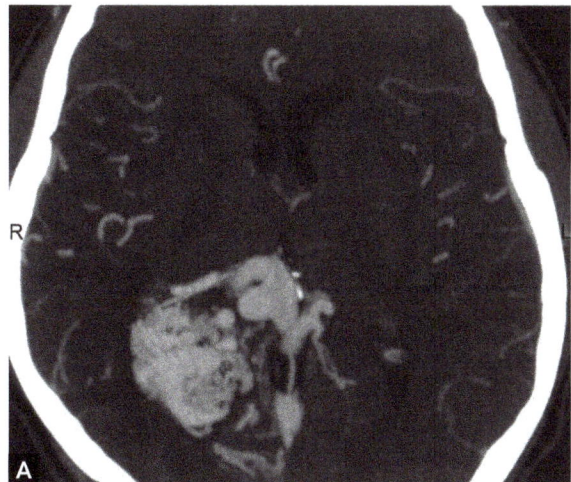

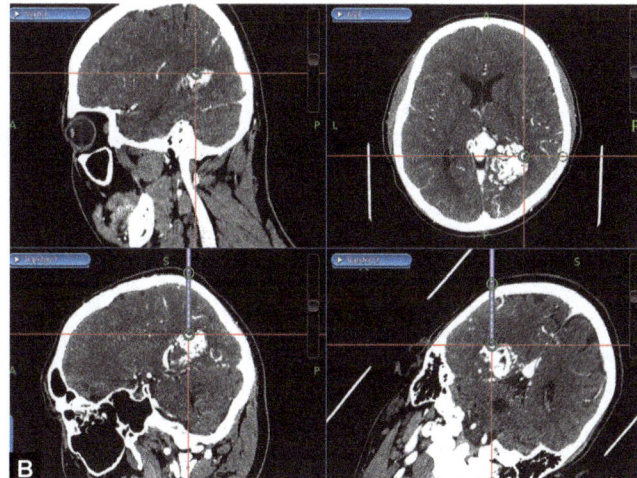

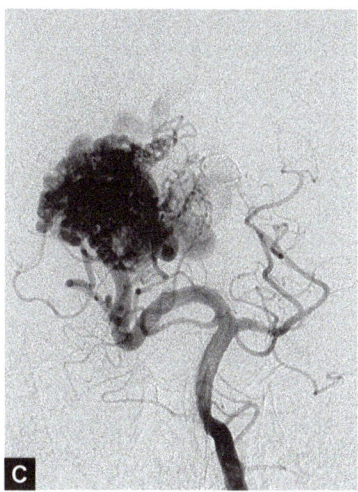

Figures 16.2A to C Image guidance for a deep arteriovenous malformation. (A) Axial computed tomography angiography (CTA) demonstrates the deep location; (B) CTA-based image guidance can be helpful to establish an operative trajectory that may not be as simple to determine from angiography alone, and (C) Anteroposterior vertebral artery injection shown
Source: Used with permission from Barrow Neurological Institute, USA.

standard cerebrovascular neurosurgical techniques enables surgeons to better resect lesions with the least amount of tissue manipulation and smaller craniotomies.[23] Functional MRI (fMRI) is currently approved for clinical use to determine the location of eloquent cortex. For surface AVMs, fMRI may better localize regional functionality than would traditional surface-based anatomy, as the AVM may induce reorganization or transfer of important cortical functions to neighboring or distant brain regions.[24] However, because no functional cortex exists within the AVM itself, our institution has had clinical success in the resection of AVMs using fMRI, even those located immediately adjacent to critical speech and motor regions. For deep-seated AVMs, fMRI helps to localize eloquent cortical functions and use these as seed points to reconstruct white matter tractography.[25] For many patients with eloquent cortex or deep-seated AVMs, their potential for future neurological catastrophe from rupture can be eliminated by successful surgical intervention. Modern neuronavigational techniques when merged with DTI and/or functional imaging can reduce the perioperative risk of treating these lesions.

Intraoperative Imaging Acquisition

Indocyanine green videoangiography is a safe and quick method to map the angioarchitecture of superficially located AVMs. ICGA is most helpful in identifying the major draining veins and how quickly they fill, as well as in delineating the nidus on the surface and highlighting superficial arterial inputs. It is less useful for deep-seated lesions where there is poor light penetration and the entire nidus may not be visible. The modality does not detect residual AVMs, except when the draining vein and associated nidus are superficial and free from overlying blood or brain tissue. ICGA should, therefore, not be used as an isolated imaging modality to confirm complete resection of the AVM or to identify en passage vessels. In our practice, ICGA is used to assess basic anatomy for AVMs with a nidus located superficially, and it is no longer used for deep-seated lesions. Caution should be exercised in relying solely on this imaging modality for any AVM surgery, especially for assessing lesion obliteration; intraoperative or immediate postoperative DSA remains the preferred modality for the confirmation of total AVM surgical resection.[26]

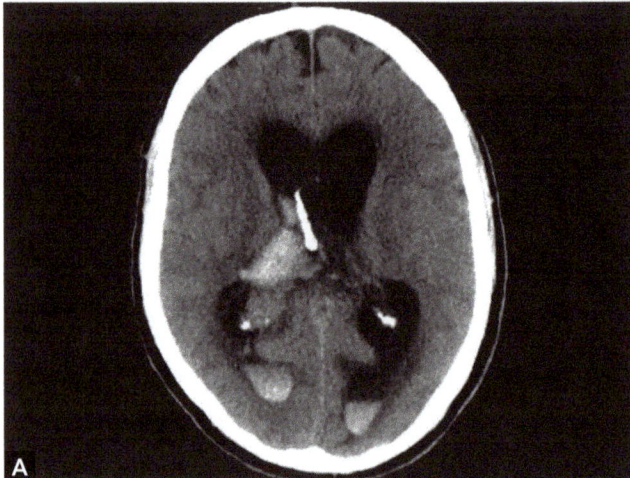 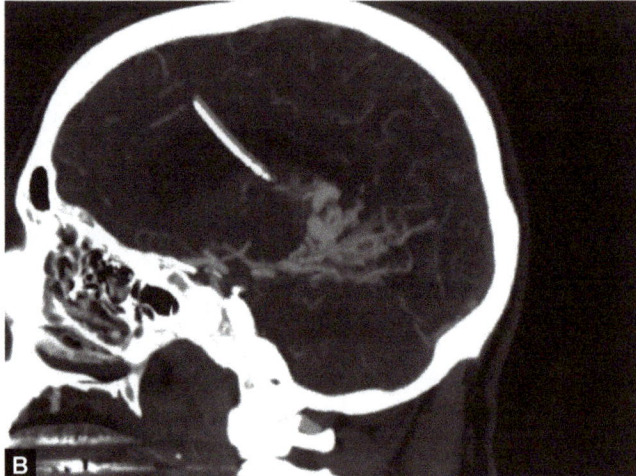

Figures 16.3A and B Image guidance may be helpful for placing a ventriculostomy in the presence of a ruptured arteriovenous malformation (AVM) with hematoma. (A) Axial and (B) sagittal views may be helpful for surgical excision of the AVM
Source: Used with permission from Barrow Neurological Institute, USA.

DURAL ARTERIOVENOUS FISTULA MICROSURGERY

Intracranial dural arteriovenous fistulas (DAVFs) are abnormal arteriovenous connections from a dural artery to a dural venous sinus or to a leptomeningeal vein, with a nidus lying within the dural leaflets. They account for 15% of all intracranial AVMs. DAVFs cause a considerable degree of clinical morbidity and mortality. The annual risks of hemorrhage or nonhemorrhagic neurological deficits for patients with DAVFs with cortical venous drainage are 8.1% and 6.9%, respectively.[27-30] Endovascular embolization and microsurgical obliteration are the main two therapeutic modalities used to treat DAVFs.[30]

Traditional frameless stereotactic image guidance is useful for approach planning and general navigation to these lesions. However, colocalization of the fistulous point as identified on preoperative imaging, such as a catheter angiography image, with the corresponding position on stereotactic MRI or CTA can be challenging. Preoperative diagnosis and characterization of DAVFs is still mostly based on DSA results. Until recently, DSA was not routinely integrated in neuronavigation workstations. Unlike AVMs, DAVFs are often small in size and may consist of only a few pathological vessels that are not easily identified on MRI. Thus, neuronavigation is more effective in assisting surgeons treating superficial rather than deep DAVFs, as brain shift and retraction is minimal. Image guidance can be used to identify arterial feeders and draining veins visible on preoperative MRA. Other modalities, such as dynamic contrast-enhanced MRA and time-of-flight MRA that can also be easily transferred to the workstation, allow visualization of pathological vessels and provide accurate localization of the DAVF.[31,32] Image guidance for the surgical treatment of DAVFs is, therefore, best applied to the precision and accuracy of positioning and surgical approaches, and less so the identification of the fistulous point itself.

For intraoperative DAVF identification as well as confirmation of fistula obliteration, we have found ICGA to be a highly useful tool **(Figures 16.4A to E)**. Our recent institutional experience with DAVF surgery (in press)[33] has demonstrated ICGA to be just as useful as intraoperative DSA for the identification of the fistulous transition as well as successful fistula ligation. However, both ICGA and intraoperative DSA fall short of the "gold standard" of postoperative DSA to demonstrate fistula obliteration (each has a false-negative rate of approximately 5–10%), and so we continue to recommend formal postoperative catheter angiography for these patients.

INTRACEREBRAL HEMORRHAGE EVACUATION

Nontraumatic intracerebral hemorrhage (ICH) can occur from a variety of causes. Those that are related to an underlying vascular pathology are most often resolved in the course of treating the primary pathology. The incidence of spontaneous ICH is 10–30 cases per 100,000 worldwide and affects approximately 67,000 people yearly in the United States.[34] The most common cause of nontraumatic, nonaneurysmal ICH is hypertension. These hemorrhages typically occur in several locations, including the basal ganglia, thalamus and deep white matter.[34,35] Surgical management of ICHs remains a matter of debate. Minimally invasive techniques have shown a trend toward improved outcomes when compared with medical management.[36,37]

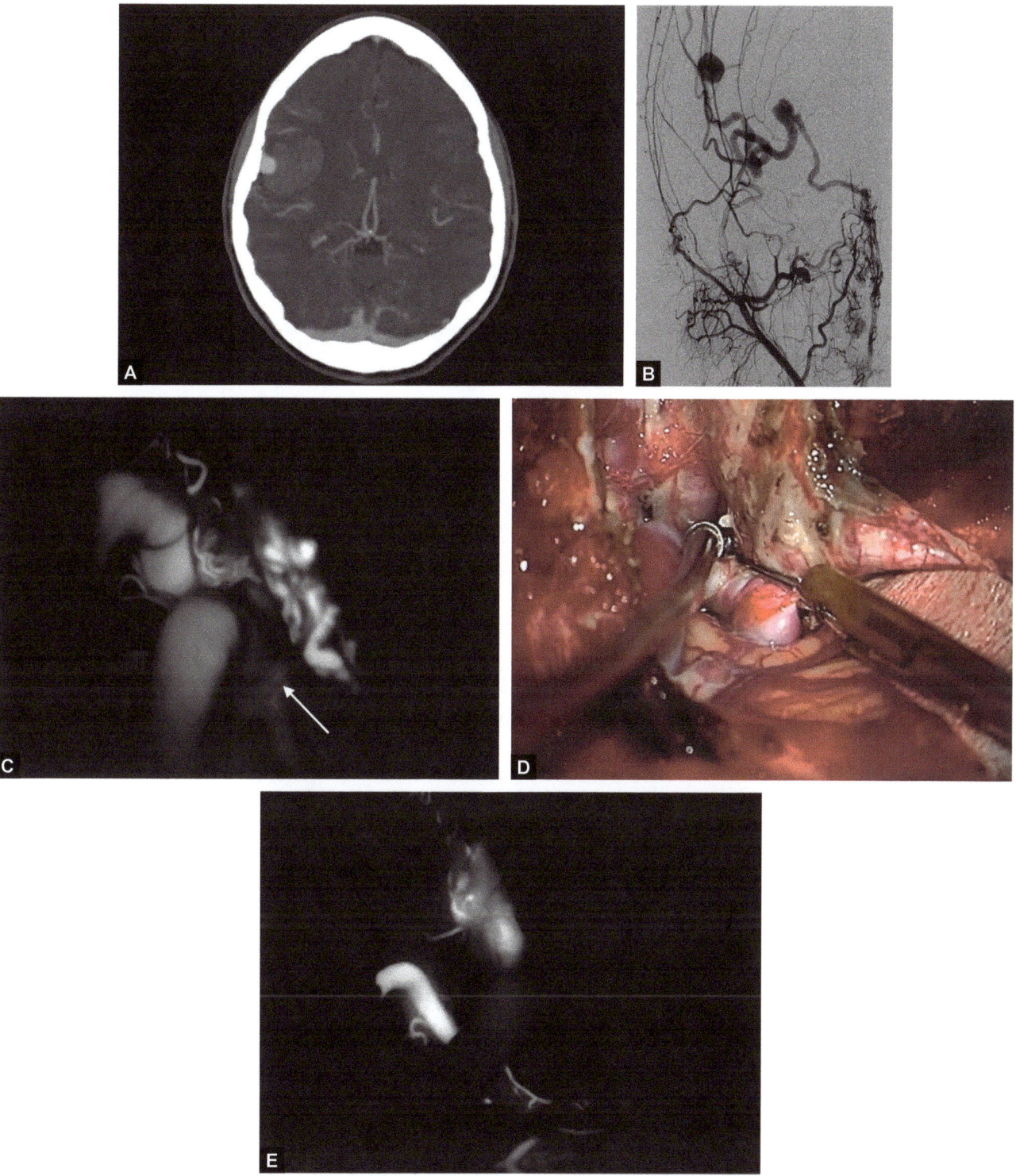

Figures 16.4A to E Arteriovenous fistula (ethmoidal fistula). (A) Preoperative axial CTA showing a right frontal hematoma and venous pouch; (B) Preoperative lateral DSA view shows an ethmoidal fistula that originates from the ethmoidal branches of the ophthalmic artery; (C) Intraoperative ICG angiogram shows the main arteriovenous fistula feeder (arrow) coming up through the ethmoidal bone defect; (D) Intraoperative microscope view of the arterial feeder after simple clipping of the fistula at the midline skull base, and (E) Intraoperative ICG angiogram after clip ligation of the fistula demonstrates complete obliteration (compare to Fig. 16.4C)

Source: Used with permission from Barrow Neurological Institute, USA.

Abbreviations: CTA, computed tomography angiography; DSA, digital subtraction angiography; ICG, indocyanine green.

Vespa et al. described the use of frameless stereotactic catheter aspiration with the use of tissue plasminogen activator in a group of 28 patients and reported more than a 75% reduction of hematoma volume with significant improvement in National Institutes of Health (NIH) Stroke Scale Score.[38] An ongoing NIH trial (MISTIE-III) is rigorously examining this technique **(Figures 16.5A to D)**. Image-guided keyhole evacuation has been reported by multiple authors, with an average hematoma reduction of 93–100%.[39,40] Cho et al. compared three different surgical modalities for ICH management including craniotomy, stereotactic aspiration and endoscopy.[41] They concluded that stereotactic aspiration and endoscopic surgery are both effective procedures with low complication and mortality rates. More recently, Dye et al. described a minimally invasive alternative for image-guided endoscopic evacuation of ICH.[42] They showed a reduction in hematoma volume of almost 80%. Clinically, the patients exhibited a trend toward improvement with better postprocedure scores on the Glasgow Coma Scale in all patients.

Stereotactic image guidance is vital in these minimally invasive procedures. Hattori et al. conducted a randomized study of the impact of stereotactic ICH evacuation on daily living after spontaneous ICH.[37] Their results confirmed the benefits of neuronavigation-based evacuation of hematomas for reducing the incidence of mortality and improving functional outcome in spontaneous ICH.[36,37] Intraoperative image acquisition during ICH evacuation is usually unnecessary, although CT or MRI can be used to verify adequate evacuation prior to leaving the operating

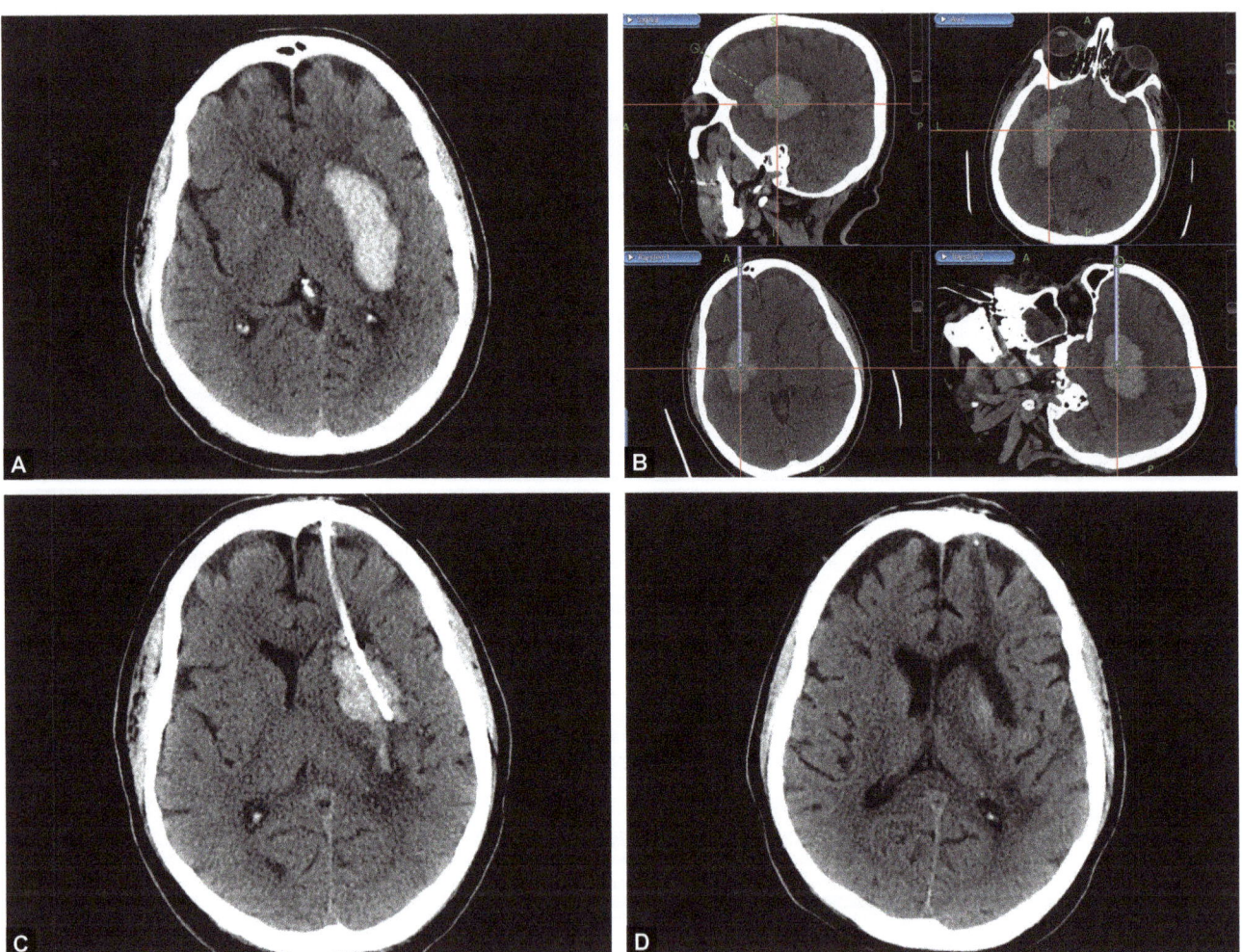

Figures 16.5A to D (A) A deep-seated basal ganglia intracerebral hematoma is seen preoperatively on axial computed tomography (CT); (B) Image guidance is used to plan a direct trajectory down the long axis of the hematoma; (C) Postoperative images show the evacuation of the hematoma and placement of a ventriculostomy catheter in the hematoma bed, and (D) A substantial resolution of the clot is visualized on axial CT taken 9 days after the surgery
Source: Used with permission from Barrow Neurological Institute, USA.

room; this may be of additional benefit in minimally invasive image-guided aspiration procedures where the surgical cavity cannot be fully visually inspected.

SUPRATENTORIAL CAVERNOUS MALFORMATION MICROSURGERY

Most cavernous malformations occur in the supratentorial white matter. The use of T2-weighted stereotactic MRI sequences for image guidance in the microsurgical resection of these lesions is now commonplace **(Figures 16.6A to E)**. In addition to standard intraoperative neuronavigation, the use of DTI in surgery for cavernous malformations has been reported.[43-46] However, DTI does not accurately represent the crossing of multiple fibers or definitively determine their cortical and subcortical termination. High-definition fiber tractography (HDFT) tracks fiber pathways more accurately than DTI, and the use of HDFT in cavernous malformation surgery provides qualitative data with respect to the relevant

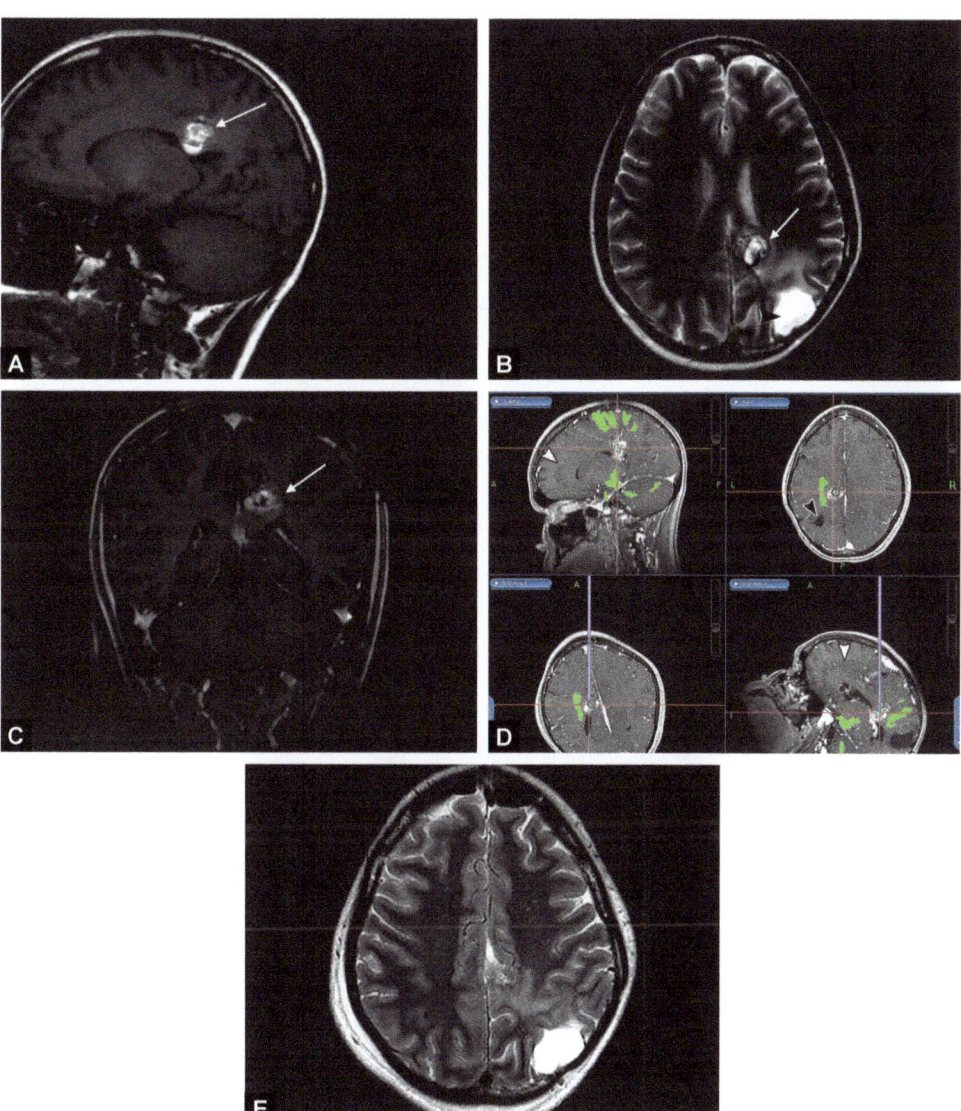

Figures 16.6A to E A deep-seated cavernous malformation of the brain in a 26-year-old woman who presented with a small hemorrhage and seizure. The cavernous malformation (light arrowhead) is seen to lie below a prior glioma resection bed (dark arrowhead) on T2-weighted magnetic resonance (MR) images in (A) sagittal, (B) axial, (C) coronal views; (D) Functional MRI of the brain in the same patient integrated into image guidance shows that the sensorimotor tracts (in green, upper right panel) lay between the prior tumor resection bed (dark arrowhead) and the cavernous malformation. Therefore, an anterior interhemispheric approach was chosen instead of a direct transcortical approach, and (E) Postoperative axial T2-weighted MR image shows a complete resection of the cavernous malformation. There was no postoperative deficit
Source: Used with permission from Barrow Neurological Institute, USA.

perilesional tracts. HDFT has allowed surgeons to assess tract position precisely with respect to cavernous malformations, facilitating decision making and appropriate surgical planning and thus, minimizing morbidity from surgical approaches.[23] In addition to adequate visualization of eloquent areas, other tracts such as the uncinate fasciculus, thalamopostcentral fibers, nondominant arcuate fasciculus, and superior longitudinal fasciculus can be identified and their anatomical relation to the cavernous malformations can be understood.[23] Images from all these modalities can be fused with MRI-based stereotactic neuronavigation when planning the surgical trajectory and entry point into the parenchyma. Lastly, the use of intraoperative MRI with preoperative functional neuronavigation imaging such as DTI, HDFT, or fMRI can update the surgeon as to the extent of residual lesion with respect to the nearby critical tracts, allowing modification of the surgical plan.[47,48]

BRAINSTEM AND DEEP-SEATED CAVERNOUS MALFORMATION MICROSURGERY

The use of stereotactic image guidance has dramatically changed the management and surgical results of cavernous malformation surgery, especially for patients with deep-seated cavernous malformations. The use of operative image guidance is absolutely indispensable in the treatment of brainstem cavernous malformations. Neuronavigation guides intraoperative decision making for the surgical trajectory to a cavernous malformation that lies deep to a normal pial surface without obvious hemosiderin staining.[49] The two-point method is used as an objective means to

guide the selection of the surgical approach **(Figures 16.7A and B)**.[49,50] With this technique, one point is placed in the center of the cavernous malformation, and a second point is placed where the lesion comes closest to the pial surface or where the safest entry point is determined. A line is drawn connecting these two points and extended to the skull, and this trajectory is used to select the most optimal surgical corridor. Abla et al. reported the outcome of a large series of patients with brainstem cavernous malformation in whom image guidance was used, and they found that this technology was essential in the surgical management of these lesions.[49] Furthermore, the use of image guidance has changed the surgical practice of our institution via a decrease in the use of more extensive skull base approaches. For example, for cerebellopontine angle cavernous malformations, the two-point method suggests a lateral trajectory. This lesion might have been previously approached through a transpetrosal approach. However, a lateral trajectory can be achieved with gentle cerebellar retraction and a less extensive retrosigmoid approach **(Figures 16.8A to D)**.[51]

SUMMARY

Stereotactic image guidance and intraoperative imaging have become commonplace within neurosurgery in the last decades, and both technologies have roles within cerebrovascular neurosurgery. Preoperatively, stereotactic image guidance has given rise to virtual reality-based simulations of cerebrovascular procedures for both education and patient care. Intraoperative stereotactic neuronavigation is especially useful in AVM and cavernous malformation resection, as well as in minimally invasive ICH evacuation. Intraoperative ICGA and other intraoperative

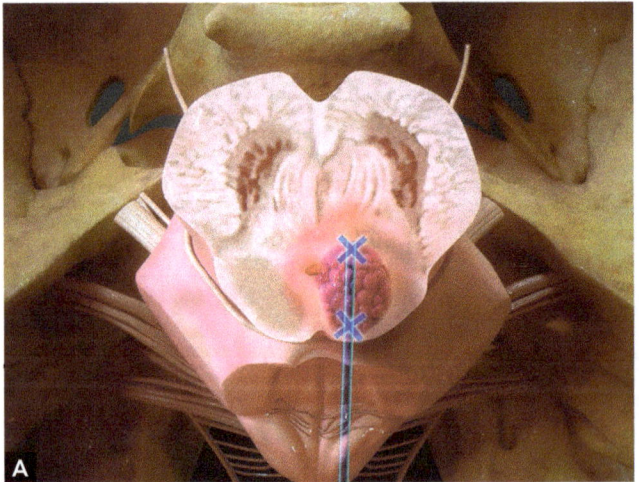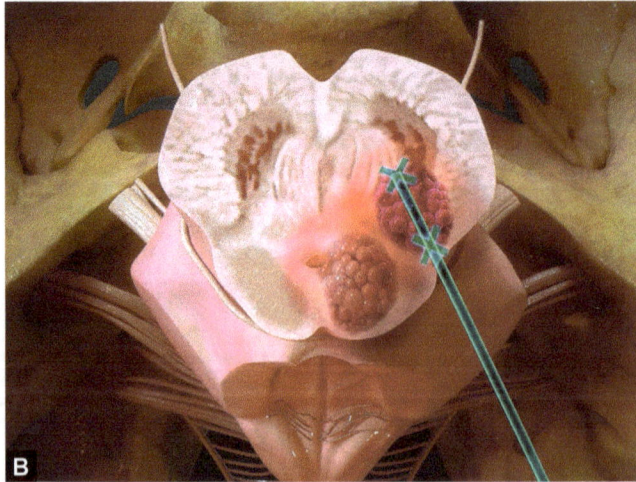

Figures 16.7A and B Two-point method to brainstem and deep-seated cavernous malformation microsurgery. A line is drawn through the center of the lesion and the most superficial point on the lesion to the surface. Therefore, a lesion oriented in the (A) sagittal plane should be approached posteriorly whereas one more (B) laterally oriented should be approached from a commensurately more lateral trajectory
Source: Used with permission from Barrow Neurological Institute, USA.

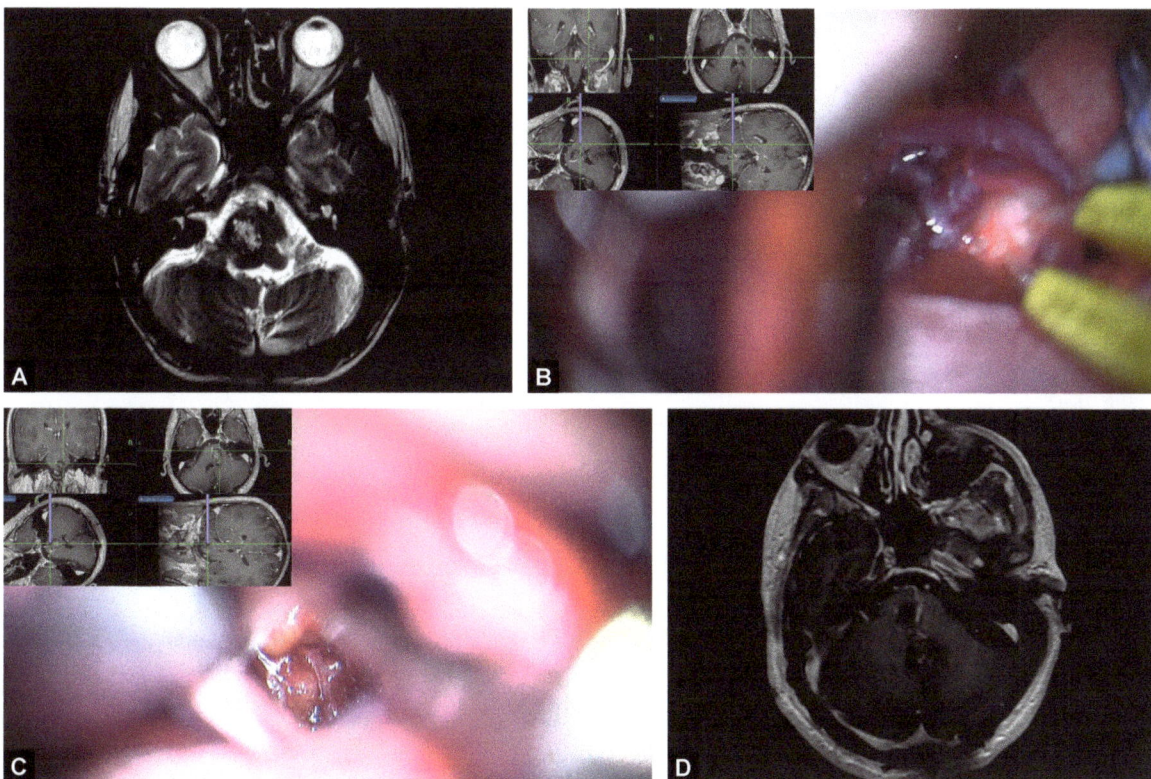

Figures 16.8A to D Brainstem cavernous malformation. (A) T2-weighted axial magnetic resonance (MR) image shows a large right pontine cavernous malformation; (B and C) Intraoperative image-guided neuronavigation depicts the chosen best entry point (middle cerebellar peduncle) into the brainstem lesion. In this case, the best entry point (C, green cross) is through the middle cerebellar peduncle just above the cranial nerves VII and VIII and posterior to the large developmental venous anomaly; and (D) Postoperative axial T1-weighted MR image shows complete resection of the cavernous malformation
Source: Used with permission from Barrow Neurological Institute, USA.

modalities to assess intraluminal flow have become routine in microsurgical aneurysm clipping and DAVF ligation. The addition of advanced neuronavigation modalities such as merged 3D catheter angiography, DTI and fMRI will continue to improve patient outcomes in cerebrovascular surgery.

REFERENCES

1. Black PM, Moriarty T, Alexander E, et al. Development and implementation of intraoperative magnetic resonance imaging and its neurosurgical applications. Neurosurgery. 1997;41(4):831-42.
2. Tronnier VM, Wirtz CR, Knauth M, et al. Intraoperative diagnostic and interventional magnetic resonance imaging in neurosurgery. Neurosurgery. 1997;40(5):891-900.
3. Wirtz CR, Tronnier VM, Bonsanto MM, et al. Image-guided neurosurgery with intraoperative MRI: update of frameless stereotaxy and radicality control. Stereotact Funct Neurosurg. 1997;68(1-4 Pt 1):39-43.
4. Zimmermann M, Seifert V, Trantakis C, et al. Open MRI-guided microsurgery of intracranial tumours in or near eloquent brain areas. Acta Neurochir (Wien). 2001;143(4):327-37.
5. Berger MS, Hadjipanayis CG. Surgery of intrinsic cerebral tumors. Neurosurgery. 2007;61(1 Suppl):279-304.
6. González-Darder JM, González-López P, Talamantes F, et al. Multimodal navigation in the functional microsurgical resection of intrinsic brain tumors located in eloquent motor areas: role of tractography. Neurosurg Focus. 2010;28(2):E5.
7. Tee JW, Dally M, Madan A, et al. Surgical treatment of poorly visualised and complex cerebrovascular lesions using preoperative angiographic data as angiographic DynaCT datasets for frameless stereotactic navigation. Acta Neurochir (Wien). 2012;154(7):1159-67.
8. Schaller K, Kotowski M, Pereira V, et al. From intraoperative angiography to advanced intraoperative imaging: the Geneva experience. Acta Neurochir Suppl. 2011;109:111-5.
9. Leng LZ, Rubin DG, Patsalides A, et al. Fusion of intraoperative three-dimensional rotational angiography and flat-panel detector computed tomography for cerebrovascular neuronavigation. World Neurosurg. 2013;79(3-4):504-9.
10. Gu SX, Yang DL, Cui DM, et al. Anatomical studies on the temporal bridging veins with Dextroscope and its application in tumor surgery across the middle and posterior fossa. Clin Neurol Neurosurg. 2011;113(10):889-94.
11. Du ZY, Gao X, Zhang XL, et al Preoperative evaluation of neurovascular relationships for microvascular decompression

in the cerebellopontine angle in a virtual reality environment. J Neurosurg. 2010;113(3):479-85.

12. Yang de L, Xu QW, Che XM, et al. Clinical evaluation and follow-up outcome of presurgical plan by Dextroscope: a prospective controlled study in patients with skull base tumors. Surg Neurol. 2009;72(6):682-9.

13. Marinho P, Thines L, Verscheure L, et al. Recent advances in cerebrovascular simulation and neuronavigation for the optimization of intracranial aneurysm clipping. Comput Aided Surg. 2012;17(2):47-55.

14. Shuhaiber JH. Augmented reality in surgery. Arch Surg. 2004;139(2):170-4.

15. Cabrilo I, Bijlenga P, Schaller K. Augmented reality in the surgery of cerebral aneurysms: a technical report. Neurosurgery. 2014;10 Suppl 2:252-60.

16. Pirotte B, Wikler D, David P, et al. Magnetic resonance angiography image guidance for the microsurgical clipping of intracranial aneurysms: a report of two cases. Neurol Res. 2004;26(4):429-34.

17. Dinesh SK, Thomas J, Ng I. Intraoperative computed tomographic angiography in cerebral aneurysm surgery: a pilot feasibility study. Neurosurgery. 2010;66(2):349-52.

18. Raabe A, Beck J, Gerlach R, et al. Near-infrared indocyanine green video angiography: a new method for intraoperative assessment of vascular flow. Neurosurgery. 2003;52(1):132-9.

19. Hardesty DA, Thind H, Zabramski JM, et al. Safety, efficacy, and cost of intraoperative indocyanine green angiography compared to intraoperative catheter angiography in cerebral aneurysm surgery. J Clin Neurosci. 2014;21(8):1377-82.

20. Russell SM, Woo HH, Joseffer SS, et al. Role of frameless stereotaxy in the surgical treatment of cerebral arteriovenous malformations: technique and outcomes in a controlled study of 44 consecutive patients. Neurosurgery. 2002;51(5):1108-16.

21. Raza SM, Papadimitriou K, Gandhi D, et al. Intra-arterial intraoperative computed tomography angiography guided navigation: a new technique for localization of vascular pathology. Neurosurgery. 2012;71(2 Suppl Operative):ons240-52.

22. Gonzalez LF, Albuquerque FC, Boom S, et al. Image-guided resection of embolized cerebral arteriovenous malformations based on catheter-based angiography. Neurosurgery. 2010;67(2):471-5.

23. Abhinav K, Pathak S, Richardson RM, et al. Application of high-definition fiber tractography in the management of supratentorial cavernous malformations: a combined qualitative and quantitative approach. Neurosurgery. 2014;74(6):668-80.

24. Prakash N, Uhlemann F, Sheth SA, et al Current trends in intraoperative optical imaging for functional brain mapping and delineation of lesions of language cortex. Neuroimage. 2009;47(Suppl 2):T116-26.

25. Ellis MJ, Rutka JT, Kulkarni AV, et al. Corticospinal tract mapping in children with ruptured arteriovenous malformations using functionally guided diffusion-tensor imaging. J Neurosurg Pediatr. 2012;9(5):505-10.

26. Zaidi HA, Abla AA, Nakaji P, et al. Indocyanine green angiography in the surgical management of cerebral arteriovenous malformations: lessons learned in 130 consecutive cases. Neurosurgery. 2014;10(Suppl 2):246-51.

27. Awad IA, Little JR, Akarawi WP, et al. Intracranial dural arteriovenous malformations: factors predisposing to an aggressive neurological course. J Neurosurg. 1990;72(6):839-50.

28. Ghobrial GM, Marchan E, Nair AK, et al. Dural arteriovenous fistulas: a review of the literature and a presentation of a single institution's experience. World Neurosurg. 2013;80(1-2):94-102.

29. Natarajan SK, Ghodke B, Kim LJ, et al. Multimodality treatment of intracranial dural arteriovenous fistulas in the Onyx era: a single center experience. World Neurosurg. 2010;73(4):365-79.

30. Rangel-Castilla L, Barber SM, Klucznik R, et al. Mid and long term outcomes of dural arteriovenous fistula endovascular management with Onyx. Experience of a single tertiary center. J Neurointerv Surg. 2014;6(8):607-13.

31. Klisch J, Strecker R, Hennig J, et al. Time-resolved projection MRA: clinical application in intracranial vascular malformations. Neuroradiology. 2000;42(2):104-7.

32. Vougioukas VI, Coulin CJ, Shah M, et al. Benefits and limitations of image guidance in the surgical treatment of intracranial dural arteriovenous fistulas. Acta Neurochir (Wien). 2006;148(2):145-53.

33. Thind H, Hardesty, DA, Zabramski, JM, et al. The role of microscope-integrated near-infrared indocyanine green videoangiography in the surgical treatment of intracranial dural arteriovenous fistulas. J Neurosurg. 2015;122(4):876-82.

34. Broderick J, Connolly S, Feldmann E, et al. Guidelines for the management of spontaneous intracerebral hemorrhage in adults: 2007 update: a guideline from the American Heart Association/American Stroke Association Stroke Council, High Blood Pressure Research Council, and the Quality of Care and Outcomes in Research Interdisciplinary Working Group. Circulation. 2007;116(16):e391-413.

35. Anik I, Secer HI, Anik Y, et al. Meta-analyses of intracerebral hematoma treatment. Turk Neurosurg. 2011;21(1):6-14.

36. Auer LM, Deinsberger W, Niederkorn K, et al. Endoscopic surgery versus medical treatment for spontaneous intra-cerebral hematoma: a randomized study. J Neurosurg. 1989;70(4):530-5.

37. Hattori N, Katayama Y, Maya Y, et al. Impact of stereotactic hematoma evacuation on activities of daily living during the chronic period following spontaneous putaminal hemorrhage: a randomized study. J Neurosurg. 2004;101(3):417-20.

38. Vespa P, McArthur D, Miller C, et al. Frameless stereotactic aspiration and thrombolysis of deep intracerebral hemorrhage is associated with reduction of hemorrhage volume and neurological improvement. Neurocrit Care. 2005;2(3):274-81.

39. Barlas O, Karadereler S, Bahar S, et al. Image-guided keyhole evacuation of spontaneous supratentorial intracerebral hemorrhage. Minim Invasive Neurosurg. 2009;52(2):62-8.

40. Carvi Y Nievas M, Toktamis S, et al. Evaluation of invasiveness and efficacy of 2 different keyhole approaches to large basal ganglia hematomas. Surg Neurol. 2005;64(3):253-9.

41. Cho DY, Chen CC, Chang CS, et al. Endoscopic surgery for spontaneous basal ganglia hemorrhage: comparing endoscopic surgery, stereotactic aspiration, and craniotomy in noncomatose patients. Surg Neurol. 2006;65(6):547-55.

42. Dye JA, Dusick JR, Lee DJ, et al. Frontal bur hole through an eyebrow incision for image-guided endoscopic evacuation

of spontaneous intracerebral hemorrhage. J Neurosurg. 2012;117(4):767-73.

43. Jhawar S, Nadkarni T, Goel A. Giant cerebral cavernous hemangiomas: a report of two cases and review of the literature. Turk Neurosurg. 2012;22(2):226-32.

44. Mai JC, Ramanathan D, Kim LJ, et al. Surgical resection of cavernous malformations of the brainstem: evolution of a minimally invasive technique. World Neurosurg. 2013;79(5-6):691-703.

45. Nimsky C, Ganslandt O, Fahlbusch R. Implementation of fiber tract navigation. Neurosurgery. 2007;61(1 Suppl):306-17.

46. Royo A, Utrilla C, Carceller F. Surgical management of brainstem-expanding lesions: the role of neuroimaging. Semin Ultrasound CT MR. 2013;34(2):153-73.

47. Sun GC, Chen XL, Zhao Y, et al. Intraoperative MRI with integrated functional neuronavigation-guided resection of supratentorial cavernous malformations in eloquent brain areas. J Clin Neurosci. 2011;18(10):1350-4.

48. Nimsky C, Ganslandt O, Kober H, et al. Integration of functional magnetic resonance imaging supported by magnetoencephalography in functional neuronavigation. Neurosurgery. 1999;44(6):1249-55.

49. Abla AA, Lekovic GP, Turner JD, et al. Advances in the treatment and outcome of brainstem cavernous malformation surgery: a single-center case series of 300 surgically treated patients. Neurosurgery. 2011;68(2):403-14.

50. Abla AA, Turner JD, Mitha AP, Lekovic G, et al. Surgical approaches to brainstem cavernous malformations. Neurosurg Focus. 2010;29(3):E8.

51. Russin J, Fusco DJ, Spetzler RF. Left retrosigmoid craniotomy for cavernous malformation of the middle cerebellar peduncle. Neurosurg Focus. 2014;36(1 Suppl):1.

17

Multimodality Image-guided Neurosurgery

Olutayo Olubiyi, Roy Torcuator, Alexandra J Golby

INTRODUCTION

Complete surgical resection of a tumor of the central nervous system carries little value to the patient, if it results in permanently impaired neurologic function. A surgically acquired neurological deficit may be due to inadvertent injury to eloquent cortical or subcortical white matter areas in close proximity to a lesion or encountered along the surgical approach. There have been rapid advances in neuroimaging and brain mapping, with a host of new techniques with corresponding improvement in neurosurgical outcomes.[1,2] Neurosurgeons have long employed invasive brain mapping techniques; however, recent technological advances have introduced less invasive functional brain mapping methods. In addition, intraoperative imaging has gained acceptance as a useful surgical tool for guiding surgery, particularly of low-grade primary glial neoplasms. This chapter briefly presents the emergence of image-guided techniques in neurosurgery as well as the multimodality image-guided operating suite.

GENERAL CONSIDERATIONS IN BRAIN SURGERY

As with general surgical oncology practice, the ultimate goal of brain tumor surgery is to achieve complete resection of the lesion. However, unlike general surgical practice, a clear wide margin is not plausible in brain tumor surgery because the surrounding tissue is functionally important, and its removal or traumatization may result in profound morbidity.[3] Similarly, extensive exposure for direct visualization of deeply located lesions is often not practicable. In addition, gliomas are infiltrative in nature, making it difficult to identify a clear boundary, especially in low-grade tumors, which may contain functional tissue within the tumor.[3-5] Also, it is important to note that because the brain lacks intrinsic rigid support, it changes shape with disruption of its surrounding structures (including the dura matter, drainage of CSF, and resection of tumor) during surgery. Therefore, methods of navigation that use images to guide the neurosurgeon through a safe path to the tumor have become the standard of care.[6] It is also important for the neurosurgeon to visualize the patient-specific functionally critical areas of the brain in order to protect and preserve them during surgery.

IMAGE-GUIDED SURGERY

Image-guided techniques are used widely in surgical practice, with significant application in the different subspecialties of surgery including abdominal, orthopedic, urology, cardiothoracic, obstetrics/gynecology and neurosurgery. Neurosurgery, however, may utilize this technology more often than any other surgical specialty for obvious reasons as highlighted in the section above [general considerations in brain surgery]. Many preoperative and intraoperative imaging methods have been utilized, including ultrasound (US)-guided biopsies and abscess drainage, magnetic resonance image (MRI)-guided biopsies and ablative therapies; and computed tomography (CT) image-guided procedures. More often these procedures utilize preoperatively acquired images, either singly or a combination of different images to provide better visualization of structures, guidance and outcome.

In neurosurgery, preoperative imaging strategies employ structural imaging to delineate tumors or lesions from surrounding structures. Structural imaging commonly used includes modalities such as CT, MRI and MR spectroscopy, all of which are largely non-invasive. Addition of contrast agents to facilitate visualization and delineation of lesions is the standard practice. Positron emission tomography (PET) is a molecular imaging technique which uses the differential uptake of a radiotracer (most commonly radioactively labeled glucose) to define the area of neoplasm.

Another important and growing area of imaging is functional mapping, which utilizes non-invasive methods to visualize functional cortex and advanced structural imaging techniques for visualization of white mater fiber tracts. These include the following:

- *Functional magnetic resonance imaging (fMRI)* can demonstrate eloquent cortical areas in relation to the tumor. fMRI measures cerebral blood flow changes as a surrogate for neuronal activity, often as blood oxygen level-dependent (BOLD) changes in MR signal. Neuronal activity is followed by increased perfusion of local capillaries which outstrips the increased demand, resulting in increased ratio of oxyhemoglobin (oxy-Hb) to deoxyhemoglobin (deoxy-Hb).[7] Since the iron in deoxy-Hb is paramagnetic, it reduces T2* signal on MRI. In summary, neuronal activity produces a relative increase in oxy-Hb concentration and consequent increase in T2* (BOLD) signal;[8]

- *Diffusion tensor imaging (DTI)* is utilized to outline white matter tract fiber bundles in the brain. DTI measures the direction of diffusion of water molecules as a marker for the axis of these tracts with an assumption that axonal membranes and myelin directionally restrict free diffusion of water. Water diffuses more readily in the direction parallel to fiber tracts, while diffusion is constrained perpendicular to tracts, producing anisotropic diffusion in regions of tightly packed white matter.[9] Magnetic field gradients are applied in multiple orientations and a mathematical model, e.g. the diffusion tensor, is used to estimate the direction of dominant diffusivity of water molecules for every voxel, which corresponds to the principal axis of white mater tracts in that voxel. Cerebrospinal fluid (CSF) and water within gray matter diffuses equally in all directions (isotropic) in contrast to the pattern in white matter **(Figures 17.1A and B)**.[10-12]

- Preoperative mapping with fMRI involves multiple functions including motor, sensory, language, vision and memory. Adequate mapping of each of these functional tasks may require use of multiple task paradigms. It also requires the patient to be able to perform the tasks. Each of these paradigms is often viewed in 3 planes; axial, coronal and sagittal for reconstruction into 3D format for anatomical correlate.[30-33]

- *Diffusion tensor imaging* of white matter anatomy demonstrates white matter location and trajectory *in vivo*.[34-37] Tractography is suitable for three-dimensional reconstruction and anatomical correlation.[37] Its quality is dependent on algorithms, which can be either single tensor or double-tensor, and utilize unscented Kalman fiber (UKF) tracking or a streamline method. There are still unresolved challenges of tracking within areas of brain edema and regions of crossing fibers and therefore there is need for validation of these methods, within these regions **(Figures 17.2A to D)**.[11,12,37-40]

- *Magnetoencephalography:* Magnetoencephalography (MEG) maps functional activity in the cortical area by measuring the magnetic fields that accompany neuronal activity. MEG is similar to electroencephalography (EEG), but

Diffusion imaging of white matter anatomy

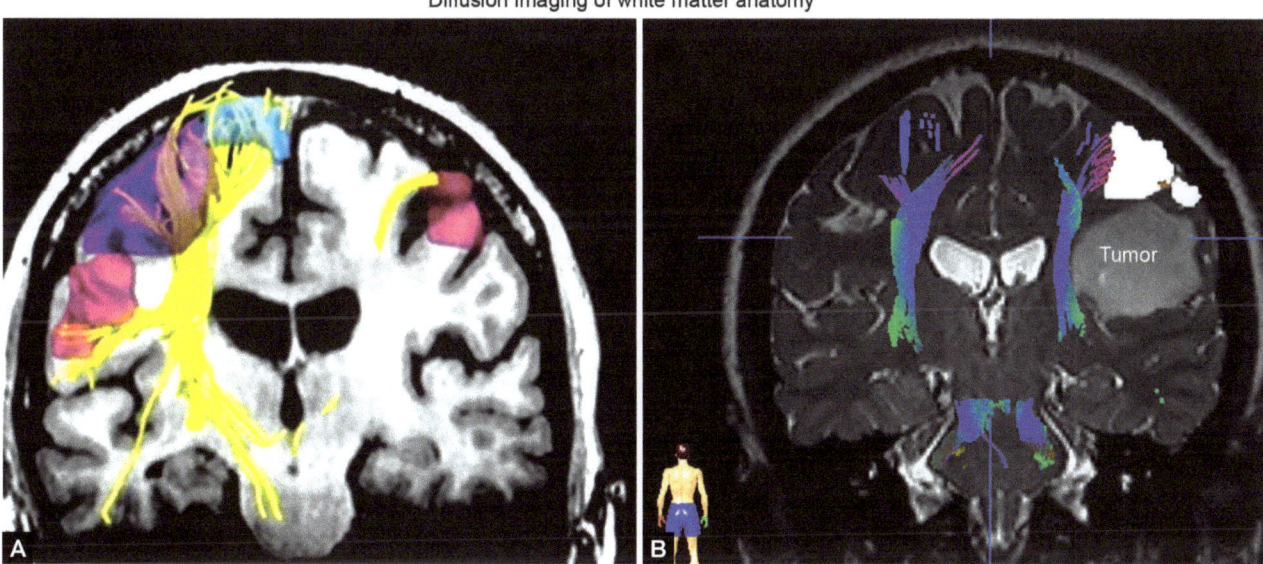

Figures 17.1A and B Diffusion tensor image showing the corticospinal tracts in relation to eloquent motor areas mapped by functional MRI. Figure A shows the CST including lateral projections to the hand and face areas (pink, purple and blue solids) in a normal subject using two tensor modeling [*Adapted with permission from* Qazi et al. Resolving crossings in the corticospinal tract by two-tensor streamline tractography: Method and clinical assessment using fMRI Neuroimage 2009]. Figure B shows the CST in a patient with hemispheric glioma (the white solid represents fMRI activations from the hand-clenching task)

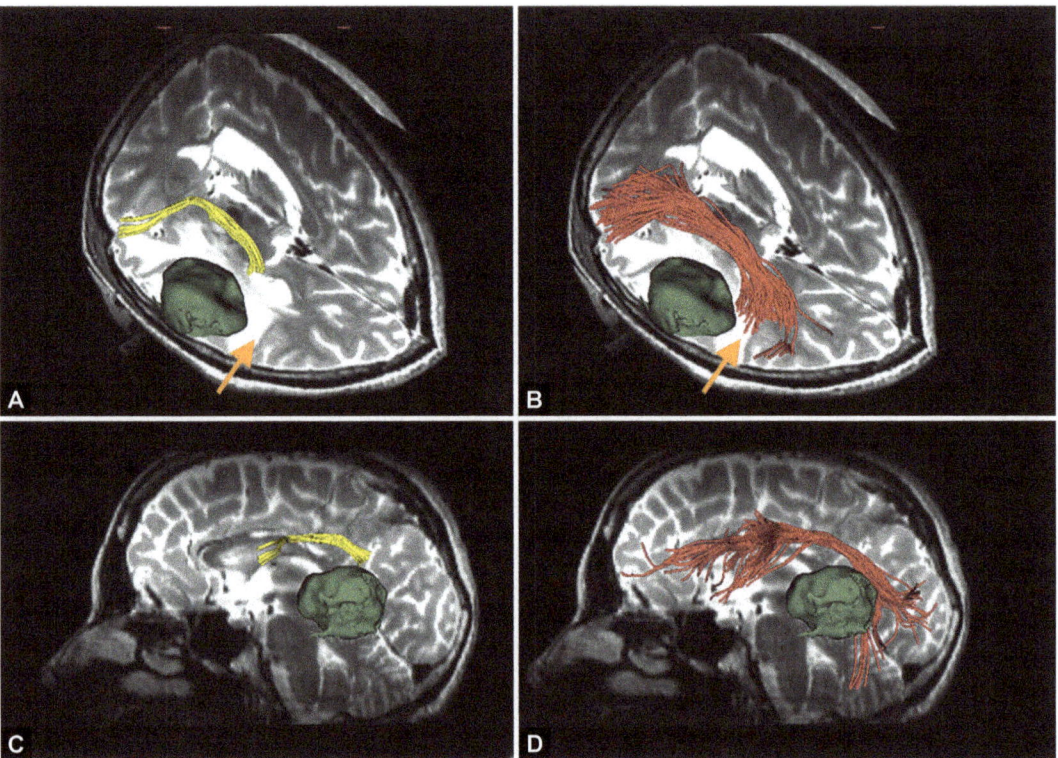

Figures 17.2A to D DTI fiber tracking within peritumoral edema showing single-tensor streamline tractography (yellow) appears to indicate a disrupted AF, terminating in the vicinity of the peritumoral edema margin (arrow). (B and D) Two-tensor UKF tractography produces a frontotemporally arching tract running through the T2-bright area (arrow). [*Reprinted with permission from* Chen et al. Reconstruction of the arcuate fasciculus for surgical planning in the setting of peritumoral edema using two-tensor unscented Kalman filter tractography. NeuroImage: Clinical 2015]

is based on magnetic field changes rather than voltage changes and is thus less affected by the scalp and the skull.[13,14]

- *Transcranial magnetic stimulation (TMS)*, is a non-invasive method used to map functional brain areas by delivering a strong magnetic pulses to the scalp which, in turn, stimulates or inhibits neuronal electrical activity in the underlying cortex.[13,15-17] TMS has been shown to reliably map motor and sensory cortex with close correspondences to direct electrical cortical stimulation testing (ECS).

Invasive methods of functional mapping include:

- *Electrical cortical stimulation (ECS)* is applied intra-operatively and uses the direct application of current (either bipolar or monopolar) to the cortical surface to either stimulate function (as in motor mapping) or to temporarily block function (as in language mapping). This is the oldest and most proven brain mapping method, although its use is limited to centers which perform a fairly high volume of the techniques, since it requires expertise by all members of the team to assure reliable

and safe performance. The ECS is usually performed in conjunction with Electrocorticography (ECoG) which records electrical activity directly from cerebral cortical surface and is essential for detecting after discharges or seizures.

- *Wada testing also known as the intracarotid amytal test (IAT)* is used for identification of the language-dominant cerebral hemisphere and is often used in preparation for epilepsy surgeries.[6,18-22]
- Utilization of the above-mentioned functional mapping methods has been shown to improve surgical outcomes.[23-26] Surgical outcomes in neurosurgery have also correlated significantly with achieved extent of tumor resection (EOR).[27,28] However, a resection that is carried too far may damage critical tissues and result in neurologic morbidity; therefore efficient functional mapping is needed to maximize EOR while sparing eloquent brain tissues. In dominant temporal lobe epilepsy surgery, preoperatively acquired fMRI and DTI combined with intraoperative neuro-navigation and MRI produces excellent neurological outcome with low complication rate.[29]

INTRAOPERATIVE IMAGE-GUIDED NEUROSURGERY

Intraoperative Imaging

Neurosurgical intraoperative imaging in various forms has been in use for many decades. Ultrasound-based methods have been in use since the 1960s,[41] and are particularly useful in cases of brain abscess and cystic lesions. CT-based methods have been in use primarily for stereotactic surgeries since the 1980s.[42]

Why intraoperative MRI?

Neuronavigation using preoperatively acquired images has added tremendous advantage to neurosurgical practice, but it is not without major challenges. This kind of navigation is significantly compromised by brain shift, which inevitably occurs during the course of the operation, and markedly degrades the precise alignment between the preoperative MR data and the intraoperative outline of the brain structures.[43] This shift could reach up to 10 mm or more within an hour of dural opening.[44-50]

Similarly, intraoperative overestimation of extent of tumor resection (EOR) by the surgeon has frequently resulted in inadvertent retention of residual tumor from surgically resectable lesions, especially for intrinsic tumors.[51] Therefore, there is a need to objectively update the changes occurring in the brain and tumor during the course of surgery. Intraoperative imaging provides a point update on these changes. Intraoperative MRI (IoMRI) is the preferred method as the acquired data are of higher resolution and better soft tissue contrast than most other imaging methods.[3,52-55]

With IoMRI, improved placement and tracking of operative tools is possible. Being able to precisely track tools and monitor therapy (e.g. temperature mapping via MR thermometry) has allowed the development of minimally invasive procedures such as thermal ablation of lesions.[56,57] IoMRI also enhances monitoring for treatment complications intraoperatively for prompt intervention **(Figures 17.3A and B)**.

Intraoperative Guidance

Introduction of intraoperative MRI to neuronavigation has improved several aspects of brain tumor surgeries: the surgeon can better locate the lesion in the operative field, distinguish tumor margins from often similar-appearing healthy brain tissue, and identify occurrence of brain shift. This results in more informed adjustment as needed to achieve a safer and more complete resection. It equally informs the surgeon of the location and extent residual tumor.[58] All these benefits culminate in helping neurosurgeons achieve maximal extent of resection with highest level of safety **(Figures 17.4A to C)**.[50,59]

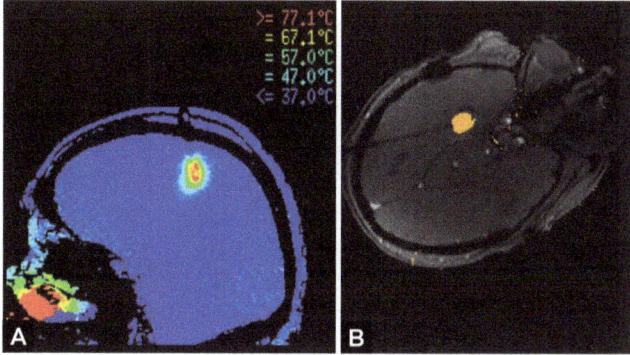

Figures 17.3A and B Intraoperative images of Laser interstitial thermal ablation therapy. Figure A shows a color map representing temperature; Figure B shows axial T1 MRI anatomic image from a different patient overlaid with a damage estimate calculated from temperature under the time curve

Multimodal Neuronavigation

In an attempt to adequately answer the question "Where are the critical structures relative to a tumor?" an optimum navigation method can be uses that combines preoperatively acquired images from different imaging modalities, including: structural imaging (MRI and/or CT sequences), functional cortical mapping (fMRI, or electro-cortical mapping), subcortical fiber tracking (DTI), angiography (either conventional or cross sectional (CT or MR-based arteriograms or venograms), and metabolic imaging with PET. This can then also be combined with intraoperative imaging, such as ultrasound which has been in use decades before the introduction of low-field (0.5 T) intraoperative MRI in the early 1990s.[60] Subsequently, modern intraoperative navigation suites have emerged with integration of high-field MRI, 3D ultrasound, PET/CT, fluoroscopy, and intraoperative molecular diagnostic capabilities and electrical mapping.

Intraoperative high-field MR machines offer unique opportunities for detailed anatomic resolution, fiber tracking, and novel research endeavors aimed towards solving many long-standing challenges.[61-63] For example, intraoperatively acquired functional data, including intraoperative DTI may be able to provide additional insight into functional brain networks during tumor resection.[64-67] In addition, variable shifting of white matter tracts has been seen in preoperatively acquired DTI data compared to intraoperatively acquired data, from 8 mm inward to 15 mm outward, during resection of adjacent mass lesions.[64] Resection of contrast-enhancing lesions is associated with significantly larger shift in the tumor to corticospinal tract distance than removal of non-contrast-enhancing lesions.[68] In such cases of significant intraoperative shift in location of adjacent eloquent brain tissues, direct electrocortical stimulation (ECS) is often used to re-orientate the surgeon and enhance preservation of these important structures.

Intraoperative monitoring of residual tumor

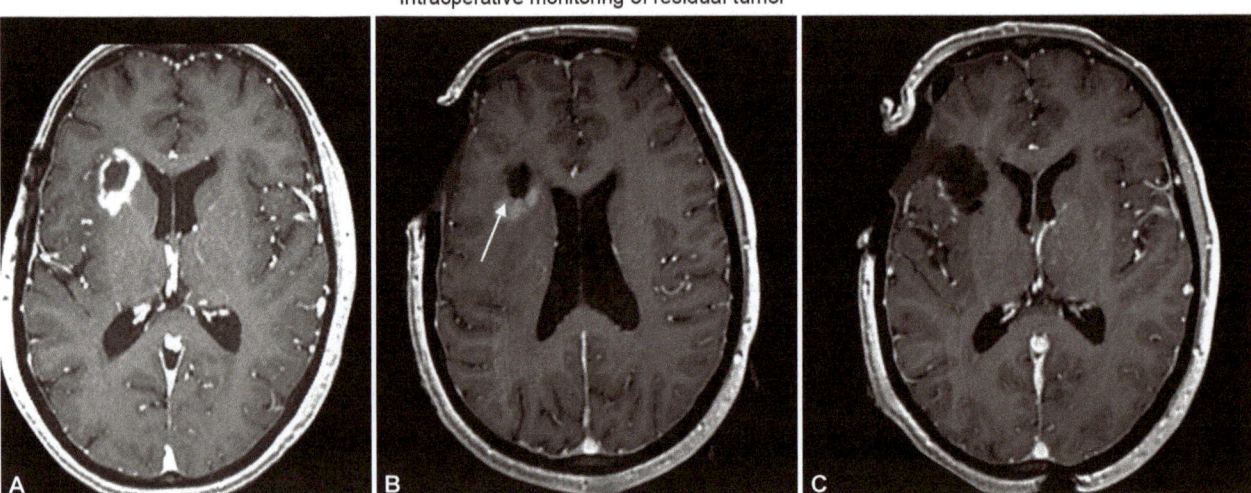

Figures 17.4A to C Pre- and intraoperative magnetic resonance imaging showing enhanced axial T1-images. (A) Preoperative image; (B) intraoperative MRI after initial resection showing residual (arrow); and (C) after further tumor resection showing complete resection

However, the use of intraoperative direct ECS sometimes fails to provide diagnostically useful data due to seizures,, non-compliance of the patient, or ambiguous results. Furthermore, difficult airway and pain may account for ECS failure. Preoperative fMRI- mapping may be used as a fallback option in cases of failed ECS (20–30% failure rate), or whenever it is unworkable due to any of the reasons stated above.[70,71] Both low-field and higher-field intraoperative fMRI have also been employed by several groups, but these have been limited by time constraints and low sensitivity.[66,67,69]

MAGNETIC RESONANCE THERAPY TO ADVANCED MULTIMODALITY IMAGE-GUIDED OPERATING (MRI TO AMIGO)

The world's first intraoperative MR was conceived by Ferenc Jolesz, MD and his team at the Brigham and Women's Hospital/Harvard Medical School, Departments of Radiology and Neurosurgery in collaboration with General Electric (GE) USA. This significant step was prompted by the great advances provided by preoperative MRI and early neuronavigation efforts. With the MRI located within the operating room (OR), any MR-based imaging modality became possible. After successful implementation of MRI within the OR, it then became conceivable that CT-scan, mass-spectrometry and other imaging methods could be adapted intraoperatively as well. All these imaging techniques have been integrated into the OR that is now known as the Advanced Multimodality Image-Guide Operating AMIGO suite at Brigham and Women's Hospital. Similar operating suite are now available in several centers across the globe.

An integrated platform by which all these different imaging modalities would be efficiently handled intraoperatively has become indispensable. This led to introduction of different software platforms into surgical practice, some of which are licensed for clinical use, including neuronavigation platforms, and many others which presently remain research tools including 3D-slicer [*www.slicer.org*]. These software packages are capable of processing and displaying different imaging modalities for a near real-time guidance of surgical procedures.

Implementation of these technological tools requires expertise from radiology, computer science, engineering, as well as dedicated clinical champions.

Increasingly, gains in neurosurgery are being adopted by other surgical and interventional specialists who are using this technology to visualize multiple organs within the body and to guide therapeutic interventions. Intraoperative MRI has been adapted into different surgical specialties and interventional medicine or radiology, and has been well integrated for use in urology, hepatic surgery, cardiothoracic surgery, and gynecology.

Advanced Multimodality Image-guided Operating: A Translational Laboratory

Due to a wealth of technical resources and expert personnel, the AMIGO suite is an ideal platform for translating laboratory discoveries into clinical tools. It is now possible to integrate functional mapping images as well as preoperatively and intraoperatively acquired DTI for fiber tracking intraoperatively to further enhance surgical guidance.

In addition, accurate registration of image-to-image and image-to-patient has seen significant improvement via the use of mathematical geometry-based rigid and non-rigid image registration methods that have been developed **(Figures 17.5A and B)**.

Registration of intraoperative ultrasound, (iUS) to MRI is another on-going project with great promises of converting MRI-guidance into "real-time" intraoperative guidance.

Updated localization of structures has provided ability for real-time tracking of operative devices and target areas, all of which have culminated into better definition of organ and tissue anatomy.

Meanwhile, successful running of this OR requires extensive collaborations between many investigators, clinicians, companies, medical centers, government and non-governmental agencies, funders and researchers due to the enormous resources required for its proper setup, utilization and maintenance. This includes equipment and materials, services and expertise, cost, space, and especially subjects with the clinical conditions for which new therapy approach is desired.

Development and Validation of Tissue Biomarkers in AMIGO

This research effort aims at improving the accuracy of defining tumor margins by confirming the cellular composition of tissue intraoperatively. In an effort to better understand the relationship between imaging and tissue composition, we integrate data from different imaging modalities including MRI, PET, CT, US, mass spectrometry, histopathology slides, and stimulated Raman spectroscopy (SRS) **(Figure 17.6)**.

Mass spectrometry (MS) is an analytical tool used for detailed chemical analysis of a wide range of samples with the required sensitivity and specificity for biomedical applications. Molecules must be introduced into the instrument, ionized, and further separated from other molecules according to unique mass to charge ratio (m/z). This can provide accurate information on elemental composition and structure of molecules. Tissue analysis by MS is performed directly via different desorption/ionization techniques including matrix assisted laser desorption ionization (MALDI),[72-74] desorption electrospray ionization (DESI),[75,76] and others. Use of MS in a near-real-time fashion during surgery comes with a requirement for minimal to no sample preparation.[77,78] There are ongoing efforts on validation of MS against histopathology, and implementation of real-time and near real-time MS approaches to support surgical decision-making in the AMIGO suite. With the aid of neuro-navigation, sampling sites are digitally registered and the coordinates later used to overlay molecular characterization results from MS with 3D images from structural and functional MRIs using in house developed, open access image analysis software (3D Slicer).[79]

MS analysis of tissue has been shown to distinguish between viable glioblastoma and necrotic tissue.[80] It has also been found to be valid in the classification of human gliomas and meningiomas according to their subtypes. Recently, MS was used to detect tumor metabolites including 2-hydroxyglutarate (2-HG) found in glial tumors harboring a mutation in the Krebs cycle enzyme isocitrate dehydrogenase (IDH1 and IDH2).[81] Providing surgeons with 2-HG analysis during surgery could provide diagnostic and prognostic information, and detailed stereotactic analysis of metabolite can be used to delineate the tumor.

Current work on newer interfaces for the introduction of surgical material into MS either from a stereotactic sample or direct and continuously from within the surgical cavity will further facilitate adoption of MS as an intraoperative real-time tissue characterization tool.

Other Neurosurgical Procedures in Advanced Multimodality Image-guided Operating

Neurosurgery is one of the major users of the AMIGO suite. In addition to popular neurosurgical procedures discussed above, other procedures undertaken in this suite include MRI-guided deep brain stimulation (DBS), validation of brain deformation estimates, development of tissue markers, and delivery of drugs (and other therapeutics).

Drug delivery to the brain involves a somewhat unique mechanism. It is especially important in oncologic treatment of brain tumors due to the challenge posed by the blood-brain barrier on drug access to the tumor tissue. These methods ensure that the chemical agent (chemotherapeutic agents, large molecule, or biologic agents) reaches the tumor tissue.[82-85] The commonly employed methods are focus ultrasound (FUS) targeted drug delivery, and convection-enhanced (CE) drug delivery

Focused ultrasound is a novel noninvasive method for enhancing delivery of therapeutic agents (or gene therapy) into targeted areas in the brain through focal, reversible, and safe disruption of the blood-brain barrier (BBB).[82,83] FUS at quite low power can be used also to target release of chemotherapeutic agents from nano-encapsulated drug carriers for targeted drug delivery.[86] FUS uses microbubbles controlled by ultrasound as a vehicle for the drug (or gene therapy) and to increase membrane permeability. These microbubbles focus ultrasound energy by lowering the threshold for ultrasound bioeffects.[87] Interstitial drug administration via convection-enhanced delivery (CED) is an alternative route for chemotherapy that potentially circumvents systemic toxicities and ensures CNS delivery challenges by directly bypassing the BBB. This approach both allows for both directed administration of therapeutic agents and newer, tumor-selective agents which were usually excluded from the CNS due to their large molecular

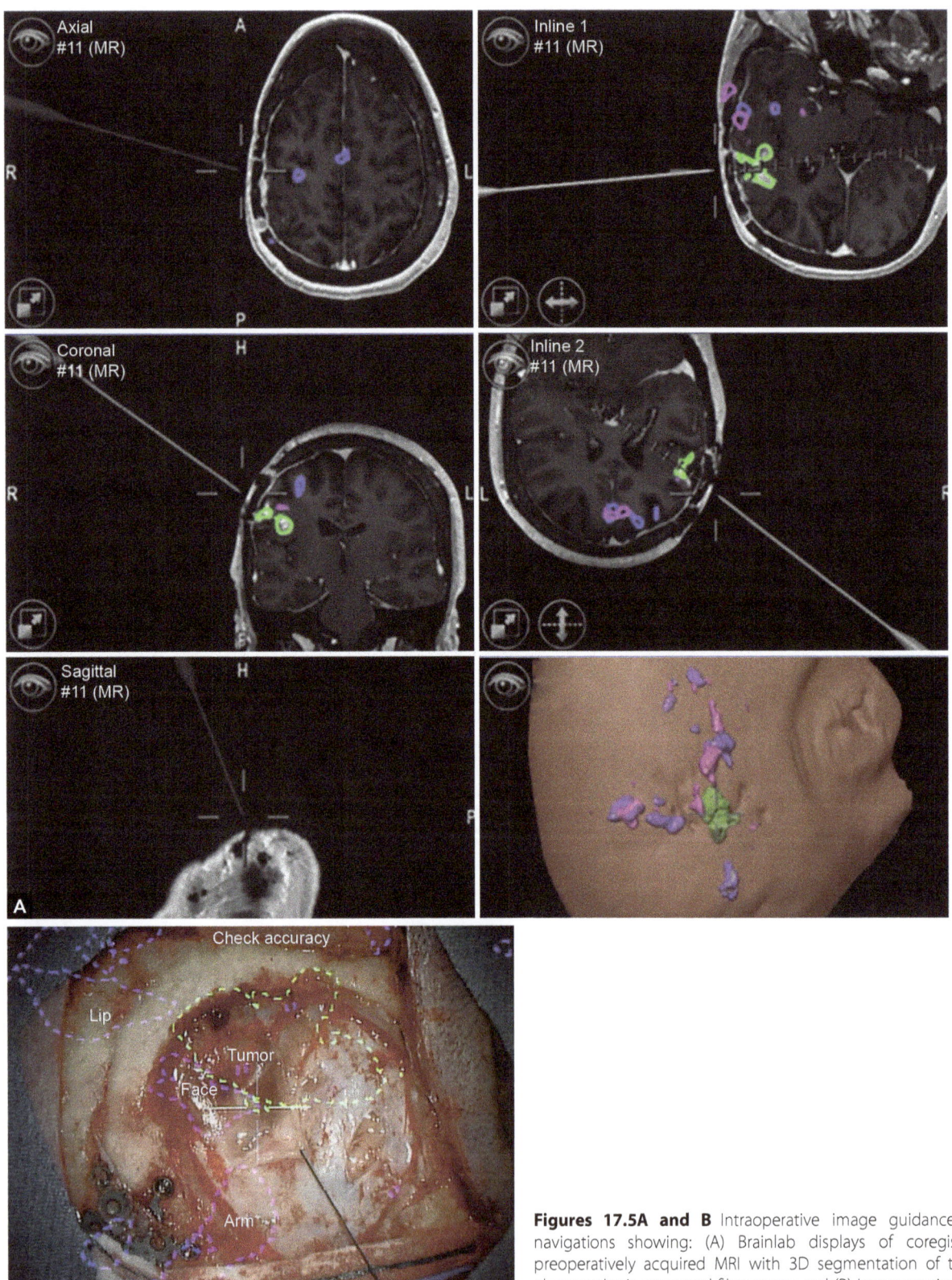

Figures 17.5A and B Intraoperative image guidance and navigations showing: (A) Brainlab displays of coregistered preoperatively acquired MRI with 3D segmentation of tumor, eloquent brain areas and fiber tracts; and (B) Intraoperative view of overlaid images for surgical guidance

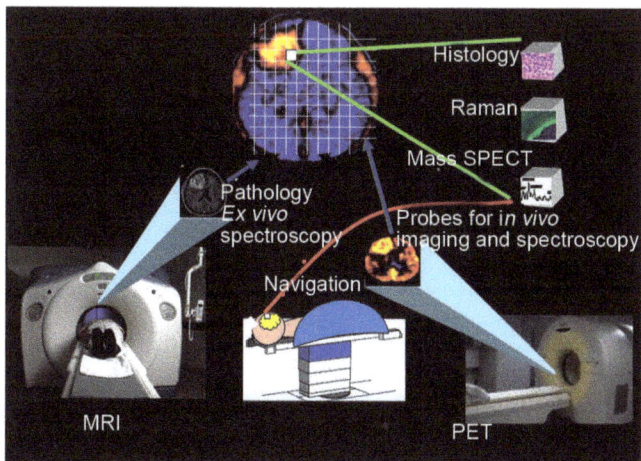

Figure 17.6 A cartoon of development and validation of tissue biomakers in the advanced multimodality image-guided operating (AMIGO) suite

size alone.[88] In this method, drugs are delivered via one to several catheters which are stereotactically placed directly within or around the tumor mass or resection cavity. This technology is suitable for administration of several classes of therapeutic agents, including approved chemotherapeutics and some experimental drugs.[89]

CHALLENGES, LIMITATIONS AND FUTURE DIRECTIONS

Maturation and wide acceptance of intraoperative navigation and imaging modalities continues, however, several challenges need to be addressed to maximize the impact of these technologies. IoMRI introduces major restrictions on compatible instruments, intraoperative neurophysiologic monitoring, and safety precautions. Also, acquisition of intraoperative images and functional mapping can increase procedure time by up to 90 minutes. Judicious resource utilization for access, the multimodality image-guided operative room time allotment, staffing, and dedicated equipment is required to maintain this expensive technology.

CONCLUSION

Multimodality image-guided surgery has brought great improvement to neurosurgery. It is rapidly evolving, and promises a brighter future for the practice of neurosurgery. However, lots of work remains to be done in overcoming the new and often complex challenges and in validation of these techniques in order to achieve a future of "an ideal world" in neurosurgery.

ACKNOWLEDGMENTS

The authors wish to acknowledge Laura Rigolo (MS); Neurosurgical Brain Mapping Laboratory, Department of Neurosurgery, Brigham and Women's Hospital, Boston MA, for her contribution to this work.

REFERENCES

1. Pouratian, N, et al. Shedding light on brain mapping: advances in human optical imaging. Trends in Neurosciences. 2003; 26(5):277-82.
2. Lenroot RK, Giedd JN. Brain development in children and adolescents: insights from anatomical magnetic resonance imaging. Neuroscience and Biobehavioral Reviews. 2006. 30(6):718-29.
3. Schneider JP, et al. Gross-total surgery of supratentorial low-grade gliomas under intraoperative MR guidance. American Journal of Neuroradiology. 2001;22(1):89-98.
4. Skirboll SS, et al. Functional cortex and subcortical white matter located within gliomas. Neurosurgery. 1996;38(4):678-84; discussion 684-5.
5. Ojemann JG, Miller JW, Silbergeld DL. Preserved function in brain invaded by tumor. Neurosurgery. 1996;39(2):253-8; discussion 258-9.
6. Tate MC. Surgery for Gliomas, in Current Understanding and Treatment of Gliomas 2015, Springer. p. 31-47.
7. Fox PT, Raichle ME. Focal physiological uncoupling of cerebral blood flow and oxidative metabolism during somatosensory stimulation in human subjects. Proc Natl Acad Sci USA. 1986;83(4):1140-4.
8. Ogawa S, et al. Brain magnetic resonance imaging with contrast dependent on blood oxygenation. Proc Natl Acad Sci USA. 1990;87(24):9868-72.
9. Moseley ME, et al. Diffusion-weighted MR imaging of anisotropic water diffusion in cat central nervous system. Radiology. 1990;176(2):439-45.
10. Jellison BJ, et al. Diffusion tensor imaging of cerebral white matter: a pictorial review of physics, fiber tract anatomy, and tumor imaging patterns. Am J Neuroradiol. 2004;25(3): 356-69.
11. Qazi AA, et al. Resolving crossings in the corticospinal tract by two-tensor streamline tractography: Method and clinical assessment using fMRI. Neuroimage. 2009;47:T98-106.
12. Golby AJ, et al. Interactive diffusion tensor tractography visualization for neurosurgical planning. Neurosurgery. 2011; 68(2):496.
13. Baillet S, Mosher JC, Leahy RM. Electromagnetic brain mapping. Signal Processing Magazine, IEEE. 2001;18(6):14-30.
14. Cook IA, et al. Assessing the accuracy of topographic EEG mapping for determining local brain function. Electroencephalography and clinical neurophysiology. 1998; 107(6):408-14.
15. Barker AT, Jalinous R, Freeston IL. Non-invasive magnetic stimulation of human motor cortex. Lancet. 1985;1(8437): 1106-7.
16. Rossini PM, et al. Non-invasive electrical and magnetic stimulation of the brain, spinal cord and roots: basic principles and procedures for routine clinical application. Report of

an IFCN committee. Electroencephalography and Clinical Neurophysiology. 1994;91(2):79-92.

17. George JS, et al. Mapping function in the human brain with magnetoencephalography, anatomical magnetic resonance imaging, and functional magnetic resonance imaging. Journal of Clinical Neurophysiology. 1995;12(5):406-31.

18. Binder J, et al. Determination of language dominance using functional MRI: a comparison with the Wada test. Neurology. 1996;46(4):978-84.

19. Lachaux JP, Rudrauf D, Kahane P. Intracranial EEG and human brain mapping. Journal of Physiology-Paris. 2003;97(4):613-28.

20. Lachaux JP, et al. Relationship between task-related gamma oscillations and BOLD signal: New insights from combined fMRI and intracranial EEG. Human brain mapping. 2007; 28(12):1368-75.

21. Ojemann G, et al. Cortical language localization in left, dominant hemisphere: an electrical stimulation mapping investigation in 117 patients. Journal of neurosurgery. 1989; 71(3):316-26.

22. Lee H, et al. Mapping of functional organization in human visual cortex: electrical cortical stimulation. Neurology. 2000; 54(4):849-54.

23. Duffau H, et al. Usefulness of intraoperative electrical subcortical mapping during surgery for low-grade gliomas located within eloquent brain regions: functional results in a consecutive series of 103 patients. Journal of Neurosurgery. 2003;98(4):764-78.

24. Rössler K, et al. Evaluation of preoperative high magnetic field motor functional MRI (3 Tesla) in glioma patients by navigated electrocortical stimulation and postoperative outcome. Journal of Neurology, Neurosurgery and Psychiatry. 2005;76(8):1152-7.

25. Nimsky C, et al. Preoperative and intraoperative diffusion tensor imaging-based fiber tracking in glioma surgery. Neurosurgery. 2005;56(1):130-8.

26. Nimsky C, et al. Integration of functional magnetic resonance imaging supported by magnetoencephalography in functional neuronavigation. Neurosurgery. 1999;44(6):1249-55.

27. Sanai N, Berger MS. Glioma extent of resection and its impact on patient outcome. Neurosurgery. 2008;62(4):753-66.

28. Smith JS, et al. Role of extent of resection in the long-term outcome of low-grade hemispheric gliomas. Journal of Clinical Oncology. 2008;26(8):1338-45.

29. Rössler K, et al. Risk Reduction in Dominant Temporal Lobe Epilepsy Surgery Combining fMRI/DTI Maps, Neuronavigation and Intraoperative 1.5-Tesla MRI. Stereotactic and Functional Neurosurgery. 2015;93(3):168-77.

30. LI, J-c, J-l LI, and Q-c ZHUGE. Functional magnetic resonance imaging mapping of the motor cortex in patients with cerebral tumors. Journal of Wenzhou Medical College. 2001;6:009.

31. Mueller WM, et al. Functional magnetic resonance imaging mapping of the motor cortex in patients with cerebral tumors. Neurosurgery. 1996;39(3):515-21.

32. Voyvodic JT, Petrella JR, Friedman AH. fMRI activation mapping as a percentage of local excitation: consistent presurgical motor maps without threshold adjustment. Journal of Magnetic Resonance Imaging. 2009;29(4):751-9.

33. Holodny AI, et al. Motor and sensory mapping. Neurosurgery Clinics of North America. 2011;22(2):207-18.

34. Witwer BP, et al. Diffusion-tensor imaging of white matter tracts in patients with cerebral neoplasm. Journal of Neurosurgery. 2002;97(3):568-75.

35. Mori S, Oishi K, Faria AV. White matter atlases based on diffusion tensor imaging. Current opinion in neurology. 2009; 22(4):362.

36. Itagiba VGA, et al. Use of diffusion tensor magnetic resonance imaging in the assessment of patterns of white matter involvement in patients with brain tumors: is it useful in the differential diagnosis? Radiologia Brasileira. 2010;43(6):362-8.

37. Mori S, Tournier JD. Introduction to Diffusion Tensor Imaging: And Higher Order Models 2013: Academic Press.

38. Chen Z, et al. NI-13 resolving the challenges of peritumoral edema in tracing arcuate fasciculus for surgical planning using two-tensor unscented Kalman filter tractography. Neuro-oncology. 2014;16(suppl 5):v140-v140.

39. Chen Z, et al. Reconstruction of the arcuate fasciculus for surgical planning in the setting of peritumoral edema using two-tensor unscented Kalman filter tractography. NeuroImage: Clinical. 2015;7:815-22.

40. Cheng G, et al. Tractography from HARDI using an Intrinsic Unscented Kalman Filter, 2015.

41. Schlagenhauff R, Glasauer F. Experience with intraoperative echoencephalography in cerebral mass lesions. Acta radiologica: diagnosis. 1971;13:735-42.

42. Lunsford L, Leksell L, Jernberg B. Probe holder for stereotactic surgery in the CT scanner a technical note. Acta neurochirurgica. 1983;69(3-4):297-304.

43. Archip N, et al. Non-rigid alignment of pre-operative MRI, fMRI, and DT-MRI with intra-operative MRI for enhanced visualization and navigation in image-guided neurosurgery. Neuroimage. 2007;35(2):609-24.

44. Nimsky C, et al. Quantification of, visualization of, and compensation for brain shift using intraoperative magnetic resonance imaging. Neurosurgery. 2000;47(5):1070-80.

45. Roberts DW, et al. Intraoperative brain shift and deformation: a quantitative analysis of cortical displacement in 28 cases. Neurosurgery. 1998;43(4):749-58.

46. Barnett GH. The role of image-guided technology in the surgical planning and resection of gliomas. Journal of Neuro-oncology. 1999;42(3):247-58.

47. Nabavi A, et al. Serial intraoperative magnetic resonance imaging of brain shift. Neurosurgery. 2001;48(4):787-98.

48. Gering DT, et al. An integrated visualization system for surgical planning and guidance using image fusion and an open MR. Journal of Magnetic Resonance Imaging. 2001;13(6):967-75.

49. Mori S, et al. Brain white matter anatomy of tumor patients evaluated with diffusion tensor imaging. Annals of Neurology, 2002;51(3):377-80.

50. Olubiyi OI, et al. Intra-operative Magnetic Resonance Imaging In Intracranial Glioma Resection: A Single Center Retrospective Blinded Volumetric Study. World Neurosurgery, 2015.

51. Orringer D, et al. Extent of resection in patients with glioblastoma: limiting factors, perception of resectability, and effect on survival. J Neurosurg. 2012;117(5):851-9.

52. Aisen AM, et al. MRI and CT evaluation of primary bone and soft-tissue tumors. American Journal of Roentgenology. 1986; 146(4):749-56.

53. Lunsford LD, Martinez AJ, Latchaw RE. Stereotaxic surgery with a magnetic resonance- and computerized tomography-compatible system. Journal of Neurosurgery. 1986;64(6):872-8.

54. Schmidt F, et al. Technological and logistic problems and first clinical results of an interventional 0.5-T MRI system used by various medical specialities. Der Radiologe. 1998;38(3):173-84.

55. Black PM, et al. Development and implementation of intra-operative magnetic resonance imaging and its neurosurgical applications. Neurosurgery. 1997;41(4):831-45.

56. Carpentier A, et al. Real-time magnetic resonance-guided laser thermal therapy for focal metastatic brain tumors. Neurosurgery. 2008;63(1):ONS21-9.

57. Tovar-Spinoza Z, et al. The use of MRI-guided laser-induced thermal ablation for epilepsy. Child's Nervous System. 2013; 29(11):2089-94.

58. Schneider JP, et al. Intraoperative MRI to guide the resection of primary supratentorial glioblastoma multiforme: a quantitative radiological analysis. Neuroradiology. 2005;47(7): 489-500.

59. Senft C, et al. Intraoperative MRI guidance and extent of resection in glioma surgery: a randomised, controlled trial. The Lancet Oncology. 2011;12(11):997-1003.

60. Black PM, et al. Development and implementation of intra-operative magnetic resonance imaging and its neurosurgical applications. Neurosurgery. 1997;41(4):831-42; discussion 842-5.

61. Lichy, MP, et al. Magnetic resonance imaging of the body trunk using a single-slab, 3-dimensional, T2-weighted turbo-spin-echo sequence with high sampling efficiency (SPACE) for high spatial resolution imaging: initial clinical experiences. Investigative Radiology. 2005;40(12):754-60.

62. Reichenbach JR, et al. High-resolution MR venography at 3.0 Tesla. Journal of Computer Assisted Tomography. 2000;24(6): 949-57.

63. Fujii Y, Nakayama N, Nakada T. High-resolution T2-reversed magnetic resonance imaging on a high magnetic field system: technical note. Journal of Neurosurgery. 1998;89(3):492-5.

64. Nimsky C, et al. Preoperative and intraoperative diffusion tensor imaging-based fiber tracking in glioma surgery. Neurosurgery. 2005;56(1):130-7; discussion 138.

65. Nimsky C, et al. Intraoperative visualization of the pyramidal tract by diffusion-tensor-imaging-based fiber tracking. Neuroimage. 2006;30(4):1219-29.

66. Azmi H, et al. Functional imaging in a low-field, mobile intraoperative magnetic resonance scanner: expanded paradigms. Neurosurgery. 2007;60(1):143-8; discussion 148-9.

67. Gasser T, et al. Intraoperative MRI and functional mapping. Acta Neurochir Suppl. 2011;109:61-5.

68. Shahar T, et al. Preoperative imaging to predict intraoperative changes in tumor-to-corticospinal tract distance: an analysis of 45 cases using high-field intraoperative magnetic resonance imaging. Neurosurgery. 2014;75(1):23-30.

69. Gasser T, et al. Intraoperative functional MRI: implementation and preliminary experience. Neuroimage. 2005;26(3):685-93.

70. Rigolo L, et al. Development of a Clinical Functional Magnetic Resonance Imaging Service. Neurosurgery Clinics of North America. 2011;22(2):307-14.

71. Rushmore RJ, et al. Age-dependent sparing of visual function after bilateral lesions of primary visual cortex. Behavioral Neuroscience. 2008;122(6):1274.

72. Ait-Belkacem R, et al. MALDI imaging and in-source decay for top-down characterization of glioblastoma. Proteomics; 2014; 14(10):1290-301.

73. Stoeckli M, et al. Imaging mass spectrometry: a new technology for the analysis of protein expression in mammalian tissues. Nature Medicine. 2001;7(4):493-6.

74. McDonnell LA, et al. Peptide and protein imaging mass spectrometry in cancer research. Journal of Proteomics. 2010; 73(10):1921-44.

75. Chen H, et al. Desorption electrospray ionization mass spectrometry for high-throughput analysis of pharmaceutical samples in the ambient environment. Analytical Chemistry, 2005;77(21):6915-27.

76. Wiseman JM, et al. Tissue imaging at atmospheric pressure using desorption electrospray ionization (DESI) mass spectrometry. Angewandte Chemie International Edition, 2006;45(43):7188-92.

77. Cooks RG, et al. Ambient mass spectrometry. Science. 2006; 311(5767):1566-70.

78. Eberlin LS, et al. Ambient mass spectrometry for the intraoperative molecular diagnosis of human brain tumors. Proceedings of the National Academy of Sciences. 2013;110(5): 1611-6.

79. Fedorov A, et al. 3D Slicer as an image computing platform for the Quantitative Imaging Network. Magnetic Resonance Imaging. 2012;30(9):1323-41.

80. Calligaris D, et al. Mass spectrometry imaging as a tool for surgical decision-making. Journal of Mass Spectrometry. 2013; 48(11):1178-87.

81. Santagata S, et al. Intraoperative mass spectrometry mapping of an onco-metabolite to guide brain tumor surgery. Proceedings of the National Academy of Sciences. 2014;111(30):11121-6.

82. Etame AB, et al. Focused ultrasound disruption of the blood brain barrier: a new frontier for therapeutic delivery in molecular neuro-oncology. Neurosurgical Focus. 2012;32(1): E3.

83. O'Reilly MA, et al. Focused-ultrasound disruption of the blood-brain barrier using closely-timed short pulses: influence of sonication parameters and injection rate. Ultrasound in Medicine and Biology. 2011;37(4):587-94.

84. Garg T, et al. Current strategies for targeted delivery of bio-active drug molecules in the treatment of brain tumor. Journal of Drug Targeting. 2015;(10):1-23.

85. Azad TD, et al. Therapeutic strategies to improve drug delivery across the blood-brain barrier. Neurosurgical Focus. 2015; 38(3):E9.

86. Gourevich D, et al. Ultrasound activated nano-encapsulated targeted drug delivery and tumour cell poration, in Nano-Biotechnology for Biomedical and Diagnostic Research. 2012, Springer. pp. 135-44.

87. Juffermans L, et al. Ultrasound and microbubble-targeted delivery of therapeutic compounds. Netherlands Heart Journal. 2009;17(2):82-6.

88. Healy AT, Vogelbaum MA. Convection-enhanced drug delivery for gliomas. Surgical Neurology International. 2015;6(Suppl 1): S59.

89. Debinski W, Tatter SB. Convection-enhanced delivery for the treatment of brain tumors, 2009.

18

Future of Navigation and Intraoperative Imaging

Richard Bucholz

INTRODUCTION

In its short history since inception in the early 1990s neuronavigation, also known as image-guided surgery or frameless stereotactic surgery, has had a major impact on enabling new techniques in neurosurgery. By coupling the act of surgery with imaging in a real-time fashion, neuronavigation allows the surgeon to be minimally invasive, restricting the surgical intervention to a small surgical corridor, while maintaining efficacy, by enhancing the vision of the surgeon using information supplied by advanced imaging. The power of the technique stems from the considerable developments in magnetic resonance imaging (MRI), computed tomography, and a variety of other information sources that can improve the outcome of surgery while reducing complications. The increased use of intraoperative imaging was a logical result of the use of neuronavigation, as surgeons who have become reliant on imaging to guide surgery logically demand that imaging be updated as needed to reflect the current location of critical structures in the operating room which can be modified by the resection of tissue, retraction, and drainage of cerebrospinal fluid (CSF). It can be assumed that neuronavigation and intraoperative imaging will remain tightly coupled and should be construed as being one in the same thing.

Given the use of imaging technology in neuronavigation, it is to be expected that the field will continue to rapidly evolve. Although predicting the future is always difficult and prone to error, it can be assumed that technology will improve to address all areas of neuronavigation. This chapter will focus on seven areas of neuronavigation shared by all applications which are logical targets for improvement in the near future. These areas are: (1) preoperative imaging, studies obtained prior to surgery to improve surgical planning; (2) image registration, the process by which images are precisely related to the surgical field; (3) intraoperative tracking, the mechanism by which instruments are tracked during surgery;

(4) visualization, the technique by which the surgeon is notified of information created by the imaging technology; (5) system control, the means by which the surgeon controls the technology being used to assist surgery; (6) effectors, the instruments used by the surgeon to perform the surgery; and (7) intraoperative imaging, those imaging technologies used in the operating room to update the information used to guide surgery.

PREOPERATIVE IMAGING

As imaging will be directly employed by neuronavigation to perform surgery, the outcome of surgery will, in part, depend on the quality and fidelity of the imaging employed. Therefore, preoperative imaging, regardless of modality, must be current and provide an accurate layout of critical relationships between the pathology at hand and normal anatomy to be spared to allow the planning of an appropriate approach to the surgical target. With the continued development of technology the amount of information gained in preoperative imaging studies has dramatically increased. Compounding this planning process is the simple fact that the human brain is the most complex structure known, that its connections are known only in very crude terms, that there is considerable variability even between normal brains, and surgery is usually performed on anatomy distorted by the presence of space-occupying pathology. There is a need to determine not only the connections present in the area of the planned surgical approach, but also a technique to determine the importance of each connection to the patient, in order to create a surgical plan with the least risk of debilitating neurological deficit. To address the need, current research is focused on delineating the human connectome and its role in neurosurgery. A connectome refers to the complete structural connectivity of an organism's nervous system and identification of specific areas of the brain so connected. The field of connectomics refers to the collection of data, mapping and analysis of neural connections. A basic connectome has been completed in a population of normal twins using functional MRI (fMRI), diffusion tensor imaging (DTI) with tractography and magnetoencephalography (MEG), and the techniques developed are being rapidly deployed to study multiple populations of patients with neurological conditions. It can be assumed that identification of specific abnormal pathways will allow greater understanding of neuropathology, particularly in psychiatry, and this objective technology will allow more specific interventions to be performed, including surgical procedures, to treat such disease.

Elucidation of connections within the brain is not limited to functional imaging alone. The localization of targets for deep brain stimulation (DBS) at present is primarily based upon axial high resolution stereotactic MRI with the addition of intraoperative microelectrode recordings and stimulation for confirmation of successful lead placement. An article by Pouratian et al. examined thalamic connections in six patients with bilateral DBS leads (12 leads total) inserted for the treatment of tremor. The goal of the study was to investigate the role of tractography-based thalamic segmentation for DBS targeting. It was found that the thalamic region associated with greatest efficacy for relief of tremor had a high probability of connecting with the premotor area.[1] It was also observed that there was high variability of the location of this thalamic region in relation to the anterior and posterior commissures which serve as common landmarks for DBS planning. This implies a potential for improved success with selection of DBS targets based on the individual patient's connectivity as determined by connectivity analysis using DTI.

Another study by Barkhoudarian et al. investigated three patients who underwent DBS placement for movement disorders. The subthalamic nucleus, globus pallidus interna, and ventral intermediate nucleus targets were studied with DTI tractography at various parameters which demonstrated reproducible fiber connections to the frontal eye field, premotor, primary motor, and primary sensory cortices via corticospinal tracts and corticopontocerebellar tracts.[2,3] They found that with increasing the size of the field of interest, the connections to other structures increased as well. The potential implication is that with better understanding of the connectivity of different DBS targets with preoperative connectivity maps, one can the more accurately predict the benefits and side effects of the specific area targeted.

Recently, Banks et al. aimed to use preoperative imaging to identify responders and nonresponders to dorsal anterior cingulotomy for obsessive compulsive disorder (OCD). In the study, 15 patients underwent the aforementioned procedure with a response rate of 53%.[4] Preoperative MRI voxel-based morphometry and DTI were used to identify structural and connectivity variations between patients. Local variations in grey matter architecture and hemispheric differences in connectivity were found to correlate with patient response.[4]

These are a few examples of how DTI can be employed as an information source for image-guided surgery. Tractography is complex and subject to multiple variables and sources of noise, and as image resolution and computer techniques improve, DTI will allow this technique to be employed clinically. Our understanding of the human connectome will continue to advance rapidly and will lead to improved patient selection, surgical target selection, and improved outcomes.

Functional MRI is an imaging modality useful in the preoperative period by identifying areas of eloquent cortex (primary motor, speech areas, etc.) by measuring blood oxygen level dependent (BOLD) signal change while patients perform specific tasks. This technique is highly dependent on patient understanding and accurate participation in the image acquisition. This can unfortunately make obtaining accurate fMRI difficult in patients with neurologic pathology. A recent study by Tie et al. looks to circumvent this issue by examining resting-state fMRI (rs-fMRI). The premise is that there is a low frequency fluctuation of BOLD signal that occurs at rest, regardless of consciousness, that can assist in identifying the language network.[5] This technique may allow connectivity analysis using preoperative fMRI even in the comatose, confused, or aphasic patients that accurately maps their language pathways.

The combination of high resolution tractography and fMRI can further help the surgeon plan the most optimal surgical approach and safest extent of resection of tumors in eloquent areas. One study by Jia et al. involved 13 patients with gliomas involving the motor cortex who underwent preoperative fMRI and high-resolution DTI. The corticospinal tracts were successfully identified in all patients, aiding in surgical planning and subsequent resection of their lesions. The average Karnofsky performance status increased by more than 10 points postoperatively.[6]

While fMRI, improved tractography and connectomics provide critical structural information, positron emission tomography-computed tomography (PET-CT) provides metabolic information based on differences in substrate metabolism between normal and pathologic tissues. A commonly used tracer in PET-CT imaging is F-fluorodeoxyglucose (FDG). An issue with PET-CT evaluation of cerebral masses arises due to the brain's high background rate of glucose metabolism, making tumor delineation difficult. A study by Venneti et al. evaluated the in vivo use of a glutamate-based tracer to reduce background metabolism from the normal brain tissue.[7] Compared with FDG, there appeared to be similar uptake of the glutamate tracer by tumor cells but a reduction in uptake by normal brain tissue. Another study by Christensen et al. examined the alpha-[11C] methyl-L-tryptophan (AMT) tracer as a method of better delineating high grade gliomas when compared with standard contrasted MRI when planning extent of resection. They found that a gross tumor volume defined by AMT-PET produced similar volume, but superior recurrence coverage than the treated standard MRI-determined volume.[8] With further research into the metabolic activity of tumors and capabilities of PET-CT, it is theoretically possible to delineate tumors anatomically in the preoperative period based on their metabolic activity. This could potentially aid in surgical planning, especially when considering extent of resection and postoperative radiation targets.

In addition to providing information regarding the location and margins of tumors, PET-CT may have utility in providing clues as to the histologic grade of tumors as well. Ferdova et al. compared standard uptake values (SUV) of 18F-fluorothymidine (18FLT) with the histologic WHO grade of glioma tissue samples in 26 patients. Their data suggest that increased uptake of 18FLT is associated with higher tumor grade.[9] Previous studies document a similar correlation with FDG uptake and tumor grade.[10,11] With this assumption, fusion of PET "hot spots" with contrasted MRI can help guide surgical resection as well as provide targets for biopsy.[12-14]

Information obtained preoperatively for surgical planning does not need to be limited to imaging. Transcranial magnetic stimulation (TMS) has the potential to largely replace intraoperative mapping with direct cortical stimulation. This would allow more careful and precise mapping of critical areas to be avoided during surgical intervention in a completely awake patient with no time limitation imposed by surgical restraints. By mapping TMS to structural imaging these results can be overlaid on the surgical plan and the information employed to optimize surgical planning.

It is apparent that as the sources of information increase, and their value to the planning process is delineated, that surgical planning will become far more rigorous and important that what is commonly employed. Fortunately, the advent of inexpensive networked computer resources should allow such planning to be performed at leisure prior to surgical intervention with optimization of the surgical approach and uploading of the finalized plan to the navigational system employed during the procedure.

Image Registration

Preoperative imaging has to be precisely related to the surgical field through the process of image registration. Different modalities to achieve this include frame-based, frameless point merge, and surface-based registration (SBR). With the use of frameless fiducial-based registration, fiducials are affixed to the patient, and imaged during a fine slice, stereotactic CT or MRI preoperatively. In the operating room, a tracked probe touches these points on the patient, merging the preoperative images with the intraoperative environment. SBR relies on the 3D surface anatomy of the patient to align with preoperative imaging. Prior studies have concluded that SBR is less accurate than that of fiducial-based registration while others claim they are comparable. An advantage of SBR is that dedicated imaging studies with

fiducial markers in place are not needed, reducing cost and time needed for preoperative coordination. A study by Shamir et al. suggests that for targets in close proximity to the face (the point of registration in most SBR), the accuracy is higher than those located more posterior.[15] In an attempt to increase the accuracy of surface based for posterior-based targets, Fan et al. have proposed a portable 3D scanner to acquire point registration of the entire head.[16] With current trends, the time it takes to perform registration is decreasing while maintaining an acceptable level of accuracy.

Currently, existing forms of SBR and facial tracing are being applied to different imaging modalities than traditionally used. For example, Stidd et al. demonstrated acceptable registration error using facial tracing registration in a cadaver model based off of 3D digital subtraction angiography (DSA).[17] DSA is considered the gold standard imaging study for cerebral vasculature but typically lacks the soft tissue information needed to appropriately register the images to the patient. In this study, a 3D spin obtained during angiography as well as the contrasted runs were uploaded to the StealthStation S7 Surgical Navigation System (Medtronic). A pterional craniotomy was performed and vascular landmarks were checked with the navigation probe and measurement errors were taken. This study is interesting in that it shows how different methods of registration allow for the incorporation of a wider range of imaging modalities to increase the accuracy and utility of neuronavigation.

Another form of SBR was proposed by Jiang et al.[18] In their study, a structured light technique was used to reconstruct the faces of 10 volunteers. This real-time facial reconstruction was then merged with a segmented facial reconstruction based on preoperative CT or MRI. The authors claim a minimal reduction in registration accuracy but a large reduction in run time for the registration process. Surgical instruments would then be tracked using an optical system as in other existing systems.

In a study by Lefranc et al., the ROSA® (Medtech) robot was used to perform frameless stereotactic biopsies in 100 patients.[19] When surface registration was used, the robot was affixed to the MAYFIELD® (Integra) headrest and automatic registration was performed using automatic robotic movements and a nontouch laser system which used around 5,000–8,000 points of registration. Once complete, accuracy was confirmed by the surgeon by checking anatomical landmarks. Frameless biopsy using fiducial marker registration was also performed using the robot. Safe biopsies with acceptable diagnostic yield were performed on the patients in this series. More will be discussed on the use of robotics and intraoperative instrument tracking below. The ROSA® is a useful tool in that it allows for the surgeon to not only use automatic, hands-free registration with the option of using frame-based and frameless fiducial registration as well.

Today, image registration in spinal surgery is primarily performed as a reference frame connected to spinous processes or the iliac crest after initial exposure has been obtained or through small incisions during minimally invasive surgery. Automatic registration is performed with an intraoperative CT or fluoroscopic images obtained with the reference frame in place.[20] Many studies have evaluated the accuracy of hardware placement in spinal surgery using neuronavigation with free hand or robot-assisted techniques.[21-26] According to Shin et al., pedicle screws placed using neuronavigation had a significantly lower risk of pedicle perforation than those placed using free-hand technique alone.[27] Rahmathulla et al. mentions several considerations regarding the accuracy of frameless registration. Similarly to cranial procedures, the farther the distance from the reference frame, the less accurate the registration becomes.[28] A reference frame is easily attached during the exposure for open spinal procedures but this presents an issue however when procedures like stereotactic radiosurgery are performed and there is no open surgical field. In fiducial-based systems, screws are anchored into the spinous processes of the levels to be treated, providing a potential for morbidity to the patient. Several studies have demonstrated how a frameless, autoregistration system can provide similar accuracy to a fiducial-based system during spinal radiosurgery without the invasiveness of implanted fiducials.[29,30]

Current image registration trends are leaning toward faster and more automated techniques that require less input from the surgeon without sacrificing accuracy.[31] The availability of high-resolution imaging in the operating room, consisting of either CT or MRI, will allow automated registration with an accuracy that exceeds any contour or fiducial-based technique.

INTRAOPERATIVE TRACKING

Maximum utilization of a registered preoperative image requires accurate, real-time tracking of the instruments being used. Several intraoperative tracking methods include magnetic tracking, optical tracking, direct visualization with real-time image acquisition, and robotic assistance. Optical tracking of instruments is based on the surgical instrument or probe being visualized by a camera that also sees a reference frame rigidly fixed to the patient. In contrast, magnetic tracking does not require rigid fixation as it does not require a line of sight between instrument, reference point, and receiver.[32] Circumventing the need for rigid pin fixation has allowed electromagnetic (EM) neuronavigation to become a useful tool in pediatric patients or other scenarios where rigid fixation is contraindicated. When compared to free-hand technique, EM has been shown to increase ventricular catheter placement accuracy, potentially leading to decreased shunt revision rates.[33,34] EM navigation also uses smaller, flexible tools that allow for subsurface tracking.[35] This allows for the potential tracking of various instruments, including suction catheters, needles and endoscopes.[35-39] In contrast

to optical tracking, EM instruments are tracked at their tip rather than their tail. A study by Wray et al., emphasizes this point while using EM for the free-hand placement of depth electrodes.[40] Despite the advantage of not requiring a line of site trajectory for instrument tracking, EM navigation can be impacted by ferromagnetic interference. Newer systems can detect the magnetic interference and will disable localization if the detected interference is at an unacceptable level.[35] Different available EM systems have also been compared in regards to their magnetic susceptibility.[41] The increased resistance to ferromagnetic interference and potential for tracking with different surgical instruments make magnetic navigation a versatile tool.

As mentioned earlier, robots are finding increased utility in cranial and spinal surgical procedures. In addition to being involved in the image registration process via frame-based, frameless fiducial-based and autoregistration processes, robots also play a role in the tracking of instruments in the surgical field. Many robots use an optical system to track instrument position. Newer technologies include haptic feedback as well. A study by Comparetti et al. involved an optically sensed three robot system which assisted with probe insertion on a model to simulate a key-hole neurosurgical procedure. The act of probe insertion involved a haptic interface with good accuracy to the predetermined target.[42] With increasing technology, robots are being used in increasing numbers of areas of neurosurgery, including open cranial procedures, spinal surgery and endovascular neurosurgery. A recent study by Lu et al. examined the Vascular Intervention Robot-2 system (VIR-2) in 15 patients who underwent robot-assisted cerebral angiography. In this system, vascular access is obtained and the robot is then integrated in the field. A remote operator then controls the robot, visualizing catheter placement and advancement directly using standard fluoroscopy. Results of this study showed adequate and safe angiography with reduced radiation exposure to the operator.[43] There are several devices available for robot-assisted pedicle screw placement. Mentioned earlier for its performance of autoregistration, the ROSA® robot (Medtech) has also been used in spinal procedures. Lonjon et al. looked at its accuracy and safety in pedicle screw placement when compared with conventional methods. The system uses an optical tracking system with a reference frame fixed to the patient's iliac crest. The robot uses an optical system to track the reference frame in relation to the patient. This allows for trajectory adjustments to account for subtle patient movements like during respirations.[24] SpineAssist and the Mazor robot are robotic systems which guide the trajectory of pedicle screw placement using an optical system.[44,45] Other uses of these robotic systems in spinal procedures include biopsies, deformity cases and vertebroplasties. Optical systems are also being explored as a means of instrument tracking in other settings. Kantelhardt et al. experimented with connecting a standard operating microscope to robotic controls. In this study, the microscope was moved using several motors which recorded constant positional information. The relationship of the microscope to the operative field was obtained using optical navigation as well as optical coherence tomography. This allowed for the microscope to perform autofocus activities as well as automatic positioning to desired targets within 1 mm.[46]

The earlier mentioned methods of tracking all involve a probe or instrument related to a reference frame on the patient which is correlated with a pre- or intraoperative related image. Although accuracy with these methods is high, situations can arise where the physical operating field changes in relation to the acquired images, creating an increase in error. Some changes commonly encountered or tissue deformation, brain shift, CSF loss and pneumocephalus.[47] Direct visualization techniques are being developed that obtain intraoperative MRI to help plan and guide the procedure, allowing adaptation to the live operating environment. Without the production of ionizing radiation, MRI can run continuously during the procedure, giving constant feedback. One such system is ClearPoint* by MRI Interventions, Inc. This system is designed to perform minimally invasive neurosurgical procedures under real-time visualization using MRI. The system involves an MRI compatible SmartFrame* trajectory frame that allows for MRI-guided alignment and insertion of various devices depending on the procedure at hand. The ClearPoint* software allows for intraoperative surgical planning, changes to device alignment, navigation to the target, monitoring during the procedure, and a postprocedure report. Current therapeutic uses for this system advertised by the company are electrode placement, catheter placement, laser ablation catheters, drug infusion catheters and brain biopsy.

Deep brain stimulation is dependent on a high degree of accuracy when placing electrodes. In adult patients, awake testing during surgical implantation can provide information related to stimulation efficacy and presence of side effects. Microelectrode recordings can also assist with ensuring accurate lead placement.[48] In children undergoing DBS electrode placement, awake surgery is much less feasible. A study by Starr et al. examined the accuracy of lead placement in children undergoing surgery for dystonia as well as their clinical outcomes. They suggest that the ClearPoint® system provides acceptable accuracy with similar clinical results.[49] Another study by Chabardes et al. evaluated the ClearPoint® system in two adult patients with Parkinson's disease (PD) who were unable to undergo awake lead placement. They reported a slight increase in accuracy of lead placement in addition to safety, efficacy and ease of use.[50]

A recent study by Chittiboina et al. examined the precision and feasibility of the ClearPoint® system in three patients undergoing placement of convection-enhanced delivery (CED) cannula placement. Two patients with brainstem gliomas and one patient with PD were selected for cannula placement with the ClearPoint® system. The authors concluded that the interventional-MRI based targeting and CED cannula placement is a safe and accurate technique with a minimal, acceptable amount of error.[51]

VISUALIZATION

So far we have discussed the acquisition of images in the preoperative settings, how those images are linked to the operative field, and the means by which surgical instruments are tracked during navigation. This section will focus on the injection of navigational information into the view of the surgical field as seen by the surgeon. Whether spinal or cranial, current navigational techniques strive to provide the most accurate relation of surgical tools to a desired target. Augmented reality aims to provide a means of utilizing navigation and intraoperative imaging techniques to visualize hidden surgical targets by directly projecting them on the surgical field. In this setting, the surgeon would be directly looking at the surgical field with navigational information displayed directly on the patient rather than having to turn to a monitor. Several previous studies have examined augmented reality techniques in various models and operative scenarios.[52-57] Below, we will look at some recent clinical applications.

Besharati Tabrizi and Mahvash recently published a study showing intraoperative application of augmented reality during five neurosurgical cases. They also compared the accuracy of the augmented reality tumor projection on the patient with standard navigation. In their study, 3D reconstructions of the patient's brains based on MRI imaging with tumor segmentation were projected onto the patient during their operations. They claim that accurate visualization of region of interest locations from start to finish allows for better incision, craniotomy and resection performance.[58] They compared the projected location of the tumors with that identified by navigation and found minimal difference. One limitation mentioned by the authors includes a need for projector line of sight to the field, an issue with current optical tracking as well. Cabrilo et al. utilized augmented reality during extracranial-intracranial (ECIC) bypass procedures in four patients. They used 3D image sets with the desired vessels sectioned out and projected on the patient via the microscope eyepiece. The authors suggest that this system gives accurate, real-time visualization of target vessels, allowing for precise and minimally invasive procedures.[59] Another study by Cabrilo examined the use of augmented reality on a skull base case where a patient underwent transoral and transnasal resection of a recurrent clival chordoma. In this case, the patient's head was placed in a head holder with reference frame. The microscope also had a reference frame attached and was registered to the patient. Various structures including skin, bone, blood vessels, nerves and the tumor were all selectively displayed or removed during the case. The goal of this case report was to demonstrate the feasibility and usefulness of augmented reality during a skull base case.[60] The same author also examined the utility of augmented reality during aneurysm surgery in a study involving 30 operations. They discussed how augmented reality seemed to help with head positioning to produce the best surgical corridor, minimizing dissection, visualizing vascular architecture, and allow for confirmation of accuracy of neuronavigation.[61] Kersten-Oertel and colleagues examined the benefits of using augmented reality during arteriovenous malformation (AVM) surgery.[62]

Augmented reality has also been examined as an aid for training various procedures. Yudkowsky et al. used an augmented reality simulator with haptic feedback as a training tool for ventriculostomy insertion. Normal and abnormal virtual brains were used for the simulations. Participants were able to remove different virtual layers of the head to get visual feedback of their virtual "catheter" placement.[63] Mitha et al. discuss how augmented reality can aid in the training of residents and fellows in the performance of endovascular procedures.[64] Another study by Alaraj et al. examined virtual and augmented reality in both cranial and spinal simulated procedures.[65] Shenai et al. used a form of "teleimmersion" and virtual reality with the Virtual Interactive Presence and Augmented Reality (VIPAR) system during a cadaveric carotid endarterectomy and pterional craniotomy to demonstrate how a remote surgeon can inject audio and visual information to the local, operating surgeon.[66] In this model, the remote surgeon is able to view the same field as the operating surgeon and is able to, in turn, relate information visually, back to the operating surgeon. As novel techniques continue to be developed, augmented reality and the injection of visual information into the operative field and training environment will contribute to the evolution of minimally invasive neurosurgery. A recent study by Marcus et al. compared no image guidance, triplanar display of axial, sagittal and coronal images, always on solid overlay augmented reality, always on wire mesh overlay augmented reality, and on-demand inverse realism augmented reality during treatment of a basilar tip aneurysm on a model head. The authors claim that the augmented reality arm significantly reduced the time to task completion.[67]

A key issue with all of these technologies is the risk of overwhelming the surgeon with information not immediately applicable to the stage of the procedure being performed. For example, visualization of deep arterial branches is not needed when planning the bone opening for a tumor resection, but would be applicable for an aneurysm clipping. As information sources continue to develop, it will be key to use machine intelligence to comprehend the current stage of the procedure and tailor the information being displayed to show only that information needed for that stage of the procedure.

SYSTEM CONTROL

As various additional systems are added to the surgical environment, a need arises to operate, manipulate and update the systems involved. Examples of commonly encountered system control issues include but are not limited to: a sterile surgeon needing to interact with nonsterile equipment, need for the surgeon to look away from the operating field to visualize and operate a device, and the need for the surgeon to remove their hands from the operating field to operate a device. Assistants may be able to circumvent some of these issues, but future technologies aim to provide seamless surgeon control of the operating environment without interrupting the natural flow.

Endoscopic transsphenoidal approaches to the sella are a common operation in neurosurgery and otolaryngology. During these procedures, an assistant often holds the endoscope while the primary surgeon performs the procedure. Hand tremor and lack of skill operating the endoscope are potential difficulties faced during these procedures. Robot arm holders of the endoscope or even complete robot performed procedures have been investigated.[68] In 2006, Nathan et al. studied the voice command capabilities of the Automated Endoscopic System for Optimal Positioning (AESOP). In this study, the robot arm would hold the endoscope during a standard transphenoidal approach to the sella. The authors claim that the voice commands allowed for one surgeon to operate with both hands while the robot arm provided steady control of the endoscope.[69] Criticism of this system is that the constant vocal input from the surgeon to keep the voice recognition software listening can be distracting. As with any voice recognition software, errors in command recognition may arise as well. Recently, the Swarup Robotic Arm (SWARM) has sought to improve upon the voice recognition capabilities of the AESOP.[70] Though primarily studies in the fields of general surgery, urology and gynecological surgery, endoscopy is becoming increasingly popular in minimally invasive skull base neurosurgery. Voice-controlled robot assistance has the potential to improve upon current techniques. It can be anticipated that the rapid development of voice recognition devices in the consumer market will lead to improved utilization in the operating room.

Frequently during neurosurgical procedures, the operating surgeon needs to review relevant imaging. This act can be awkward and interrupt the flow of surgery if the surgeon has to verbally direct an assistant to open and navigate to the appropriate image series. The surgeon may also leave the immediate operating field to use a designated tool to interact with a touch screen, potentially risking contamination. This highlights the need for a surgeon-computer interface where sterility can be maintained that causes minimal interruption to the operating room setup. In 2008, Wachs et al. tested a gesture-based control system called "Gestix" during a brain biopsy procedure. The system is designed to recognize surgeon's hand gestures to navigate imaging software in real time, without changing their position in the operating room or risking sterility.[71] A myriad of gesture control systems exist commercially, but studies documenting its utility in the operating room is sparse. Feied et al. also propose a similar, gesture-based control system of an electronic health record, primarily geared for intraoperative use.[72] Once again consumer developments of devices like the Microsoft Kinect may be surgically applicable.

Also in the realm of endoscopy, gaze has been investigated as a means of camera control. Previous studies have looked at eye movements, dwell times and blink commands as a means of operation.[73-75] Natural eye movements and dwell times can lead to inadvertent input and blink-related commands would require periods of the surgeon to keep their eyes closed for brief periods while operating. Fujii et al. proposed a gaze-based gesture control system for laparoscopic surgery. In their study, specific eye movements are used to carry out different camera movements commands. They reported an accuracy rate of 97% and false-positive rate of 1.4%.[76] As means of system control are refined, they will likely continue to increase their use in the realm of surgery. Microscopes that change their focus and position based on the surgeon's voice or eye movements and navigation systems with 3D gesture controls may be realities in the near future.

EFFECTORS

Innovations in neuronavigation allow for less invasive techniques to access target regions. Improved access to surgical targets, coupled with new therapeutic technologies, allows for the precise delivery of novel treatments. This section will briefly touch on recent therapies enhanced by neuronavigation.

Ultrasound as a lesioning tool has been in existence for decades. Neurosurgical applications of high-intensity focused ultrasound (HIFU) first appeared in 1940.[77] Prior limitations of this therapy included inability to target and monitor treatments as well as heating of the skull. Advances in neuronavigation and intraoperative imaging have made an assortment of ultrasonic applications possible, including: tissue ablation/lesioning, drug delivery, clot lysis and coagulation.[77,78] Neuronavigation and improved target localization have made it possible to explore the benefits of HIFU. Several studies have demonstrated the feasibility and safety of transcranial MRI-guided focused ultrasound (tcMRgFUS) in various functional neurosurgical procedures.[79-83] During these procedures, the patient undergoes stereotactic ablation of a selected target with focused ultrasonography. Intraoperative MRI allows for thermal monitoring during sonication to prevent damage to surrounding brain tissue. Coluccia et al. present a case report

demonstrating successful tumor ablation using tcMRgFUS.[84] Their patient had a recurrent glioblastoma located near the basal ganglia. The deep location (away from bone) made it suitable for current tcMRgFUS. The patient was awake for the procedure and discharged the next day without change in neurologic examination. Postoperative imaging demonstrated discrete lesioning of the tumor as planned.[84] TcMRgFUS highlights the role of neuronavigation in providing accurate delivery of a lesional therapeutic modality while sparing surrounding brain tissue. Focused ultrasound can also induce desired, transient changes in intracranial structures. One such application of this concept is the ability of FUS to induce transient permeability in the blood-brain barrier (BBB) without harming surrounding tissue.[85-89] Current studies are investigating FUS-induced BBB disruption and its effect on the delivery of chemotherapeutic agents.[90-92] The addition of microbubbles has been shown to allow for lower ultrasound intensity and, therefore, reduce thermal effects and neuronal damage.[93] Regardless of the therapy applied, MRI-guided ultrasound remains highly coupled with neuronavigation to utilize some of its most appealing traits; the delivery of highly focused therapy without disruption of surrounding brain tissue. Current research continues to improve its accuracy.[94]

Like HIFU, stereoelectroencephalography (SEEG) has been used for many decades, but with advances in neuronavigation, is now experiencing a marked increase in utilization. SEEG involves the implantation of electrodes into deep brain structures to help determine the location of an epileptogenic focus. This can provide localization when standard noninvasive means (video EEG, SPECT, MEG, etc.) are unable to do so, or the lesion is located in an eloquent region.[95] As neuronavigation improves, the accuracy of electrode insertion will also improve, thus enhancing the diagnostic yield of SEEG. This technique requires a burr hole for electrode insertion rather than a large craniotomy as with traditional subdural electrode mapping, making it less invasive.[95] Various techniques are currently being used for electrode insertion, including frame-based, frameless and robot-assisted insertion.[96-98] Meng et al. propose a robot-assisted technique for SEEG electrode insertion to expedite multiple electrodes deployment. The authors claim that the robotic-guided trajectories can save time while maintaining the accuracy afforded by optically tracked neuronavigation.[99] Serletis et al. utilized both frame-based and robot-assisted lead insertion for SEEG.[100] Balanescu et al. propose a system for electrode insertion using a custom-made frame which attaches to implanted skull fiducials. The trajectories are crafted into the frame using laser sintering and attached to the patient via the fiducials. The authors report reduced operating time and high accuracy with this system.[101] Dorfer et al. propose a percutaneous bolt method for SEEG electrode insertion using frameless stereotactic navigation.[102] Munyon et al. utilize multiple electrodes inserted for SEEG recording to make a 3D grid to localize epileptogenic foci. They also mention being able to use these multiple electrodes as navigational points of reference during surgical resection.[103] Neuronavigation allows for increasingly less intrusive access to deeper structures allowing more targeted interventions; the multiplicity of suggested solutions imply that an optimal solution has yet to be found.

Stem cell transplantation has been and continues to be an exciting area of research in the treatment of a myriad of pathologic conditions. In the realm of neurosurgery, neurotransplantation of stem cells shows potential for the treatment of various degenerative neurologic diseases. Here, we will touch more on the technical considerations and their impact on neurotransplantation. Several small studies regarding Huntington's Disease (HD) have suggested motor and cognitive improvements and stabilization as well as increased PET activity at the graft site, however efficacy is not established conclusively.[104-108] PD is another neurodegenerative disease that shows promise for neural transplantation.[109] Studies have also shown that transplanted tissue has limited migratory capacity, further underlining the need for accurate placement of the donor graft.[104,110] Stereotactic insertion of stem cells into the striatum for Huntington's disease has been reported since the early 1990s.[111,112]. Whether transplanting tissue into the caudate and putamen for HD or into the substantia nigra for PD, there are special considerations to be made for these patient populations. For instance, the therapeutic targets are significantly atrophic as is the overall brain. These considerations make accurate transplantation paramount to maximize safety and efficacy of the therapy.[113] Lopez et al. discuss software that allows for model-based and mirrored coordinates to allow for faster stereotactic surgical planning for the patients in their series who underwent bilateral striatal neurotransplantation for Huntington's Disease.[114] The authors used a frame-based trajectory arm that was adjusted based on preplanned coordinates using their software. Depending on the individual patient, multiple target locations were selected for tissue transplantation. The right side was typically done first, with the left side done at a staged fashion. The programmed coordinate mapping and ability to mirror the coordinates allow for decreased planning time according to the authors.[114] Lopez et al. also report a technique using the Riechert-Mundinger frame-based system.[115] An interesting concept proposed by Rowland et al. is the combination of DBS therapy in addition to cell transplantation for the treatment of PD.[116] Most current techniques for neurotransplantation appear to be frame-based techniques, but it would be reasonable to foresee frameless techniques and intraoperative MRI tracking techniques to replace the framed version.

Focused delivery of chemotherapy and biologic agents in oncologic and neurodegenerative disorders is another area of ongoing investigation. The BBB is an obstacle to systemic treatment of CNS disease. Current areas of research focus on different delivery methods of therapeutics to the desired site of action in an attempt to circumvent the BBB. This section will touch briefly on different delivery methods rather than focus on the mechanism and successes of current treatment strategies which are described elsewhere.[89,117-121] CED involves stereotactic catheter placement within a brain tumor or the surrounding resection cavity to facilitate local delivery of chemotherapy.[89,122,123] Several important considerations during placement of CED catheters have been described which include: taking the longest possible route through parenchyma, placement within enhancing tissue, and avoidance of adjacent cavities (ventricles, resection cavity, etc.).[124] The necessity for strategic catheter placement emphasizes the need for accurate neuronavigation to optimize utilization of these new therapies.[125] Barua et al. discuss using a robotic arm for catheter placement[126] while Lonser et al. describe a method of using frameless, stereotactic placement of an MRI compatible catheter for infusion of chemotherapy in two patients.[127] Using intraoperative MRI and a chemotherapeutic agent mixed with Gd-diethylenetriamine pentaacetic acid, they were able to watch infusion of the treatment in real time into the target region.[127] Lewis et al. demonstrated increase in Evans blue dye distribution using a low profile transducer cannula assembly during CED infusion in a rat module with the addition of ultrasound as well as microbubble infusion.[128] Using a frame-based technique Anderson et al. placed CED catheters within pontine gliomas of two children and demonstrated high infusion rates of chemotherapeutic agent.[129] In addition to chemotherapeutic agents, image-guided neurosurgery has expanded the range of treatment options, allowing for exciting new possibilities, including nanoparticles, stem cells, viral vectors, and gene therapy deliver directly to the site of intended action.[130-138]

INTRAOPERATIVE IMAGING

As previously mentioned, the advancement of neuronavigation and intraoperative imaging is tightly coupled, as are the new technologies made possible by these entities. Although we have touched on intraoperative imaging unavoidably throughout this chapter, this final section will focus more on some of the recent advancements in the intraoperative acquisition of imaging information. Intraoperative CT and MR imaging are now routinely available and used in high volume centers. One use for intraoperative MRI is to assess extent of tumor resection while still in the operating room. Multiple studies have demonstrated an improvement in survival with increased extent of resection in glioma surgery.[139,140] 5-aminolevulinic acid (5-ALA) is a compound given orally several hours prior to surgery which accumulates in various epithelia and cancerous tissues.[141,142] Several studies and trials report an increase in extent of resection using 5-ALA.[143,144] Li et al. found that "5-ALA-guided surgery is more effective than conventional neuronavigation-guided surgery in increasing diagnostic accuracy and extent of tumor resection, enhancing quality of life, or prolonging survival in patients with high-grade malignant gliomas" based on available literature.[145] However, Hefti et al. claim that in lower grade tumors with satellite lesions, neuronavigation with intraoperative imaging may be necessary to obtain maximum resection rather than just using 5-ALA for tumor fluorescence alone.[146] Several other studies report success using a combination of intraoperative fluorescence and neuronavigation.[147-149] Other tracers are also under investigation.[150] Once again neuronavigation will provide the required information infrastructure to make maximal use of information obtained during surgery and presenting that information in a useful fashion to the surgeon.

We have previously mentioned the role of intraoperative MRI in the setting of functional neurosurgery and real-time visualization of catheter or electrode insertion. Sun et al. also report intraoperative MRI for monitoring during a frame-based stereotactic biopsy of a lesion near the basal ganglia.[151] MRI has become an increasingly valuable tool during lesion resection whether it be neoplasm or epileptogenic focus. A randomized controlled trial by Senft et al. claims level 1 evidence that using intraoperative MRI improves extent of resection and progression-free survival during glioma surgery.[152,153] Zhang et al. discuss a technique of using intraoperative MRI in addition to functional neuronavigation. The authors of their study indicate improved extent of resection with preservation of function of eloquent cortex.[154] Sommer et al. discuss the use of intraoperative MRI during resection of gangliogliomas for the treatment of drug resistant epilepsy. They found that the combination of neuronavigation and intraoperative MRI led to increase in extent of resection and subsequent improvement in seizure control.[155] Kurwale et al. also report an increase in extent of resection in lesional epilepsy surgery using intraoperative MRI.[156] In addition to monitoring the extent of target lesion resection, intraoperative fMRI allows for monitoring of intraoperative changes during functional procedures. Hiss et al. propose a method for using blood oxygenation level-dependent fMRI intraoperatively for monitoring the effects of DBS on the nucleus accumbens and internal capsule during DBS for OCD.[157] Sun et al. utilize intraoperative MRI in addition to microscope-based functional neuronavigation with augmented reality in the resection of cavernous malformations within the centrum semiovale in 12 pediatric patients. They conclude that the combination of these modalities allows for safe resection of these lesions.[158] Bond et al. have investigated the use of intraoperative MRI during Chiari decompression in an attempt to perform the least aggressive surgery needed to obtain adequate decompression. Their results were limited due to positioning issues but still represent another potential use for intraoperative MRI in the future.[159]

Intraoperative ultrasound provides an inexpensive, quick and real-time image during neurosurgical procedures. When compared to intraoperative MRI during glioma resection, Gerganov et al. claim that intraoperative MRI provides superior information throughout various stages of the operation but that ultrasound allows for good initial delineation and characterization of the tumor but image quality decreased during resection.[160] The authors propose a technique of initial, ultrasound-guided resection followed by intraoperative MRI assessment for residual tumor. Mari et al. claim in their study that intraoperative ultrasound helped increase the extent of resection during brain tumor surgery.[161] A study by Coburger et al. compared traditional intraoperative ultrasound with a linear array ultrasound and compared the two with intraoperative MRI. The authors claim that the linear array is superior to standard ultrasound and comparable to MRI with the linear array being more sensitive but less specific than intraoperative MRI.[162] When dealing specifically with low-grade gliomas, Petridis et al. claim that tumor identification is improved using intraoperative ultrasound and neuronavigation when compared to neuronavigation alone.[163] They retrospectively analyzed patients who underwent surgery for low-grade gliomas. They found the surgical target was not missed in any patients where ultrasound and neuronavigation were used as opposed to a missed target in 5 out of 19 cases when neuronavigation alone was used.[163] The addition of intravenous ultrasound contrast agents has aimed to further increase the information obtained with intraoperative ultrasound. Prada et al. evaluated contrasted ultrasound with microbubbles in the resection of brain tumors in 71 patients. The authors claim that the contrast-enhanced ultrasound (CEUS) helped to highlight the lesion at hand, demonstrate vascular anatomy of the tumor, show hyperperfused areas and differentiate from edematous brain tissue.[164] In addition to anatomical and spatial evaluation of brain tumors, Chauvet et al. recorded Shear Wave Elastographic (SWE) data regarding the elasticity of different brain tissues and normal brain parenchyma intraoperatively. They found differences in elasticity between different tumor types as well as normal brain. This suggests a potential diagnostic role for intraoperative ultrasound.[165] Intraoperative ultrasound also has been shown to have applications in vascular neurosurgery. Podlesek et al. used high-resolution 3D intraoperative ultrasound registered to DSA as a reference. They claim that this method provides real-time information on the vascular tree at hand pre- and post-clip application during aneurysm surgery with coregistration to DSA as a confirmation of anatomical assignment.[166] Prada et al. also describes a technique of performing intraoperative angiography using CEUS.[167] A study by Park et al. also suggests that intraoperative ultrasound may be a useful tool to diagnose etiology of cerebral swelling during ruptured aneurysm clipping.[168] Ultrasonography has also been proposed as a method for real-time assessment of

DBS lead insertion. Ahmadi et al. examined the accuracy of transcranial ultrasound localization of DBS lead placement in eight patients. They reported a mean accuracy of 4.8 mm and stated that although this is not currently acceptable for use as intraoperative confirmation of lead placement, it poses an area for future research and refinement.[169] Prior to the investigation of MRI as a means to assess the extent of decompression and/or durotomy during Chiari decompression, intraoperative ultrasound using Doppler flow has been used in several studies.[170-173] Narenthiran et al. suggest that tailoring level of decompression using intraoperative ultrasound does not compromise outcomes.[173] Also within the realm of spine surgery, Nishimura et al. utilized intraoperative ultrasound during decompression of symptomatic thoracic disk herniation in 16 patients. They claim that ultrasound allowed for real-time visualization of the spinal cord during surgery, therefore, improving safety while operating in the tight thoracic central canal.[174] In addition to therapeutic effects of ultrasonography, intraoperative ultrasound continues to evolve and improve.

Intraoperative use of CT has also become an increasingly common modality in modern neurosurgery. This section will focus on recent advances and utilizations of intraoperative CT. Various modalities including angiography, perfusion and incorporation into intraoperative navigation are currently in use.[175-178] Judicious use of intraoperative CT is typically practiced due to awareness of the ionizing radiation produced.[179,180] This has led to intraoperative CT typically being used in a snap-shot fashion for confirmation of instrument location or as a quick assessment of the operative environment for variables such as hemorrhage. Many studies have been performed to evaluate the usefulness of intraoperative CT combined with neuronavigation to aid in spinal instrumentation.[181-192] Data from these studies suggests increase in accuracy of hardware placement, extent of decompression and reduction of complications. Arishima et al. describe two cases of intraoperative assessment of foramen magnum decompression in patients with achondroplasia.[193] The utility of intraoperative CT in spine surgery is expanding in the number of procedures where it is utilized.[194,195] This coincides with the current trend towards minimally invasive procedures. Kim et al. report their success using percutaneous pedicle screw placement with intraoperative CT.[196] Intraoperative CT is also being increasingly used in functional neurosurgery. In 2010, Patil et al. described using intraoperative CT to confirm placement using frame-based stereotactic insertion of a probe at the trigeminal ganglion.[197] Shahlaie et al. and later Burchiel et al. describe using intraoperative CT to compare actual DBS lead location with preoperative planning based on fused CT and MRI. They suggest this method gives intraoperative confirmation of lead placement which achieves accuracy similar to other current lead placement techniques.[198,199] Collins et al. describe using intraoperative CT to guide

percutaneous radiofrequency cordotomy for the treatment of pain.[200] Thompson and coauthors also describe CT-guided tractotomy-nucleotomy in facial postherpetic neuralgia and postoperative hemicranial neuralgia. In their series, they describe their technique as providing confirmation of probe placement, reducing the need for the procedure to be performed on an awake patient, which can be difficult in this group secondary to allodynia.[201] Bohnstedt et al. also describe intraoperative CT used during foramen ovale cannulation during a rhizotomy procedure.[202] As touched on previously, intraoperative CT can also aid in confirmation of electrode implantation in epilepsy surgery.[203] Intraoperative CT angiography (CTA) and perfusion studies may provide benefit during vascular neurosurgical cases according to some studies. In 2010, Schichor et al. looked at intraoperative CTA and perfusion studies. The quality of images obtained was evaluated by a neurosurgeon and radiologist. They also mention how in their series, one patient underwent clip adjustment based on perfusion changes.[204] Hybrid operating rooms where microsurgical and endovascular interventions are available in the same operative setting are becoming increasingly popular. Leng et al. describe the acquisition of intraoperative CT as well as angiographic information in this setting to accurately update neuronavigation during vascular neurosurgical cases.[205] Schnell et al. describe the complementary roles of classic indocyanine green (ICG) angiography and intraoperative CT perfusion capabilities to aid in aneurysm surgery.[206] Coil/clip artifact was said to obscure the intraoperative CT images when compared to ICG angiography, but CTA allowed for visualization of vessels otherwise obscured by brain parenchyma during ICG.[206] Intraoperative CTA using an arterial injection for the treatment of small vascular pathology is described by Raza et al.[207] They claim that visualization is improved with this modality when compared to other preoperative studies used for neuronavigation. Tsuruta et al. also describe intraoperative CT with contrast material for vascular evaluation in the setting of stent placement.[208] Intraoperative imaging modalities currently in use are summarized nicely by Goren et al.[209] Much like intraoperative MRI, intraoperative CT has been used in the setting in tumor resection as well as evacuation of cerebral hematomas. Mori et al. describe the use of contrast-enhanced intraoperative CT to provide updated neuronavigation with vascular information during transphenoidal surgery. They claim this imaging modality is easy to perform and provides a useful adjunct to surgery, resulting in increased tumor resection and added safety.[210] In a study by Fujisawa et al., 58 patients underwent evacuation of lobar hemorrhages using intraoperative CT. Imaging was used to assess extent of evacuation as well as evaluate for abnormal vasculature with contrast administration.[211] Taddei et al. present a case report in which intraoperative CT was used in the trauma setting to uncover a contralateral hematoma during evacuation of the ipsilateral subdural. They claim the quickly obtained imaging allowed for quick action to be taken to address the contralateral pathology.[212] As with other intraoperative imaging modalities, CT allows for quick assessment of the operative situation to help guide surgical decision making.

CONCLUSION

Advances in neuronavigation continue to spread into all areas of neurosurgery and all phases of patient care. With advances in preoperative imaging techniques, surgeons will be able to plan more sophisticated approaches based on increasingly detailed understanding of individual patient anatomy. Less invasive surgical corridors bypassing eloquent structures will likely become more and more commonplace. Augmented reality and other advances in neuronavigation will assist the surgeon in delivering novel therapies to previously inaccessible regions of the central nervous system. Refinement of intraoperative imaging acquisition will add information important to decision making, allowing intraoperative adjustments to the surgical plan. Although the future is difficult to predict, recent history and current research point to exciting advances in neuronavigation and image-guided neurosurgery that will likely lead to the most important measure of all: improved patient care.

REFERENCES

1. Pouratian N, Zheng Z, Bari AA, et al. Multi-institutional evaluation of deep brain stimulation targeting using probabilistic connectivity-based thalamic segmentation: Clinical article. J Neurosurg. 2011;115(5):995-1004.
2. Barkhoudarian G, Klochkov T, Sedrak M, et al. A role of diffusion tensor imaging in movement disorder surgery. Acta Neurochir (Wien). 2010;152(12):2089-95.
3. Clelland CD, Zheng Z, Kim W, et al. Common cerebral networks associated with distinct deep brain stimulation targets for cluster headache. Cephalalgia. 2014;34(3):224-30.
4. Banks GP, Mikell CB, Youngerman BE, et al. Neuroanatomical characteristics associated with response to dorsal anterior cingulotomy for obsessive-compulsive disorder. JAMA Psychiatry. 2015;72(2):127-35.
5. Tie Y, Rigolo L, Norton IH, et al. Defining language networks from resting-state fMRI for surgical planning--a feasibility study. Hum Brain Mapp. 2014;35(3):1018-30.
6. Jia XX, Yu Y, Wang XD, et al. fMRI-driven DTT assessment of corticospinal tracts prior to cortex resection. Can J Neurol Sci. 2013;40(4):558-63.
7. Venneti S, Dunphy MP, Zhang H, et al. Glutamine-based PET imaging facilitates enhanced metabolic evaluation of gliomas in vivo. Sci Transl Med. 2015;7(274):274ra17.
8. Christensen M, Kamson DO, Snyder M, et al. Tryptophan PET-defined gross tumor volume offers better coverage of initial progression than standard MRI-based planning in glioblastoma patients. J Radiat Oncol. 2014;3(2):131-8.
9. Ferdová E, Ferda J, Baxa J, et al. Assessment of grading in newly-diagnosed glioma using 18F-fluorothymidine PET/CT. Anticancer Res. 2015;35(2):955-9.
10. Padma MV, Said S, Jacobs M, et al. Prediction of pathology and survival by FDG PET in gliomas. J Neurooncol. 2003;64(3):227-37.
11. Jacobs AH, Kracht LW, Gossmann A, et al. Imaging in neurooncology. NeuroRx. 2005;2(2):333-47.
12. Preuss M, Werner P, Barthel H, et al. Integrated PET/MRI for planning navigated biopsies in pediatric brain tumors. Childs Nerv Syst. 2014;30(8):1399-403.
13. Pirotte B, Goldman S, Massager N, et al. Combined use of 18F-fluorodeoxyglucose and 11C-methionine in 45 positron emission tomography-guided stereotactic brain biopsies. J Neurosurg. 2004;101(3):476-83.
14. Pauleit D, Floeth F, Hamacher K, et al. O-(2-[18F]fluoroethyl)-L-tyrosine PET combined with MRI improves the diagnostic assessment of cerebral gliomas. Brain. 2005;128(Pt 3):678-87.
15. Shamir RR, Freiman M, Joskowicz L, et al. Surface-based facial scan registration in neuronavigation procedures: a clinical study. J Neurosurg. 2009;111(6):1201-6.
16. Fan Y, Jiang D, Wang M, et al. A new markerless patient-to-image registration method using a portable 3D scanner. Med Phys. 2014;41(10):101910.
17. Stidd DA, Wewel J, Ghods AJ, et al. Frameless neuronavigation based only on 3D digital subtraction angiography using surface-based facial registration. J Neurosurg. 2014;121(3):745-50.
18. Jiang L, Zhang S, Yang J, et al. A robust automated markerless registration framework for neurosurgery navigation. Int J Med Robot. 2015;11(4):436-47.
19. Lefranc M, Capel C, Pruvot-Occean AS, et al. Frameless robotic stereotactic biopsies: a consecutive series of 100 cases. J Neurosurg. 2015;122(2): 342-52.
20. Drazin D, Kim TT, Polly DW Jr, et al. Introduction: Intraoperative spinal imaging and navigation. Neurosurg Focus. 2014; 36(3): p: Introduction.
21. Holly LT, Bloch O, Johnson JP. Evaluation of registration techniques for spinal image guidance. J Neurosurg Spine. 2006;4(4):323-8.
22. Moses ZB, Mayer RR, Strickland BA, et al. Neuronavigation in minimally invasive spine surgery. Neurosurg Focus. 2013;35(2):E12.
23. Devito DP, Kaplan L, Dietl R, et al. Clinical acceptance and accuracy assessment of spinal implants guided with SpineAssist surgical robot: retrospective study. Spine (Phila Pa 1976). 2010;35(24):2109-15.
24. Lonjon N, Chan-Seng E, Costalat V, et al. Robot-assisted spine surgery: feasibility study through a prospective case-matched analysis. Eur Spine J. 2016;25(3):947-55.
25. Roser F, Tatagiba M, Maier G. Spinal robotics: current applications and future perspectives. Neurosurgery. 2013;72 Suppl 1:12-8.
26. Bertelsen A, Melo J, Sánchez E, et al. A review of surgical robots for spinal interventions. Int J Med Robot. 2013;9(4):407-22.
27. Shin BJ, James AR, Njoku IU, et al. Pedicle screw navigation: a systematic review and meta-analysis of perforation risk for computer-navigated versus freehand insertion. J Neurosurg Spine. 2012;17(2):113-22.

28. Rahmathulla G, Nottmeier EW, Pirris SM, et al. Intraoperative image-guided spinal navigation: technical pitfalls and their avoidance. Neurosurg Focus. 2014. 36(3):E3.

29. Muacevic A, Staehler M, Drexler C, et al. Technical description, phantom accuracy, and clinical feasibility for fiducial-free frameless real-time image-guided spinal radiosurgery. J Neurosurg Spine. 2006;5(4):303-12.

30. Fürweger C, Drexler C, Kufeld M, et al. Patient motion and targeting accuracy in robotic spinal radiosurgery: 260 single-fraction fiducial-free cases. Int J Radiat Oncol Biol Phys. 2010;78(3):937-45.

31. Serej ND, Ahmadian A, Mohagheghi S, et al. A projected landmark method for reduction of registration error in image-guided surgery systems. Int J Comput Assist Radiol Surg. 2015;10(5):541-54.

32. Hayhurst C, Byrne P, Eldridge PR, et al. Application of electro-magnetic technology to neuronavigation: a revolution in image-guided neurosurgery. J Neurosurg. 2009;111(6):1179-84.

33. Jung N, Kim D. Effect of electromagnetic navigated ventriculoperitoneal shunt placement on failure rates. J Korean Neurosurg Soc. 2013;53(3):150-4.

34. Hermann EJ, Capelle HH, Tschan CA, et al. Electromagnetic-guided neuronavigation for safe placement of intraventricular catheters in pediatric neurosurgery. J Neurosurg Pediatr. 2012;10(4):327-33.

35. Mert A, Gan LS, Knosp E, et al. Advanced cranial navigation. Neurosurgery. 2013;72 Suppl 1:43-53.

36. Glossop ND. Advantages of optical compared with electromagnetic tracking. J Bone Joint Surg Am. 2009;91 Suppl 1:23-8.

37. Atsumi H, Matsumae M, Hirayama A, et al. Newly developed electromagnetic tracked flexible neuroendoscope. Neurol Med Chir (Tokyo). 2011;51(8):611-6.

38. Harrisson SE, Shooman D, Grundy PL. A prospective study of the safety and efficacy of frameless, pinless electromagnetic image-guided biopsy of cerebral lesions. Neurosurgery. 2012;70(1 Suppl Operative):29-33; discussion 33.

39. McMillen JL, Vonau M, Wood MJ. Pinless frameless electromagnetic image-guided neuroendoscopy in children. Childs Nerv Syst. 2010;26(7):871-8.

40. Wray CD, Kraemer DL, Yang T, et al. Freehand placement of depth electrodes using electromagnetic frameless stereotactic guidance. J Neurosurg Pediatr. 2011;8(5):464-7.

41. Schicho K, Figl M, Donat M, et al. Stability of miniature electromagnetic tracking systems. Phys Med Biol. 2005;50(9):2089-98.

42. Comparetti MD, Vaccarella A, Dyagilev I, et al. Accurate multi-robot targeting for keyhole neurosurgery based on external sensor monitoring. Proc Inst Mech Eng H. 2012;226(5):347-59.

43. Lu WS, Xu WY, Pan F, et al. Clinical application of a vascular interventional robot in cerebral angiography. Int J Med Robot. 2016;12(1):132-6.

44. Schatlo B, Molliqaj G, Cuvinciuc V, et al. Safety and accuracy of robot-assisted versus fluoroscopy-guided pedicle screw insertion for degenerative diseases of the lumbar spine: a matched cohort comparison. J Neurosurg Spine. 2014; 20(6):636-43.

45. Dreval' ON, Rynkov IP, Kasparova KA, et al. Results of using Spine Assist Mazor in surgical treatment of spine disorders. Zh Vopr Neirokhir Im N N Burdenko. 2014;78(3):14-20.

46. Kantelhardt SR, Finke M, Schweikard A, et al. Evaluation of a completely robotized neurosurgical operating microscope. Neurosurgery. 2013;72 Suppl 1:19-26.

47. Elias WJ, Fu KM, Frysinger RC. Cortical and subcortical brain shift during stereotactic procedures. J Neurosurg. 2007;107(5):983-8.

48. Larson PS, Starr PA, Bates G, et al. An optimized system for interventional magnetic resonance imaging-guided stereotactic surgery: preliminary evaluation of targeting accuracy. Neurosurgery. 2012;70(1 Suppl Operative):95-103; discussion 103.

49. Starr PA, Markun LC, Larson PS, et al. Interventional MRI-guided deep brain stimulation in pediatric dystonia: first experience with the ClearPoint system. J Neurosurg Pediatr. 2014;14(4):400-8.

50. Chabardes S, Isnard S, Castrioto A, et al. Surgical implantation of STN-DBS leads using intraoperative MRI guidance: technique, accuracy, and clinical benefit at 1-year follow-up. Acta Neurochir (Wien). 2015;157(4):729-37.

51. Chittiboina P, Heiss JD, Lonser RR. Accuracy of direct magnetic resonance imaging-guided placement of drug infusion cannulae. J Neurosurg. 2015:1-7.

52. Mahvash M, Besharati Tabrizi L. A novel augmented reality system of image projection for image-guided neurosurgery. Acta Neurochir (Wien). 2013;155(5):943-7.

53. Inoue D, Cho B, Mori M, et al. Preliminary study on the clinical application of augmented reality neuronavigation. J Neurol Surg A Cent Eur Neurosurg. 2013;74(2):71-6.

54. Low D, Lee CK, Dip LL, et al. Augmented reality neurosurgical planning and navigation for surgical excision of parasagittal, falcine and convexity meningiomas. Br J Neurosurg. 2010;24(1):69-74.

55. Kockro RA, Tsai YT, Ng I, et al. Dex-ray: augmented reality neurosurgical navigation with a handheld video probe. Neurosurgery. 2009. 65(4):795-807; discussion 807-8.

56. Lovo EE, Quintana JC, Puebla MC, et al. A novel, inexpensive method of image coregistration for applications in image-guided surgery using augmented reality. Neurosurgery. 2007;60(4 Suppl 2):366-71; discussion 371-2.

57. Martins C, Ribas EC, Rhoton AL Jr, et al. Three-dimensional digital projection in neurosurgical education: technical note. J Neurosurg. 2015:1-4.

58. Besharati TL, Mahvash M. Augmented reality-guided neurosurgery: accuracy and intraoperative application of an image projection technique. J Neurosurg. 2015:1-6.

59. Cabrilo I, Schaller K, Bijlenga P. Augmented Reality-Assisted Bypass Surgery: Embracing Minimal Invasiveness. World Neurosurg. 2015;83(4):596-602.

60. Cabrilo I, Sarrafzadeh A, Bijlenga P, et al. Augmented reality-assisted skull base surgery. Neurochirurgie. 2014;60(6):304-6.

61. Cabrilo I, Bijlenga P, Schaller K. Augmented reality in the surgery of cerebral aneurysms: a technical report. Neurosurgery. 2014;10 Suppl 2:252-60; discussion 260-1.

62. Kersten-Oertel M, Chen SS, Drouin S, et al. Augmented reality visualization for guidance in neurovascular surgery. Stud Health Technol Inform. 2012;173:225-9.

63. Yudkowsky R, Luciano C, Banerjee P, et al. Practice on an augmented reality/haptic simulator and library of virtual brains improves residents' ability to perform a ventriculostomy. Simul Healthc. 2013;8(1):25-31.

64. Mitha AP, Almekhlafi MA, Janjua MJ, et al. Simulation and augmented reality in endovascular neurosurgery: lessons from aviation. Neurosurgery. 2013;72 Suppl 1:107-14.

65. Alaraj A, Charbel FT, Birk D, et al. Role of cranial and spinal virtual and augmented reality simulation using immersive touch modules in neurosurgical training. Neurosurgery. 2013;72 Suppl 1:115-23.

66. Shenai MB, Dillavou M, Shum C, et al. Virtual interactive presence and augmented reality (VIPAR) for remote surgical assistance. Neurosurgery. 2011;68(1 Suppl Operative):200-7; discussion 207.

67. Marcus HJ, Pratt P, Hughes-Hallett A, et al. Comparative effectiveness and safety of image guidance systems in neurosurgery: a preclinical randomized study. J Neurosurg. 2015;123(2):307-13.

68. Chauvet D, Missistrano A, Hivelin M, et al. Transoral robotic-assisted skull base surgery to approach the sella turcica: cadaveric study. Neurosurg Rev. 2014;37(4):609-17.

69. Nathan CO, Chakradeo V, Malhotra K, et al. The voice-controlled robotic assist scope holder AESOP for the endoscopic approach to the sella. Skull Base. 2006;16(3):123-31.

70. Deshpande SV. Innovation in robotic surgery: the Indian scenario. J Minim Access Surg. 2015;11(1):106-10.

71. Wachs JP, Stern HI, Edan Y, et al. A gesture-based tool for sterile browsing of radiology images. J Am Med Inform Assoc. 2008;15(3):321-3.

72. Feied C, Gillam M, Wachs J, et al. A real-time gesture interface for hands-free control of electronic medical records. AMIA Annu Symp Proc. 2006:920.

73. Fejtova M, Fejt J, Lhotska J. Controlling a PC by eye movements: The MEMREC project. Computers Helping People with Special Needs: Proceedings. 2004;3118:770-3.

74. Mylonas GP, Darzi A, Yang GZ. Gaze-contingent control for minimally invasive robotic surgery. Comput Aided Surg. 2006;11(5):256-66.

75. Stoyanov D, Mylonas GP, Yang GZ. Gaze-contingent 3D control for focused energy ablation in robotic assisted surgery. Med Image Comput Comput Assist Interv. 2008;11(Pt 2):347-55.

76. Fujii K, Salerno A, Sriskandarajah K, et al. Gaze Contingent Cartesian Control of a Robotic Arm for Laparoscopic Surgery. Rep U S. 2013;2013:3582-9.

77. Jagannathan J, Sanghvi NT, Crum LA, et al. High-intensity focused ultrasound surgery of the brain: part 1--A historical perspective with modern applications. Neurosurgery. 2009;64(2):201-10; discussion 210-1.

78. Jolesz FA, McDannold NJ. Magnetic resonance-guided focused ultrasound: a new technology for clinical neurosciences. Neurol Clin. 2014;32(1):253-69.

79. Martin E, Jeanmonod D, Morel A, et al. High-intensity focused ultrasound for noninvasive functional neurosurgery. Ann Neurol. 2009;66(6):858-61.

80. Elias WJ, Huss D, Voss T, et al. A pilot study of focused ultrasound thalamotomy for essential tremor. N Engl J Med. 2013;369(7):640-8.

81. Moser D, Zadicario E2, Schiff G2, et al. MR-guided focused ultrasound technique in functional neurosurgery: targeting accuracy. J Ther Ultrasound. 2013;1:3.

82. Dallapiazza R, Khaled M, Eames M, et al. Feasibility and Safety of MR-guided Focused Ultrasound Lesioning in the Setting of Deep Brain Stimulation. Stereotact Funct Neurosurg. 2015;93(2):140-6.

83. Wang TR, Dallapiazza R, Elias WJ. Neurological applications of transcranial high intensity focused ultrasound. Int J Hyperthermia. 2015:1-7.

84. Coluccia D, Fandino J, Schwyzer L, et al. First noninvasive thermal ablation of a brain tumor with MR-guided focused ultrasound. J Ther Ultrasound. 2014;2:17.

85. Blanchette M, Pellerin M, Tremblay L, et al. Real-time monitoring of gadolinium diethylenetriamine penta-acetic acid during osmotic blood-brain barrier disruption using magnetic resonance imaging in normal wistar rats. Neurosurgery. 2009;65(2):344-50; discussion 350-1.

86. Baseri B, Choi JJ, Tung YS, et al. Multi-modality safety assessment of blood-brain barrier opening using focused ultrasound and definity microbubbles: a short-term study. Ultrasound Med Biol. 2010;36(9):1445-59.

87. Arvanitis CD, Livingstone MS, Vykhodtseva N, et al. Controlled ultrasound-induced blood-brain barrier disruption using passive acoustic emissions monitoring. PLoS One. 2012;7(9):e45783.

88. Beccaria K, Canney M, Goldwirt L, et al. Opening of the blood-brain barrier with an unfocused ultrasound device in rabbits. J Neurosurg. 2013;119(4):887-98.

89. Azad TD, Pan J, Connolly ID, et al. Therapeutic strategies to improve drug delivery across the blood-brain barrier. Neurosurg Focus. 2015;38(3):E9.

90. Aryal M, Vykhodtseva N, Zhang YZ, et al. Multiple treatments with liposomal doxorubicin and ultrasound-induced disruption of blood-tumor and blood-brain barriers improve outcomes in a rat glioma model. J Control Release. 2013;169(1-2):103-11.

91. Chen PY, Hsieh HY, Huang CY, et al. Focused ultrasound-induced blood-brain barrier opening to enhance interleukin-12 delivery for brain tumor immunotherapy: a preclinical feasibility study. J Transl Med. 2015;13:451.

92. Deibert CP1, Zussman BM, Engh JA. Focused ultrasound with microbubbles increases temozolomide delivery in u87 transfected mice. Neurosurgery. 2015;76(4):N22-3.

93. Konofagou EE. Optimization of the ultrasound-induced blood-brain barrier opening. Theranostics. 2012;2(12):1223-37.

94. Eames MD, Farnum M, Khaled M, et al. Head phantoms for transcranial focused ultrasound. Med Phys. 2015;42(4):1518.

95. Gonzalez-Martinez J, Mullin J, Bulacio J, et al. Stereoelectroencephalography in children and adolescents with difficult-to-localize refractory focal epilepsy. Neurosurgery. 2014;75(3):258-68; discussion 267-8.

96. Abhinav K, Prakash S, Sandeman DR. Use of robot-guided stereotactic placement of intracerebral electrodes for investigation of focal epilepsy: initial experience in the UK. Br J Neurosurg. 2013;27(5):704-5.

97. Gonzalez-Martinez J, Mullin J, Vadera S, et al. Stereotactic placement of depth electrodes in medically intractable epilepsy. J Neurosurg. 2014;120(3):639-44.

98. Cardinale F, Cossu M, Castana L, et al. Stereoelectro-encephalography: surgical methodology, safety, and stereotactic application accuracy in 500 procedures. Neurosurgery. 2013;72(3):353-66; discussion 366.

99. Meng F, Ding H, Wang G. A stereotaxic image-guided surgical robotic system for depth electrode insertion. Conf Proc IEEE Eng Med Biol Soc. 2014;2014:6167-70.

100. Serletis D, Bulacio J, Bingaman W, et al. The stereotactic approach for mapping epileptic networks: a prospective study of 200 patients. J Neurosurg. 2014;121(5):1239-46.

101. Balanescu B, Franklin R, Ciurea J, et al. A personalized stereotactic fixture for implantation of depth electrodes in stereoelectroencephalography. Stereotact Funct Neurosurg. 2014;92(2):117-25.

102. Dorfer C, Stefanits H, Pataraia E, et al. Frameless stereotactic drilling for placement of depth electrodes in refractory epilepsy: operative technique and initial experience. Neurosurgery. 2014;10 Suppl 4:582-90; discussion 590-1.

103. Munyon C, Sweet J, Luders H, et al. The 3-dimensional grid: a novel approach to stereoelectroencephalography. Neurosurgery. 2015;11 Suppl 2:127-33; discussion 133-4.

104. Bachoud-Lévi AC, Rémy P, Nguyen JP, et al. Motor and cognitive improvements in patients with Huntington's disease after neural transplantation. Lancet. 2000;356(9246):1975-9.

105. Bachoud-Lévi AC, Gaura V, Brugières P, et al. Effect of fetal neural transplants in patients with Huntington's disease 6 years after surgery: a long-term follow-up study. Lancet Neurol. 2006;5(4):303-9.

106. Reuter I, Tai YF, Pavese N, et al. Long-term clinical and positron emission tomography outcome of fetal striatal transplantation in Huntington's disease. J Neurol Neurosurg Psychiatry. 2008;79(8):948-51.

107. Gaura V, Bachoud-Lévi AC, Ribeiro MJ, et al. Striatal neural grafting improves cortical metabolism in Huntington's disease patients. Brain. 2004;127(Pt 1):65-72.

108. Furtado S, Sossi V, Hauser RA, et al. Positron emission tomography after fetal transplantation in Huntington's disease. Ann Neurol. 2005;58(2):331-7.

109. Bjorklund A, Kordower JH. Cell therapy for Parkinson's disease: what next? Mov Disord. 2013;28(1):110-5.

110. Gallina P, Paganini M, Di Rita A, et al. Human fetal striatal transplantation in Huntington's disease: a refinement of the stereotactic procedure. Stereotact Funct Neurosurg. 2008;86(5):308-13.

111. Sramka M, Rattaj M, Molina H, et al. Stereotactic technique and pathophysiological mechanisms of neurotransplantation in Huntington's chorea. Stereotact Funct Neurosurg. 1992;58(1-4):79-83.

112. Palfi S, Nguyen JP, Brugieres P, et al. MRI-stereotactical approach for neural grafting in basal ganglia disorders. Exp Neurol. 1998;150(2):272-81.

113. Freeman TB, Cicchetti F, Bachoud-Lévi AC, et al. Technical factors that influence neural transplant safety in Huntington's disease. Experimental Neurology. 2011;227(1):1-9.

114. Lopez WO, Nikkhah G, Schültke E, et al. Stereotactic planning software for human neurotransplantation: suitability in 22 surgical cases of Huntington's disease. Restor Neurol Neurosci. 2014;32(2):259-68.

115. Lopez WO, Nikkhah G, Kahlert UD, et al. Clinical neurotransplantation protocol for Huntington's and Parkinson's disease. Restor Neurol Neurosci. 2013;31(5):579-95.

116. Rowland NC, Starr PA, Larson PS, et al. Combining cell transplants or gene therapy with deep brain stimulation for Parkinson's disease. Mov Disord. 2015;30(2):190-5.

117. Khan IS, Ehtesham M. Emerging strategies for the treatment of tumor stem cells in central nervous system malignancies. Adv Exp Med Biol. 2015;853:167-87.

118. Talibi SS, Talibi SS, Aweid B, et al. Prospective therapies for high-grade glial tumours: A literature review. Ann Med Surg (Lond). 2014;3(3):55-9.

119. Hendricks BK, Cohen-Gadol AA, Miller JC. Novel delivery methods bypassing the blood-brain and blood-tumor barriers. Neurosurg Focus. 2015;38(3):E10.

120. Lidar Z, Mardor Y, Jonas T, et al. Convection-enhanced delivery of paclitaxel for the treatment of recurrent malignant glioma: a phase I/II clinical study. J Neurosurg. 2004;100(3):472-9.

121. Hall WA, Sherr GT. Convection-enhanced delivery: targeted toxin treatment of malignant glioma. Neurosurg Focus. 2006;20(4):E10.

122. Voges J, Reszka R, Gossmann A, et al. Imaging-guided convection-enhanced delivery and gene therapy of glioblastoma. Ann Neurol. 2003;54(4):479-87.

123. Lonser RR, Sarntinoranont M, Morrison PF, et al. Convection-enhanced delivery to the central nervous system. J Neurosurg. 2015;122(3):697-706.

124. Vandergrift WA, Patel SJ, Nicholas JS, et al. Convection-enhanced delivery of immunotoxins and radioisotopes for treatment of malignant gliomas. Neurosurg Focus. 2006;20(4):E13.

125. Yin D, Valles FE, Fiandaca MS, et al. Optimal region of the putamen for image-guided convection-enhanced delivery of therapeutics in human and non-human primates. Neuroimage. 2011;54 Suppl 1:S196-203.

126. Barua NU, Lowis SP, Woolley M, et al. Robot-guided convection-enhanced delivery of carboplatin for advanced brainstem glioma. Acta Neurochir (Wien). 2013;155(8):1459-65.

127. Lonser RR, Warren KE, Butman JA, et al. Real-time image-guided direct convective perfusion of intrinsic brainstem lesions. Technical note. J Neurosurg. 2007;107(1):190-7.

128. Lewis GK Jr, Schulz ZR, Pannullo SC, et al. Ultrasound-assisted convection-enhanced delivery to the brain in vivo with a novel transducer cannula assembly: laboratory investigation. J Neurosurg. 2012;117(6):1128-40.

129. Anderson RC, Kennedy B, Yanes CL, et al. Convection-enhanced delivery of topotecan into diffuse intrinsic brainstem tumors in children. J Neurosurg Pediatr. 2013;11(3):289-95.

130. Kells AP, Forsayeth J, Bankiewicz KS. Glial-derived neurotrophic factor gene transfer for Parkinson's disease: anterograde distribution of AAV2 vectors in the primate brain. Neurobiol Dis. 2012;48(2):228-35.

131. Tobias A, Ahmed A, Moon KS, et al. The art of gene therapy for glioma: a review of the challenging road to the bedside. J Neurol Neurosurg Psychiatry. 2013;84(2):213-22.

132. Bernal GM, LaRiviere MJ, Mansour N, et al. Convection-enhanced delivery and in vivo imaging of polymeric nanoparticles for the treatment of malignant glioma. Nanomedicine. 2014;10(1):149-57.

133. Diaz RJ, McVeigh PZ, O'Reilly MA, et al. Focused ultrasound delivery of Raman nanoparticles across the blood-brain barrier: potential for targeting experimental brain tumors. Nanomedicine. 2014;10(5):1075-87.

134. Ghosh D, Bagley AF, Na YJ, et al. Deep, noninvasive imaging and surgical guidance of submillimeter tumors using targeted M13-stabilized single-walled carbon nanotubes. Proc Natl Acad Sci U S A. 2014;111(38):13948-53.

135. Martinez-Quintanilla J, He D, Wakimoto H, et al. Encapsulated stem cells loaded with hyaluronidase-expressing oncolytic virus for brain tumor therapy. Mol Ther. 2015;23(1):108-18.

136. Meisen WH, Wohleb ES, Jaime-Ramirez AC, et al. The impact of macrophage and microglia secreted TNFalpha on oncolytic HSV-1 therapy in the glioblastoma tumor microenvironment. Clin Cancer Res. 2015;21(14):3274-85.

137. Weber-Adrian D, Thévenot E, O'Reilly MA, et al. Gene delivery to the spinal cord using MRI-guided focused ultrasound. Gene Ther. 2015;22(7):568-77.

138. Kundra SN, Toward the emergence of nanoneurosurgery: part III-nanomedicine: targeted nanotherapy, nanosurgery and progress toward the realization of nanoneurosurgery. Neurosurgery. 2008;62(6):E1384; author reply E1384.

139. McGirt MJ, Chaichana KL, Gathinji M, et al. Independent association of extent of resection with survival in patients with malignant brain astrocytoma. J Neurosurg. 2009;110(1):156-62.

140. Lacroix M, Abi-Said D, Fourney DR, et al. A multivariate analysis of 416 patients with glioblastoma multiforme: prognosis, extent of resection, and survival. J Neurosurg. 2001;95(2):190-8.

141. Zhao S, Wu J, Wang C, et al. Intraoperative fluorescence-guided resection of high-grade malignant gliomas using 5-aminolevulinic acid-induced porphyrins: a systematic review and meta-analysis of prospective studies. PLoS One. 2013;8(5):e63682.

142. Diaz RJ, Dios RR, Hattab EM, et al. Study of the biodistribution of fluorescein in glioma-infiltrated mouse brain and histopathological correlation of intraoperative findings in high-grade gliomas resected under fluorescein fluorescence guidance. J Neurosurg. 2015;122(6):1360-9.

143. Stummer W, Pichlmeier U, Meinel T, et al. ALA-Glioma Study Group. Fluorescence-guided surgery with 5-aminolevulinic acid for resection of malignant glioma: a randomised controlled multicentre phase III trial. Lancet Oncol. 2006;7(5):392-401.

144. Stummer W, Tonn JC, Mehdorn HM, et al. Counterbalancing risks and gains from extended resections in malignant glioma surgery: a supplemental analysis from the randomized 5-aminolevulinic acid glioma resection study. Clinical article. J Neurosurg. 2011;114(3):613-23.

145. Li Y, Rey-Dios R, Roberts DW, et al. Intraoperative fluorescence-guided resection of high-grade gliomas: a comparison of the present techniques and evolution of future strategies. World Neurosurg. 2014;82(1-2):175-85.

146. Hefti M, von Campe G, Moschopulos M, et al. 5-aminolevulinic acid induced protoporphyrin IX fluorescence in high-grade glioma surgery: a one-year experience at a single instituion. Swiss Med Wkly. 2008;138(11-12):180-5.

147. Yamada S, Muragaki Y, Maruyama T, et al. Role of neurochemical navigation with 5-aminolevulinic acid during intraoperative MRI-guided resection of intracranial malignant gliomas. Clin Neurol Neurosurg. 2015;130:134-9.

148. Gessler F, Forster MT, Duetzmann S, et al. Combination of Intraoperative Magnetic Resonance Imaging and Intraoperative Fluorescence to Enhance the Resection of Contrast Enhancing Gliomas. Neurosurgery. 2015;77(1):16-22; discussion 22.

149. Schatlo B, Fandino J, Smoll NR, et al. Outcomes after combined use of intraoperative MRI and 5-aminolevulinic acid in high-grade glioma surgery. Neuro Oncol. 2015;17(12):1560-7.

150. Margetis K, Rajappa P, Tsiouris AJ, et al. Intraoperative stereotactic injection of Indigo Carmine dye to mark ill-defined tumor margins: a prospective phase I-II study. J Neurosurg. 2015;122(1):40-8.

151. Sun X, Chen Z, Yang S, et al. Role of high-field intraoperative magnetic resonance imaging on a multi-image fusion-guided stereotactic biopsy of the basal ganglia: A case report. Oncol Lett. 2015;9(1):223-6.

152. Senft C, Bink A, Franz K, et al. Intraoperative MRI guidance and extent of resection in glioma surgery: a randomised, controlled trial. Lancet Oncol. 2011;12(11):997-1003.

153. Barbosa BJ, Mariano ED, Batista CM, et al. Intraoperative assistive technologies and extent of resection in glioma surgery: a systematic review of prospective controlled studies. Neurosurg Rev. 2015;38(2):217-27.

154. Zhang J, Chen X, Zhao Y, et al. Impact of intraoperative magnetic resonance imaging and functional neuronavigation on surgical outcome in patients with gliomas involving language areas. Neurosurg Rev. 2015; 38(2):319-30.

155. Sommer B, Wimmer C, Coras R, et al. Resection of cerebral gangliogliomas causing drug-resistant epilepsy: short- and long-term outcomes using intraoperative MRI and neuronavigation. Neurosurg Focus. 2015;38(1):E5.

156. Kurwale NS, Chandra SP, Chouksey P, et al. Impact of intraoperative MRI on outcomes in epilepsy surgery: preliminary experience of two years. Br J Neurosurg. 2015;29(3):380-5.

157. Hiss S, Hesselmann V, Hunsche S, et al. Intraoperative functional magnetic resonance imaging for monitoring the effect of deep brain stimulation in patients with obsessive-compulsive disorder. Stereotact Funct Neurosurg. 2015;93(1):30-7.

158. Sun GC, Chen XL, Yu XG, et al. Paraventricular or centrum ovale cavernous hemangioma involving the pyramidal tract in children: intraoperative MRI and functional neuronavigation-guided resection. Childs Nerv Syst. 2015;31(7):1097-102.

159. Bond AE, Jane JA Sr, Liu KC, et al. Changes in cerebrospinal fluid flow assessed using intraoperative MRI during posterior fossa decompression for Chiari malformation. J Neurosurg. 2015;122(5):1068-75.

160. Gerganov VM, Samii A, Giordano M, et al. Two-dimensional high-end ultrasound imaging compared to intraoperative MRI during resection of low-grade gliomas. J Clin Neurosci. 2011;18(5):669-73.

161. Mari AR, Shah I, Imran M, et al. Role of intraoperative ultrasound in achieving complete resection of intra-axial solid brain tumours. J Pak Med Assoc. 2014;64(12):1343-7.

162. Coburger J, Scheuerle A, Kapapa T, et al. Sensitivity and specificity of linear array intraoperative ultrasound in glioblastoma surgery: a comparative study with high field intraoperative MRI and conventional sector array ultrasound. Neurosurg Rev. 2015;38(3):499-509; discussion 509.

163. Petridis AK, Anokhin M, Vavruska J, et al. The value of intraoperative sonography in low grade glioma surgery. Clin Neurol Neurosurg. 2015;131:64-8.

164. Prada F, Perin A, Martegani A, et al. Intraoperative contrast-enhanced ultrasound for brain tumor surgery. Neurosurgery. 2014;74(5):542-52; discussion 552.

165. Chauvet D, Imbault M, Capelle L, et al. In Vivo Measurement of Brain Tumor Elasticity Using Intraoperative Shear Wave Elastography. Ultraschall Med. 2016;37(6):584-90.

166. Podlesek D, Meyer T, Morgenstern U, et al. Improved Visualization of Intracranial Vessels with Intraoperative Coregistration of Rotational Digital Subtraction Angiography and Intraoperative 3D Ultrasound. PLoS One. 2015;10(3):e0121345.

167. Prada F, Del Bene M, Saini M, et al. Intraoperative cerebral angiosonography with ultrasound contrast agents: how I do it. Acta Neurochir (Wien). 2015;157(6):1025-9.

168. Park J, Woo H, Kim GC. Diagnostic usefulness of intraoperative ultrasonography for unexpected severe brain swelling in ultra-early surgery for ruptured intracranial aneurysms. Acta Neurochir (Wien). 2012;154(10):1869-75.

169. Ahmadi SA, Milletari F, Navab N, et al. 3D transcranial ultrasound as a novel intra-operative imaging technique for DBS surgery: a feasibility study. Int J Comput Assist Radiol Surg. 2015;10(6):891-900.

170. Milhorat TH, Bolognese PA. Tailored operative technique for Chiari type I malformation using intraoperative color Doppler ultrasonography. Neurosurgery. 2003;53(4):899-905; discussion 905-6.

171. Yeh DD, Koch B, Crone KR. Intraoperative ultrasonography used to determine the extent of surgery necessary during posterior fossa decompression in children with Chiari malformation type I. J Neurosurg. 2006;105(1 Suppl):26-32.

172. McGirt MJ, Attenello FJ, Datoo G, et al. Intraoperative ultrasonography as a guide to patient selection for duraplasty after suboccipital decompression in children with Chiari malformation Type I. J Neurosurg Pediatr. 2008;2(1):52-7.

173. Narenthiran G, Parks C, Pettorini B. Management of Chiari I malformation in children: effectiveness of intra-operative ultrasound for tailoring foramen magnum decompression. Childs Nerv Syst. 2015;31(8):1371-6.

174. Nishimura Y, Thani NB, Tochigi S, et al. Thoracic discectomy by posterior pedicle-sparing, transfacet approach with real-time intraoperative ultrasonography: Clinical article. J Neurosurg Spine. 2014;21(4):568-76.

175. Tonn JC, Schichor C, Schnell O, et al. Intraoperative computed tomography. Acta Neurochir Suppl. 2011;109:163-7.

176. Gasiński P, Zieliński P, Harat M, et al. Application of intraoperative computed tomography in a neurosurgical operating theatre. Neurol Neurochir Pol. 2012;46(6):536-41.

177. Costa F, Dorelli G, Ortolina A, et al. Computed tomography-based image-guided system in spinal surgery: state of the art through 10 years of experience. Neurosurgery. 2015;11 Suppl 2:59-67; discussion 67-8.

178. Carlson AP, Phelps J, Yonas H. et al. Alterations in surgical plan based on intraoperative portable head computed tomography imaging. J Neuroimaging. 2012;22(4):324-8.

179. O'Donnell C, Maertens A, Bompadre V, et al. Comparative radiation exposure using standard fluoroscopy versus cone-beam computed tomography for posterior instrumented fusion in adolescent idiopathic scoliosis. Spine (Phila Pa 1976). 2014;39(14):E850-5.

180. Bandela JR, Jacob RP, Arreola M, et al. Use of CT-based intraoperative spinal navigation: management of radiation exposure to operator, staff, and patients. World Neurosurg. 2013;79(2):390-4.

181. Tormenti MJ, Kostov DB, Gardner PA, et al. Intraoperative computed tomography image-guided navigation for posterior thoracolumbar spinal instrumentation in spinal deformity surgery. Neurosurg Focus. 2010;28(3):E11.

182. Oertel MF, Hobart J, Stein M, et al. Clinical and methodological precision of spinal navigation assisted by 3D intraoperative O-arm radiographic imaging. J Neurosurg Spine. 2011;14(4):532-6.

183. Karandikar M, Mirza SK, Song K, et al. Complex pediatric cervical spine surgery using smaller nonspinal screws and plates and intraoperative computed tomography. J Neurosurg Pediatr. 2012;9(6):594-601.

184. Steudel WI, Nabhan A, Shariat K. Intraoperative CT in spine surgery. Acta Neurochir Suppl. 2011;109:169-74.

185. Yu X, Li L, Wang P, et al. Intraoperative computed tomography with an integrated navigation system in stabilization surgery for complex craniovertebral junction malformation. J Spinal Disord Tech. 2014;27(5):245-52.

186. Dinesh SK, Tiruchelvarayan R, Ng I. A prospective study on the use of intraoperative computed tomography (iCT) for image-guided placement of thoracic pedicle screws. Br J Neurosurg. 2012;26(6):838-44.

187. Lee MH, Lin MH, Weng HH, et al. Feasibility of Intra-operative Computed Tomography Navigation System for Pedicle Screw Insertion of the Thoraco-lumbar Spine. J Spinal Disord Tech. 2012. [Epub ahead of print].

188. Mathew JE, Mok K, Goulet B. Pedicle violation and Navigational errors in pedicle screw insertion using the intraoperative O-arm: A preliminary report. Int J Spine Surg. 2013;7:e88-94.

189. Bydon M, Xu R, Amin AG, et al. Safety and efficacy of pedicle screw placement using intraoperative computed tomography: consecutive series of 1148 pedicle screws. J Neurosurg Spine. 2014;21(3):320-8.

190. Hsieh JC, Drazin D, Firempong AO, et al. Accuracy of intraoperative computed tomography image-guided surgery in placing pedicle and pelvic screws for primary versus revision spine surgery. Neurosurg Focus. 2014;36(3):E2.

191. Jeswani S, Drazin D, Hsieh JC, et al. Instrumenting the small thoracic pedicle: the role of intraoperative computed tomography image-guided surgery. Neurosurg Focus. 2014;36(3):E6.

192. Shevelev IN, Konovalov NA, Starchenko VM, et al. [Experience of using an intraoperative cone beam computed tomography scanner and the modern navigation system in surgical treatment of spine and spinal cord disorders]. Zh Vopr Neirokhir Im N N Burdenko. 2014;78(3):21-9.

193. Arishima H, Tsunetoshi K, Kodera T, et al. Intraoperative computed tomography for cervicomedullary decompression of foramen magnum stenosis in achondroplasia: two case reports. Neurol Med Chir (Tokyo). 2013;53(12):902-6.

194. Park P. Three-Dimensional Computed Tomography-based Spinal Navigation in Minimally Invasive Lateral Lumbar Interbody Fusion: Feasibility, Technique, and Initial Results. Neurosurgery. 2015;11 Suppl 2:259-67.

195. Ling JM, Tiruchelvarayan R, Seow WT, et al. Surgical treatment of adult and pediatric C1/C2 subluxation with intraoperative computed tomography guidance. Surg Neurol Int. 2013;4(Suppl 2):S109-17.

196. Kim TT, Drazin D, Shweikeh F, et al. Clinical and radiographic outcomes of minimally invasive percutaneous pedicle screw placement with intraoperative CT (O-arm) image guidance navigation. Neurosurg Focus. 2014;36(3):E1.

197. Patil AA. Stereotactic approach to the trigeminal ganglion using a stereotactic frame and intraoperative computed

tomography scans: technical note. Stereotact Funct Neurosurg. 2010;88(5):277-80.

198. Burchiel KJ, McCartney S, Lee A, et al. Accuracy of deep brain stimulation electrode placement using intraoperative computed tomography without microelectrode recording. J Neurosurg. 2013;119(2):301-6.

199. Shahlaie K, Larson PS, Starr PA. Intraoperative computed tomography for deep brain stimulation surgery: technique and accuracy assessment. Neurosurgery, 2011. 68(1 Suppl Operative):114-24; discussion 124.

200. Collins KL, Patil PG. Flat-panel fluoroscopy O-arm-guided percutaneous radiofrequency cordotomy: a new technique for the treatment of unilateral cancer pain. Neurosurgery. 2013;72(1 Suppl Operative):27-34; discussion 34.

201. Thompson EM, Burchiel KJ, Raslan AM. Percutaneous trigeminal tractotomy-nucleotomy with use of intraoperative computed tomography and general anesthesia: report of 2 cases. Neurosurg Focus. 2013;35(3):E5.

202. Bohnstedt BN, Tubbs RS, Cohen-Gadol AA. The use of intraoperative navigation for percutaneous procedures at the skull base including a difficult-to-access foramen ovale. Neurosurgery. 2012;70(2 Suppl Operative):177-80.

203. Lee DJ, Zwienenberg-Lee M, Seyal M, et al. Intraoperative computed tomography for intracranial electrode implantation surgery in medically refractory epilepsy. J Neurosurg. 2015;122(3):526-31.

204. Schichor C, Rachinger W, Morhard D, et al. Intraoperative computed tomography angiography with computed tomography perfusion imaging in vascular neurosurgery: feasibility of a new concept. J Neurosurg. 2010;112(4):722-8.

205. Leng LZ, Rubin DG, Patsalides A, et al. Fusion of intraoperative three-dimensional rotational angiography and flat-panel detector computed tomography for cerebrovascular neuro-navigation. World Neurosurg. 2013;79(3-4):504-9.

206. Schnell O, Morhard D, Holtmannspötter M, et al. Near-infrared indocyanine green videoangiography (ICGVA) and intra-operative computed tomography (iCT): are they complementary or competitive imaging techniques in aneurysm surgery? Acta Neurochir (Wien). 2012;154(10):1861-8.

207. Raza SM, Papadimitriou K, Gandhi D, et al. Intra-arterial intraoperative computed tomography angiography guided navigation: a new technique for localization of vascular pathology. Neurosurgery. 2012;71(2 Suppl Operative): ons240-52; discussion ons252.

208. Tsuruta W, Matsumaru Y, Hamada Y, et al. Analysis of closed-cell intracranial stent characteristics using cone-beam computed tomography with contrast material. Neurologia Medico-Chirurgica. 2013;53(6):403-8.

209. Goren O, Monteith SJ, Hadani M, et al. Modern intraoperative imaging modalities for the vascular neurosurgeon treating intracerebral hemorrhage. Neurosurg Focus. 2013;34(5):E2.

210. Mori R, Joki T, Matsuwaki Y, et al. Initial experience of real-time intraoperative C-arm computed-tomography-guided navigation surgery for pituitary tumors. World Neurosurg. 2013;79(2):319-26.

211. Fujisawa M, Yamashita S, Katagi R. Usefulness of intraoperative computed tomography for the evacuation of lobar hemorrhage. Acta Neurochir Suppl. 2013;118:175-9.

212. Taddei G, Ricci A, Cola FD, et al. The usefulness of intraoperative mobile computed tomography in severe head trauma. Turk Neurosurg. 2013;23(3):401-3.

Index

Page numbers followed by *f* refer to figure and *t* refer to table

CLINICAL CASES IN GLAUCOMA
An Evidence-based Approach

CLINICAL CASES IN GLAUCOMA
An Evidence-based Approach

Editors

Shibal Bhartiya MS
Senior Consultant
Department of Ophthalmology
Fortis Memorial Research Institute
Gurgaon, Haryana, India

Parul Ichhpujani MS
Associate Professor
Glaucoma Services
Department of Ophthalmology
Government Medical College and Hospital
Chandigarh, India

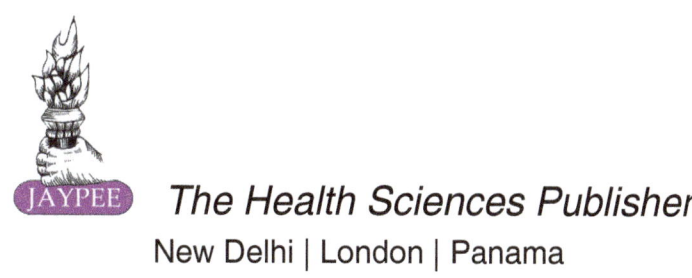

JAYPEE *The Health Sciences Publisher*
New Delhi | London | Panama

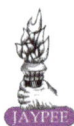

Jaypee Brothers Medical Publishers (P) Ltd

Headquarters

Jaypee Brothers Medical Publishers (P) Ltd
4838/24, Ansari Road, Daryaganj
New Delhi 110 002, India
Phone: +91-11-43574357
Fax: +91-11-43574314
E-mail: jaypee@jaypeebrothers.com

Overseas Offices

JP Medical Ltd
83 Victoria Street, London
SW1H 0HW (UK)
Phone: +44 20 3170 8910
Fax: +44 (0)20 3008 6180
E-mail: info@jpmedpub.com

Jaypee-Highlights Medical Publishers Inc
City of Knowledge, Bld. 235, 2nd Floor, Clayton
Panama City, Panama
Phone: +1 507-301-0496
Fax: +1 507-301-0499
E-mail: cservice@jphmedical.com

Jaypee Brothers Medical Publishers (P) Ltd
17/1-B, Babar Road, Block-B, Shaymali
Mohammadpur, Dhaka-1207
Bangladesh
Mobile: +08801912003485
E-mail: jaypeedhaka@gmail.com

Jaypee Brothers Medical Publishers (P) Ltd
Bhotahity, Kathmandu, Nepal
Phone: +977-9741283608
E-mail: kathmandu@jaypeebrothers.com

Website: www.jaypeebrothers.com
Website: www.jaypeedigital.com

Inquiries for bulk sales may be solicited at: jaypee@jaypeebrothers.com

Clinical Cases in Glaucoma: An Evidence-based Approach

First edition: 2017

ISBN: 978-93-86056-96-2

Printed at

Dedicated

To those, who will read this book
And to Aradhya, who will only ever read the dedication.

Contributors

Youssef Abdelmassih MD
Beirut Eye and ENT Specialist Hospital
Al-Mathaf Square
Beirut, Lebanon

Oscar Albis-Donado MD
OMESVI Diagnostic Group
Mexico City, Mexico
Instituto Mexicano de Oftalmología
Querétaro, México

Jorge Vila Arteaga MD FEBO
Glaucoma Consultant
Innova Ocular, Clinica Vila
Valencia, Spain

Shibal Bhartiya MS
Senior Consultant
Department of Ophthalmology
Fortis Memorial Research Institute
Gurgaon, Haryana, India

Madhu Bhoot DNB
Consultant
Glaucoma and Anterior Segment
Dr Shroff Charity Eye Hospital
New Delhi, India

Giovanna Casale-Vargas MD
Cornea, OMESVI, Mexico
Glaucoma, Glaucos
Zacatecas, Mexico

M Chockalingam DO DNB FRCS (Glasgow)
PGDHHM
Consultant
Apollo Hospital, Chennai
Senior Consultant
Apollo Specialty Hospital
Vanagaram, Chennai
Visiting Faculty
Apollo Institute of Hospital Management
and Allied Sciences, Chennai and
KMCH Institute of Hospital
Administration, Coimbatore
Chief Consultant
Vignesh Meenu Eye Clinic
Chennai, Tamil Nadu, India

Nikhil S Choudhary MS
Consultant
Seetha Lakshmi Glaucoma Center
Anand Eye Institute
Hyderabad, Telangana, India

Paaraj Dave MS
Consultant
Dr TV Patel Eye Institute and
Sheth ML Vaduwala Eye Hospital
Vadodara, Gujarat, India

Jasleen Dhillon MS
Consultant
Glaucoma and Cataract Services
Centre for Sight
New Delhi, India

Syril Dorairaj MD
Associate Professor
Department of Ophthalmology
Mayo Clinic
Jacksonville, Florida, USA

Suneeta Dubey MS
Consultant
Glaucoma Services
Dr Shroff Charity Eye Hospital
New Delhi, India

Sylvain el-Khoury MD
Beirut Eye and ENT Specialist Hospital
Al-Mathaf Square
Beirut, Lebanon

Monica Gandhi MS
Consultant
Glaucoma Services
Dr Shroff Charity Eye Hospital
New Delhi, India

Ivan Goldberg MD FRANZCO
Clinical Associate Professor
Ophthalmologist and
Head of Glaucoma Unit
Sydney Eye Hospital
Sydney, Australia

Alejandra Hernandez-Oteyza MD
OMESVI Diagnostic Group
Mexico City, Mexico
Instituto Mexicano de Oftalmología
Querétaro, México

Gábor Holló MD PhD DSc
Director
Glaucoma Services and Perimetry Unit
Department of Ophthalmology
Semmelweis University
Budapest, Hungary

Parul Ichhpujani MS
Associate Professor
Glaucoma Services
Department of Ophthalmology
Government Medical College and Hospital
Chandigarh, India

Fabio Kanadani PhD
Head of the IOCM's
Ophthalmology Department
Full Professor of the Medical Science
College of Minas Gerais
Minas Gerais, Brazil

Pankaj Kataria MS
Senior Resident
Glaucoma Services
Advanced Eye Centre
Postgraduate Institute of Medical
Education and Research
Chandigarh, India

Sushmita Kaushik MS
Additional Professor
Glaucoma Services
Advanced Eye Centre
Postgraduate Institute of Medical
Education and Research
Chandigarh, India

Ziad Khoueir MD MSEd (Ophthalmology)
Diseases and Surgery of the Eye
Beirut Eye and ENT Specialist Hospital
Al-Mathaf Square
Beirut, Lebanon

Mona Khurana MS
Consultant
Glaucoma Services
Sankara Nethralaya
Chennai, Tamil Nadu, India

Suresh Kumar MS
Professor
Glaucoma Services
Department of Ophthalmology
Government Medical College and Hospital
Chandigarh, India

Gabriel Lazcano-Gómez MD
Glaucoma Department
Asociación para Evitar la
Ceguera en México IAP
San Lucas Coyoacan
Mexico DF, Mexico

André Mermoud MD
Professor
Glaucoma Center, Montchoisi Clinic
Lausanne, Switzerland

Gowri J Murthy DO DNB FRCO (Lon) FRCS (Edin)
Senior Consultant
Glaucoma Services
Prabha Eye Clinic and Research Centre
Vittala International Institute of
Ophthalmology
Bengaluru, Karnataka, India

Praveen R Murthy MS DNB FMRF
Senior Consultant
Vitreoretinal and Cataract Services
Prabha Eye Clinic and Research Centre
Vittala International Institute of
Ophthalmology
Bengaluru, Karnataka, India

Aditya Neog DO DNB FMRF
Glaucoma Consultant
Centre for Sight
Superspeciality Eye Hospital
Hyderabad, Telangana, India

Julie Pegu MS
Consultant
Dr Shroff Charity Eye Hospital
New Delhi, India

Tiago Prata MD PhD
Associate Professor
Glaucoma Services
Department of Ophthalmology
Federal University of São Paulo
São Paulo, Brazil

Nadia Ríos-Acosta MD
Resident in Ophthalmology
Mexican Institute of
Ophthalmology
Querétaro, Mexico

Sylvain Roy MD PhD
Swiss Federal Institute of
Technology
Glaucoma Center
Montchoisi Clinic
Lausanne, Switzerland

Tarek Shaarawy MD PD
Head
Glaucoma Unit
Geneva University Hospital
Geneva, Switzerland

Dushyant Sharma MS
Glaucoma Fellow
Dr Shroff Charity Eye Hospital
New Delhi, India

Nishtha Singh MS
Glaucoma Fellow
Dr Shroff Charity Eye Hospital
New Delhi, India

Simon Skalicky MMed MPhil FRANZCO
Discipline of Ophthalmology
University of Sydney, Sydney
Department of Ophthalmology and
Surgery
Royal Melbourne Hospital
Centre for Eye Research Australia
Royal Victorian Eye and Ear Hospital
University of Melbourne
Melbourne, Australia

Oana Stirbu MD FEBO
Glaucoma Consultant
Instituto Condal de Oftalmologia
Barcelona, Spain

Sahil Thakur MBBS
Junior Resident
Department of Ophthalmology
Government Medical College and
Hospital
Chandigarh, India

Augusto Vieira MD
Glaucoma Staff
Eye Institute of Minas Gerais
Minas Gerais, Brazil

Preface

There is some stuff that we love to read, and then there is some stuff that we have to read: to remain relevant in our clinical practice, to be responsible citizens, to be who we want to be. The *Journal of Current Glaucoma Practice, Journal of Glaucoma, Survey of Ophthalmology, American Journal of Ophthalmology, British Journal of Ophthalmology, Annals of Ophthalmology, National Geographic, New York Times, Guardian, Times of India, Leo Tolstoy, Harry Potter, Orson Scott Card, Calvin and Hobbes, Vogue...*The list is not half complete, we have not mentioned even one of the zillion prescribed textbooks, and we already have three hundred hours of reading, to be crammed into a twenty-four hour day, if we read every day. A twenty-four hour day that also needs us to work, sleep, and go about the general business of living.

So what we have done, in this beautiful little book, is to condense all of the current published glaucoma evidence into tiny bite-sized pieces, relevant to your everyday glaucoma practice. Some of the best minds in glaucoma who have been reading and writing glaucoma for very many years, have got together and picked up representative cases from their own clinics, and delineated the preferred practice pattern in the light of the available evidence-base. We have sifted the information on glaucoma that is currently available, chosen the one which actually stands up to scrutiny, removed the statistical jargon and concentrated on the lowest common denominator: evidence-based clinical practice of glaucoma.

Clinical Cases in Glaucoma: An Evidence-based Approach is therefore an easy read, and gives you a real world feel of how the early manifest glaucoma trial (EMGT) or the tube versus trabeculectomy (TVT) or the ocular hypertension treatment study (OHTS) actually translate into the last patient you saw on Thursday. Reading the book will help you make better clinical judgments, if you are a veteran clinician-surgeon. It will help you understand the science of glaucoma better, if you are a researcher, and it will help you take care of your patients better, if you are just stepping into clinical practice.

All of us who have worked on this book together have at various points in our career missed having a book such as this in the front pockets of our lab coats. We are, therefore, delighted to have actually put it together for you, and for ourselves, when the fingerprints of the newly available minimally invasive glaucoma surgery (MIGS) escape us, as we scratch our heads over a 52-year-old patient who keeps forgetting to use his glaucoma medication.

Happy reading, and our best wishes for taking care of your glaucoma patients better. Each day.

Shibal Bhartiya MS
Parul Ichhpujani MS

Acknowledgments

We would like to acknowledge the efforts of all our authors and contributors. Without their continued support and dedication, this book would not have been possible.

We would also like to thank our publishers, Jaypee Brothers Medical Publishers (P) Ltd for their valued support and faith in us. A special word of gratitude for Ms Chetna Malhotra Vohra (Associate Director—Content Strategy) and our extremely competent and capable Development Editor, Ms Nedup Denka Bhutia.

It would have impossible to take on this project without the continued and unwavering support of our family, friends and colleagues. A very special thanks to them too.

Contents

15A. Clinical Trials in Glaucoma   165

Suneeta Dubey, Madhu Bhoot, Nishtha Singh, Dushyant Sharma, Monica Gandhi

15B. Basics of a Trial Design for Glaucoma   175

Shibal Bhartiya, Parul Ichhpujani

CHAPTER 1

Ocular Hypertension

Shibal Bhartiya, Parul Ichhpujani

▌ INTRODUCTION

Ocular hypertension (OHT) is defined as the presence of elevated intraocular pressure (IOP) measured more than 21 mm Hg on at least two occasions, in subjects with normal, open anterior chamber angles, no glaucomatous optic nerve changes or retinal nerve fiber layer (RNFL) defects or visual field abnormalities. The elevation of IOP must not be secondary to steroid use, uveitis, neovascularization, etc.

Case 1: No treatment required for ocular hypertension

Mr X, a 42-year-old gentleman, was found to have persistently elevated IOPs on three visits [oculus uterque (OU) 24, 25, 24 mm Hg]. The cup-to-disc (C:D) ratio was 0.3:1 and 0.2:1, with a healthy neuroretinal rim. The visual field did not show any changes suggestive of glaucomatous damage. The central corneal thickness (CCT) was 531 microns and 522 microns for the right and left eyes, respectively. The optical coherence tomography RNFL did not show any RNFL defects and gonioscopy showed wide open angles. The risk of developing glaucoma in one eye, over 5 years was found to be less than 15% as per the OHT risk calculator. Risks and benefits of initiating glaucoma therapy were discussed with Mr X, and he agreed that a continuous yearly follow-up was better for managing his condition.

Some patients do not like the unknown desire therapy, while others are comfortable in being followed. If therapy is commenced and adverse effects are noted or the medications are ineffective, then going back to careful monitoring is indicated.

Case 2: Treatment for ocular hypertension required depending on age

An optometrist referred a 25-year-old African-American male for an applanation IOP. Subject's IOP measured 34 mm Hg OU on the noncontact tonometer at his initial visit with the optometrist. His applanation IOP was 34 mm Hg oculus dexter (OD) and 32 mm Hg oculus sinister (OS) and his C:D ratios measured 0.4 OU. His neuroretinal rim (NRR) was healthy with no nerve fiber layer defects. Automated visual field testing and nerve fiber analysis revealed no glaucomatous defects. Gonioscopy reveals open angles with no pigmentation. His grandfather had been operated for glaucoma.

Considering patient's young age, high IOP, race and a positive family history; he was labeled as a "high-risk" ocular hypertensive (Fig. 1.1); therefore, he was started on glaucoma medication.

Case 3: Treatment for ocular hypertension required depending on central corneal thickness

A healthy 50-year-old Caucasian male presented for a routine exam. His IOP measured 24 mm Hg OU and his C:D ratios measure 0.4:0.45 OU. His NRR is healthy and no nerve fiber layer defects are detected. Automated visual field testing and nerve fiber analysis reveal no glaucomatous defects. Gonioscopy reveals open angles with trace trabecular meshwork pigmentation with no peripheral anterior synechiae. He has no family history of glaucoma.

Factors	Points for factors				
	0	1	2	3	4
Age (years)	<45	45 to <55	55 to <65	65 to <75	≥75
Intraocular pressure (mm Hg) means (3 measurements per eye and average of 2 eyes)	<22	22 to <24	24 to <26	26 to <28	≥28
Central corneal thickness (μ) means (3 measurements per eye and average of 2 eyes)	≥600	576–600	551–575	526–550	≤525
Vertical cup/disc ratio by contour means (3 measurements per eye and average of 2 eyes)	<0.3	0.3 to <0.4	0.4 to <0.5	0.5 to <0.6	≥0.6
Visual field: Humphrey pattern standard deviation (dB) means (2 measurements per eye and average of 2 eyes)	<1.8	1.8 to <2.0	2 to <2.4	2.4 to <2.8	≥2.8
OR Octopus loss variance means (2 measurements per eye and average of 2 eyes)	<3.24	3.24<4.0	4.0<5.76	5.78<7.84	≥7.84
Sum of points estimated 5-year risk of developing POAG					
Sum of points	0–6	7–8	9–10	11–12	>12
Estimated 5-year risk of developing POAG	≤4.0%	10%	15%	20%	≥33%

Fig. 1.1: Patient's risk of converting to primary open-angle glaucoma (POAG) as calculated on http://ohts.wustl.edu/risk.

How to Manage this Patient if His Central Corneal Thickness Measured 480 Microns or 610 Microns?

If the patient has a thick CCT (>600 m) and an IOP of 24 mm Hg, his true IOP is likely lower than the Goldmann tonometer measurement and has a negative family history of glaucoma, so we can monitor him. On the other hand, if the patient has a CCT of 480 microns, consideration of medical therapy may be warranted prophylactically.

Physicians must remember that one CCT measurement may not be satisfactory for long-term patient follow-up. It is suggested to perform at least one repeat measurement at a follow-up appointment to ascertain whether the initial CCT value was accurate, and then to repeat it once every year. A helpful strategy while doing pachymetry is to take five measurements, disregard the first and the last measurements and select the lowest of the remaining three measurements.

Interpretation of CCT measurements varies amongst physicians. Some practitioners alter measurements based on a pachymeter adjustment factor, whereas others classify measurements as thin, average or thick. Currently, no single algorithm for adjusting IOP based on pachymetry measurements is accepted because the relationship between IOP and CCT is believed to be nonlinear.

	9 AM	1 PM	5 PM	9 PM	1 AM	5 AM	9 AM
OD	24	27	29	30	34	37	29
OS	28	25	25	30	32	36	30

Fig. 1.2: Phasing for Case 4.

Case 4: Treatment for ocular hypertension required depending on DV and high peak pressures

Mr A, a 44-year-old Asian-Indian man, was found to have persistently elevated IOPs on three visits (OU 26, 30, 24 mm Hg). His CCT was 560 OD and 555 microns OS. The C:D ratio was 0.3:1 OU, with a healthy neuroretinal rim. He was planned for phasing. The maximum IOP was 37 mm Hg OD and 36 mm Hg OS. The peak IOP was in the morning at 5 AM in both the eyes. The difference between the maximum and minimum IOPs was 13 mm Hg OD and 11 mm Hg OS (Fig. 1.2). In view of significant fluctuation in IOP throughout the day and the fact that the patient was a frequent international traveller and had difficulty visiting the clinic for frequent follow-up, he was started on G Travoprost HS.

A study has demonstrated that portions of the lamina cribrosa move maximally during pressure changes of

5–7 mm Hg, in contrast to minimal movement at pressure changes exceeding 15 mm Hg. Kinking of the axons may occur in small pockets of the lamina cribrosa, which move maximally at small pressure changes while other pockets remain relatively stationary. Another proposed theory is that fluctuations may result in an ischemia reperfusion injury.

Diurnal fluctuations in IOP increase the risk of visual field loss for patients with glaucoma. For patients with significant IOP fluctuation, it is suggested to monitor IOP closely and prescribe medication that best controls IOP with the least amount of fluctuation.

Investigations

Every patient of OHT requires a careful and comprehensive eye examination to rule out early signs of glaucoma or secondary causes of elevated IOP.

Mandatory tests include:

Visual acuity and refraction

Tonometry (applanation): On at least two different occasions, at different times of the day, with IOP more than 21 mm Hg is mandatory for diagnosing OHT.

Gonioscopy: Anatomically normal and open angles are mandatory for diagnosing OHT.

Optic nerve assessment: A dilated assessment of the optic nerve head is essential together with a red free evaluation of the peripapillary RNFL. The optic nerve head (ONH) can be documented using a hand drawn, labeled diagram (special emphasis on C:D ratio, notching, RNFL defects, and/or hemorrhage) and/or a clinical picture. A colored photo and a red-free photo of the ONH are essential for serial follow-up.

Visual field testing: Reliable visual fields provide a baseline for future follow-up.

Central corneal thickness or pachymetry is required to make therapeutic decisions.

In addition, the following tests, if performed help in managing the condition better, in case the facilities exist, and are affordable to the patient.

Stereo optic disc photographs to confirm normal optic nerve parameters and document baseline

Imaging of the optic nerve with RNFL analysis (ocular coherence tomography, Heidelberg retinal tomography or scanning laser polarimetry) provide a statistical comparison with the normative database, thereby providing additional information for subsequent management.

Diurnal variation of IOP curve may provide additional information and influence treatment protocol.

Water drinking test (WDT): A WDT with 10 mL/kg body weight of water over five minutes, may be performed as a surrogate for diurnal variation of IOP to provide a rough idea of IOP peaks and fluctuation.

Follow-up Protocol

Follow-up protocol is to be customized to the individual patient, depending on the risk of developing glaucoma, risk factors present, and whether treatment has been initiated or not. Initially, a follow-up may be scheduled every 3–6 months for IOP checks. Repeat visual field and optic nerve testing may be performed annually or sooner, if changes are suspected.

Commentary

The definitive study that influences management of OHT in the current evidence-based practice of glaucoma is the OHT treatment study. The study is described in brief in the Box 1.1, while Box 1.2 describes the European Glaucoma Prevention Study.

POINTS TO REMEMBER

- Intraocular pressure must be measured two or more times on separate occasions, before labeling a patient as having OHT.
- A gonioscopy must be performed to rule out angle closure, and a slit lamp biomicroscopy, and/or imaging studies of the ONH must be performed to rule out optic nerve damage. A reliable visual field is essential for ruling out field changes.
- A pachymetry is required to give an indication of the eyes ability to withstand higher pressures. There are no validated normograms for IOP correction on the basis of CCT. IOP corrected for corneal thickness, therefore, does not provide a valid basis for initiating or not initiating therapy.
- The threshold for starting treatment for OHT must be lower for patients with increased risk factors (Fig. 1.3). These include:
  - African or Hispanic ancestry
  - Family history of glaucoma or glaucoma induced blindness
  - Younger patients
  - Patients with myopia

Box 1.1: Ocular hypertension treatment study.

Objectives: Role of topical hypotensives in preventing onset of POAG
Risk factors in development of POAG
Participants: 1636 patients, Age group 40–80 years; IOP 24–32 mm Hg in one eye and 21–32 in fellow eye
Intervention: Randomized to observation versus 20% IOP reduction (to IOP ≤24) using topical medication
End point: Optic nerve glaucomatous change or visual field abnormality
Conclusions:

- 5-year glaucoma risk is 4.4% in treated versus 9.5% in untreated eyes
- Risk factors for developing glaucoma include:
  - *Old age*: 10 years older → 22% more risk
  - African-American race (only univariate analysis)
  - Higher IOP: 1 mm Hg rise in IOP corresponds to a 10% increase in risk Thinner CCT (< 555 um): 40 um decrease corresponds to a 81% increase in risk Higher PSD: 0.2 change corresponds to a 22% increase in risk Higher baseline C:D: Increase in vertical C:D ratio by 0.1 corresponds to a 32% increase in risk not family history (though most other studies say yes)
- 13-year follow-up: Treatment initiated after 7.5 years of observation, monitored for 5.5 more years:
  - 16% treated versus 22% untreated eyes develop glaucoma
  - No further increase in risk once treatment is started.

(C:D: Cup-to-disc; CCT: Central corneal thickness; IOP: Intraocular pressure; POAG: Primary open-angle glaucoma; PSD: Pattern standard deviation).

Box 1.2: European glaucoma prevention study.

Objectives: To evaluate the efficacy of reduction of IOP, by means of dorzolamide, in preventing patients affected by ocular hypertension from developing glaucoma.
Participants: 1,077 patients >30 years old, at 18 European centers. IOP 22–29 mm Hg; two normal and reliable visual fields (on the basis of mean deviation and corrected PSD); and a normal optic disc.
Intervention: Treatment with dorzolamide or a placebo (the vehicle of dorzolamide) in one or both eyes.
End point: Optic nerve glaucomatous change or visual field abnormality
Conclusions:

- Mean percent reduction in IOP in the dorzolamide group was 15% after 6 months and 22% after 5 years
- Mean IOP declined by 9% after 6 months and by 19% after 5 years in the placebo group
- At 60 months, the cumulative probability of converting to an efficacy end point was 13.4% in the dorzolamide group and 14.1% in the placebo group
- Dorzolamide reduced IOP by 15–22% throughout the 5 years of the trial
- The EGPS failed to detect a statistically significant difference between medical therapy and placebo in reducing the incidence of POAG among a large population of OHT patients at moderate risk for developing POAG, because placebo also significantly and consistently lowered IOP.

Three significant differences with the OHTS may explain the failure of the EGPS to find a therapy benefit:
1. Its commitment to dorzolamide therapy alone, regardless of IOP lowering with placebo control
2. A major regression to the mean in IOP at 6 months; and
3. Selective loss to follow-up of persons with higher IOP.

(EGPS: European glaucoma prevention study; IOP: Intraocular pressure; OHT: Ocular hypertension; OHTS: Ocular hypertension treatment study; POAG: Primary open-angle glaucoma; PSD: Pattern standard deviation).

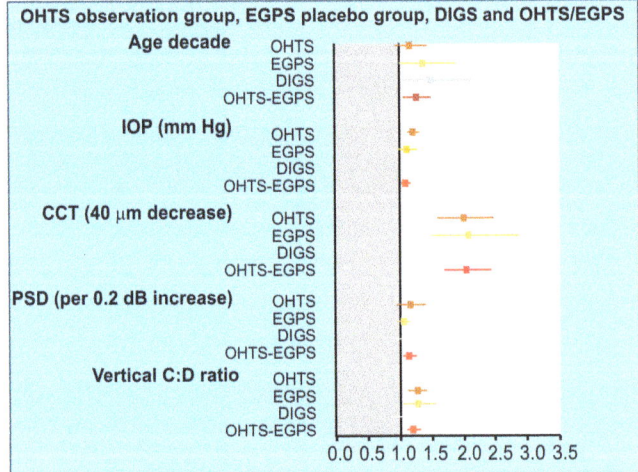

Fig. 1.3: Multivariate hazard ratios for predictors of POAG. (C:D: Cup-to-disc; CCT: Central corneal thickness; DIGS: Diagnostic innovations in glaucoma study; EGPS: European glaucoma prevention study; IOP: Intraocular pressure; OHT: Ocular hypertension; OHTS: Ocular hypertension treatment study; POAG: Primary open-angle glaucoma; PSD: Pattern standard deviation).

- Patients with poor access to repeat glaucoma investigations
- Patients with decreased corneal thickness, high C:D ratio and/or visual fields with high pattern standard deviation.
- It is important to consider the economics of glaucoma therapy as also compliance issues. Quality of life costs of treatment versus no treatment must be weighed for the individual patient.
- The risks and benefits of selective laser trabeculoplasty versus topical glaucoma therapy must be discussed with the patient.

SUGGESTED READING

1. Asrani S, Zeimer R, Wilensky J, Gieser D, Vitale S, Lindenmuth K. Large diurnal fluctuations in IOP are an independent risk factor in glaucoma patients. J Glaucoma. 2000;9:134-42.

2. European Glaucoma Prevention Study (EGPS) Group; Miglior S, Pfeiffer N, Torri V, Zeyen T, Cunha-Vaz J, et al. Predictive factors for open-angle glaucoma among patients with ocular hypertension in the European Glaucoma Prevention Study. Ophthalmology. 2007;114(1):3-9.

3. Gordon MO1, Beiser JA, Brandt JD, Heuer DK, Higginbotham EJ, Johnson CA, et al. The Ocular Hypertension Treatment Study: baseline factors that predict the onset of primary open-angle glaucoma. Arch Ophthalmol. 2002;120(6):714-20.

4. Herndon LW, Weizer JS, Stinnett SS. Central corneal thickness as a risk factor for advanced glaucoma damage. Arch Ophthalmol. 2004;122(1):17-21.

5. Kass MA, Heuer DK, Higginbotham EJ, Johnson CA, Keltner JL, Miller JP, et al. The Ocular Hypertensive Treatment Study: a randomized trial determines that topical ocular hypotensive medication delays or prevents the onset of primary open-angle glaucoma. Arch Ophthalmol. 2002; 120(6):701-13.

CHAPTER 2

Glaucoma Suspect

Augusto Vieira, Tiago Prata, Fabio Kanadani, Syril Dorairaj

WHO IS A GLAUCOMA SUSPECT?

Glaucoma is defined as a progressive optic neuropathy of characteristic appearance and corresponding visual field loss that may be associated with a raised intraocular pressure (IOP) and where all other possible causes have been ruled out.

Patients are generally designated as glaucoma suspects if:

- IOP is higher than normal
- The optic discs have large cup-to-disc (C:D) ratios
- There is asymmetry between the size or shape of the optic disc rim or cup between the two eyes
- There is a suspicious visual field abnormality that corroborates glaucomatous optic neuropathy
- Associated risk factors for glaucoma arousing strong suspicion.

Case 1: Strong risk factors

A 67-year-old Caucasian woman was referred to outpatient clinic due to a strong family history. Her parents were glaucomatous, and other risk factors for glaucoma such as systemic hypertension and type II diabetes. Her first ophthalmic examination was in 2009 and based on her risk factors, a complete glaucoma evaluation was performed. Her IOP was 15 mm Hg on both eyes oculus uterque (OU) during the morning. Her central corneal thickness (CCT) was 512 microns and 509 microns on the right oculus dexter (OD) and left oculus sinister (OS) eyes, respectively. The gonioscopy presented an open angle (ciliary band) and pigmentation of 1+/4+ OU. Her diurnal curve of IOP ranged between 15 mm Hg and 13 mm Hg. Computerized visual field, stereophotos and optical coherence tomography (OCT) showed no significant changes. Her follow-up was lost and she turned to the clinic only after 6 years. She had undergone phacoemulsification on both eyes and her new glaucoma evaluation showed no progression regarding her previous condition. She was once again counseled and the importance of a proper follow-up was reinforced.

Learning Points

- Normal exam findings should not be considered as a solid reason to disregard proper follow-up when it comes to patients with significant risk factors.[1]
- As glaucoma usually does not present with pain or acute vision loss, patients struggle to understand the high risk of presenting with this pathology. Thus, a doctor-patient relationship is important to treat each patient individually.[2]
- Glaucoma presents a scenario of a complex interplay of factors in which a detailed anamnesis is paramount.[3]

Case 2: Disc hemorrhage

A 70-year-old systemic hypertensive man presented to the clinic in 2014 to investigate whether a previous laser procedure was correctly performed or not. He did not know which procedure was done or why, but referred that a doctor once told him he had a "different optic disc". He had previous peripheral laser iridotomy and was pseudophakic OU, showed an open angle (scleral spur) with pigmentation of 2+/4+, IOP of 19 mm Hg and 18 mm Hg on his OD and OS, respectively, during the morning. Diurnal

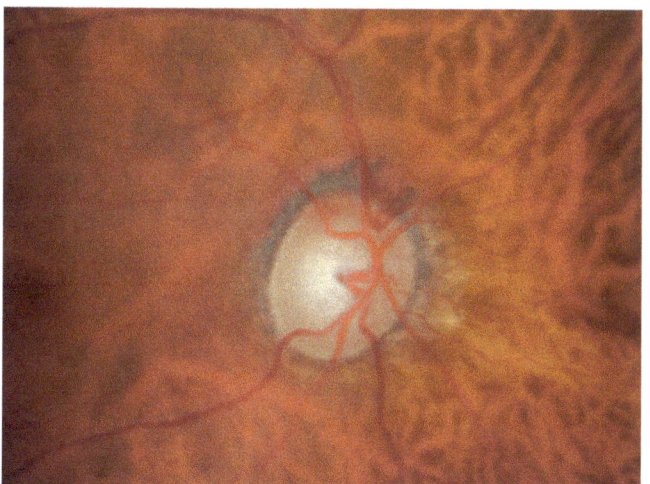

Fig. 2.1: Small disc hemorrhage at superior margin of the right optic disc.

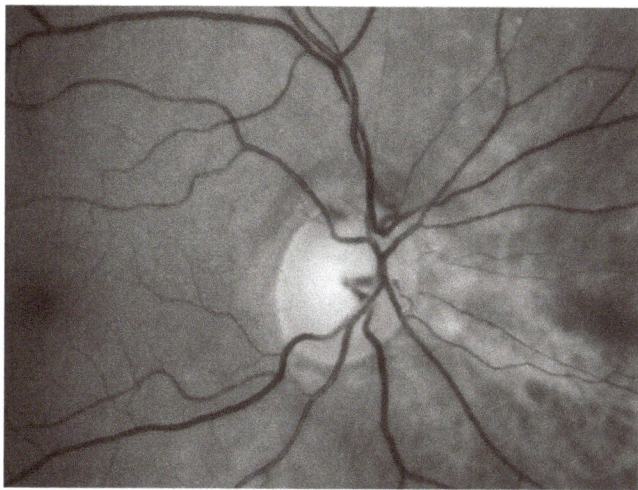

Fig. 2.2: Red free photo showing a small disc hemorrhage at superior margin of the right optic disc, with no nerve fiber layer defect.

curve ranged between 19 mm Hg and 17 mm Hg. OCT, slit lamp fundoscopy, computerized visual field and stereophotos showed no significant aspects. During his follow-up in 2016, his right disc photos and red free photos exhibited a disc hemorrhage (Figs. 2.1 and 2.2). The other exams showed no alterations. The patient was counseled regarding his presentation and proper treatment was initiated.

Learning Points

- Disc hemorrhages can be very subtle and delicate being a challenging sign for the doctor to observe on a daily practice where time and noncooperative patients are important issues to manage.[1]
- Disc hemorrhages are both a diagnostic and a progression marker for glaucoma, so immediate action to address this sign is mandatory.[4]
- Disc hemorrhages per se are not pathognomonic of glaucoma damage.

Case 3: Low central corneal thickness

A 55-year-old woman presented to the clinic with previous exams. There was a significant variance on the CCT—478 microns and 480 microns on her OD and OS, respectively, in 2013. During examination, she was diagnosed with a high myopia. Her CCT in 2016 was 460 microns and 465 microns; the gonioscopy showed an open angle and pigmentation of 2+/4+. Her other exams were not altered. Such a CCT demands appropriate investigation and close attention to her follow-ups.

Learning Points

- Central corneal thickness is both a progression and diagnostic marker; low CCT has been demonstrated to be cardinal regarding glaucoma management.[5,6]
- Although the CCT exam is not difficult to perform, its measurements may vary, leading to some misunderstanding.[7]
- The natural history of glaucoma guides the doctor to watch for progression in such cases; hence, follow-ups are imperative.

Case 4: Disc asymmetry

A 59-year-old woman was admitted at the clinic for an annual evaluation. She had a relevant disc asymmetry, small discs, and a deep cupping showing prominent lamina cribrosa pores. Her clinical history was negative for traumas, comorbidities and vascular events. C:D ratio was 0.2 in the right eye (Figs. 2.3 and 2.4) the OS had bigger C:D ratio and higher IOP value during a 4-year-follow-up (Figs. 2.5 and 2.6). The IOP ranged between 12 mm Hg and 15 mm Hg in the OD and 15–19 mm Hg in the OS with a CCT of 561 micra and 567 micra, on the OD and OS, respectively. Her other exams did not reveal notable alterations. She is still being annually assessed at the clinic and her stereophotos, OCT and computerized visual fields show no sign of progression.

Learning Points

- Deep disc cupping and focal lamina cribrosa defects may be associated with glaucoma progression.[8]

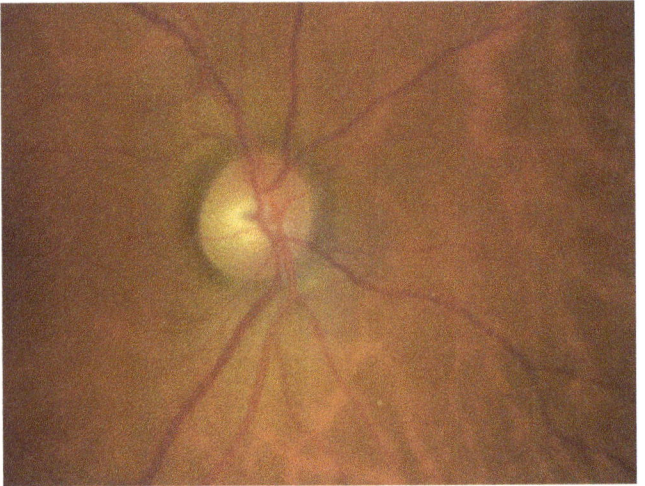

Fig. 2.3: OD optic disc C:D ratio 0.2.

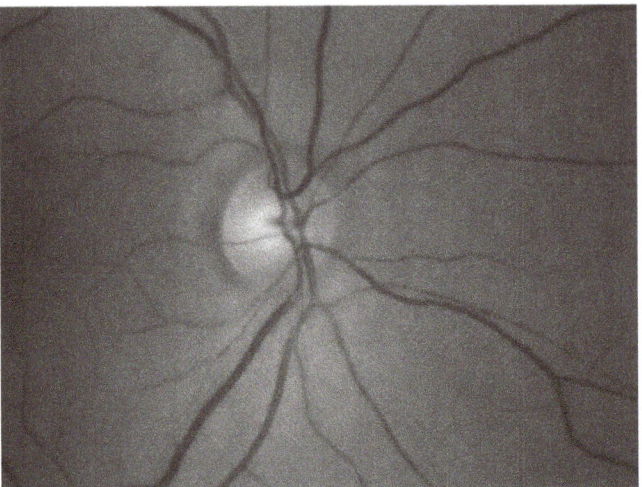

Fig. 2.4: Red free photo showing OD Optic disc C:D ratio 0.2 with no nerve fiber layer defects.

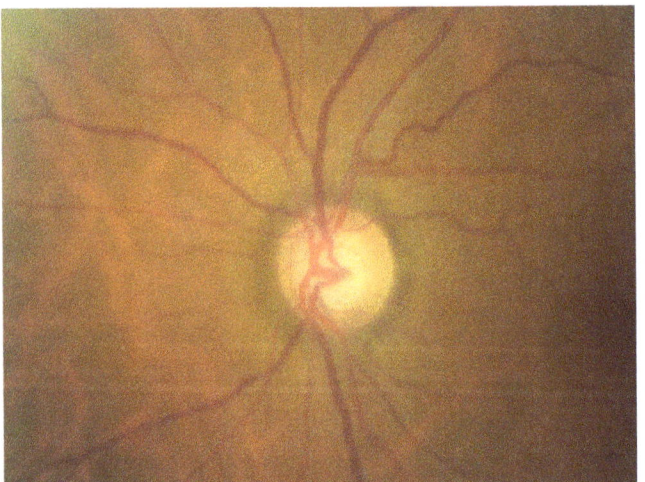

Fig. 2.5: OS C:D ratio of 0.6.

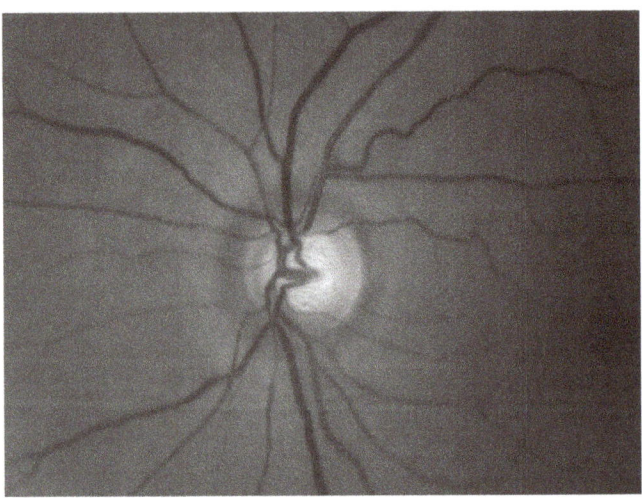

Fig. 2.6: Red free photo showing OD Optic disc C:D ratio 0.7 with no nerve fiber layer defects.

- Disc asymmetry is an essential marker for glaucoma diagnosis and should be closely and thoroughly studied.[3]
- Glaucoma is a chronic and progressive pathology, which can take years, even decades, to be pronounced. A consistent investigation is decisive to evaluate your patient risk for developing glaucoma.

Case 5: Diurnal variation of intraocular pressure

In 2013, a 75-year-old man was recommended to our clinic to be evaluated due to a diurnal IOP variation. He was under systemic hypertension treatment. He had a CCT of 534 microns and 544 microns on his OD and OS, respectively, open angle and pigmentation of 1+/4+. His OCT, stereophotos and computerized visual fields did not indicate relevant findings. His diurnal IOP curve ranged from 22 mm Hg to 13 mm Hg on his OD and from 21 mm Hg to 12 mm Hg on his OS. Another doctor performed his diurnal curve again on the same day on other Goldmann applanation tonometer to exclude any external interference. The IOP data was the similar on both tonometers. After a follow-up of 3 years, his diurnal curves continued to show a substantial variation in spite of not demonstrating any sign of glaucoma in his other exams.

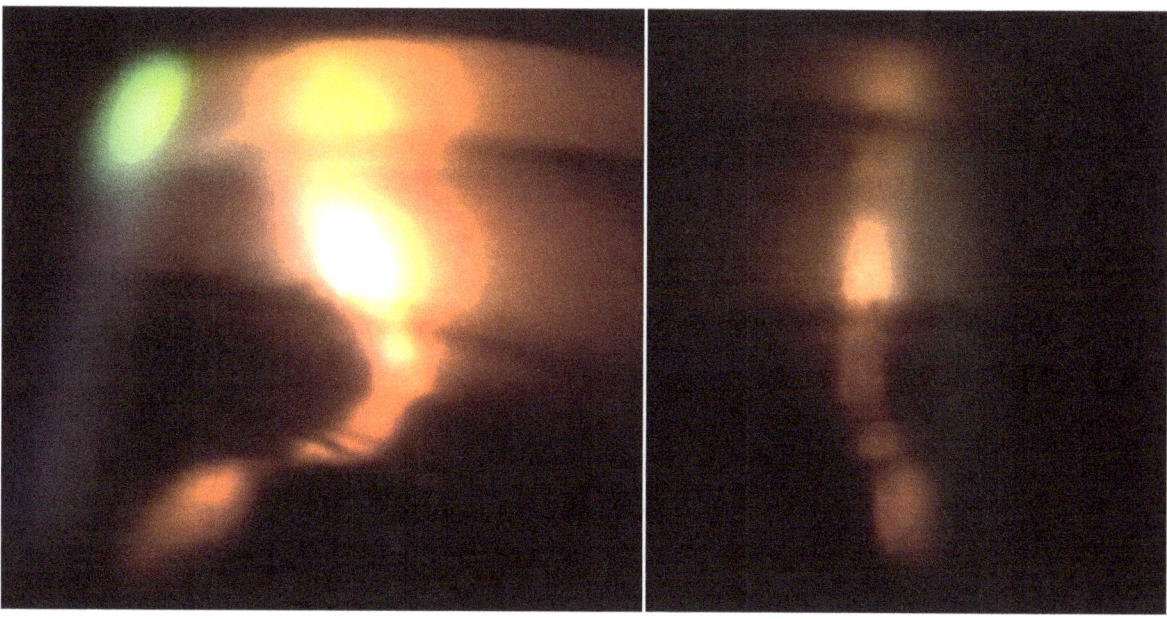

Fig. 2.7: Concave configuration of the iris.

Learning Points

- Cyclic fluctuations in IOP happen throughout the day. IOP measurement can vary depending on multiple factors, such as the patient's position, time of the day, drugs being used, and food and water intake and so on.[9,10]
- Glaucomatous patients can have IOP fluctuations higher than 10 mm Hg during the day whereas healthy subjects usually present fluctuations ranging between 2 mm Hg and 6 mm Hg. IOP variation is an important aspect of glaucoma management although its specific role concerning glaucoma progression has to be better studied and evaluated.[11,12]

Case 6: Glaucoma suspect at a young age

A young 24-year-old male was referred to the clinic to investigate for Krukenberg's spindle. In 2015, the patient's records show acute eye pain after strenuous exercises. His paternal uncle was suffering from glaucoma. His gonioscopy revealed a concave iris (Fig. 2.7) and 4+/4+ pigmented wide angle (Fig. 2.8) and slit lamp biomicroscopy confirmed the Krukenberg's spindle. His optic nerve heads were physiological. Other exams, such as OCT, stereophotos and computerized visual fields presented no significant changes. We performed a peripheral laser iridotomy on both eyes with controlled IOPs thereafter. His

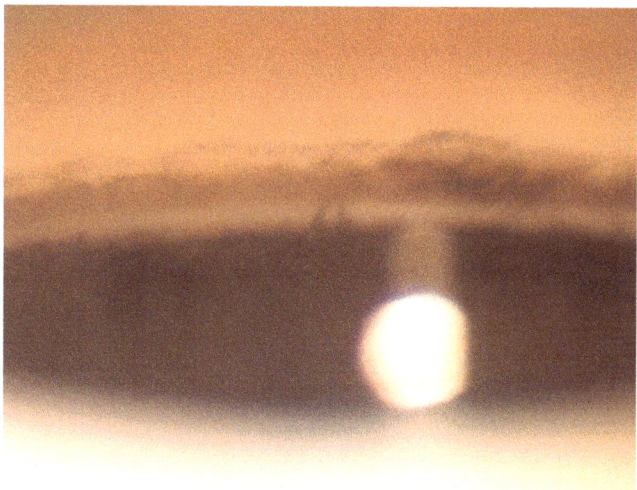

Fig. 2.8: Marked pigmentation in the angle on gonioscopy.

chances of developing glaucoma were a cause of constant anxiety for him. A very thorough advice and instructions were given and proper follow-up was planned.

Learning Points

- Tendency analysis over time, sometimes decades, is one of the most important aspects of managing glaucoma. This is not a single event pathology, and the patient has to be informed about this challenging reality.

- Most patients underestimate their chance of developing glaucoma, but anxious and more informed patients tend to over-react and have difficulties coping with a chronic pathology. Doctor-patient relationship builds up trust and provides the patient with a feeling of security, which, in turn, may ensure proper adherence to future treatments.

LITERATURE REVIEW

Intraocular Pressure

Intraocular pressure, a remarkable risk factor, is pivotal to the onset and development of glaucoma. Prevalence and incidence of glaucoma strongly increases when IOP is above 22 mm Hg.[11,13-18] Patients presenting with asymmetric IOPs were studied and findings had consistently demonstrated a more severe visual field loss in the eye with higher IOP when compared to the adelpho-eye.[19] IOPs ranging from 20 mm Hg to 30 mm Hg caused visual field loss in 6–12 % of the eyes in a study by Armaly.[20] Moreover, when the IOP exceeds 30 mm Hg the visual field loss reached 30% of the studied population. Patients presenting with IOPs of 22 mm Hg comprise 5% of the general population and it was found that amongst this ocular hypertensive population, 1–34% develop glaucoma in their lifetime.[21,22] Since elevated IOP is usually asymptomatic the ophthalmologist should perform a comprehensive examination and careful anamnesis in order to exclude other causes of this presentation. Different IOP readings can be yielded depending on the patient's cooperation, doctor's ability, tonometer's type and time of the day (higher in the early morning).[23] Thus, ocular hypertensive patients build up a heterogeneous group where both healthy and glaucomatous individuals are to be thoroughly examined to provide a proper treatment for each of them.

Optic Nerve Head

Optic nerve head features regarding glaucoma are strongly related to nerve fiber layer thinning. Retinal ganglion cells death leads to visible structural changes such as large C:D ratio, notch or notching, peripapillary atrophies and disc hemorrhages.[23]

Optic nerve head analysis is one of the most important steps for glaucoma diagnosis and its morphometric evaluation must include diffuse enlargement of the optic disc cup, focal optic disc damage, generalized and/or localized nerve fiber layer thinning.[24,25]

The disc cup is, in more than 93% of the patients, larger horizontally; but size, configuration and appearance of the optic nerve head have profound interindividual variations.[24,26]

Imaging techniques for structural evaluation are essential for follow-up, diagnosis and treatment of glaucoma. Stereoscopic optic disc head photos and OCT are pivotal to the challenging management of glaucoma suspects (Flowchart 2.1). Studies show that nerve fiber layer changes may occur until 5 years before any visual filed defect could be detected.[27-29]

Some reports state that 40% loss of ganglion cells may occur without any detection of functional defects.[30]

A retrospective study analyzed patients' data from 1950 to 2013 and found that disc hemorrhages, increasing C:D ratio above 0.7 and disc asymmetry above 0.3 provide a strong likelihood of diagnosing the patient with glaucoma.[31]

Disc hemorrhages are usually flame-shaped and occur at the edge of the optic nerve head. They are reported to be a strong independent risk factor regarding the development and progression of glaucoma and more related to normal tension glaucoma. Their transient characteristic provide us with a challenging sign to document, thus a comprehensive ophthalmoscopic examination and stereoscopic photographs are paramount. These hemorrhages develop at the border of the nerve fiber layer defect or at the edges of notches, and are often found in the inferotemporal and superotemporal areas. Patients presenting IOP higher than 22 mm Hg and disc hemorrhage are six times more likely to develop glaucoma than a patient which does not present such a hemorrhage. Large beta zones of atrophy, female sex, local vasospasm at the optic nerve head, blood flow autoregulation, migraine, nocturnal hypotension, increased age and small neuroretinal rims are risk factors for disc hemorrhages. Therefore, the simple presence of a disc hemorrhage in a previously glaucoma suspect patient must set a red flag and trigger a more aggressive treatment.[2-4]

Central Corneal Thickness

Central corneal thickness as an independent predictive factor for the development of glaucoma must be carefully assessed during examination.[5] Thinner corneas are present in the glaucomatous population and are both a risk factor and a progression factor.[6] CCT below 555 μm had a threefold higher risk for developing glaucoma when compared to patients with a CCT higher than 588 μm as showed by the ocular hypertension treatment study (OHTS).[7]

Flowchart 2.1: Glaucoma suspect management.

```
Elevated IOP I          Optic disc II         Visual field III        Angle analysis IV
     |                       |                      |                       |
     |                       |                      |                       v
     |                       |                      |                  Dark room
     |                       |                      |                  indentation
     |                       |                      |                  gonioscopy
     |                       |                      |                       |
     v        v              v                      v                       v
IOP > 24   21 < IOP <24  Disc asymmetry > 0.2  Neurologic cause?    Closed/Occludable/
(no risk   + Risk        Cup-to-disc ratio     Media opacity?       non-pupillary block
 factors*)   factors*    > 0.6                 Refractive error?    mechanism
                         Disc hemorrhage       Learning curve?
```

- Recheck IOP
- Gonioscopy
- OCT (RNFL thickness/GCC)
- Stereoscopic photography
- Visual field

Laser iridotomy

*Risk factors: race, myopia, age, family history, peripapillary atrophy, low central corneal thickness, pigment dispersion syndrome, pseudoexfoliation syndrome, Flammer syndrome, Alzheimer syndrome, migraine, ocular hypertension

Follow-up

Group I
Every 6 months

Treat (25-30%
IOP reduction)

Low or moderate risk   high-risk

Groups II and III
Every year

Groups I, II, III
Every 6 months

Groups I, II, III
Every 4 months

(IOP: Intraocular pressure; OCT: Optical coherence tomography; RNFL: Retinal nerve fiber layer; GCC: Ganglion cell complex).

Risk Factors for Glaucoma

Patients with glaucomatous first-degree relatives have a two to four times increase in their risk of developing glaucoma. An accurate glaucoma diagnosis deeply relies on anamnesis. Family history, advanced age, black race and myopia are well-established risk factors, migraine and vascular diseases are risk factors regarding normal tension glaucoma.[1,3] Low systolic blood pressure and vasospastic disorders were found to related and play a significant role in the pathogenesis of discs hemorrhages. Optic nerve hypoperfusion is a contributing factor for progression of normal tension glaucoma. Migraine is both a predictor for disc hemorrhage and a risk factor, as demonstrated in the collaborative normal tension glaucoma study.[2,32]

The burden of blindness must always be taken into account when it comes to glaucoma. Clinical acumen and technology embarked in our daily practice are the foundation of a solid glaucoma management.

REFERENCES

1. Sousa MC, Biteli LG, Dorairaj S, Maslin JS, Leite MT, Prata TS. Suitability of the visual field index according to glaucoma severity. J Curr Glaucoma Pract. 2015;9(3):65-8.
2. Fan N, Wang P, Tang L, Liu X. Ocular blood flow and normal tension glaucoma. Biomed Res Int. 2015;2015:308505.
3. Weinreb RN, Aung T, Medeiros FA. The pathophysiology and treatment of glaucoma: a review. JAMA. 2014;311(18): 1901-11.
4. Uhler TA, Piltz-Seymour J. Optic disc hemorrhages in glaucoma and ocular hypertension: implications and recommendations. Curr Opin Ophthalmol. 2008;19(2):89-94.
5. Saenz-Frances F, Jañez L, Berrozpe-Villabona C, Borrego-Sanz L, Morales-Fernández L, Acebal-Montero A, et al. Corneal segmentation analysis increases glaucoma diagnostic ability of optic nerve head examination, heidelberg retina tomograph's moorfield's regression analysis, and glaucoma probability score. J Ophthalmol. 2015;2015:215951.
6. Rashid RF, Farhood QK. Measurement of central corneal thickness by ultrasonic pachymeter and oculus pentacam in patients with well-controlled glaucoma: hospital-based comparative study. Clin Ophthalmol. 2016;10:359-64.

7. Pan CW, Li J, Zhong H, Shen W, Niu Z, Yuan Y, et al. Ethnic variations in central corneal thickness in a rural population in China: The Yunnan minority eye studies. PLoS One. 2015;10(8):e0135913.

8. Faridi OS, Park SC, Kabadi R, Su D, De Moraes CG, Liebmann JM, et al. Effect of focal lamina cribrosa defect on glaucomatous visual field progression. Ophthalmology. 2014;121(8):1524-30.

9. Syam PP, Mavrikakis I, Liu C. Importance of early morning intraocular pressure recording for measurement of diurnal variation of intraocular pressure. Br J Ophthalmol. 2005;89(7):926-7.

10. Liu JH, Zhang X, Kripke DF, Weinreb RN. Twenty-four-hour intraocular pressure pattern associated with early glaucomatous changes. Invest Ophthalmol Vis Sci. 2003;44(4):1586-90.

11. Rhee DJ. (2009). IOP Fluctuation: what's the connection? [online] Available from http://www.reviewofophthalmology.com/content/d/glaucoma_management/i/1217/c/22924/ [Accessed July, 2016].

12. Asrani S. (2014). Diurnal IOP control: how important is it? [online] Available from http://glaucomatoday.com/2014/08/diurnal-iop-control-how-important-is-it/ [Accessed July, 2016].

13. Sapienza A, Raveu AL, Reboussin E, Roubeix C, Boucher C, Dégardin J, et al. Bilateral neuroinflammatory processes in visual pathways induced by unilateral ocular hypertension in the rat. J Neuroinflammation. 2016;13:44.

14. Buhrmann RR, Quigley HA, Barron Y, West SK, Oliva MS, Mmbaga BB, et al. Prevalence of glaucoma in a rural East African population. Invest Ophthalmol Vis Sci. 2000;41(1):40-8.

15. Ramakrishnan R, Nirmalan PK, Krishnadas R, Thulasiraj RD, Tielsch JM, Katz J, et al. Glaucoma in a rural population of Southern India: the Aravind comprehensive eye survey. Ophthalmology. 2003;110(8):1484-90.

16. Sommer A, Tielsch JM, Katz J, Quigley HA, Gottsch JD, Javitt J, et al. Relationship between intraocular pressure and primary open angle glaucoma among white and black Americans. The Baltimore Eye Survey. Arch Ophthalmol. 1991;109(8):1090-5.

17. Kass MA, Heuer DK, Higginbotham EJ, Johnson CA, Keltner JL, Miller JP, et al. The ocular hypertension treatment study: a randomized trial determines that topical ocular hypotensive medication delays or prevents the onset of primary open-angle glaucoma. Arch Ophthalmol. 2002;120(6):701-13.

18. Leske MC, Heijl A, Hussein M, Bengtsson B, Hyman L, Komaroff E, et al. Factors for glaucoma progression and the effect of treatment: the early manifest glaucoma trial. Arch Ophthalmol. 2003;121(1):48-56.

19. Cartwright MJ, Anderson DR. Correlation of asymmetric damage with asymmetric intraocular pressure in normal-tension glaucoma (low-tension glaucoma). Arch Ophthalmol. 1988;106(7):898-900.

20. Armaly MF. Interpretation of the tonometry and ophthalmoscopy. Invest Ophthalmol. 1972;11(2):75-9.

21. Armaly MF. Ocular pressure and visual fields. A ten-year follow-up study. Arch Ophthalmol. 1969;81(1):25-40.

22. Klein BE, Klein R, Sponsel WE, Franke T, Cantor LB, Martone J, et al. Prevalence of glaucoma. The Beaver Dam Eye Study. Ophthalmology. 1992;99(10):1499-504.

23. Giuffrè G, Giammanco R, Dardanoni G, Ponte F. Prevalence of glaucoma and distribution of intraocular pressure in a population. The Casteldaccia Eye Study. Acta Ophthalmol Scand. 1995;73(3):222-5.

24. Dielemans I, Vingerling JR, Wolfs RC, Hofman A, Grobbee DE, de Jong PT. The prevalence of primary open-angle glaucoma in a population based study in The Netherlands. The Rotterdam Study. Ophthalmology. 1994;101(11):1851-5.

25. Jonas JB, Gusek GC, Naumann GO. Optic disc, cup and neuroretinal rim size, configuration and correlations in normal eyes. Invest Ophthalmol Vis Sci. 1988;29(7):1151-8.

26. Tuulonen A, Airaksinen PJ. Initial glaucomatous optic disc and retinal nerve fiber layer abnormalities and their progression. Am J Ophthalmol. 1991;111(4):485-90.

27. Garway-Heath DF, Ruben ST, Viswanathan A, Hitchings RA. Vertical cup/disc ratio in relation to optic disc size: its value in the assessment of the glaucoma suspect. Br J Ophthalmol. 1998;82(10):1118-24.

28. Damms T, Dannheim F. Sensitivity and specificity of optic disc parameters in chronic glaucoma. Invest Ophthalmol Vis Sci. 1993;34(7):2246-50.

29. Quigley HA. Open-angle glaucoma. N Engl J Med. 1993;328(15):1097-106.

30. Harasymowycz P, Kamdeu Fansi A, Papamatheakis D. Screening for primary open-angle glaucoma in the developed world: are we there yet? Can J Ophthalmol. 2005;40(4):477-86.

31. Hollands H, Johnson D, Hollands S, Simel DL, Jinapriya D, Sharma S. Do findings on routine examination identify patients at risk for primary open-angle glaucoma? The rational clinical examination systematic review. JAMA. 2013;309(19):2035-42.

32. Chung HJ, Hwang HB, Lee NY. The association between primary open-angle glaucoma and blood pressure: two aspects of hypertension and hypotension. Biomed Res Int. 2015;2015:827516.

CHAPTER 3

Primary Open-Angle Glaucoma

Shibal Bhartiya, Parul Ichhpujani

▌ INTRODUCTION

Primary open-angle glaucoma (POAG) is a chronic progressive optic neuropathy defined by an open, normal appearing anterior chamber angle and raised intraocular pressure (IOP), with no other underlying disease, in the presence of the characteristic cupping of the optic disc with corresponding visual field defects, due to retinal ganglion cell loss. If there is an identifiable underlying cause for raised IOP, this is termed secondary glaucoma. If the IOP is within normal limits, this is termed normal-tension glaucoma (NTG) or low-tension glaucoma (LTG).

Case 1: No treatment required for early primary open-angle glaucoma

Mr X, a 72-year-old gentleman, was found to have persistently elevated IOPs on three visits [oculus uterque (OU) 23, 24, 24 mm Hg]. The cup-to-disc (C:D) ratio was 0.5:1 and 0.45:1 with slightly eccentric cup with inferior > superior > nasal > temporal (ISNT) maintained (Fig. 3.1). The visual field [humphrey visual field (HVF) 30–2, Swedish Interactive Threshold Algorithms standard] showed early changes suggestive of glaucomatous damage (Fig. 3.2). The central corneal thickness (CCT) was 531 microns and

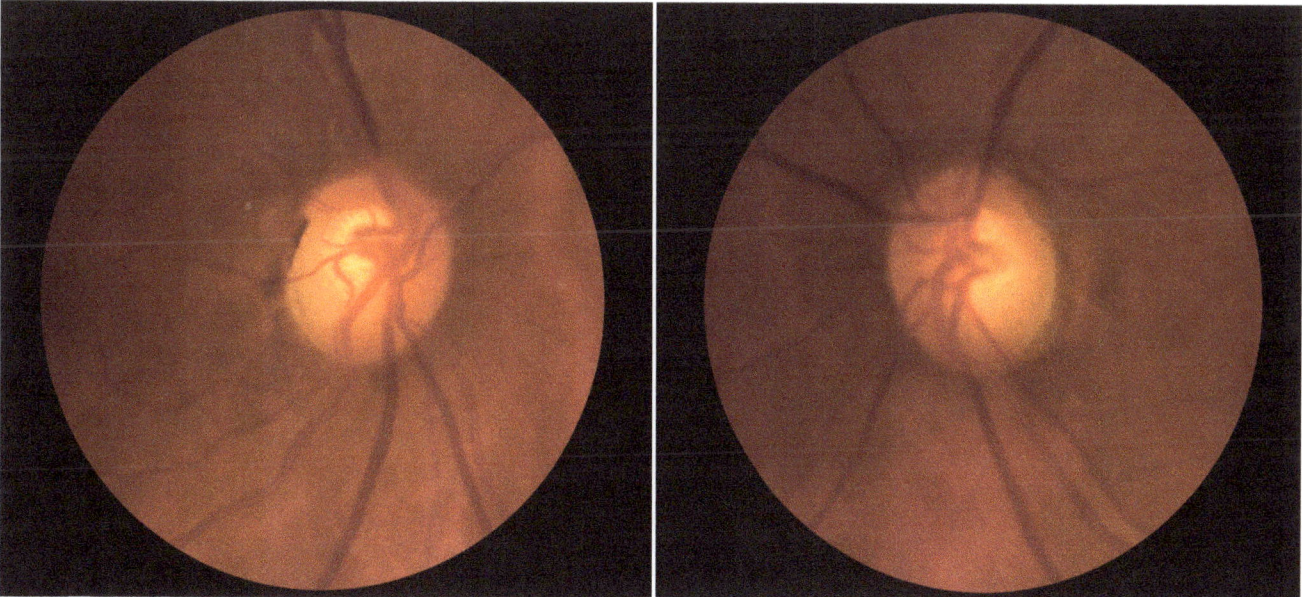

Fig. 3.1: Vertical cup-to-disc ratio of 0.5:1 and 0.45:1, with slightly eccentric cup with ISNT rule maintained.

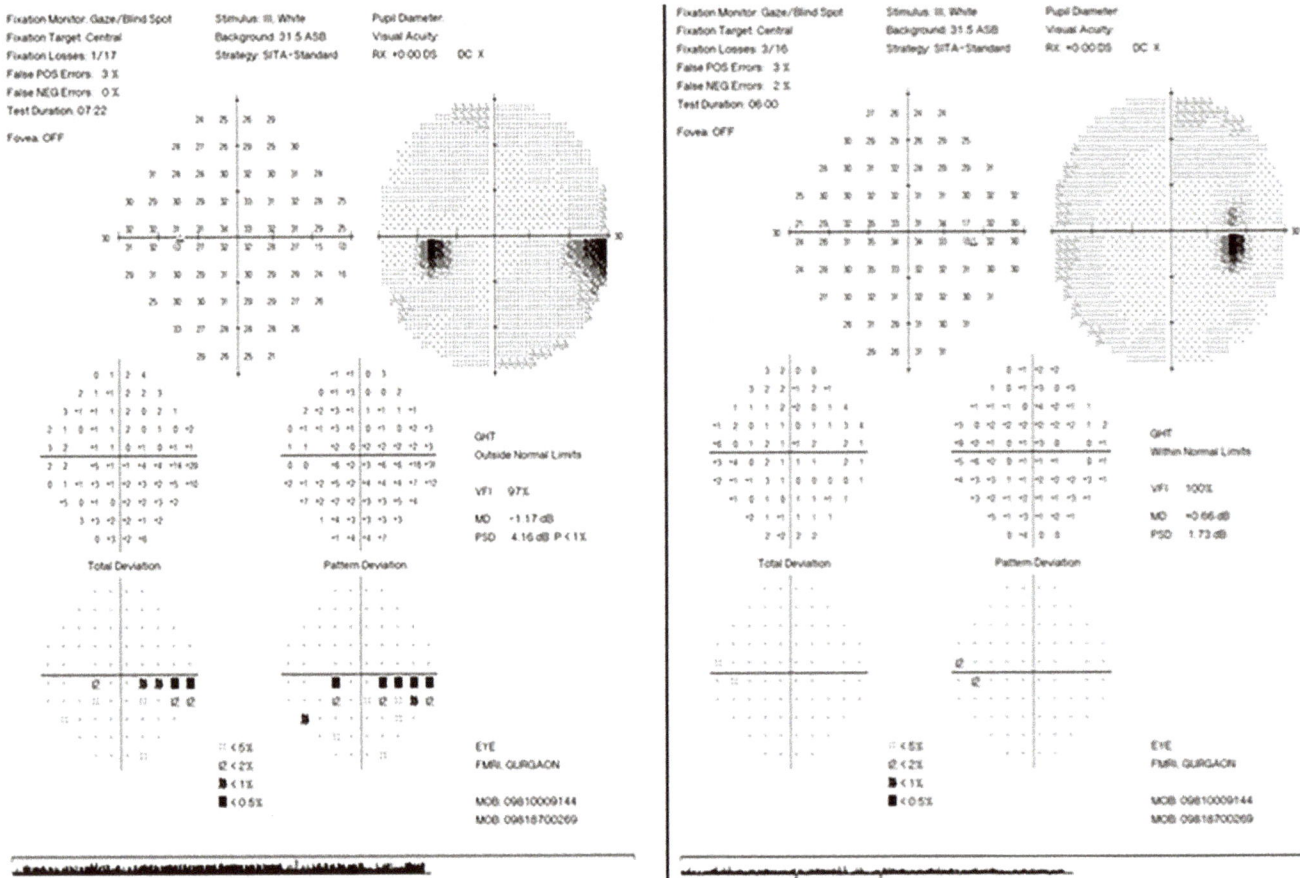

Fig. 3.2: Early glaucomatous damage in left eye.

522 microns for the right and left eyes, respectively. The retinal nerve fiber layer (RNFL) optical coherence tomography (OCT) (CIRRUS) did show early RNFL thinning (Fig. 3.3), and gonioscopy showed wide open angles with no pigmentation. He had a coronary artery bypass surgery 6 years ago and was a hypertensive on medication. There was no family history of glaucoma or blindness.

Risks and benefits of initiating glaucoma therapy were discussed with Mr X, keeping in mind the following:
- Life expectancy
- Early field defects
- Slightly elevated eye pressures
- Pre-existing dry eye due to old age which would probably get exacerbated with antiglaucoma medication.

He agreed that deferring treatment was better than initiating treatment immediately on diagnosis. He was asked to follow-up every 4–6 months for 2 years. His visual fields did not show any significant change on serial monitoring. The visual field evaluation was thereafter scheduled for once a year.

Case 2: Treatment for early primary open-angle glaucoma required depending on age

Ms A, a 53-year-old lady, was found to have persistently elevated IOPs on three visits (OU 28, 24, 25 mm Hg) with a diurnal fluctuation of 8 mm Hg in both the eyes. The cup: disc ratio was 0.6:1 and 0.55:1 with a focal neuroretinal rim thinning. The visual field showed early changes suggestive of glaucomatous damage (Fig. 3.4). The CCT was 532 and 526 for the right and left eyes, respectively. The RNFL OCT (Cirrus) showed RNFL thinning (Fig. 3.5), and gonioscopy showed wide open angles. She had no comorbidities. There was no family history of glaucoma or blindness.

Risks and benefits of initiating glaucoma therapy were discussed with Ms A, keeping in mind the following:
- Long-life expectancy
- Early field defects
- Slightly elevated eye pressures.

ONH and RNFL OU Analysis: Optic Disc Cube 200 × 200   OD ⬤ | ⬤ OS

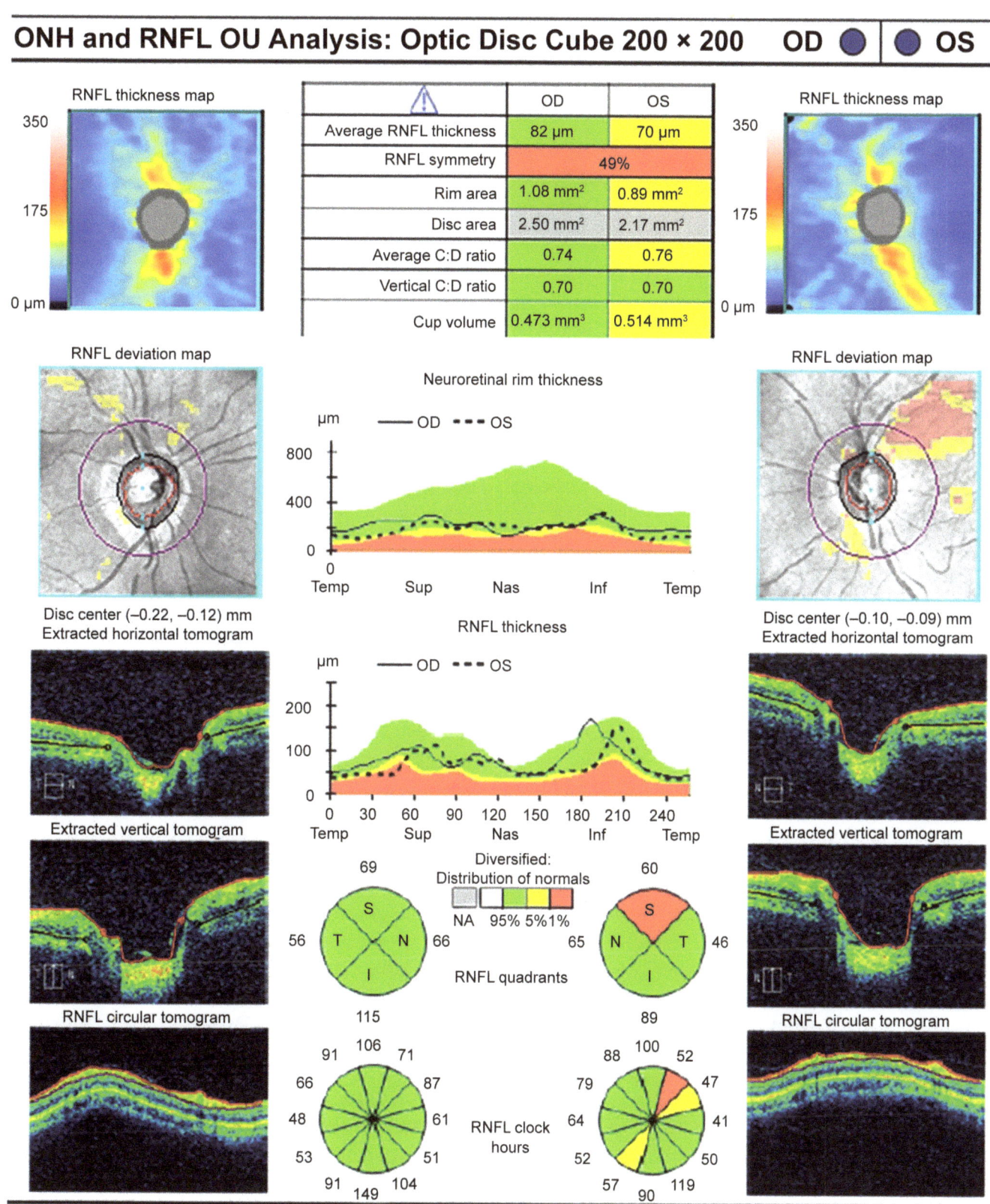

⚠	OD	OS
Average RNFL thickness	82 µm	70 µm
RNFL symmetry	49%	
Rim area	1.08 mm²	0.89 mm²
Disc area	2.50 mm²	2.17 mm²
Average C:D ratio	0.74	0.76
Vertical C:D ratio	0.70	0.70
Cup volume	0.473 mm³	0.514 mm³

Fig. 3.3: Early RNFL thinning in the left eye on SDOCT.
(ONH: Optic nerve head; RNFL: Retinal nerve fiber layer; SDOCT: Spectral domain optical coherence tomography).

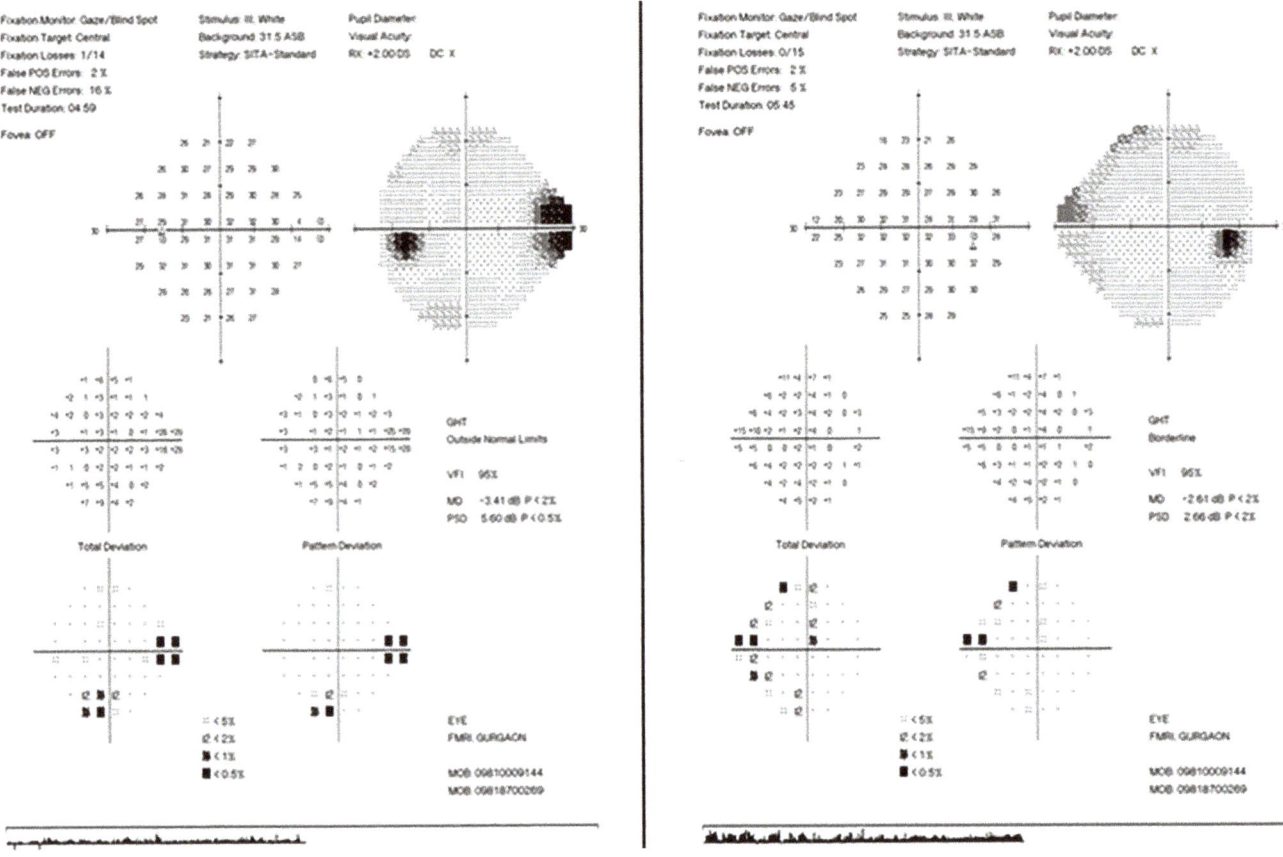

Fig. 3.4: Early glaucomatous visual field defects.

She agreed that it was better to initiate treatment immediately on diagnosis. She was prescribed travoprost eye drops, one drop each eye, once at bedtime in both eyes and asked to follow-up after 6 weeks. The IOP was found to be 18 mm Hg OU with a diurnal fluctuation of 4 mm Hg and 5 mm Hg, respectively. She was advised to repeat fields after 6 months, and no significant change on serial monitoring was noted for over 2 years. She was advised to continue drops as prescribed.

Case 3: Treatment for early primary open-angle glaucoma required depending on central corneal thickness

Mrs X, a 68-year-old lady was found to have persistently elevated IOPs on three visits (OU 24, 25, 25 mm Hg), with a diurnal fluctuation of 9 mm Hg and 8 mm Hg, respectively. The cup: disc ratio was 0.7 and 0.65 with corresponding early changes on visual fields suggestive of glaucomatous damage. The CCT was 472 μ and 482 μ for the right and left eyes, respectively. The RNFL OCT (CIRRUS) showed early RNFL thinning (Fig. 3.6), and gonioscopy showed wide open angles. She had no comorbidities. There was no family history of glaucoma or blindness.

Risks and benefits of initiating glaucoma therapy were discussed with Ms X, keeping in mind the following:
- Life expectancy
- Early field defects
- Elevated eye pressures
- Increased chances of progression in CCT less than 520 microns.

She agreed that it was better to initiate treatment immediately on diagnosis. She was prescribed bimatoprost eye drops, one drop each eye, once at bedtime in both eyes and asked to follow-up after 6 weeks. The IOP was found to be 16 OU with a diurnal fluctuation of 4 mm Hg and 3 mm Hg, respectively. She was advised to repeat fields after 6 months and no significant change on serial monitoring for over 2 years. She complained of dryness in both eyes and was prescribed carboxymethylcellulose eye drops, thrice a day, which obviated her symptoms. She was advised to continue drops as prescribed, and the visual field evaluation was thereafter scheduled for once a year.

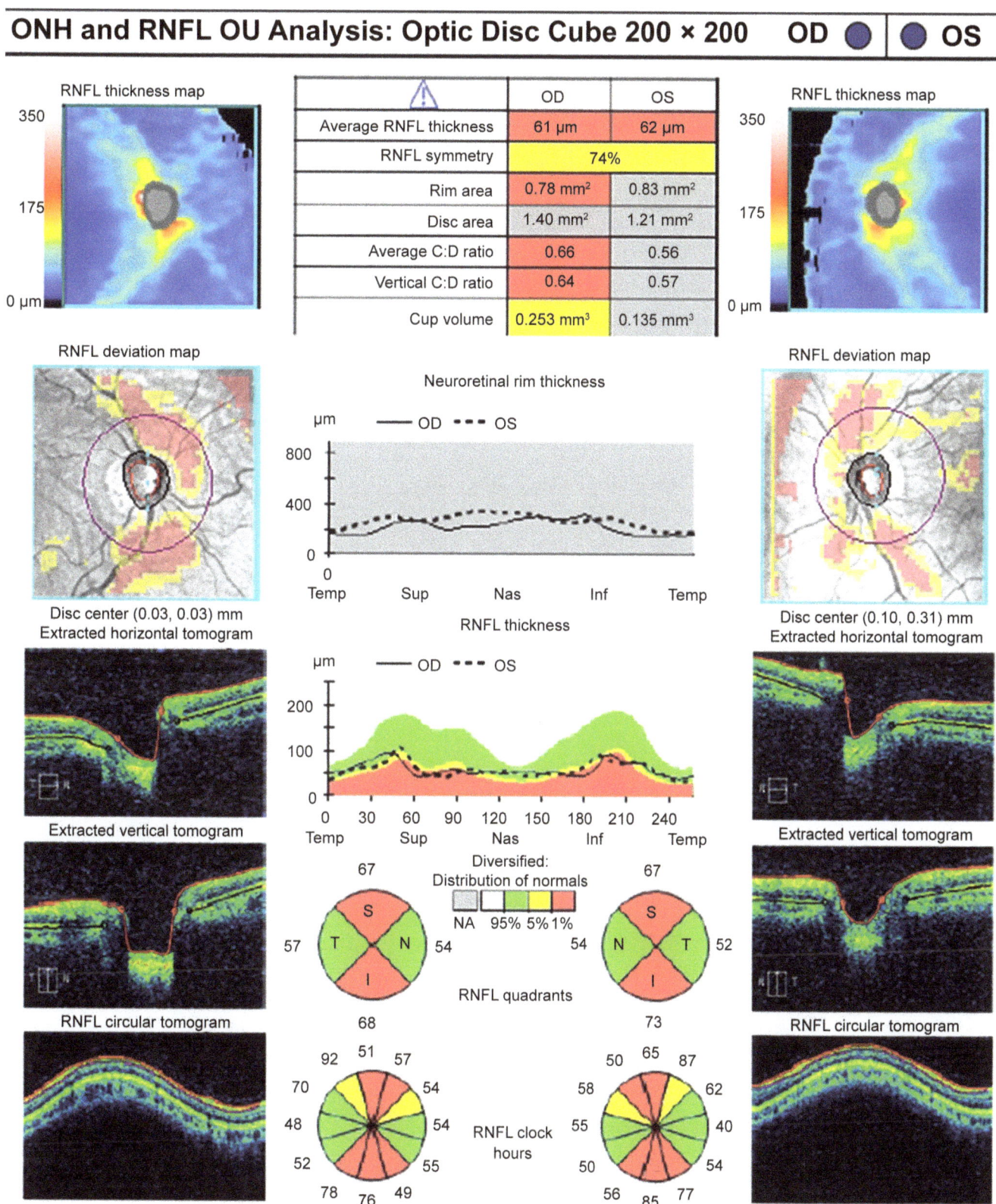

Fig. 3.5: Flattening of retinal nerve fiber layer humps on SDOCT.
(ONH: Optic nerve head; RNFL: Retinal nerve fiber layer; SDOCT: Spectral domain optical coherence tomography).

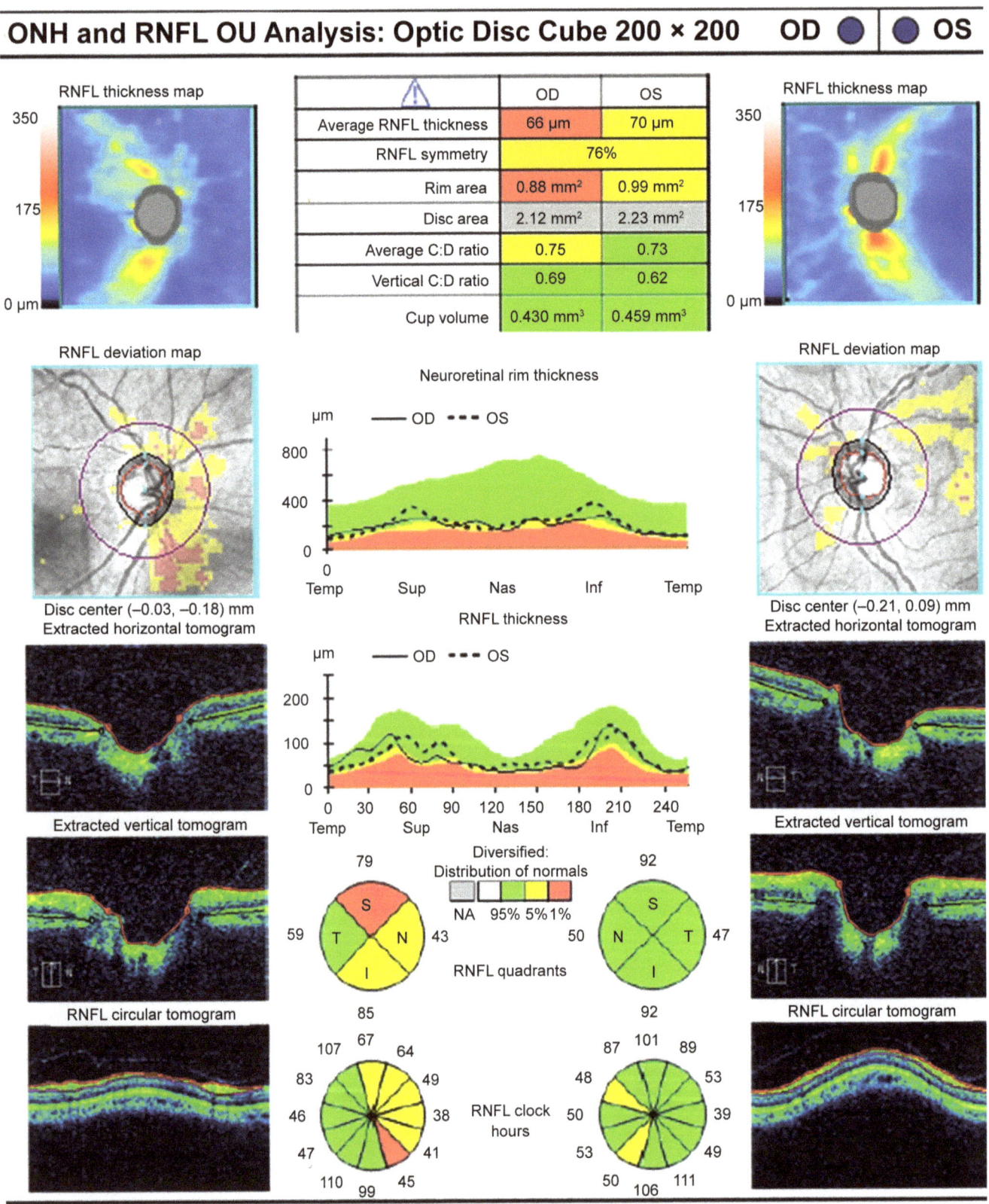

Fig. 3.6: SDOCT showing thinning of retinal nerve fibre layer in right eye.
(ONH: Optic nerve head; RNFL: Retinal nerve fiber layer; SD OCT: Spectral domain optical coherence tomography).

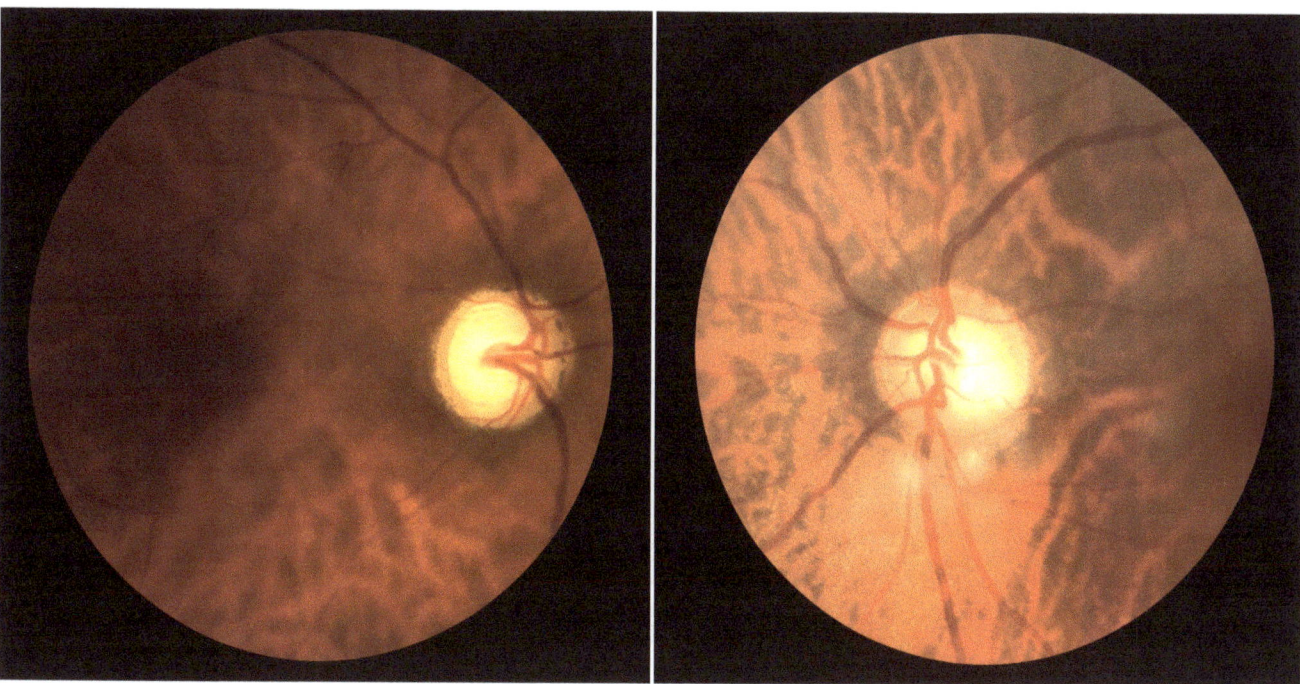

Fig. 3.7: Vertical cup-to-disc ratio of 0.85 and 0.7, with broken ISNT rule.

Case 4: Treatment for moderate primary open-angle glaucoma requiring more than one antiglaucoma medication

Mr X, a 67-year-old gentleman, was diagnosed with moderate POAG with persistently elevated IOPs on two visits (OD and OS: 34, 35 mm Hg) with a diurnal fluctuation of 8 mm Hg OU. The C:D ratio was 0.85 and 0.7 with broken ISNT rule and corresponding moderate glaucomatous damage on visual fields (Fig. 3.7). The CCT was 522 and 512 for the right and left eyes, respectively. The RNFL OCT also showed flattening of RNFL humps and gonioscopy showed wide open angles.

Risks and benefits of initiating glaucoma therapy were discussed with him, keeping in mind the following:
- Life expectancy
- Field defects
- Elevated eye pressures
- Increased chances of progression in CCT less than 520 microns.

He agreed that it was better to initiate treatment immediately on diagnosis and to try a single medication for efficacy and safety rather than combination therapy. He was prescribed bimatoprost eye drops, one drop each eye, once at bedtime in both eyes, and asked to follow-up after 2 days. The IOP was found to be 24 mm Hg OU, and he was thereafter asked to report for a water drinking test (WDT) after 4 weeks. The IOP was found to be 22 mm Hg OU with a diurnal fluctuation of 4 mm Hg and 6 mm Hg, respectively.

Since the target IOP was not reached with one drug, a fixed dose combination of bimatoprost and timolol was advised, once at bedtime. The fact that the efficacy of timolol is less at night was weighed against the chances of reduced compliance with addition of a second bottle. This was discussed with the patient and he preferred to use a fixed-dose combination (FDC) in view of convenience of use. At 4 weeks follow-up, the IOP was found to be 16 mm Hg OU with a diurnal fluctuation of 3 mm Hg and 5 mm Hg, respectively.

He was advised to repeat fields after 4 months and no significant change was observed on serial monitoring for over 2 years. He was advised to continue drops as prescribed and the visual field evaluation was thereafter rescheduled for once every 6 months, with a RNFL OCT performed annually.

Case 5: Treatment of severe primary open-angle glaucoma requiring surgery since not controlled on maximal tolerable medical therapy

Mr X, a 69-year-old pseudophakic gentleman, was on treatment for advanced POAG over the last 6 years with persistently elevated IOPs on two visits (OD and OS: 26, 25)

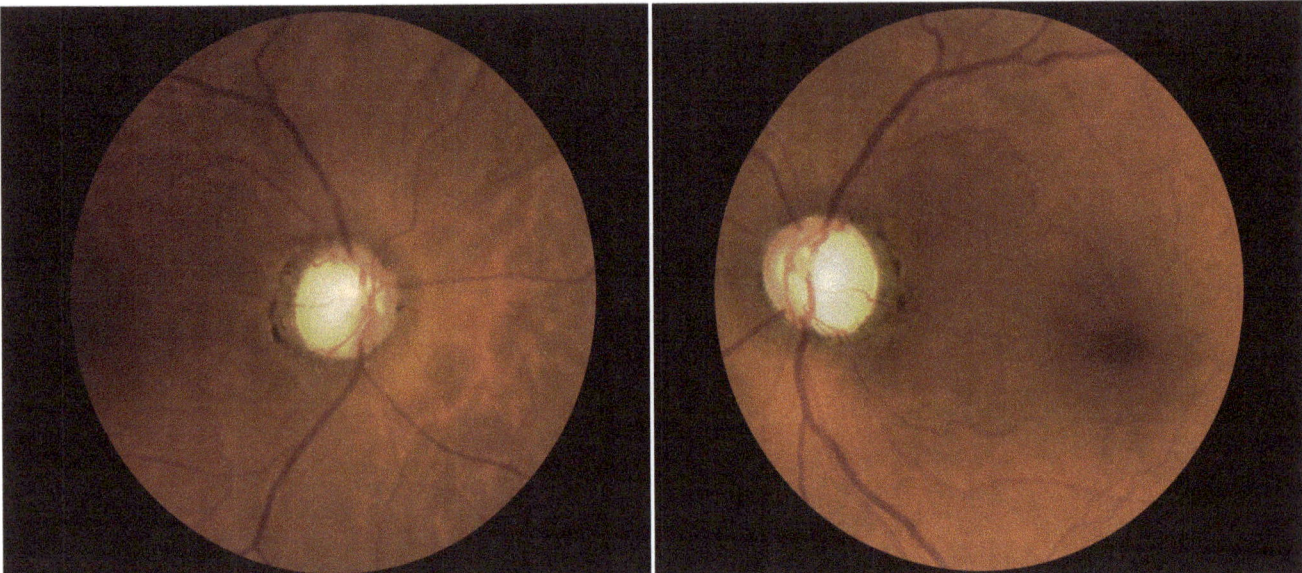

Fig. 3.8: Vertical cup-to-disc ratio of 0.9 OU with a marked concentric neuroretinal rim loss.

with a diurnal fluctuation of 8 mm Hg OU on treatment [bimatoprost harmonized system (HS), brimonidine + timolol FDC BD, brinzolamide BD]. The C:D ratio was 0.9 OU with a marked concentric neuroretinal rim (NRR) loss (Fig. 3.8). The visual field could not be performed to poor visual acuity. The CCT was 532 and 541 for the right and left eyes, respectively. Risks and benefits of glaucoma surgery were discussed with him and he agreed that it was better to go ahead with surgery since even maximal topical therapy was insufficient to control his IOP.

He was advised trabeculectomy augmented with mitomycin C, for the right eye first, followed by the left eye. After surgery his IOP was 16 and 18, respectively, without any medication, despite release of the releasable sutures in the early postoperative period. He required the addition of a prostaglandin analog (bimatoprost HS, OU) to achieve target pressure of 11 mm Hg and 12 mm Hg, respectively. He attained the target IOP and then he was advised to continue drops as prescribed.

Case 6: Treatment of severe primary open-angle glaucoma requiring surgery at first diagnosis due to severe visual field loss

Mrs X, a 65-year-old pseudophakic lady with diabetes, presented to the outpatients clinic with IOP of 32 both eyes, and a near total optic atrophy in the right eye, and a C:D ratio of 0.85 OD and 0.9:1 OS. Her best-corrected visual acuity in right eye was 6/60 and 3/60 in the left eye.

A 24-2 HVF OD was predictably showing a severe visual field loss encroaching fixation and a 10-2 test was there after advised, which showed split fixation. Visual field in left eye could not be performed due to poor vision.

The possibility of imminent visual loss was discussed with her and the risks and benefits of primary surgery were also discussed with the patient and her family. Given the advanced stage of glaucomatous damage, high IOP, it was decided to perform a primary trabeculectomy on both eyes at an interval of 4 weeks. In the interim, she was referred to an internist for euglycemic control and prescribed bimatoprost HS, brimonidine + timolol FDC BD and brinzolamide BD eye drops for both eyes. After surgery, her IOP was 12 and 11, respectively, without any medication following release of the releasable sutures in the early postoperative period for the left eye only. A repeat field was ordered after 4 months for the right eye and no significant change was observed on serial monitoring for over a year.

INVESTIGATIONS

Every patient of glaucoma requires a careful and comprehensive eye examination. Mandatory tests include:
- **Visual Acuity and Refraction**
- **Tonometry (Applanation)**
  On at least two different occasions, at different times of the day, with IOP more than 21 mm Hg is mandatory for diagnosing POAG. IOP less than 21 mm Hg does not rule out glaucoma.

- **Slit Lamp Examination**
  A through slit lamp evaluation is mandatory to rule out any secondary reasons for elevated IOP.
- **Gonioscopy**
  Anatomically normal and open angles are mandatory for diagnosing POAG.
- **Optic Nerve Assessment**
  A dilated assessment of the optic nerve head (ONH) is essential together with a red-free evaluation of the peripapillary RNFL. The ONH can be documented using a hand-drawn, labeled diagram (special emphasis on cup/disc ratio, notching, RNFL defects and/or hemorrhage) and/or a clinical picture. A color photo and a red-free photo of the ONH are essential for serial follow-up.
- **Visual Field Testing**
  Reliable visual fields provide a baseline for future follow-up. The first visual fields are usually discarded as unreliable or having a learning curve.
- **Central Corneal Thickness (Pachymetry)**
  It is an adjunct that helps to make therapeutic decisions.
- **Imaging of the Optic Nerve with Retinal Nerve Fiber Layer Analysis**
  Imaging of the optic nerve with RNFL analysis (ocular coherence tomography, Heidelberg retinal tomography or scanning laser polarimetry) provides a statistical comparison with the normative database, thereby providing additional objective information for subsequent management.

  In addition, the following tests, if performed, help in managing the condition better in case the facilities exist and are affordable to the patient.
- **Diurnal Variation of Intraocular Pressure**
  A 24-hour diurnal variation of IOP includes IOP recording every 2 hours, preferably using the same Goldmann applanation tonometry, by the same observer, whenever possible. A diurnal variation of more than 8 mm over 24 hours is considered indicative of glaucoma. Diurnal variation of IOP curve may provide additional information and influence treatment protocol.
- **Water Drinking Test**
  A WDT with 10 mL/kg body weight of water over 5 minutes may be performed as a surrogate for diurnal variation of IOP to provide a rough idea of IOP peaks and fluctuation.
- Stereo-optic disc photographs to confirm normal optic nerve parameters and document baseline.

Table 3.1: Severity of primary open-angle glaucoma.

Severity	Description
Mild	GON + normal visual field on SAP
Moderate	GON + VFD in one hemifield, but not within 5° of fixation on SAP
Severe	GON + VFD in both hemifields ± loss within 5° of fixation in at least one hemifield on SAP

(GON: Glaucomatous optic neuropathy; VFD: Visual field defect; SAP: Standard automated perimetry).
Source: American Academy of Ophthalmology Glaucoma Panel. (2010). Preferred practice pattern guidelines. Primary open-angle glaucoma. [online] Available from www.aao.org/ppp. [Accessed July, 2016].

- Based on the above investigations POAG severity can be graded as mentioned in Table 3.1.

FOLLOW-UP PROTOCOL

Follow-up protocol is to be customized to the individual patient depending on the risk of developing glaucoma, risk factors present and whether treatment has been initiated or not. Initially, a follow-up may be scheduled after 4–6 weeks for safety and efficacy checks after initiating topical antiglaucoma therapy. Six fields, done over 2 years, are required for establishing the rate of progression.

Repeat visual field and optic nerve testing may be performed annually or sooner if changes are suspected.

WHAT IS THE NATURAL COURSE OF THE DISEASE?

- Of approximately 1.2 million RGC at birth, about 25% are naturally lost over 75 years.
- With POAG retinal ganglion cell loss is accelerated with a generally slow, but variable rate of loss.
- Up to 40% of optic nerve fibers need to be lost before a visual field defect appears on automated perimetry usually progressing from paracentral or mid-peripheral defect in the earlier stages to temporal visual field loss and loss of central fixation points in advanced disease.
- On comparing the mean age at presentation of patients with early relative visual field loss to those with absolute field loss within 5° of fixation, the estimated average time for untreated early disease to progress to end-stage blindness substratified by IOP levels 21–25 mm Hg, 25–30 mm Hg, and more than 30 mm Hg was 14.4 years, 6.5 years and 2.9 years, respectively.

Table 3.2: Randomized clinical trials in primary open angle glaucoma establishing the role of intraocular pressure lowering in reducing development and progression of disease.

Trial	No. of patients	Follow-up years	Study	Intervention	Outcome
OHTS	1,636	10	Eyes without POAG and IOP 24–32 mm Hg 20% IOPR	Medications	POAG risk: 4.4% treated vs. 9% untreated 10% increased risk for every mm Hg increase
CNTGS	230	7	POAG in eyes with IOP< 24 mm Hg 30% IOPR	Medications and surgery	POAG progression: 12% treated vs. 35% untreated
EMGT	255	7–11	Newly diagnosed early stage POAG. IOPR protocol driven	Betaxolol and laser trabeculoplasty or no treatment	POAG progression: 45% treated vs. 62% untreated
CIGTS	607	5+	Newly diagnosed POAG. IOPR protocol driven	Medications and surgery	No significant difference in visual field loss with initial trabeculectomy (−46%) vs. medical therapy (−38%)
AGIS	591	10–13	Advanced POAG. IOPR protocol driven	Argon laser trabeculoplasty (A) and trabeculectomy (T): ATT and TAT sequences	Visual function outcomes better with ATT in blacks and TAT in whites. Mean visual field loss 3 times greater when IOP 14.0–17.5 mm Hg vs.< 14.0 mm Hg.

(POAG: Primary open-angle glaucoma; OHTS: Ocular hypertension treatment study; IOPR: Intraocular pressure reduction; CNTGS: Collaborative normal-tension glaucoma study; EMGT: Early manifest glaucoma trial; CIGTS: Collaborative initial glaucoma treatment study; AGIS: Advanced glaucoma intervention study; ATT: Argon trabeculoplasty followed by trabeculectomy followed by trabeculectomy; TAT: Trabeculectomy followed by argon trabeculoplasty followed by trabeculectomy).

- Early manifest glaucoma trial (EMGT) has shown that progression was faster in older than in younger patients ($p = 0.002$), and those with newly diagnosed untreated pseudoexfoliative glaucoma (PXFG) (93%) compared with high-tension glaucoma (HTG) (74%) or NTG (56%) ($p = 0.012$) over 5 years. Median time to progression also differed considerably among groups: 19.5 months in pseudoexfoliation glaucoma, 44.8 months in HTG and 61.1 months in NTG (p less than 0.0001).
- Table 3.2 enlists the trials, which show the beneficial effect of IOP lowering in reducing the disease progression.

BROAD GUIDELINES FOR MANAGEMENT

The goals of treatment in POAG are to control IOP in a target range and to maintain stable optic nerves, RNFL and visual fields. The target IOP is different for each patient and is the pressure at which it is thought that the patient will not sustain further damage. Table 3.3 enlists the risk categories, which guide treatment targets.

POINTS TO REMEMBER

1. Intraocular pressure must be measured two or more times on separate occasions before labeling a patient as having elevated eye pressures. The risk for ONH damage increases 10 times when IOP more than or equal to 24 mm Hg, more than 40 times when IOP more than 30 mm Hg.

2. A gonioscopy must be performed to rule out angle closure and a slit lamp biomicroscopy, and/or imaging studies of the ONH must be performed to document optic nerve damage. A reliable visual field is essential for diagnosing glaucoma.

3. A pachymetry is required to give an indication of the eyes ability to withstand higher pressures. There are *no* validated nomograms for IOP correction on the basis of CCT. IOP corrected for corneal thickness, therefore, does not provide a valid basis for initiating or not initiating therapy.

4. The threshold for starting treatment and establishing target IOP for POAG must be lower for patients with increased risk factors. These include:
   - *Race:* West Africans, Afro-Caribbeans and Hispanics have the highest predilection for disease as well as blindness
   - *Family history:* Family history of glaucoma, or glaucoma-induced blindness: a first-degree relative with POAG increases the risk 9 times, and increases the risk of disease to and 23%
   - *Age:* Younger patients

Table 3.3: Risk categories to guide treatment targets for primary open angle glaucoma.

Risk category*	Description	Treatment targets
High	• Moderate-advanced GON with VFD+ • Higher IOP • Rapid progression • Bilateral VFD • Pigmentary or pseudoexfoliative glaucoma • Advanced VFD or fixation threat • Glaucoma-related visual disability • Younger age	≥40% IOPR or 1–2 SD below population mean (9–12 mm Hg)
Moderate	• Mild GON with early VFD • Mild-moderate GON with low IOP • Younger age	>30% IOP reduction or population mean
Glaucoma suspect with moderate risk	• Fellow eye of established GON: excluding secondary unilateral glaucoma • OH with multiple risk factors: thin CCT, high IOP, suspicious discs • GLC gene mutations associated with severe POAG • Recurrent disc hemorrhages • Pseudoexfoliation • Younger age	Monitor closely for change or treat depending on risk and patient preferences Treat if risk(s) increase(s) with ≥20% IOP reduction or 1 SD above population mean
Glaucoma suspect with low risk	• OH • Older age • Pigment dispersion with normal IOP • Glaucoma suspect disc, including disc asymmetry • Glaucoma family history • Less important: 　– Steroid responder 　– Myopia 　– β-peripapillary atrophy 　– Diabetes mellitus 　– Uveitis 　– Systemic hypertension	Monitor

(GON: Glaucomatous optic neuropathy; VFD: Visual field defect; IOP: Intraocular pressure; IOPR: Intraocular pressure reduction; OH: Ocular hypertension; CCT: Central corneal thikness; GLC: Glaucoma; POAG: Primary open-angle glaucoma).
Source: Adapted from Asia-Pacific Glaucoma Guidelines, 2nd edition. 2008.

- *Patients with myopia:* Myopic eyes may have weaker scleral support, thus becoming more susceptible to damage, with an additional familial link between the two diseases.
- Patients with poor access to repeat glaucoma investigations.
- *Thin CCT:* A CCT of less than or equal to 555 μm increased the risk three times as compared with a CCT more than 588 μm. For every 40 μm decrease in CCT, the relative risk of developing POAG is 1.71
- *Optic nerve head hemorrhage:* Disc hemorrhage increases risk of POAG 3.7 times, although most eyes with the hemorrhage (87%) may not develop POAG over 5 years (OHTS)
- *Low Ocular Perfusion Pressure:* Diastolic ocular perfusion pressure (OPP) [diastolic blood pressure (BP) – IOP] less than 50 mm Hg may alter blood flow to the ONH and systolic OPP (systolic BP – IOP)

less than or equal to 125 mm Hg is known to have a higher risk of POAG progression.
- *Ancillary risk factors*:
- *Genetic:* Myocilin gene (MYOC) on chromosome 1 (3–4% of POAG)
- *Vasospasm:* Migraine, Raynaud's disease
- Long-term steroid use
- Obstructive sleep apnea.
5. It is important to consider the economics of glaucoma therapy as also compliance issues. Quality of life costs of treatment versus no treatment must be weighed for the individual patient.
6. The risks and benefits of selective laser trabeculoplasty versus topical glaucoma therapy must be discussed with the patient.
7. Advanced visual field damage must be addressed surgically whenever required. Indications for surgery are discussed later in the book.

SUGGESTED READING

1. American Academy of Ophthalmology Glaucoma Panel. (2010). Preferred practice pattern guidelines. Primary open-angle glaucoma. [online] Available from www.aao.org/ppp. [Accessed July, 2016].
2. Broman AT, Quigley HA, West SK, Katz J, Munoz B, Bandeen-Roche K, et al. Estimating the rate of progressive visual field damage among those with open-angle glaucoma from cross-sectional data. Invest Ophthalmol Vis Sci. 2008;49:66-76.
3. Heijl A, Bengtsson B, Hyman L, Leske MC; Early Manifest Glaucoma Trial Group. Natural history of open-angle glaucoma. Ophthalmology. 2009;116:2271-6.
4. Jay JL, Murdoch JR. The rate of visual field loss in untreated primary open angle glaucoma. Br J Ophthalmol. 1993;3:176-8.
5. Leske MC, Heijl A, Hussein M, Bengtsson B, Hyman L, Komaroff E, et al. Factors for glaucoma progression and the effect of treatment: the early manifest glaucoma trial. Arch Ophthalmol. 2003;121:48-56.
6. Leske MC, Heijl A, Hyman L, Bengtsson B, Dong L, Yang Z, et al. Predictors of long-term progression in the early manifest glaucoma trial. Ophthalmology. 2007;114: 1965-72.
7. Lichter PR, Musch DC, Gillespie BW, Guire KE, Janz NK, Wren PA, et al. Interim clinical outcomes in the Collaborative Initial Glaucoma Treatment Study comparing initial treatment randomized to medications or surgery. Ophthalmology. 2001;108:1943-53.
8. South East Asia Glaucoma Interest Group. Asia-Pacific Glaucoma Guidelines, 2nd edition. 2008.

CHAPTER 4

Medical Therapy: Monotherapy, Fixed Combinations, Side Effects and Quality of Life Implications

Simon Skalicky, Ivan Goldberg

▌ DEFINITION

Glaucoma is a chronic progressive optic neuropathy with characteristic optic nerve head changes, with raised intraocular pressure (IOP), its major risk factor. Medical therapy, topical ocular or systemic IOP-lowering pharmacologic agents, remains the mainstay of treatment for most types of glaucoma. Most patients are initially managed with one IOP-lowering agent (monotherapy). Over time often more than one medication is required to reduce IOP to target levels; these can be administered in fixed combination preparations to simplify regimens to improve adherence, persistence and minimize treatment-related side effects. With all treatment decisions, the need to minimize future glaucomatous progression by IOP-lowering therapies needs to be balanced against potential side effects induced by that treatment. The impact on quality of life (QoL) needs to be considered, not only from glaucomatous visual loss, but also from the glaucoma treatments.

Case 1: Monotherapy

Mrs M, a-55-year-old lady, was found to have a left optic disc inferior nerve fiber layer hemorrhage (NFLH) by her optometrist. She denied any problems with her eyes or vision, but has a family history of glaucoma. Her IOPs were elevated [22/24 mm Hg oculus dexter/oculus sinister (OD/OS)] with central corneal thickness of 525 um in each eye. Anterior chambers were deep and quiet with no evidence of pseudoexfoliation (PXF), pigment dispersion or other cause of secondary glaucoma. Gonioscopy showed open

angles. Near the NFLH there was left inferotemporal rim loss associated with thinning of the retinal nerve fiber layer (RNFL) and macular ganglion cell complex (Figs. 4.1A and B). The visual field (VF) did not show any changes suggestive of glaucomatous damage.

The nature of glaucoma, including the significance of a NFLH near the disc, was discussed with Mrs M. In addition, the importance of ongoing regular monitoring was emphasized. The benefits of IOP lowering therapy to reduce the risk of glaucomatous progression were discussed and IOP-lowering treatment was recommended. Mrs M commenced with a prostaglandin analog once every evening (e.g. travoprost 0.004%, latanoprost 0.005%, bimatoprost 0.03% or tafluprost 0.0015%). Potential treatment side effects of ocular discomfort, red eyes, darkening in iris color and lengthening of eyelashes were discussed. Drop administration technique, including digital occlusion of the lacrimal sac, was discussed and demonstrated, as was the importance of good adherence and persistence with the therapy. For further information and support, Mrs M was recommended to connect with Glaucoma Australia (telephone 1800-500-880). Mrs M returned 6 weeks later to assess her IOP response (ideally 25–30% from baseline) and to discuss issues related to side effects, drop technique and adherence.

Case 2: Fixed drug combinations

Mr G, aged 72, had been diagnosed with primary open-angle glaucoma 10 years previously. Pretreatment IOPs were 23/26 mm Hg (OD/OS), with pachymetry of 532/545 um (OD/OS). He was initially treated with a prostaglandin

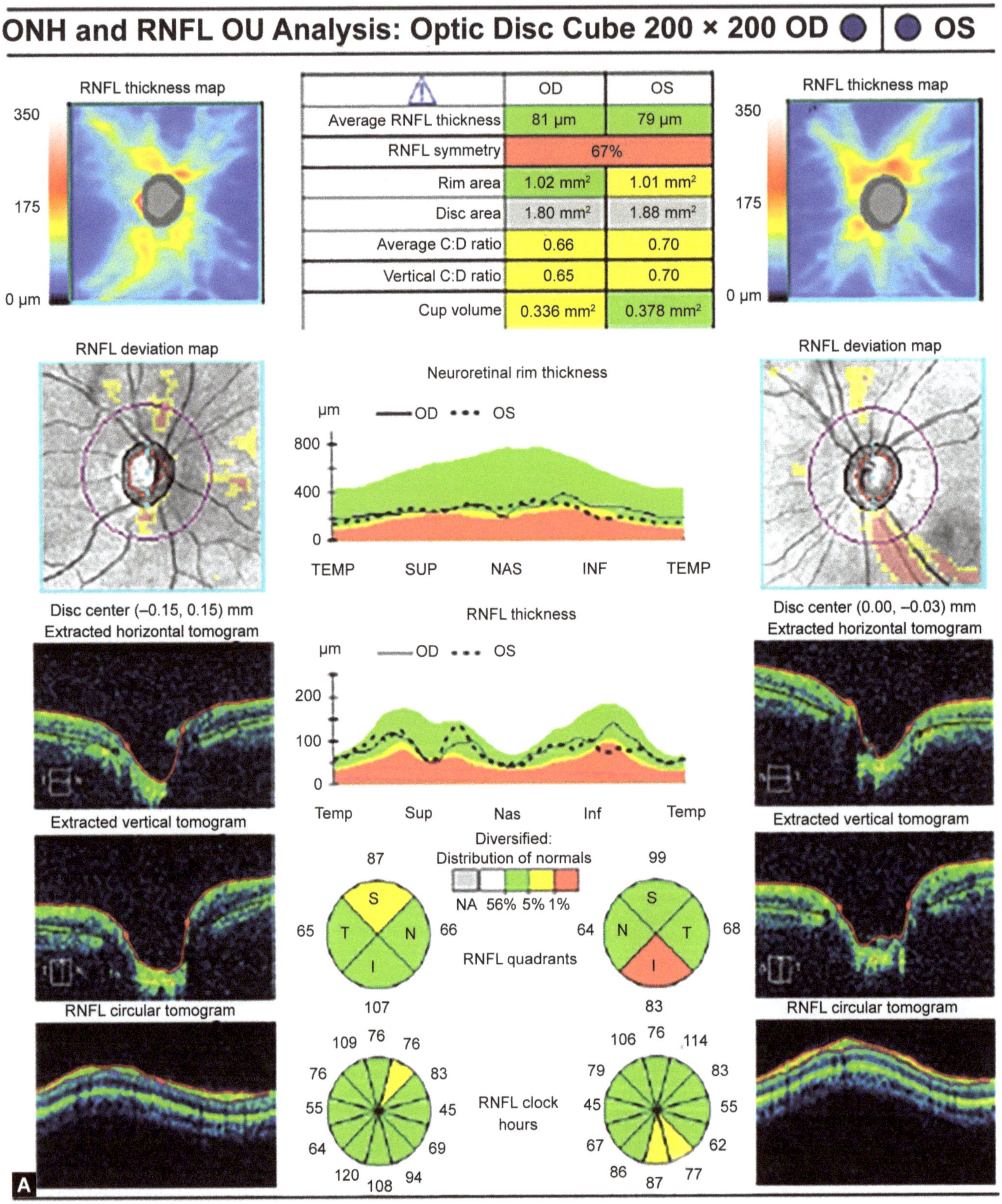

ONH and RNFL OU Analysis: Optic Disc Cube 200 × 200 OD ● | ● OS

RNFL thickness map

	⚠	OD	OS
Average RNFL thickness		81 µm	79 µm
RNFL symmetry		67%	
Rim area		1.02 mm²	1.01 mm²
Disc area		1.80 mm²	1.88 mm²
Average C:D ratio		0.66	0.70
Vertical C:D ratio		0.65	0.70
Cup volume		0.336 mm²	0.378 mm²

RNFL thickness map

RNFL deviation map

Neuroretinal rim thickness

RNFL deviation map

Disc center (−0.15, 0.15) mm
Extracted horizontal tomogram

RNFL thickness

Disc center (0.00, −0.03) mm
Extracted horizontal tomogram

Extracted vertical tomogram

Diversified:
Distribution of normals

NA 56% 5% 1%

RNFL quadrants

Extracted vertical tomogram

RNFL circular tomogram

RNFL clock hours

RNFL circular tomogram

Fig. 4.1A: Optical coherence tomography scan of the right and left optic nerve heads, demonstrating an inferior defect of the left retinal nerve fibre layer.

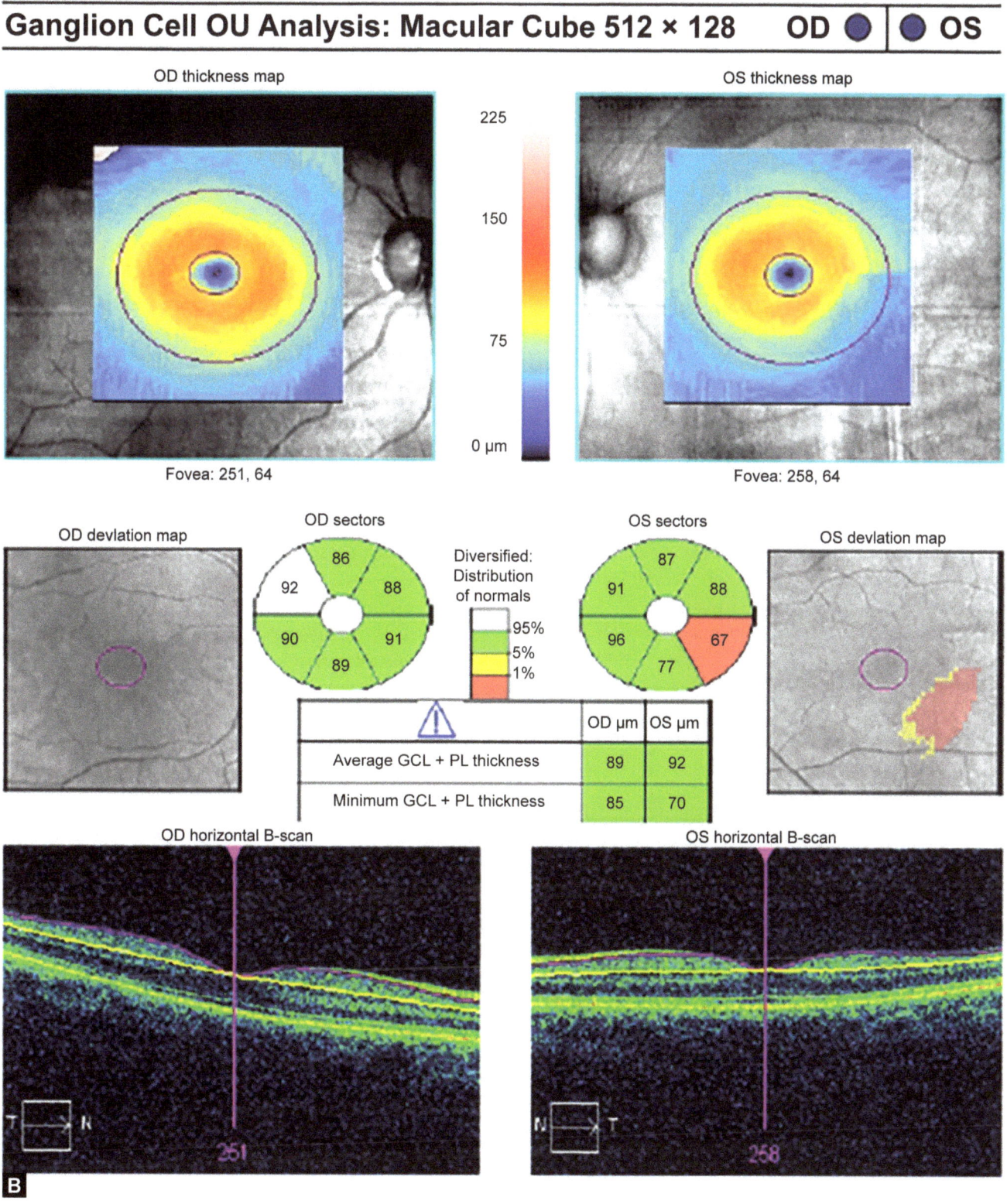

Fig. 4.1B: Optical coherence tomography scan of the right and left macular ganglion cell complexes, showing a corresponding area of left inferotemporal macular ganglion cell loss.

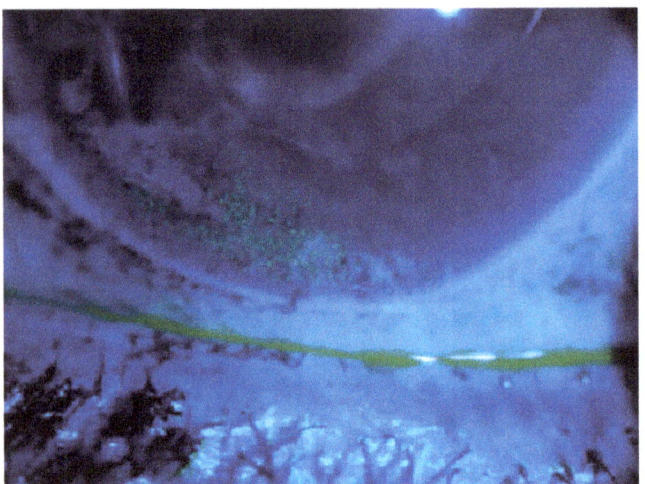

Fig. 4.2: Inferior corneal punctate epithelial erosions, detected on fluorescein staining and ultraviolet light on biomicroscopy.

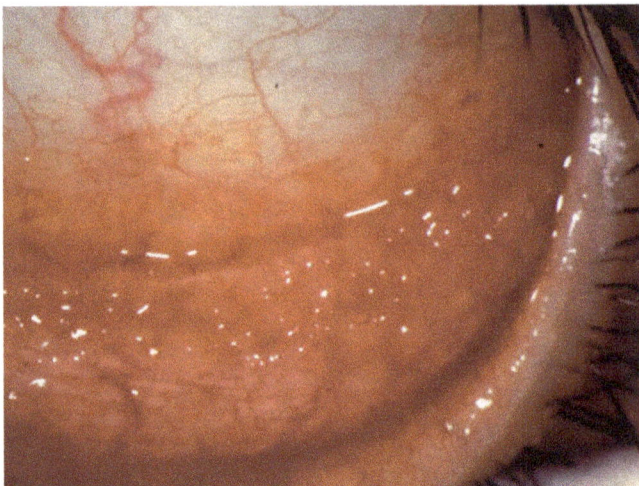

Fig. 4.3: Inferior forniceal and palpebral follicular conjunctivitis of the left eye.

analog once daily in both eyes which reduced his IOPs to 15/16 mm Hg. He tolerated this medicine well with minimal side effects and had good stated adherence to and persistence with the therapy. He was monitored 6 monthly, with annual VF tests and optical coherence tomography (OCT) scans of the retinal nerve fiber layer.

After 5 years of controlled IOPs and no progression IOPs began to rise, reaching 21/22 mm Hg. In addition, some progressive thinning of the RNFL was noted on serial OCT scans. He denied a history of asthma, systemic hypotension, uncontrolled diabetes, bradycardia or other cardiac issues. He was commenced on timolol 0.05% mane both eyes in addition to evening prostaglandin. This reduced his IOPs to 14/15 mm Hg and was well tolerated. After 3 years, the IOPs had crept up again to 22/23 mm Hg; brinzolamide 1% bd was added to both eyes. While this new regimen re-established IOP control, he developed red, irritated eyes on this regimen, with a reduced tear film break-up time and punctate epithelial erosions (Fig. 4.2). To facilitate his adherence, reduce the number of drops daily, and reduce the exposure to preservatives daily on the ocular surface, his regimen was simplified to the prostaglandin daily and combination brinzolamide or timolol bd in both eyes. It could as easily have been simplified to prostaglandin/timolol in the evenings with brinzolamide bd, the available fixed combinations offer choice.

Case 3: Side effects and quality of life

Eight months ago 68-year-old Mrs D, with IOPs of 15/27 mm Hg OD/OS, was diagnosed with left PXF syndrome with secondary ocular hypertension and commenced on an alpha-2 agonist (brimonidine 0.1%) twice daily in that eye. The treatment reduced IOP to 15/18 mm Hg OD/OS, but provoked a left red, watery and irritated eye with occasional blurred vision. She attended for a second opinion. Visual acuity was 6/5 oculus uterque (OU) with a left follicular conjunctivitis (Fig. 4.3). Her anterior chamber angles were open on gonioscopy with signs of left PXF. Discs appeared healthy with both sides obeying the ISNT rule and no focal thinning or notching of the neuroretinal rim. Cup-to-disc ratio was 0.5 on either side. No VF defects were evident on standard automated perimetry.

With confirmed PXF and raised IOP, she was advised that the risk for onset of glaucoma justified IOP-reducing strategies. While brimonidine is often used to reduce unilateral raised IOP, occasionally it can prove to be locally intolerance, with follicular conjunctivitis, anterior uveitis and rarely bradycardia or hypotension. Brimonidine would best be ceased and an alternative can be considered. Various treatment options include:

- *Prostaglandin analog*, with their once daily instillation (simpler and easier to remember). However, when used monocularly these medications can result in unilateral lash lengthening, iris color change and periorbital skin darkening with asymmetry of facial appearance.
- *Topical beta-blockers:* These may be used once or twice daily. They are contraindicated in certain health states (asthma, bradycardia, systemic hypotension, insulin-dependent diabetes, poorly controlled heart failure). They should be used cautiously for patients already on oral beta-blockers (in whom they are less effective topically) or calcium channel inhibitors, because of

enhanced risks of systemic side effects (in particular heart failure and hypotension). They can cause or exacerbate breathlessness, syncope, hypoglycemia, depression or nightmares.

- *Topical carbonic anhydrase inhibitors*: These are administered twice daily, and occasionally can cause a local allergy and rarely serious systemic health issues, such as Stevens-Johnson syndrome (a systemic/dermatological reaction that can be severe and even life-threatening).

- *Selective laser trabeculoplasty (SLT)*: Laser energy is applied to the trabecular meshwork) to enhance the function of the conventional outflow pathway. It can be applied to the whole drainage area (360°) or half (180°) over 1–2 sessions. While it sufficiently reduces IOP in just 65–75% or patients, it is safe, with minimal side effects. Rarely, it can provoke a transient IOP rise, corneal or intraocular inflammation that are self-limiting. Even though this effect may wear off over time, the treatment is repeatable; the second and/or third treatment is generally not as effective as the first.

Considering her options, Mrs D felt that SLT was the most suitable treatment for her. She understood that should the SLT fail to achieve the desired IOP level, another topical medication could be considered. She was grateful to have been offered these options and felt empowered to make the best possible treatment decision for herself.

Investigations

See Ocular Hypertension + Glaucoma chapters.

Follow-up Protocol

In general patients with glaucoma should be monitored 4–6 monthly with at least annual VF testing and RNFL imaging. Patients with ocular hypertension or glaucoma suspects should be monitored 6–12 monthly with 1–2 yearly VF testing and RNFL imaging.

However, for all patients, whenever treatment is initiated or altered, follow-up should be scheduled within 6 weeks to assess:

- Efficacy of treatment (has the treatment achieved the desired IOP level?)
- Adherence to the new therapy
- Tolerance, comfort and unwanted side effects.

BRIEF REVIEW OF LITERATURE

Raised IOP is the major modifiable risk factor for glaucomatous progression; multiple clinical trials have demonstrated that reduction in patients with ocular hypertension or glaucoma is protective.[1-4]

Despite progress in surgical and laser technology[5-9] topical hypotensive medications are the most common treatment for most forms of glaucoma today, and will likely continue to be in the future.[10,11] Topical IOP-lowering agents are suitable first line treatments as they are generally safe, effective and relatively simple to administer. Limitations of topical medications include preservative-related drop toxicity, systemic and/or ocular side effects and for some individuals physical difficulties with self-administration (arthritis, tremor).

The success of any medications to prevent progressive glaucomatous damage depends upon patient adherence to and persistence with their therapy.[12,13] Yet poor adherence and persistence remain significant barriers to effective treatment.[14,15] Glaucoma, like many chronic systemic conditions, is initially asymptomatic and generally progresses slowly; treatment can be cumbersome, uncomfortable, costly and intrusive to patients' lifestyle. All of these factors can reduce patient motivation for regular adherence to treatment regimens.[16]

Glaucoma will impact the QoL of all patients with the disease, as well as their carers and family members. Glaucoma primarily affects QoL through visual disability related to progressive glaucomatous optic neuropathy.[17] Treatment-related issues such as ocular surface discomfort, regular clinical reviews with possibly time-consuming and costly treatment contribute to the overall burden of disease.[18] The psychological burden increases as vision decreases, together with a growing fear of blindness, social withdrawal from impaired vision and depression.[19-21]

Symptoms of dry eye disease (DES) affect up to 59% of patients with glaucoma.[22,23] All classes of topical IOP-lowering medications can cause or exacerbate underlying ocular surface discomfort.[18,24,25] This can result in reduced treatment adherence.[26] DES is exacerbated by the use of multiple topical medications and can significantly reduce QoL in glaucoma patients.[18,27]

Patients on multiple topical medications who suffer from DES may benefit from combination preparations, in which active ingredients are combined in one bottle. Compared with two separate medications, a combination preparation allows similar delivery of medications with a lower dose of preservative. Additionally, altering patients' topical glaucoma medications to nonpreserved formulations or those with "gentler" preservatives may help improve symptoms and clinical signs of DES.[28,29]

Table 4.1: Intraocular pressure (IOP)-lowering agents with their efficacy, dosage and contraindications.

IOP-lowering agent	Examples	Efficacy (% IOP lowering)	Dosage	Unwanted effects	Contraindication(s)
Prostaglandin analog	Latanoprost Travoprost Bimatoprost Tafluprost	25–30	Daily	Red eyes Irritated, dry eyes Iris pigmentation Eyelid skin darkening Longer, thicker lashes	Trimester 3 pregnancy (uterine contractility) Herpes infections of the eye
β-blockers	Timolol (0.25 or 0.5%) – (nonselective) Betaxolol (0.25 or 0.5% selective β_1 receptor blocker)	20–30	BD or daily	Bradycardia Bronchospasm **Falls** Impotence Lipid disregulation Allergy	Heart block Asthma/COPD Caution in heart failure NB: Betaxolol has fewer pulmonary complications
α_2-agonists	Brimonidine (0.15 or 0.2%), Apraclonidine	20–25	BD	Allergy, tachyphylaxis Hypotension (brimonidine)	Avoid brimonidine in children
Carbonic anhydrase inhibitors	Brinzolamide Dorzolamide	15–20	TDS or BD	Blurred vision Stinging/exacerbation of dry eye Sulphonamides: Stevens-Johnson syndrome, blood dyscrasias Allergy	Sulphonamide allergy
Cholinergics	Pilocarpine (1, 2 or 4%)	10–15	BD to QID	Browache, cataract, epiphora, change in vision, increased salivation, abdominal cramps	

SUMMARY

Please see below overview of topical medications used in treatment of glaucoma or ocular hypertension:

Pharmacological Classes

- Five classes of topical IOP lowering medications are available for common clinical use
- Intraocular pressure lowering drops should be used in caution in pregnancy; brimonidine is classified as FDA category B; all other topical medications are within category C. IOP-lowering agents with their efficacy, dosage and contraindications are presented in Table 4.1.

Fixed Combination Medications

Timolol + Prostaglandin (OD):
- Xalacom (timolol/latanoprost)® Pfizer
- Duotrav (timolol/travatan)® Alcon
- Ganfort (timolol/bimatoprost)® Allergan.

Timolol + Carbonic Anhydrase Inhibitor (BD):
- Azarga (timolol/brinzolamide)® Alcon
- Cosopt (timolol/dorzolamide)®.

Timolol + Alpha-2 Agonist (BD):
- Combigan (timolol/brimonidine)® Allergan

Alpha-2 Agonist + Carbonic Anhydrase Inhibitor (BD or TDS):
- Simbrinza (brinzolamide/brimonidine)® Alcon.

Advantages of Fixed Combination Preparations

Ease of use, improved patient adherence, less preservative toxicity, better tolerability.

Disadvantages of Fixed Combination Preparations

A β_1 selective beta-blocker (betaxolol) has an advantage over nonselective beta-blockers (e.g. timolol) as it causes less bronchospasm. However, betaxolol cannot be used in combination preparations, for which timolol is the only available beta-blocker component.

Preserved versus Preservative Free Preparations

- Most glaucoma preparations are packaged in bottles that need to be discarded after 28 days.
- To prevent build-up of bacteria these preparations contain preservatives.

Box 4.1: Early manifest glaucoma trial (EMGT).

Objective: To evaluate the effect of immediately lowering IOP on the progression of newly detected open-angle glaucoma.
Design: Randomized clinical trial.
Participants: 255 patients aged 50–80 years with early glaucoma and an IOP <30 mm Hg.
Intervention: Randomized to argon laser trabeculoplasty plus topical betaxolol (n = 129) vs no initial treatment (n = 126).
Study monitoring: Humphrey full threshold 30-2 VF tests and tonometry every 3 months; optic disc photography every 6 months. Median follow-up period of 6 years (range, 51–102 months).
Main outcome measures: Glaucoma progression was defined by specific visual field deterioration on three consecutive tests and/or optic disc outcomes.
Results:
- On average, treatment reduced the IOP by 5.1 mm Hg or 25%.
- Progression was less frequent in the treatment group (45%) than in controls (62%) (P = .007) and occurred significantly later in treated patients.
Conclusion: IOP reduction in patients with open-angle glaucoma who have elevated and normal IOP significantly delayed glaucomatous progression.

(IOP: Intraocular pressure; VF: Visual field).

- The most commonly used preservative is benzalkonium chloride (BAK).
- Preservatives are often toxic to the surface of the eye, can disrupt the tear film and cause/exacerbate dry eye symptoms. The daily dose of preservative in glaucoma medications is proportional to symptoms of DES and reduced quality of life.
- Some preparations contain alternative preservatives (e.g. Purite® Allergan or PolyQuad® Alcon) that are considered "gentler" to the ocular surface than BAK.
- Some medications are available in preservative-free preparations. These can be tricky to use for patients, especially the elderly with arthritis of the hands.

Drop Instillation Technique (Instructions for New Patients)

- Wash hands
- Tilt head back or lie down and look up
- Gently pull down the lower lid to form a "pocket"
- Lightly squeeze container until a drop lands inside the lower lid. If unsure, instill a second drop
- Avoid touching the eye with the tip of the bottle
- Use a clean tissue to gently dab away excess drops
- After the drop, close eye and place a finger on the inner corner of the eye for 2–3 minutes to prevent the drop flowing down the tear sac
- Special dispensers are available for patients with compromised dexterity.

Box 4.2: UK glaucoma treatment study (UKGTS).

Objective: To assess vision preservation in patients with open-angle glaucoma treated with latanoprost compared with those treated with placebo.
Design: Randomized, triple-masked, placebo-controlled trial.
Participants: 516 patients with newly diagnosed open-angle glaucoma at ten UK centers. Baseline mean IOP was 19.6 mm Hg (standard deviation 4.6) in the latanoprost group and 20.1 mm Hg (standard deviation 4.8) in the control group.
Intervention: Eligible patients were randomized (1:1) to receive either latanoprost 0.005% (intervention group) or placebo (control group) eye drops. Drops were administered from identical bottles, once a day, to both eyes.
Study monitoring: Subjects were monitored with VF testing, quantitative disc and RNFL imaging, optic disc photography and tonometry at approximately 2-monthly intervals.
Main outcome measures: Mean reduction in IOP and deterioration in VF testing at 24 months.
Results:
- Mean reduction in IOP was 3.8 mm Hg (4.0) in the latanoprost group and 0.9 mm Hg (3.8) in in the placebo group.
- Visual field preservation was significantly longer in the latanoprost group than in the placebo group: HR 0.44 (95% CI 0.28–0.69; p = 0.0003).
Conclusion: Preservation of the VF was associated with use of an IOP-lowering drug in patients with open-angle glaucoma.

(HR: Hazard ratio; IOP: Intraocular pressure; RNFL: Retinal nerve fiber layer; VF: Visual field).

Commentary

The following studies, the Early Manifest Glaucoma Trial (EMGT) and UK Glaucoma Treatment Study (UKGTS) provide important evidence as to the role of IOP lowering from topical medications to reduce progression rate in glaucoma (Boxes 4.1 and 4.2).

▌ REFERENCES

1. Kass MA, Heuer DK, Higginbotham EJ, Johnson CA, Keltner JL, Miller JP, et al. The Ocular Hypertension Treatment Study: a randomized trial determines that topical ocular hypotensive medication delays or prevents the onset of primary open-angle glaucoma. Arch Ophthalmol. 2002;120:701-13; discussion 829-30.
2. Leske MC, Heijl A, Hyman L, Bengtsson B. Early Manifest Glaucoma Trial: design and baseline data. Ophthalmology. 1999;106:2144-53.
3. Heijl A, Leske MC, Bengtsson B, Hyman L, Bengtsson B, Hussein M, et al. Reduction of intraocular pressure and glaucoma progression: Results from the early manifest Glaucoma trial. Archives of Ophthalmology. 2002;120:1268-79.
4. Garway-Heath DF, Crabb DP, Bunce C, Lascaratos G, Amalfitano F, Anand N, et al. Latanoprost for open-angle glaucoma (UKGTS): a randomised, multicentre, placebo-controlled trial. Lancet. 2015;385:1295-304.

5. Khaw PT, Chiang M, Shah P, et al. Enhanced trabeculectomy— the Moorfields safer surgery system. Dev Ophthalmol. 2012;50:1-28.

6. Gedde SJ, Schiffman JC, Feuer WJ, et al. Tube versus Trabeculectomy Study Group. Treatment outcomes in the tube versus trabeculectomy (TVT) study after five years of follow-up. Am J Ophthalmol. 2012;153:789-803.

7. Dashevsky AV, Lanzl IM, Kotliar KE. Non-penetrating intracanalicular partial trabeculectomy via the ostia of Schlemm's canal. Graefes Arch Clin Exp Ophthalmol. 2011;249:565-73.

8. Shi JM and Jia SB. Selective laser trabeculoplasty. Int J Ophthalmol. 2012; 5: 742-9.

9. Saheb H, Ahmed II. Microinvasive glaucoma surgery: current perspectives and future directions. Curr Opin Ophthalmol. 2012;23:96-104.

10. Chae B, Cakiner-Egilmez T, Desai M. Glaucoma medications. Insight. 2013;38:5-9; quiz 10.

11. Lee AJ, Goldberg I. Emerging drugs for ocular hypertension. Expert Opin Emerg Drugs. 2011;16:137-61.

12. Lee PP, Walt JW, Rosenblatt LC, et al. Association between intraocular pressure variation and glaucoma progression: data from a United States chart review. Am J Ophthalmol. 2007;144:901-7.

13. Dreer LE, Girkin C, Mansberger SL. Determinants of medication adherence to topical glaucoma therapy. J Glaucoma. 2012;21:234-40.

14. Nordstrom BL, Friedman DS, Mozaffari E, et al. Persistence and adherence with topical glaucoma therapy. Am J Ophthalmol. 2005;140:598-606.

15. Zhou Z, Althin R, Sforzolini BS, et al. Persistency and treatment failure in newly diagnosed open angle glaucoma patients in the United Kingdom. Br J Ophthalmol. 2004; 88:1391-4.

16. Reardon G, Kotak S, Schwartz GF. Objective assessment of compliance and persistence among patients treated for glaucoma and ocular hypertension: a systematic review. Patient Prefer Adherence. 2011;5:441-63.

17. Ramulu P. Glaucoma and disability: which tasks are affected, and at what stage of disease? Curr Opin Ophtalmol. 2009: 20(2)92-8.

18. Skalicky SE, Goldberg I, McCluskey P. Ocular surface disease and quality of life in patients with glaucoma. Am J Ophthalmol. 2012;153:1-9.

19. Janz NK, Wren PA, Guire KE, et al. Fear of blindness in the Collaborative Initial Glaucoma Treatment Study: patterns and correlates over time. Ophthalmology. 2007;114:2 213-20.

20. Ramulu PY, van Landingham SW, Massof RW, et al. Fear of falling and visual field loss from glaucoma. Ophthalmology. 2012;119:1352-8.

21. Skalicky S, Goldberg, I. Depression and quality of life in patients with glaucoma: a cross-sectional analysis using the Geriatric Depression Scale-15, assessment of function related to vision, and the Glaucoma Quality of Life-15. J Glaucoma. 2008;17:546-51.

22. Leung EW, Medeiros FA and Weinreb RN. Prevalence of ocular surface disease in glaucoma patients. J Glaucoma. 2008; 17: 350-5.

23. Fechtner RD, Godfrey DG, Budenz D, Stewart JA, Stewart WC, Jasek MC. Prevalence of ocular surface complaints in patients with glaucoma using topical intraocular pressure-lowering medications. Cornea. 2010;29:618-21.

24. Saade CE, Lari HB, Berezina TL, Fechtner RD, Khouri AS. Topical glaucoma therapy and ocular surface disease: a prospective, controlled cohort study. C Can J Ophthalmol. 2015;50:132-6.

25. Servat JJ, Bernardino CR. Effects of common topical anti-glaucoma medications on the ocular surface, eyelids and periorbital tissue. Drugs Aging. 2011;28:267-82.

26. Baudouin C. Detrimental effect of preservatives in eye-drops: implications for the treatment of glaucoma. Acta Ophthalmologica. 2008;86:716-26.

27. Rossi GC, Pasinetti GM, Scudeller L, Bianchi PE. Ocular surface disease and glaucoma: how to evaluate impact on quality of life. J Ocul Pharmacol Ther. 2013;29:390-4.

28. Rossi GC, Scudeller L, Rolle T, et al. From benzalkonium chloride-preserved Latanoprost to Polyquad-preserved Travoprost: a 6-month study on ocular surface safety and tolerability. Expert opinion on drug safety. 2015;14: 619-23.

29. Goldberg I, Graham SL, Crowston JG, d'Mellow G, Australian and New Zealand Glaucoma Interest G. Clinical audit examining the impact of benzalkonium chloride-free anti-glaucoma medications on patients with symptoms of ocular surface disease. Clin Experiment Ophthalmol. 2015;43:214-20.

CHAPTER **5**

Laser Trabeculoplasty

Shibal Bhartiya, Parul Ichhpujani

INTRODUCTION

Almost 25 years ago, the Glaucoma Laser Trial (GLT) showed that primary laser trabeculoplasty using an argon laser, effectively lowers intraocular pressure (IOP) in treatment-naïve eyes. Concerns with argon laser trabeculoplasty (ALT) included a loss of efficacy over time as well as the formation of peripheral anterior synechiae (PAS) after laser treatment. These issues were addressed by Selective laser trabeculopasty (SLT), as it caused minimal structural damage to the trabecular meshwork.

SLT optimizes trabecular outflow rather than bypassing it, and is now accepted as a means to achieve moderate IOP reduction in select patients.

SLT is an excellent option for first-line therapy of glaucoma, offering several advantages including convenience, compliance and tolerability, in addition to an efficacy that is similar to prostaglandin analogs.[1] It can be performed as a replacement for eyedrops, and as an adjunct to medical therapy for open-angle glaucomas.

INDICATIONS

Selective laser trabeculoplasty may be offered to patients with open-angle glaucoma including:[2]
- Primary open-angle glaucoma (POAG)
- Ocular hypertension
- Pigmentary glaucoma
- Pseudoexfoliative glaucoma
- Steroid-induced glaucoma.

It may also be considered in cases of normal tension glaucoma (NTG) and in patients of angle-closure glaucoma with a patent laser peripheral iridotomy (LPI), in cases with sufficient access to the trabecular meshwork.

Listed below are situations in which SLT can be an integral part of glaucoma therapy for each of these patients:[1]
- As primary therapy, as "the first drop": As SLT offers several advantages including convenience, compliance and tolerability, in addition to efficacy that is similar to eyedrops
- As adjunct to medical therapy as "the second drop"
- In patients with poor compliance or tolerance with medical therapy:
  - Remember, when a patient takes drops, the SLT and drops are equivalent in terms of efficacy, but when the patient does not take drops, there is no question the laser is a better choice.
- As a temporizing measure prior to glaucoma surgery, e.g. in patients awaiting fitness for surgery during pregnancy
- In selected patients with angle-closure glaucoma with patent iridotomy (SLT can be applied to the visible areas of trabecular meshwork)
- Patients with failed ALT
- Patients considered to be suitable candidates for minimally invasive glaucoma surgery (MIGS), i.e. as an alternative to MIGS
- *Prevention of steroid-induced glaucoma:* In a study, when SLT was applied before intravitreal triamcinolone injection, none of the patients required additional antiglaucoma medication, whereas 50% of the untreated group required medications.[2]

Selective laser trabeculoplasty can be repeated and repeat SLT can be offered to both the previous SLT responders and to previous SLT nonresponders.

CONTRAINDICATIONS

It is equally important to remember the situations in which SLT may not be the procedure of choice, so as to prevent undesirable or suboptimal outcomes. The contraindications for SLT include:

- Patients of angle-closure glaucoma without a patent LPI
- Patients of angle-closure glaucoma with a patent LPI, in case there is significant synechial or appositional closure precluding access to the trabecular meshwork
- Patients who do not understand that SLT is not a permanent sure for their glaucoma, and that they will require lifelong follow-up, and probably repeat SLT
- Patients with poor access to follow-up
- Inflammatory glaucoma
- Iridocorneal endothelial (ICE) syndrome
- Developmental glaucoma
- Neovascular glaucoma
- Any conditions which preclude a clear visualization of the trabecular meshwork
- Advanced glaucoma may be a relative contraindication.

Case 1: SLT for drug induced ocular surface disease

Mr X, a 67-year-old gentleman, presented with moderate-to-severe ocular surface disease due to his antiglaucoma medication (G. Travoprost in both eyes at bedtime). He had previously been prescribed another prostaglandin (G bimatoprost) and G brimonidine tid, and had shown poor tolerance to both. His baseline IOPs were 25 mm Hg and 24 mm Hg; and the target IOP of 16–18 mm Hg OU was achieved using the eyedrops. He had mild-to-moderate glaucoma with a cup-to-disc (C:D) ratio of 0.6–0.7 OU and polar thinning of neuroretinal rim (NRR), and corresponding incomplete biarcuate visual field defects. His vision was 6/6 both eyes, with refractive correction.

He was advised SLT as a method of decreasing his dependence on eyedrops. Following the SLT both eyes achieved an IOP of 16–18 mm Hg, without any added antiglaucoma medication. This IOP drop has been maintained for the last 18 months of follow-up, with a remarkable improvement in his ocular surface disease index (OSDI) score.

Exposure to more than three drops daily of benzalkonium chloride-preserved medication has been shown to be an independent predictor of higher OSDI score.[3]

Case 2: SLT for patient unable to instill drugs

Mrs X, a 73-year-old lady, was on maximal antiglaucoma therapy (G. travoprost HS, G. brinzolamide tid and G. timolol + brimonidine BD). Her baseline IOPs were 36 mm Hg and 38 mm Hg; and the target IOP of 14–16 mm Hg OU was not achieved despite maximal medical therapy. She had severe open-angle glaucoma with a C:D ratio of 0.8:0.9 OU with concentric NRR loss and complete biarcuate defect on visual field. She was pseudophakic with a best corrected vision of 6/12 and 6/18 in the right and left eyes, respectively, due to dry age-related macular degeneration on both eyes.

Since she was arthritic, diabetic and hypertensive with severe coronary artery disease, she refused to undergo another surgery, since, in her own words, "the previous cataract surgery had not helped her glaucoma or vision". She also complained of the "hundred eyedrops she had to struggle with, despite arthritis".

After an informed consent she was taken up for SLT, with all the pre-SLT antiglaucoma medications continued as before for up to 6 weeks after the laser. Following that, individual medications were gradually withdrawn under strict medical supervision. At last follow-up, both eyes had an IOP of 14 mm Hg, with travoprost and timolol-fixed dose combination eyedrops, once at bedtime. This IOP drop has been maintained for the last 9 months.

Note: Timolol is not the first choice for patients of diabetes mellitus and Hashimoto's thyroiditis, but given the problems of drug administration with arthritic fingers, a fixed dose combination was thought to be a rational compromise.

Case 3: SLT for angle closure

Ms X, a 44-year-old lady, was diagnosed with early primary angle-closure glaucoma with baseline eye pressures of 26 mm Hg OU LPI. The optic nerve evaluation revealed a C:D ratio of 0.4:0.5 OU with broken ISNT rule (inferior ≥ superior ≥ nasal ≥ temporal) and early visual field defects (nasal step defect). A check gonioscopy following LPI showed open angles with broken posterior synechiae in two quadrants and abnormal pigmentation for about cumulative 2 clock hours. She also expressed an inability to remember eyedrops even once at bedtime due to her erratic work hours which involved a lot of travel, and was very receptive of the idea of SLT.

Selective laser trabeculoplasty was performed for her, avoiding the areas of the broken PAS and abnormal pigmentation, after counseling her that the procedure has an effect which may wane over time, and needed her to remain under constant follow-up. The target IOP of 18 mm Hg OU was achieved for Ms X within 4 weeks of SLT, without any medication, and has been maintained for the last 16 months, with stable fields. She has been counseled to remain under follow-up.

Case 4: Repeat SLT

Ms A, a 62-year-old lady, presented with moderate ocular surface disease due to her antiglaucoma medication (travoprost OU, once at bedtime; brinzolamide OU twice a day). Her baseline IOPs were 28 OU; and the target IOP of 16–18 OU was achieved using the eyedrops. She had moderate glaucoma with a C:D ratio of 0.6 OU and corresponding visual field defects. Her vision was 6/6 both eyes, with refractive correction.

She was advised SLT as a method of decreasing her dependence on eyedrops. Following the SLT both eyes achieved an IOP of 14 mm Hg, with G. travoprost HS OU, which was well tolerated. This IOP drop was maintained for about 14 months of follow-up, after which the IOP was found to creep upward to 20 mm Hg, over 4 months. She was advised a repeat SLT, and within 4 weeks of the procedure, her IOP was found to range from 14–16 OU, with travoprost OU, once at bedtime. This IOP drop has been maintained for the last 6 months of follow-up.

Repeatability of Selective Laser Trabeculoplasty

Hong et al. reported that performing repeat 360° SLT procedure is safe and effective after an initially successful 360° SLT has failed.[4] Russo and coworkers found repeated SLT to be better than ALT in lowering IOP.[5]

Selective Laser Trabeculoplasty Versus Argon Laser Trabeculoplasty

Multiple studies have demonstrated an equivalent reduction of IOP by SLT and ALT.[6,7] SLT is a gentler procedure and causes less discomfort to the patient as compared to ALT.[8] Additionally, histological studies have shown less damage with SLT than ALT, thus allowing repeat treatment with SLT.[9] ALT was typically performed after medical therapy had failed and prior to surgical intervention but SLT may be appropriate as primary therapy for patients with open-angle glaucoma.

Given its efficacy, safety, repeatability and potential cost savings, it may be prudent to suggest SLT as an alternative to medications when discussing treatment options with a newly diagnosed glaucoma patient.

REFERENCES

1. McIlraith I, Strasfeld M, Colev G, Hutnik CM. Selective laser trabeculoplasty as initial and adjunctive treatment for open-angle glaucoma. J Glaucoma. 2006;15:124-30.
2. Bozkurt E, Kara N, Yazici AT, Yuksel K, Demirok A, Yilmaz OF, et al. Prophylactic selective laser trabeculoplasty in the prevention of intraocular pressure elevation after intravitreal triamcinolone acetonide injection. Am J Ophthalmol. 2011;152:976-81.e2.
3. Skalicky SE, Goldberg I, McCluskey P. Ocular surface disease and quality of life in patients with glaucoma. Am J Ophthalmol. 2012;153:1-9.e2.
4. Hong BK, Winer JC, Martone JF, Wand M, Altman B, Shields B. Repeat selective laser trabeculoplasty. J Glaucoma. 2009; 18:180-3.
5. Russo V, Barone A, Cosma A, Stella A, Delle Noci N. Selective laser trabeculoplasty *versus* argon laser trabeculoplasty in patients with uncontrolled open-angle glaucoma. Eur J Ophthalmol 2009;19:429-34.
6. Juzych MS1, Chopra V, Banitt MR, Hughes BA, Kim C, Goulas MT, et al. Comparison of long-term outcomes of selective laser trabeculoplasty versus argon laser trabeculoplasty in open-angle glaucoma. Ophthalmology. 2004;111:1853-9.
7. Damji KF1, Shah KC, Rock WJ, Bains HS, Hodge WG. Selective laser trabeculoplasty v argon laser trabeculoplasty: a prospective randomised clinical trial. Br J Ophthalmol. 1999;83:718-22.
8. Martinez-de-la-Casa JM1, Garcia-Feijoo J, Castillo A, Matilla M, Macias JM, Benitez-del-Castillo JM, et al. Selective vs argon laser trabeculoplasty: hypotensive efficacy, anterior chamber inflammation, and postoperative pain. Eye (Lond). 2004;18:498-502.
9. Kramer TR, Noecker RJ. Comparison of the morphologic changes after selective laser trabeculoplasty and argon laser trabeculoplasty in human eye bank eyes. Ophthalmology. 2001;108:773-9.

CHAPTER 6

Angle-Closure Glaucoma

Sushmita Kaushik, Pankaj Kataria

DEFINITION

- The term "angle closure" refers to occlusion of the trabecular meshwork by the peripheral iris obstructing aqueous outflow
- Termed as primary, when it occurs in an anatomically predisposed eye, or secondary, when caused by another ocular or systemic factor
- Typically associated with greater rapidity of progression and visual morbidity than primary open-angle glaucoma (POAG)
- In India, there is a significantly high incidence of primary angle-closure glaucoma (PACG), almost half of all adult primary glaucomas seen in a hospital setting[1,2]
- Recently, its classification has moved away from a symptom-based approach (acute, subacute and chronic) to based on stages in the natural history of the disease as the majority of patients are asymptomatic and can be linked to prognosis and management
- As suggested by consensus group of the Association of International Glaucoma Societies, this new classification of primary angle closure (PAC) disease relies on three simple variables: intraocular pressures (IOP) measurements, gonioscopy and disc and visual field examination. In other words, the patient's "clinical examination" alone determines the staging of the disease.

STAGES OF ANGLE-CLOSURE DISEASE

Primary Angle-Closure Suspect

- Greater than 270° of iridotrabecular contact ("occludable" angle—posterior pigmented trabecular meshwork is not visible in more than 270° of angle)
- Absence of peripheral anterior synechiae (PAS)
- Normal IOP, disc and visual field
- In other words, the suspect eye has no signs of clinical glaucoma.

Primary Angle Closure

- Greater than 270° of iridotrabecular contact
- Either elevated IOP and/or PAS
- Normal disc and visual field examinations
- In other words, the angle is abnormal in structure (PAS) or function (elevated IOP).

Primary Angle-Closure Glaucoma

- Greater than 270° of iridotrabecular contact
- Elevated IOP
- Optic nerve and visual field damage
- In other words, angle-closure glaucoma manifests the criteria of closure above, plus demonstrable disc and/or visual field changes
- The angle is abnormal in structure and function, with optic neuropathy.

Acute Angle Closure

Acute angle closure (AAC) remains a specific observable presentation category of the disease requiring immediate recognition and intervention.

Primary Angle Closure

A 50-year-old woman, who has no eye symptoms is found during routine ophthalmic examination to have elevated

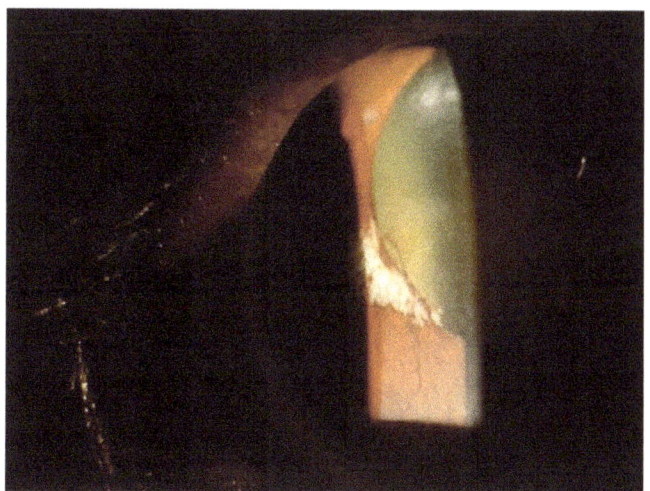

Fig. 6.1: Patchy iris atrophy in a case of primary angle closure.

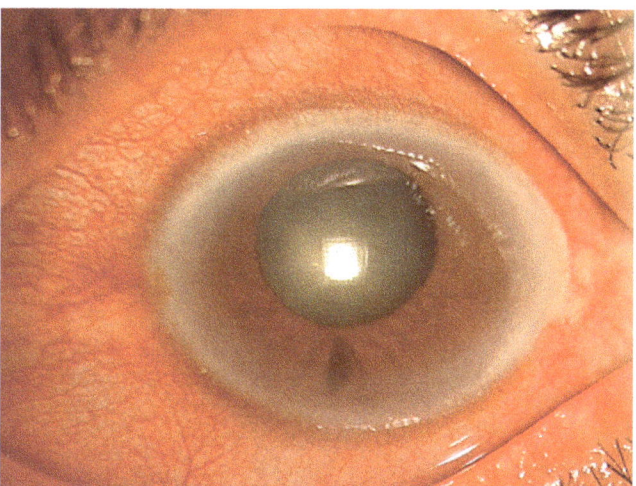

Fig. 6.2: Acute angle-closure glaucoma.

IOP of 42 mm Hg in both eyes. Fundoscopy shows that the optic nerve appears normal with no evidence of glaucomatous neuropathy. Gonioscopy shows that the anterior chamber is closed for almost the full circumference. She had patchy anterior stromal iris atrophy (Fig. 6.1). Needs bilateral laser peripheral iridotomy (LPI).

Common Vignette

A 64-year-old woman presents to the emergency room with severe pain around her right eye of 4-hour duration accompanied by blurred vision in the same eye. She is also nauseated. Examination shows a red right eye with edematous cornea and a wide pupil that is unresponsive to light. IOP is extremely elevated (60 mm Hg) only in the right eye. The anterior chamber angle is closed in both eyes. After reduction of IOP with intravenous mannitol 300 cc, cornea cleared (Fig. 6.2). Both eyes were pilocarpinesed thereafter for LPI.

Primary Angle-Closure Glaucoma (Chronic Presentation)

Patients may present with spontaneously resolving symptoms of intermittently ache and/or blurred vision with halos around lights seen from one eye. Patients may also notice a change in vision, which may represent long-standing chronic progressive visual field loss. Gonioscopy shows an occludable angle (Fig. 6.3).

The most common mechanism of angle-closure glaucoma appears to be relative pupillary block-increased resistance to aqueous flow from posterior to anterior chamber leading to forward bowing of peripheral iris and causing appositional angle closure. Prolonged or repeated, such episodes lead to PAS formation or synechial angle closure.

EPIDEMIOLOGY

- Number of people in the world affected by glaucoma is approximately 45 million. And one-third are from primary angle-closure glaucoma (PACG)
- Half of cases leading to blindness are estimated to result from PACG
- Prevalence rates highest are reported in Asian and Inuit population, and lowest rates are reported in African and European populations
- Women are 2–4 times more likely to have angle-closure glaucoma (ACG) than man
- Acute ACG is most common between 55 years and 65 years.

RISK FACTORS

Demographic Factors

- Age (more than 60 years)
- Female sex
- Southeast Asian origin
- Family history.

Anatomic Factors

- Shallow anterior chamber depth
- Thick/anteriorly positioned/increased anterior curvature of lens

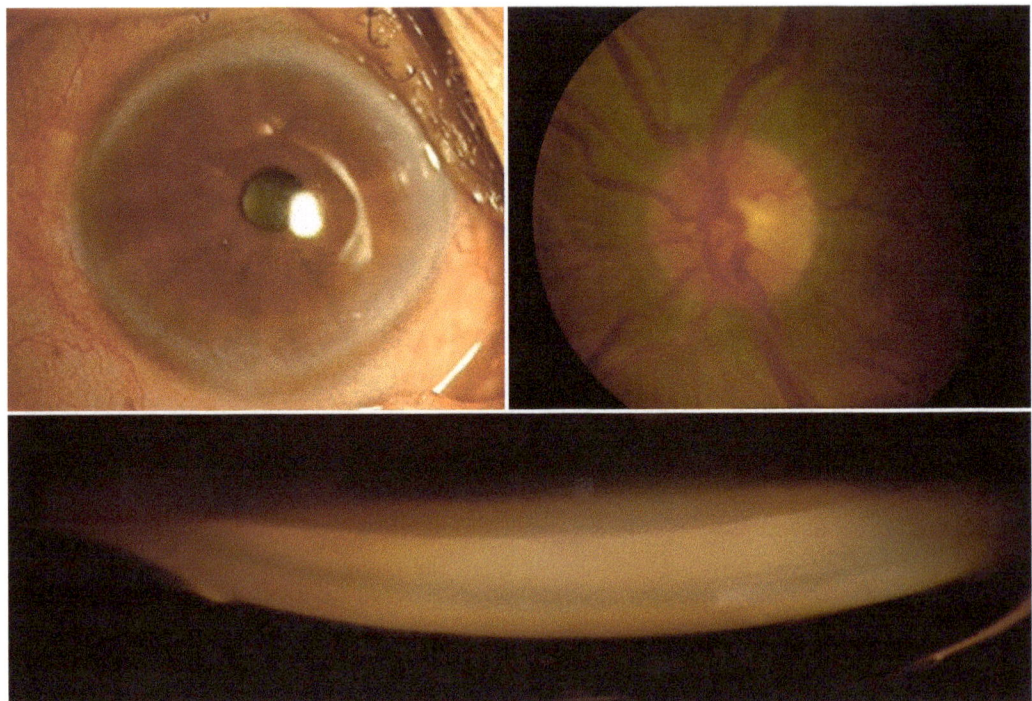

Fig. 6.3: Patient with primary angle-closure suspect showing shallow angles, normal optic disc and occludable angles.

- Short-axial length
- Small diameter/increased curvature of cornea
- Plateau iris configuration/thick peripheral iris roll.

Precipitating Factors

- Dim illumination
- Drugs:
  - Anticholinergics
  - Adrenergics
- Emotional stress.

DIAGNOSIS

External Examination

- Majority of people with PACG do not experience any symptoms, including patients with intermittently or chronically elevated IOP
- Some present acutely with colored halos around light due to corneal edema, ocular pain, redness, headache and decreased visual acuity. Digital palpation of the eye through closed eyelids reveals a firm (often rock hard) eye. Patient may also experience bradycardia or arrhythmia.

Penlight Examination

When a slit lamp or goniolens is unavailable, a penlight may be used to estimate the peripheral anterior chamber depth by shining through temporal side of the eye. An iris that is convex forwards with a corresponding shallow anterior chamber would block the illumination causing the nasal iris to be in shadow.

Slit-Lamp Examination

- Acute angle closure—hazy cornea (epithelial and stromal edema), iris bombe (pupillary block), sectoral iris stromal atrophy and lens glaukomflecken
- Peripheral anterior chamber depth:
  - Van Herick technique
  - Limbal chamber depth method (modification of Van Herick technique).

Gonioscopy

- Two or four mirror gonioscope
- Indentation gonioscopy (to rule out appositional or synechial angle closure):
  - One millimeter narrow slit beam focused, avoid any light falling on pupil

– Twenty-five times magnification

– Various grading system—Scheie, Shaffer and Spaeth.

Other Imaging Techniques

- Scheimpflug photography
- *Ultrasound biomicroscopy:* Useful for imaging cases of plateau iris, iridociliary masses causing secondary angle closure or choroidal effusions
- Anterior segment optical coherence tomography
- Scanning peripheral anterior chamber depth analyzer
- Provocative tests:
  - *Dark-room prone test:* Patient is made to stay in a dark room for 60–90 minutes to induce mydriasis. Patient must be awake to avoid sleep-induced miosis. During IOP measurement keep the light to a minimum to avoid reversal
  - *Pharmacologic pupil dilatation:* This is achieved with short-acting topical mydriatic and a rise of IOP of 8 mm Hg is considered positive.

▮ MANAGEMENT

Primary Angle-Closure Suspect

- Reported prevalence in India, 1.4% APEDS to 10.3% (the Vellore eye survey)[3,4]
- Twenty-two percent of primary angle-closure suspect (PACS) cases will progress to PAC within 5 years[2]
- Some rely on a provocative test, usually a prone dark-room test to predict progression
- Prophylactic LPI for 10.2% of Indian population over 35 years is neither feasible nor desirable
- Indications of prophylactic LPI:
  - Established PAC/PACG in fellow eye
  - Family history of PACG
  - Cannot come for regular follow-up
  - Require frequent pupillary dilatation
  - Poor access to regular ophthalmic care
  - Positive provocative tests
- If significant iridocorneal contact persists post-LPI, optimal management remains undefined: options include observation, laser iridoplasty, prophylactic with pilocarpine 1% and lens extraction
- Lens extraction:
  - Logically would result in relieving relative pupillary block, but because of ethical issues, it should be done only in case of visually significant cataract.

Primary Angle Closure

- Prophylactic LPI is recommended
- In a hospital-based study, after LPI with diurnal phasing of less than 21 mm Hg, 36.1% had chronically raised IOP of more than 22 mm Hg and 11.1% progressed to PACG even though glaucoma therapy was started to reduce IOP to less than 20 mm Hg[5]
- Thomas et al. reported that 28% of PAC went on to develop PACG after 5 years[6]
- Management is as for PACS, but with a "lower" threshold for further interventions, if there is an inadequate angle widening after LPI, particularly, if IOP remains high
- Medical treatment as for POAG may be required for substantial synechial closure or persistently elevated IOP despite an opened angle.

Acute Primary Angle Closure

- Aim is to lower IOP initially with hyperosmotic agents like intravenous mannitol, full doses of oral acetazolamide and glycerol
- Once IOP drops in about 20–30 minutes, topical pilocarpine and aqueous suppressants may be instilled
- Perform LPI as soon as possible
- Laser peripheral iridotomy can lead to a controlled IOP without any further medical or surgical therapy in about 70% of cases[2,3]
- In resistant cases, perform "laser iridoplasty" to break the attack if medical therapy fails or contraindicated and where a LPI is precluded by excessive shallowing of anterior chamber, inflammation or corneal edema
- Perform "surgical peripheral iridectomy", in case above mentioned measures fail
- Do not forget to perform LPI in other eye.

Primary Angle-Closure Glaucoma

- Treat aggressively as PACG progresses faster than POAG
- Laser peripheral iridotomy is recommended despite synechial angle closure as it can prevent further, trabecular damage and angle closure, although its role needs to be validated in randomized controlled trials
- Principles of medical therapy is similar as needed for POAG
- Most patients need trabeculectomy to control IOP
- Lens extraction:

- Various studies document significant widening of angle, lowering of postoperative medications and decrease complications as compared with surgical iridectomy or trabeculectomy
- Care should be taken during surgery as these eye are associated with high IOP, shallow anterior chamber, decreased endothelial counts, floppy iris, posterior synechiae, bulky lens, lax lens zonules and a high risk of malignant zonules
- Reports of phacoemulsification with goniosynechialysis, in presence of PAS closure, have been encouraging
- While there is currently insufficient evidence to recommend the use of cataract surgery in management of PACG, its threshold in these eyes should be lower.
- Goniosynechialysis:
  - Usually performed with lens extraction
  - Involves mechanical stripping of PAS away from the trabecular meshwork using viscoelastics or an irrigation cyclodialysis spatula
- Trabeculectomy:
  - Performed similarly to open-angle glaucoma, with the exception that surgical peripheral iridectomy should always be performed at the time of trabeculectomy
  - Use of antimetabolites should be considered.
- Trabeculectomy with cataract extraction:
  - In the absence of data as to the advantages or disadvantages of a one-stage combined versus two-stage procedure for coexistent uncontrolled PACG with cataract, the decision as to which approach to follow remains subjective.
- Glaucoma drainage implant:
  - May be considered in chronic ACG where trabeculectomy has failed to control the IOP, or in eyes that are deemed to be at high risk of failure with trabeculectomy.

REFERENCES

1. Foster PJ, Buhrmann R, Quigley HA, Johnson GJ. The definition and classification of glaucoma in prevalence surveys. Br J Ophthalmol. 2002;86:238-42.
2. Thomas R, George R, Parikh R, Muliyil J, Jacob A. Five year risk of progression of primary angle closure suspects to primary angle closure: a population based study. Br J Ophthalmol. 2003;87:450-4.
3. Dandona L, Dandona R, Mandal P, Mandal P, John RK, McCarty CA, et al. Open-angle glaucoma in an urban population in southern India: the Andhra Pradesh eye disease study. Ophthalmology. 2000;107:1702-9.
4. Jacob A, Thomas R, Koshi SP, Braganza A, Muliyil J. Prevalence of primary glaucoma in an urban south Indian population. Indian J Ophthalmol. 1998;46:81-6.
5. Sihota R, Rao A, Gupta V, Srinivasan G, Sharma A. Progression in primary angle closure eyes. J Glaucoma. 2010;19:632-6.
6. Thomas R, Parikh R, Muliyil J, Kumar RS. Five-year risk of progression of primary angle closure to primary angle closure glaucoma: a population-based study. Acta Ophthalmol Scand. 2003;81:480-5.

Trabeculectomy versus Tube

Giovanna Casale-Vargas, Oscar Albis-Donado, Gabriel Lazcano-Gómez

▌INTRODUCTION

Trabeculectomy has become the most common surgical procedure for glaucoma and is considered the gold standard for the surgical management of glaucoma.

Trabeculectomy involves removing a portion of the trabecular meshwork, and using a partial-thickness scleral flap to cover the sclerostomy.[1] This surgery requires an incomplete healing to allow the outflow of aqueous from the anterior chamber towards the subconjunctival space.[2] Success varies from 70 to 90% according to several publications.[3,4] Formation of scar tissue could cause obstruction of aqueous outflow, which is the most common reason for failure. Thus, inhibition of scar formation during the process of wound healing should promote greater success, and this goal is sought with the use of antimetabolites or multiple devices.[5]

Classically, glaucoma tube implants are indicated for eyes with previous failed glaucoma surgeries, several secondary glaucomas, in eyes with previous conjunctival scarring, and as a primary surgery for glaucomas such as neovascular glaucoma (NVG).[6,7]

Case 1: Trabeculectomy with mitomycin C

A 52-year-old man with pseudoexfoliation glaucoma was found to have an intraocular pressure (IOP) of 4 mm Hg with passive Seidel in his left eye on first postoperative day after a trabeculectomy augmented with mitomycin C (MMC) (0.5%) for 3 minutes. Visual acuity (VA) was 20/200. Fundus examination showed no choroidal detachment. Conservative management with patching and a low

dose of topical steroids was unable to stop the leak, so after 5 days additional stitches were placed. The leak became slower and after 1 month of follow-up IOP was 8 mm Hg with negative Seidel (Figs. 7A.1A and B).

Case 2: Trabeculectomy with biodegradable collagen matrix implant, and ologen

A 70-year-old female patient with a history of primary open-angle glaucoma oculus uterque (OU) and trabeculectomy with MMC 14 months ago oculus dexter (OD), was found to have avascular conjunctiva on the area of the flap with a passive leak, a well-formed anterior chamber, IOP 4 mm Hg VA 20/40 (Figs. 7A.2A and B). Transconjunctival sutures to reduce filtration were added to the scleral flap, raising the pressure to 8, but the bleb was still Seidel positive. It was decided to insert an Ologen implant over the flap, under the conjunctiva and to cover the bleb with amniotic membrane. At 12 days of follow-up IOP was 8, no leak was seen, so the remains of the amniotic membrane were removed, after which the original defect was discovered, still Seidel positive (Figs. 7A.2C to E).

Case 3: EX-PRESS mini glaucoma shunt

A 46-year-old man with pigmentary glaucoma OU was on triple hypotensive therapy since diagnosis, without adequate IOP control. An EX-PRESS mini glaucoma shunt implant OD was decided. On day 1 IOP was 9 mm Hg, VA was 20/100 and no choroidal detachment was identified. The follow-up was favorable, IOP was 12 mm Hg on timolol 0.5% bid OD at 3 months of follow-up (Figs. 7A.3A to E).

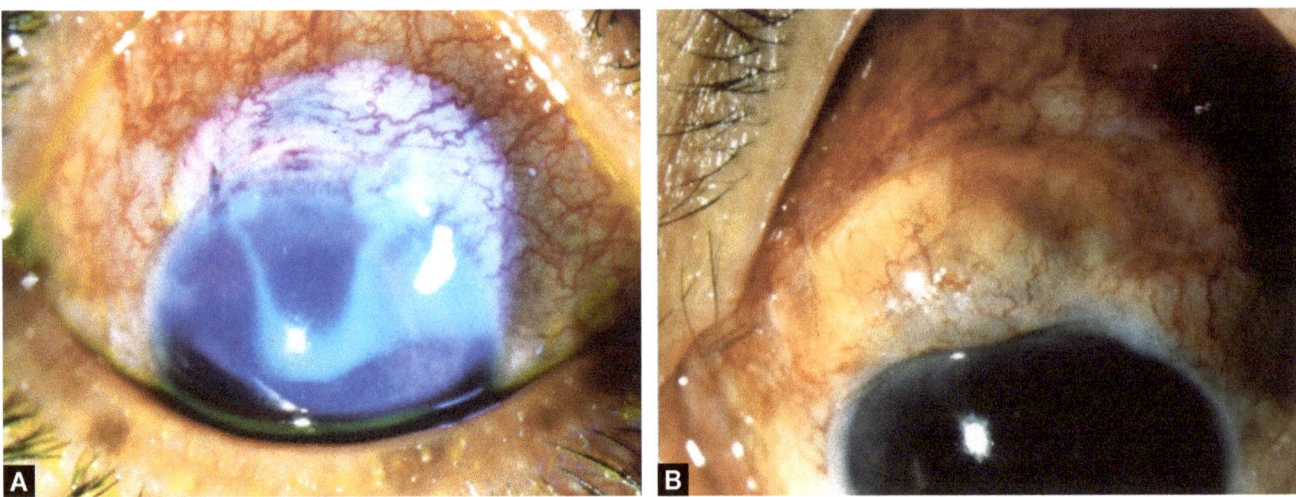

Figs. 7A.1A and B: (A) One day after surgery with a vascularized, flat bleb, with sutures in place, and passive, Seidel-positive leak. (B) One month later, the sutures have been removed and the bleb is formed with moderate vascularization and no further leak.

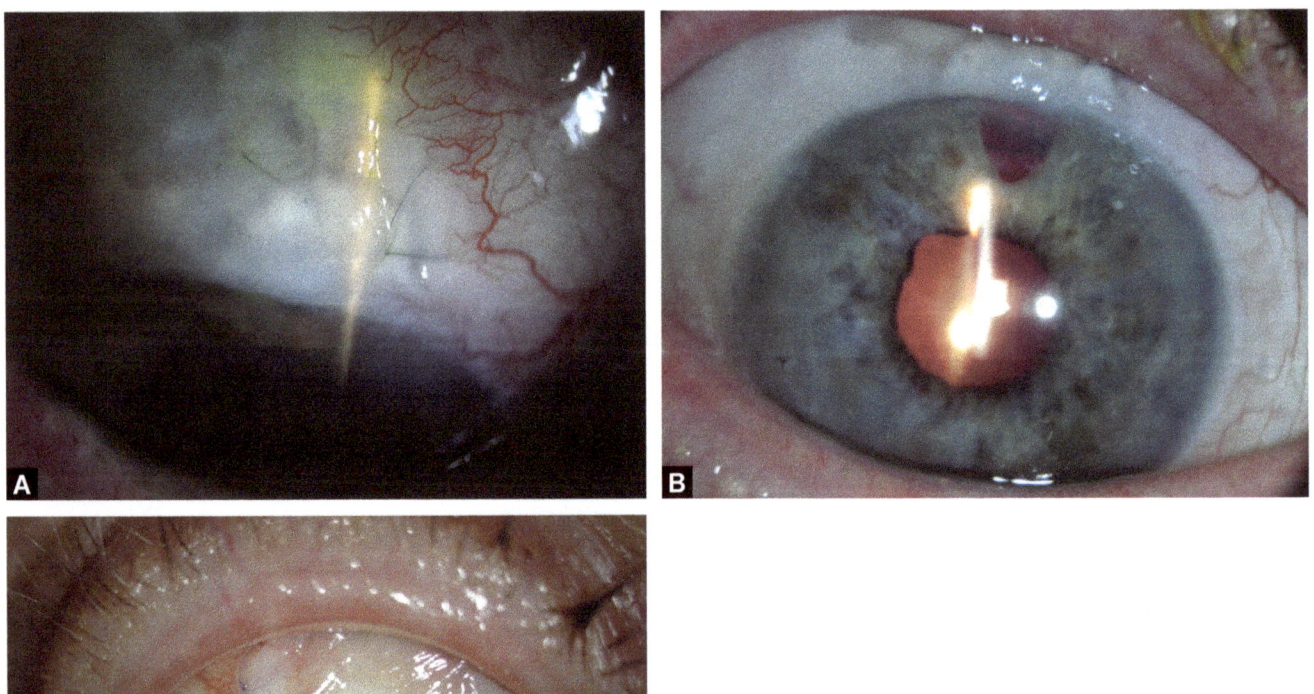

Figs. 7A.2A to C: (A) Fourteen months after a successful trabeculectomy with mitomycin C the patient has an epithelial defect at the avascular and extensive bleb, with a positive Seidel test. (B) The anterior chamber is well-formed, the iridectomy is patent, no choroidals, and no corneal or macular folds were found. (C) An Ologen implant was placed under the conjunctiva, right under the area of the leak in order to promote a scaffold for future vessel growth in the area, and the conjunctival defect was covered with amniotic membrane, held in place by several monofilament polyglactin sutures.

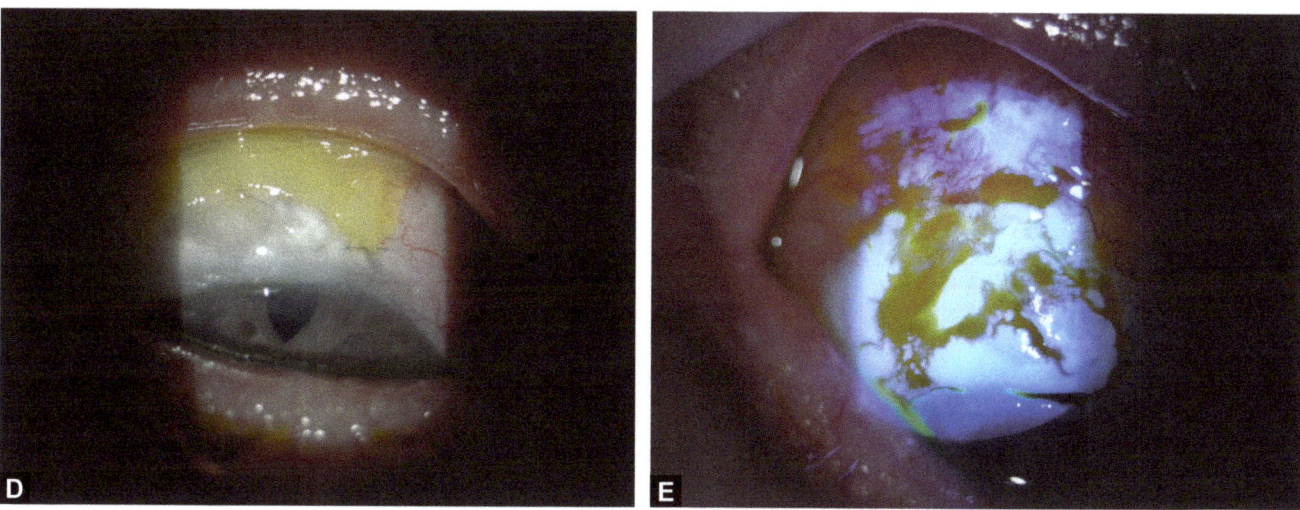

Figs. 7A.2D and E: (D) Twelve days later fluorescein staining did not reveal any aqueous leak, intraocular pressure was 8, but the sutures were causing bleeding and pain from the upper tarsus due to constant friction, so the membrane and sutures were removed. (E) Remains of the amniotic membrane were removed, and despite the Ologen implant being in place, the Seidel test was positive once more.

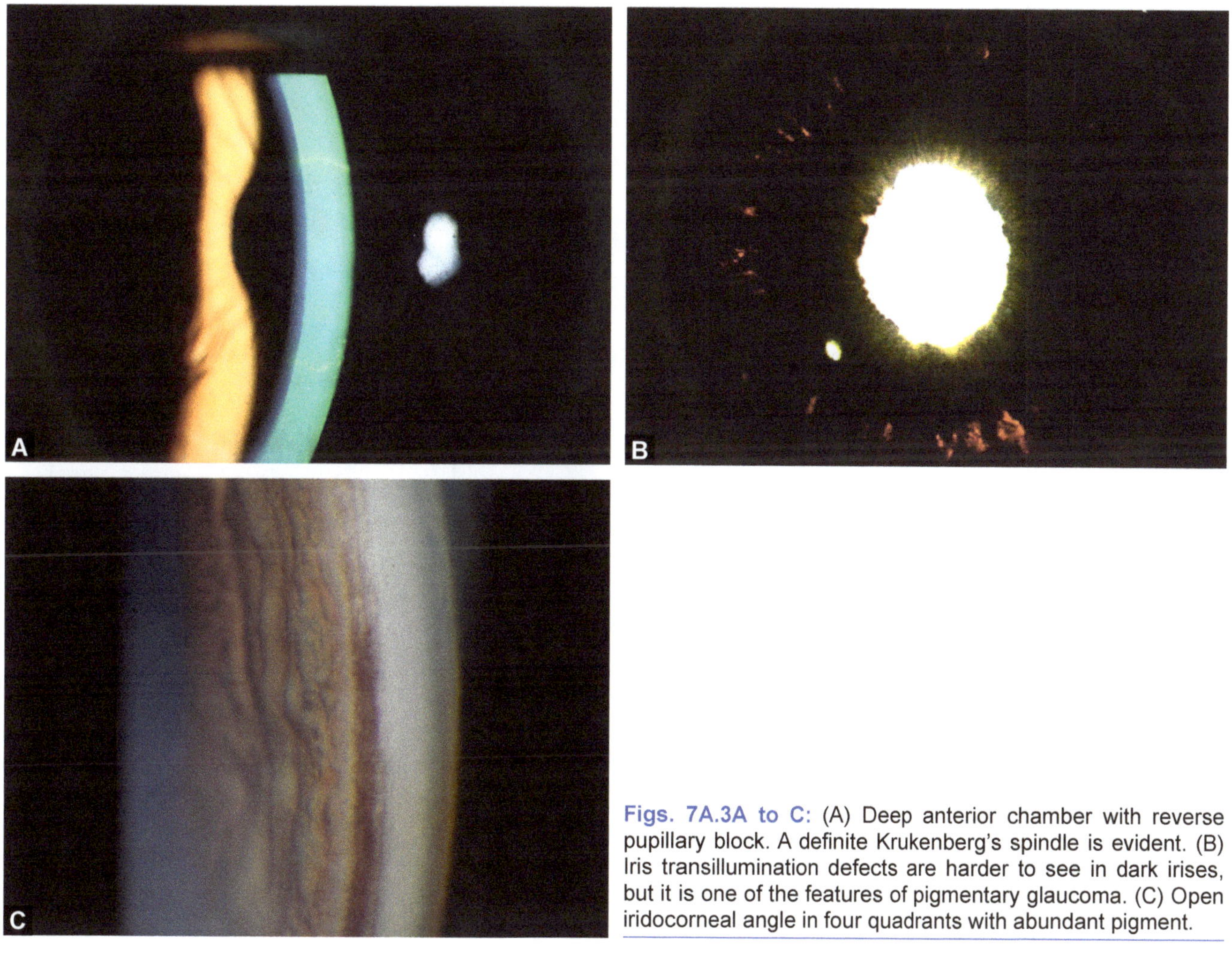

Figs. 7A.3A to C: (A) Deep anterior chamber with reverse pupillary block. A definite Krukenberg's spindle is evident. (B) Iris transillumination defects are harder to see in dark irises, but it is one of the features of pigmentary glaucoma. (C) Open iridocorneal angle in four quadrants with abundant pigment.

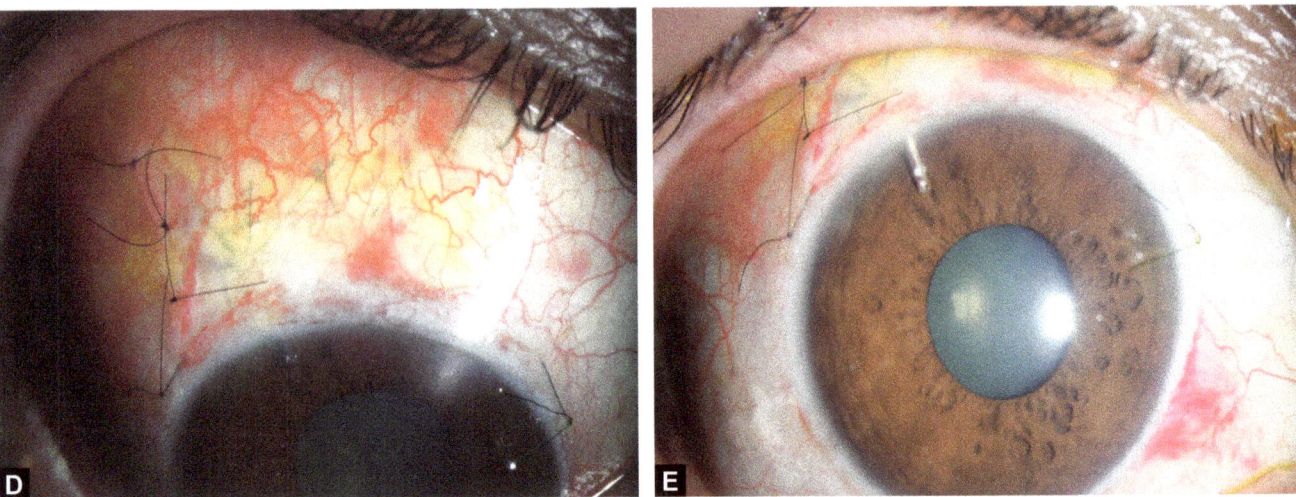

Figs. 7A.3D and E: (D) One day after surgery showing hyperemic conjunctiva with closed wound, without wound leaks, a very diffuse on low bleb. (E) The tip of the express implant can be seen at an adequate position away from both the iris and the corneal endothelium.

Case 4: Primary Ahmed valve implant

A 65-year-old patient, who had lost his right eye due to a postoperative infection of a trabeculectomy, needed a filtering surgery for his left eye. He is a farm worker and was very reluctant to having a trabeculectomy in his only remaining eye. After an explanation of the risks and costs, a primary Ahmed valve plus cataract removal was performed, viscoelastic material was left in the anterior chamber. On his last visit 2 months after surgery, IOP was 14 on 2 medications, VA was 20/20 with spectacles, and no signs of complications were seen (Fig. 7A.4).

Case 5: Ahmed valve implant and neovascular glaucoma

A 53-year-old woman with diabetes was found to have rubeosis iridis, partial angle closure due to angle rubeosis, IOP was 58, VA 20/400, mild corneal edema and proliferative diabetic retinopathy, a recent vitreous hemorrhage despite a single session of about 1200 argon laser shots 2 years previously on her OD. IOP was lowered to 32 mm Hg using oral acetazolamide plus topical timolol, brimonidine and dorzolamide. An intravitreal bevacizumab injection was administered, and 2 days later a flexible-plate Ahmed valve was placed without incidents. 3 weeks later further retinal laser therapy was performed to both eyes, IOP was 18 mm Hg, no rubeosis iridis could be seen, no further angle closure was seen, her vision was 20/40 (Figs. 7A.5A to C).

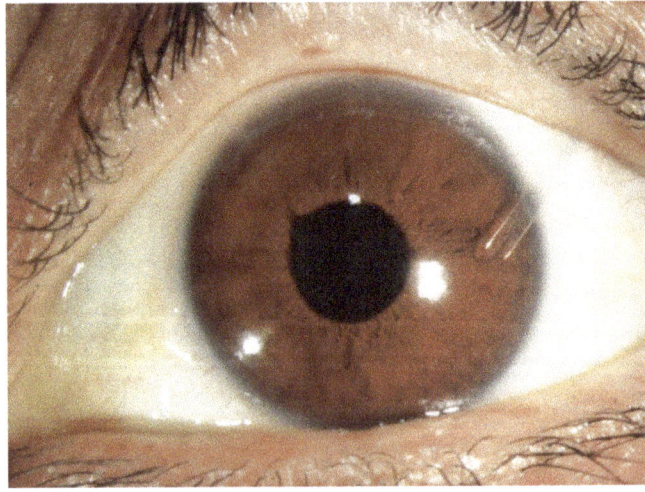

Fig. 7A.4: The tip of the tube of the Ahmed valve is closer to the iris than to the cornea. The tube was inserted through a long needle-generated tunnel without the use of a scleral patch.

INVESTIGATIONS

Follow-up Protocol

Characteristics of the bleb, anterior chamber depth, IOP, VA and posterior segment must be evaluated during follow-up of all patients submitted to a trabeculectomy with MMC, Ologen or EX-PRESS shunt implant. Patients with tubes will additionally need to have the position of the tube reviewed when the IOP becomes stable, checking for patency, distance from the endothelium, and risk of exposure.

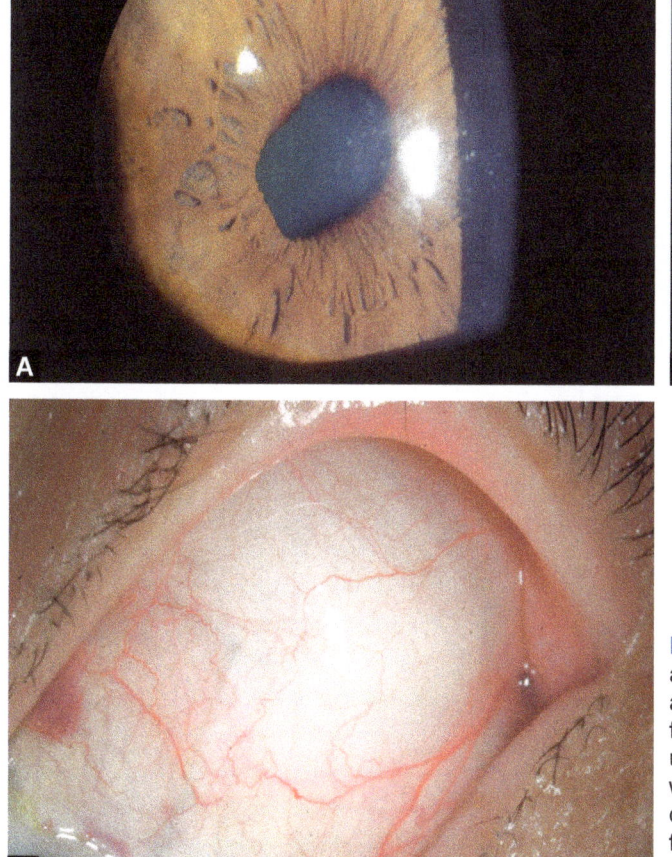

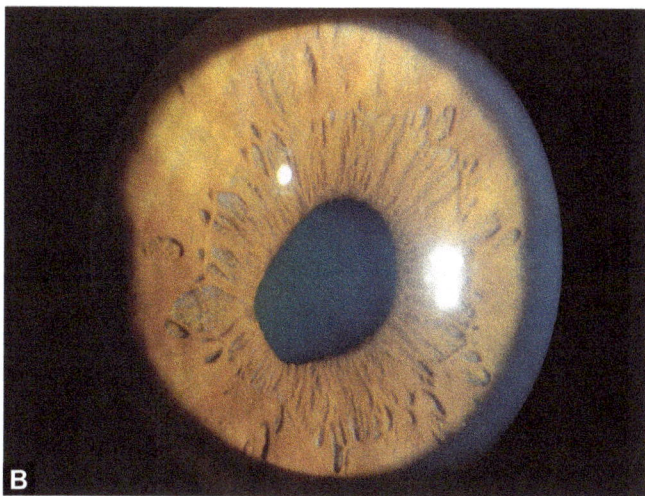

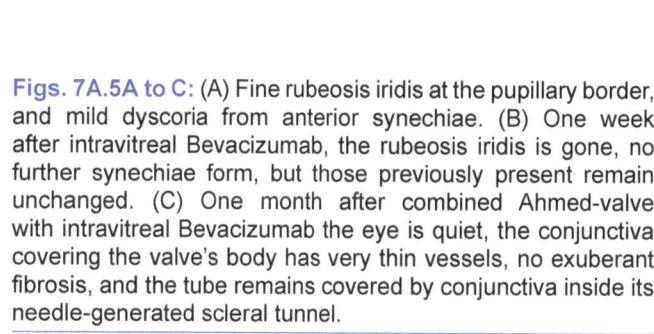

Figs. 7A.5A to C: (A) Fine rubeosis iridis at the pupillary border, and mild dyscoria from anterior synechiae. (B) One week after intravitreal Bevacizumab, the rubeosis iridis is gone, no further synechiae form, but those previously present remain unchanged. (C) One month after combined Ahmed-valve with intravitreal Bevacizumab the eye is quiet, the conjunctiva covering the valve's body has very thin vessels, no exuberant fibrosis, and the tube remains covered by conjunctiva inside its needle-generated scleral tunnel.

BRIEF REVIEW OF LITERATURE

One of the most important studies about long-term outcomes of filtering surgeries is the tube versus trabeculectomy (TVT) study. In this study, the rate of reoperation was higher following trabeculectomy with MMC (29%) than tube shunt surgery (9%), and the rate of failure was also higher after trabeculectomy (46.9% vs. 29.8%). The rate of failure after reoperations was similar (47% vs. 43%).[6,7]

The use of antimetabolites increases the success of filtering surgery, but the rate of complications such as leakage increase from 5% to 10% with their use.[8] When comparing MMC to 5 FU we can observe lower postoperative IOP with MMC, complications are similar with both drugs, except for cyst formation (MMC) and corneal decompensation (5 FU).[9]

The main complications with antimetabolites are conjunctival and corneal toxicity, hypotony maculopathy, wound leaks, endophthalmitis and cataract.[10]

Recently, tissue engineering has achieved great progress in creating biomedical devices for preventing scar formation by modifying the well-organized process of wound healing. The Ologen implant may normalize subconjuntival wound-healing and maintain good function of a more normal-looking conjunctiva and biodegrade within 30–90 days.[11]

Nevertheless, the device does not show any IOP-lowering advantage of the Ologen-augmented trabeculectomy versus trabeculectomy alone.[11] Cillino et al recently demonstrated that the Ologen implant had good efficacy in terms of IOP reduction, with a success rate quite similar to MMC.[12]

The EX-PRESS glaucoma filtration device has been approved for usage for lowering IOP in patients who have uncontrolled glaucoma, including those who have failed prior medical and conventional surgical treatments. As the device is placed in the anterior chamber angle, its usage is not recommended for phakic patients with angle-closure glaucoma.[13,14]

The results of the recent report (CPETS) suggest that the EX-PRESS implant prevented early postoperative complications like inflammation and hyphema in the anterior chamber, but that contact of this implant with the iris was more frequent.[14]

The EX-PRESS implant has not shown significant difference in success rates compared to trabeculectomy.[15] Nevertheless, some studies indicate that reduction of IOP is better with the EX-PRESS implant in comparison to trabeculectomy[16] and visual recovery to near-baseline level of vision in less time as compared with trabeculectomy.[17]

Aqueous shunts are increasingly being used in the management of glaucoma in situations where trabeculectomy is unlikely to succeed or has failed. There has been an increased use of these devices over the past years.

The Ahmed glaucoma valve and the Baerveldt glaucoma implant are two of the shunts most commonly used in clinical practice.[18] The use of these devices has been successful in refractory glaucomas or in patients with prior failed filtration surgery or cataract surgery.[7]

Results of the TVT study suggest that both the surgical and a re-operation rates are higher in patients with trabeculectomy, as compared to aqueous shunts.[7] This study also showed that both trabeculectomy and tube surgery were capable of producing sustained IOP reductions, but implants were associated with the use of more glaucoma medications during the first years.

The results of the Ahmed Baerveldt comparison (ABC) study and the Ahmed versus Baerveldt (AVB) study suggest that although glaucoma drainage implant surgery with the Baerveldt glaucoma implant may lead to better IOP outcomes, there is an increased risk of postoperative complications and reinterventions.[19-21]

SUMMARY

The adjunctive use of MMC has been a major advance in improving the efficacy of lowering IOP with trabeculectomy. However, there are complications associated with MMC use. The possible complications in the short-term and long-term include endophthalmitis hypotony, Seidel, blebitis, filtration failure, cataract, choroidal detachment or hemorrhage, hypotony maculopathy and athalamia. These complications can increase with the use of antifibrotics, which end up being a necessary evil because without them the possibility of failure in the short-term is higher.[22]

Trabeculectomy with MMC is an effective alternative in difficult to control glaucomas and those with advanced glaucoma damage. This technique should be performed with the knowledge on how to handle filtering surgery with MMC and its complications. It should not be used indiscriminately. Their use in children should be with the utmost care, and are better avoided because of the high risk of complications, blebitis and endophthalmitis in particular.

Alternatives such as Ologen might offer significant advantages when compared with trabeculectomy alone. The EX-PRESS might also offer fewer rates of complications (including maculopathy, encapsulated bleb and choroidal detachment).

Tubes can be used in almost any kind of eye, regardless of previous failed surgeries, and as such they offer a reliable means of treating the most complicated cases, although their primary use seems to have very encouraging results.

REFERENCES

1. Papaconstantinou D, Georgalas I, Karmiris E, Diagourtas A, Koutsandrea C, Ladas I, et al. Trabeculectomy with ologen versus trabeculectomy fo the treatment of glaucoma: a pilot study. Acta Ophthalmologica. 2010;88:80-5.

2. Fontana H, Nouri-Mahdavi K, Lumba J, Ralli M, Caprioli J. Trabeculectomy with Mitomycin C. Ophthalmology. 2006;113:930-6.

3. Moshaed S. Dustin L. Comparative outcomes between newer and older surgeries for glaucoma. Trans Am Ophthalmol Soc. 2009;107:127-35.

4. Sihota R, Gupta V, Agarwal HC. Long-Term evaluation of trabeculectomy in primary open angle glaucoma and chronic primary angle closure glaucoma in an Asian population. Clin Experiment Ophthalmol. 2004;32:23-8.

5. Yuan F, Li L, Chen X, Yan X, Wang L. Biodegradable 3D-Porous Collagen Matrix (ologen) Compared with Mitomycin C for treatment of primary Open-Angle Glaucoma: Results at 5 years. J Ophthalmol. 2015;2015:637537.

6. Gedde SJ, Schiffman JC, Feuer WJ, Herndon LW, Brandt JD, Budenz DL, et al. Treatment outcomes in the Tube Versus Trabeculectomy (TVT) study after five years of follow-up. Am J Ophthalmol. 2012;153(5):789-803.e2.

7. Saheb H, Gedde SJ, Schiffman JC, Feuer WJ. Outcomes of glaucoma reoperations in the tube versus trabeculectomy (TVT) study. Am J Ophthalmol. 2014;157:1179-89.

8. Francis BA, Du LT, Najafi K, Murthy R, Kurumety U, Rao N, et al. Histopathologic Features of Conjunctival Filtering Blebs. Arch Ophthalmol. 2005;123:166-70.

9. Higginbotham EJ, Stevens RK, Musch DC, Karp KO, Lichter PR, Bergstrom TJ, et al. Bleb related Endophthalmitis after Trabeculectomy with Mitomycin C. Ophthalmology. 1996; 103:650-6.

10. Shaarawy. Glaucoma: Surgical Management, Section 12, Chapter 91, Elsevier.

11. Papaconstantinou D, Georgalas I, Karmiris E, Diagourtas A, Koutsandrea C, Ladas I, et al. Trabeculectomy with ologen versus trabeculectomy for the treatment of glaucoma: a pilot study. Acta Ophthalmologica. 2010;88:80-5.

12. Cillino S, Casuccio A, Di Pace F, Cagini C, Ferraro LL, Cillino G. Biodegradable collagen matrix implant versus mitomycin-C in trabeculectomy: Five year follow-up. BMC Ophthalmol. 2016;16:24.

13. Shaarawy T, Goldberg I, Fechtner R. EX-PRESS glaucoma filtration device: Review of clinical experience and comparison with trabeculectomy. Surv Ophthalmol. 2015;60: 327-45.

14. Arimura S, Takihara Y, Miyake S, Iwasaki K, Gozawa M, Matsumura T, et al. Randomized Clinical Trial For Early Postoperative complications of EX-PRESS implantation versus Trabeculectomy: Complications Postoperative of EX-PRESS versus trabeculectomy study (CPETS). Sci Rep. 2016;6:26080.

15. Mosaed S, Dustin L, Minckler DS. Comparative outcomes between newer and older surgeries for glaucoma. Trans Am Ophthalmol Soc. 2009;107:127-33.

16. Maris PJ, Ishida K, Netland PA. Comparison of trabeculectomy with EX-PRESS miniature glaucoma device implanted under scleral flap. J Glaucoma. 2007;16:14-9.

17. Chan JE, Netland PA. EX-PRESS Glaucoma Filtration Device: efficacy, safety, and predictability. 2015;8:381-8.

18. Barton K, Feuer WJ, Budenz DL, Schiffman J, Costa VP, Godfrey DG, et al. Three-year treatment outcomes in the Ahmed Baerveldt comparison study, Ophthalmology. 2014;121:1547-57.

19. Aminlari AE, Scott IU, Aref AA. Glaucoma drainage implant surgery and evidence-based update with relevance to sub-Saharan Africa. Middle East Afr J Ophthalmol. 2013;20: 126-30.

20. Budenz DL, Barton K, Gedde SJ, Feuer WJ, Schiffman J, Costa VP, et al. Five-year treatment outcomes in the Ahmed Baerveldt comparison study. Ophthalmology. 2015;122:308-16.

21. Christakis PG, Tsai JC, Kalenak JW, Zurakowski D, Cantor LB, Kammer JA, et al. The Ahmed versus Baerveldt study: three-year treatment outcomes. Ophthalmology. 2013;120: 2232-40.

22. Rosentreter A, Schild AM, Jordan JF, Krieglstein GK, Dietlein TS. A prospective randomized trial of trabeculectomy using mitomycin C and ologen implant in open angle glaucoma. Eye (Lond). 2010;24:1449-57.

Choice of Surgery: Nonpenetrating Deep Sclerectomy

Sylvain Roy, André Mermoud

▌DEFINITION

Nonpenetrating deep sclerectomy (NPDS) is a modern surgical technique aimed at lowering the intraocular pressure (IOP) while preserving at best the drainage pathways of the eye. It was developed to prevent some of the complications occurring during penetrating procedure such as trabeculectomy. It consists in lowering the resistance to aqueous humor egress by removing most of the resistance located at the level of the juxtacanalicular meshwork and inner wall of Schlemm's canal, and allowing a thin filtering membrane to stabilize the pressure drop. Finally, aqueous humor is drained in an intrascleral space, in the subchoroidal space, and to a lesser extent in the subconjunctival space.

Case 1: Primary open-angle glaucoma

The patient presents with a target IOP not reached with neuroretinal rim thinning and hemorrhage (Fig. 7B.1) and visual field reduction despite maximally tolerated medication. The iridocorneal angle is wide. Risks and benefits of undergoing an NPDS were discussed with the patient, and such surgical procedure was performed to lower the IOP, while minimizing the risks of operative and postoperative complications (Figs. 7B.2 to 7B.6).

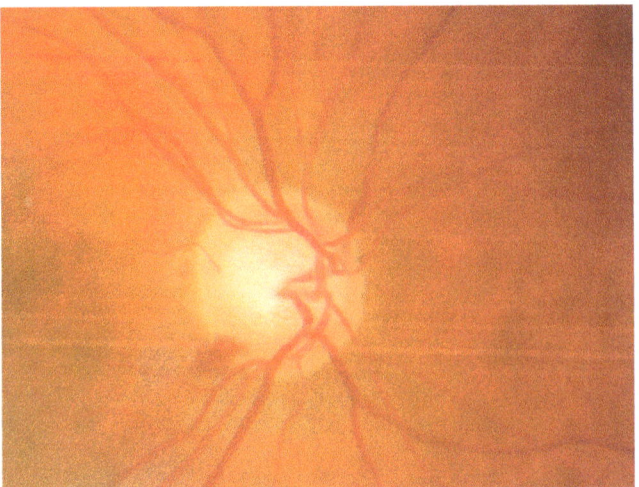

Fig. 7B.1: Optic nerve head showing a split hemorrhage in the inferior quadrant at 7 o'clock position.

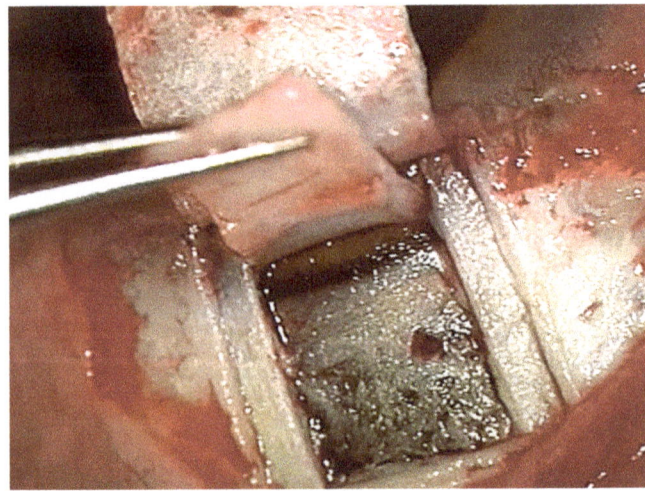

Fig. 7B.2: Surgical view showing dissection of the deep scleral flap.

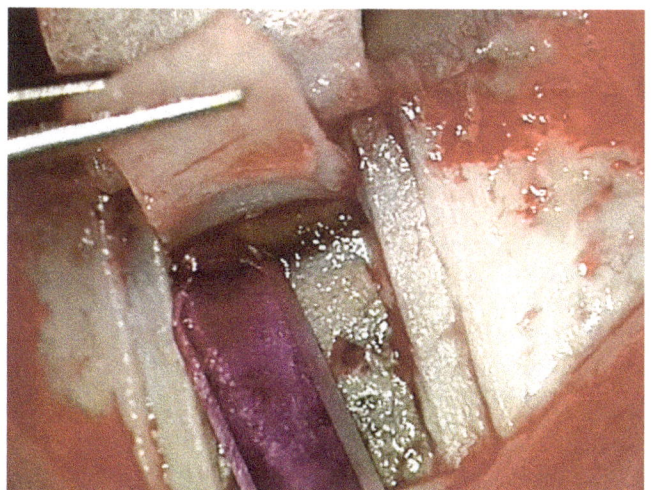

Fig. 7B.3: Surgical view showing fine dissection of the trabeculo-Descemet's membrane using a ruby crescent knife.

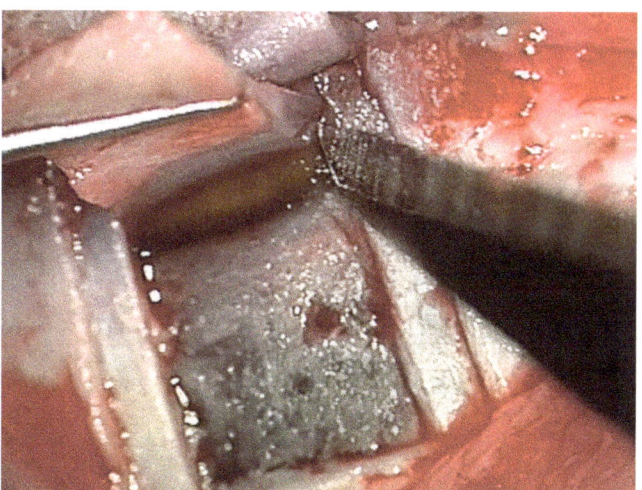

Fig. 7B.4: Surgical view showing removal of the deep scleral flap using a 11-blade.

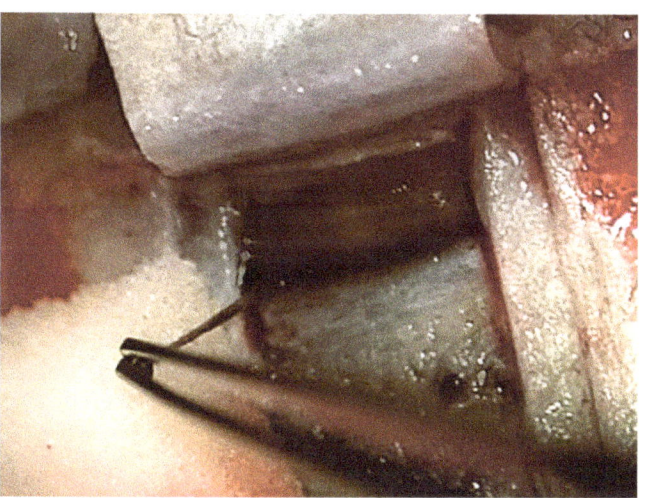

Fig. 7B.5: Surgical view showing peeling of the inner wall of Schlemm's canal using fine forceps.

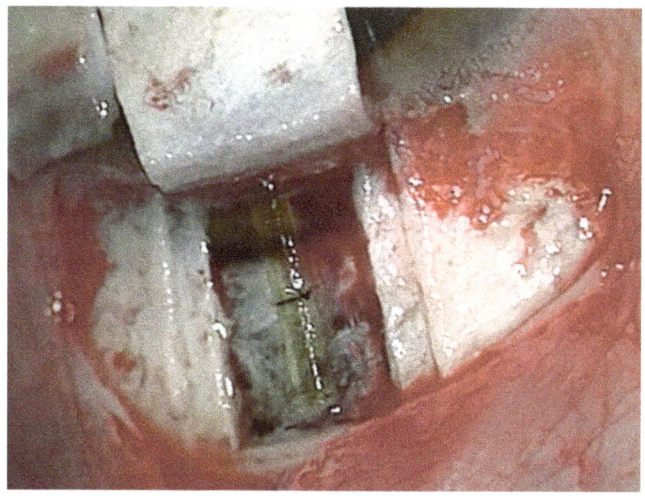

Fig. 7B.6: Surgical view showing implantation of a cylindrical collagen implant onto the scleral bed to act as a space maintainer.

Case 2: Pseudoexfoliative glaucoma

Pseudoexfoliative (PEX) glaucoma (Fig. 7B.7) can induce durable and very elevated IOP with significant optic nerve head (ONH) damages [high cup-to-disc (C:D) ratio)] and significant visual field loss (Fig. 7B.8). The aim of NPDS is to efficiently lower the IOP with a target postoperative IOP in the mid-teens (i.e. between 12 mm Hg and 16 mm Hg), without glaucoma medications. Goniopuncture may be performed more frequently in PEX glaucoma because of the thicker trabeculo-Descemet's membrane (TDM) and probably deposits of PEX material on or in the membrane (Fig. 7B.9).

Case 3: Normal tension glaucoma

The advantage of NPDS over angular procedure (e.g. iStent) is that the IOP can further be lowered at around 8–10 mm Hg, starting from 12–16 mm Hg for instance. Reduction in IOP of about 30% can even be achieved. The low complication rate and high success rate allow for a greater safety margin on these eyes with compromised ONH. The second

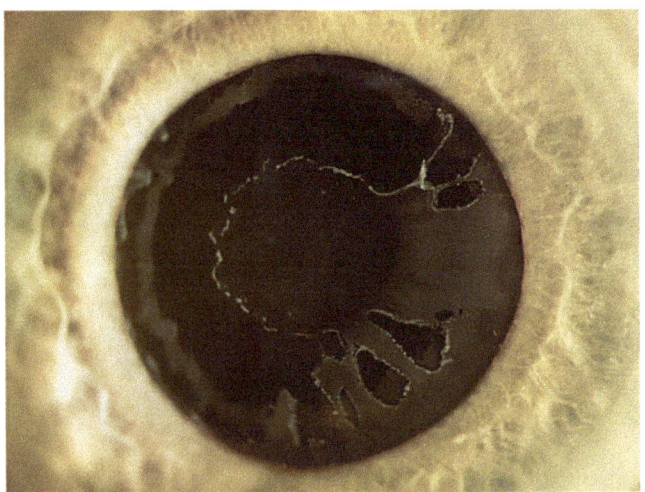

Fig. 7B.7: Slit-lamp photograph showing pseudo-exfoliation material on the anterior capsule of the lens.

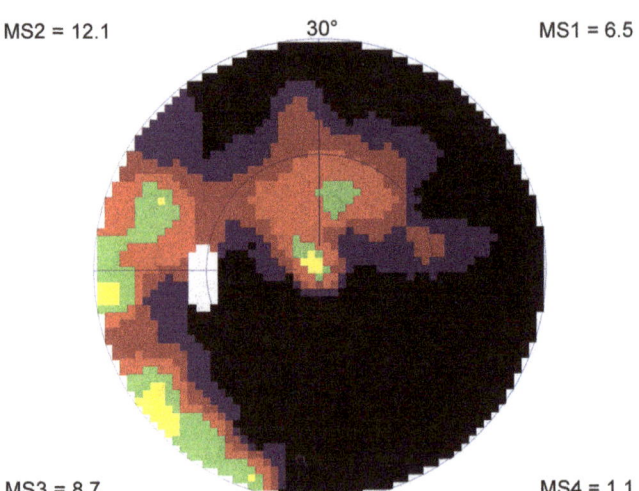

MS2 = 12.1   30°   MS1 = 6.5

MS3 = 8.7   MS4 = 1.1

Fig. 7B.8: Octopus visual field showing severe defects in the inferior and nasal quadrants. Note the central macula sparing.

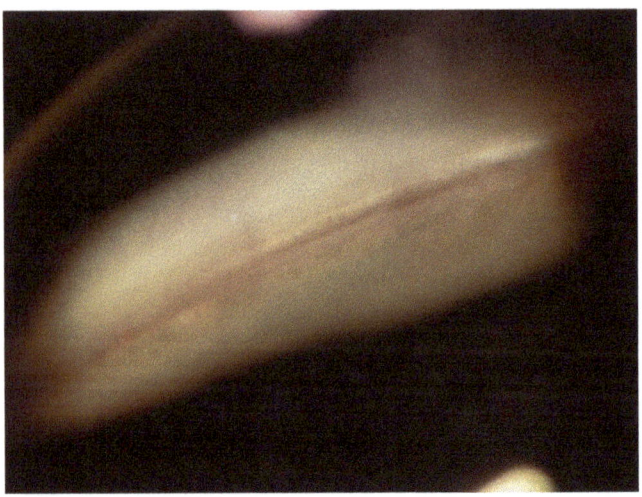

Fig. 7B.9: Gonioscopy view of the iridocorneal angle to inspect for pigment or pseudoexfoliation deposits in the angle structures.

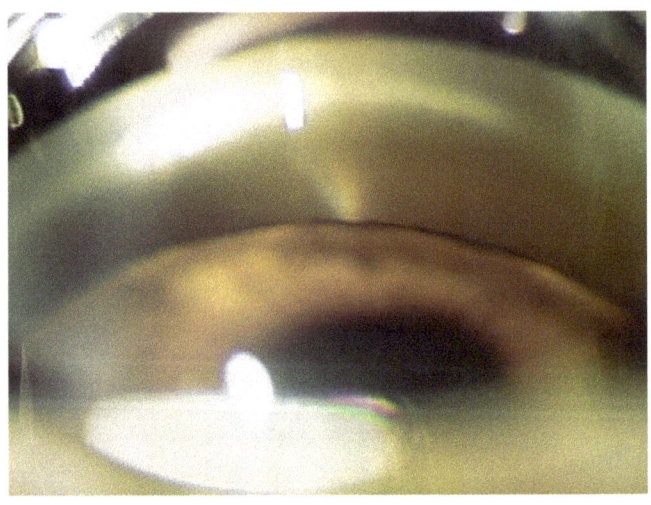

Fig. 7B.10: Gonioscopy view showing a closure of the angle in the case of closed-angle glaucoma.

advantage is that the number of antiglaucoma medications can be reduced or even suppressed.

Case 4: Angle-closure glaucoma and neovascular glaucoma

Primary and secondary angle-closure glaucomas represent relative contraindications for deep sclerectomy. Usually, the extended iris apposition against the trabeculum fully blocks aqueous outflow in the complete angle closure (Figs. 7B.10 and 7B.11). This could be prevented by performing a peripheral iridotomy and by extending further into clear cornea the dissection of the TDM (Fig. 7B.12). The new vessels growing within the angle structure in neovascular glaucoma form a bulk that also prevents aqueous humor from flowing freely towards the trabeculum represent, in that respect, an absolute contraindication for that kind of surgery (Figs. 7B.13 to 7B.15).

Case 5: Traumatic glaucoma

In case of traumatic glaucoma, the anatomy of the anterior segment is altered and normal filtration is impaired due to the structural changes resulting from the trauma

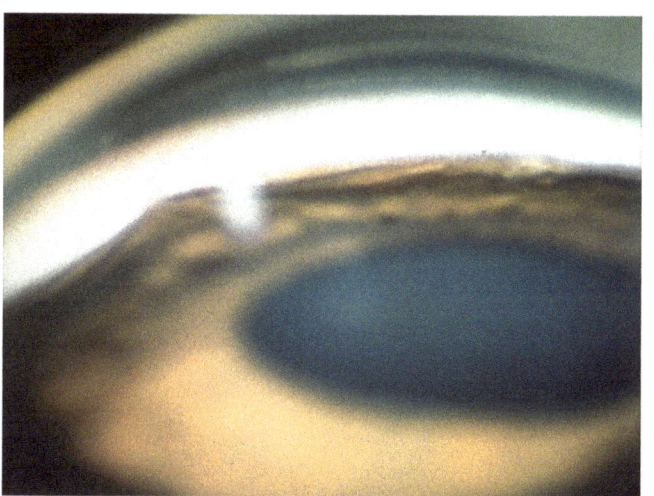

Fig. 7B.11: Gonioscopy view showing iris apposition against the trabecular meshwork in a situation of a closed-angle glaucoma.

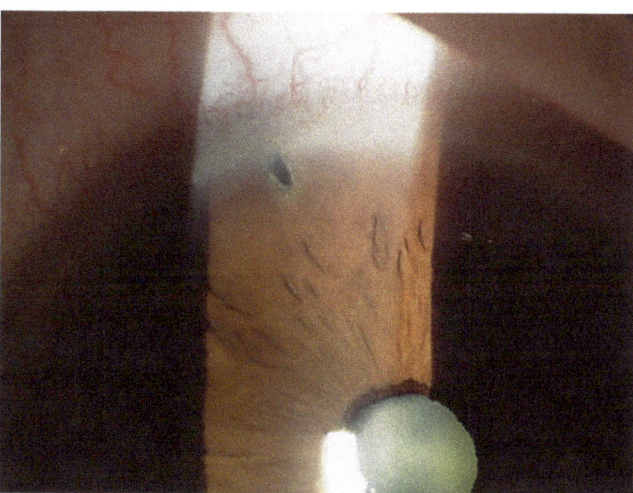

Fig. 7B.12: Slit-lamp photograph after successful laser iridotomy showing an open and patent aperture through the iris stroma.

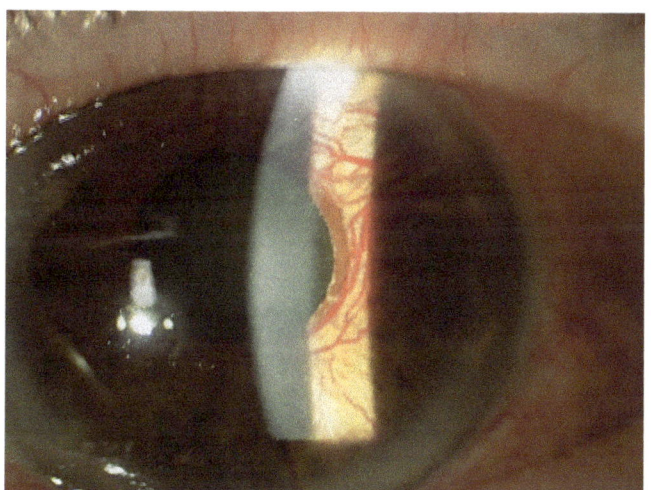

Fig. 7B.13: Slit-lamp photograph showing extensive neovascularization of the anterior surface of the iris in case of neovascular glaucoma.

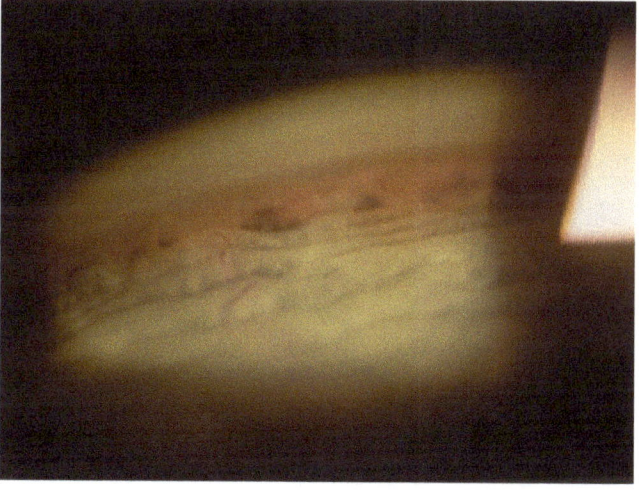

Fig. 7B.14: Gonioscopy view showing the angle structure invaded by some neovascularization running from the iris surface.

(Fig. 7B.16). NPDS aims at restoring a functional aqueous humor pathway that allows keeping the IOP in target range, thus preventing further damages to the optic nerve. The advantages of NPDS are the low rate of postoperative complications, a gentle and progressive reduction of the IOP, and less incidence of surgery-induced cataract development.

Case 6: Uveitic glaucoma

Nonpenetrating deep sclerectomy in uveitic glaucoma takes advantage in preserving the integrity of the anterior chamber by preventing opening of the trabeculum and by avoiding iris tissue from being severed when performing peripheral iridectomy, as in conventional trabeculectomy. All these maneuvers lead to increase in anterior chamber inflammation, as shown by rise in flare. Performing a filtering procedure that does not promote further anterior chamber inflammation is a real benefit for patients suffering from uveitic glaucoma, and for whom a gentle and less proinflammatory filtering procedure should be proposed.

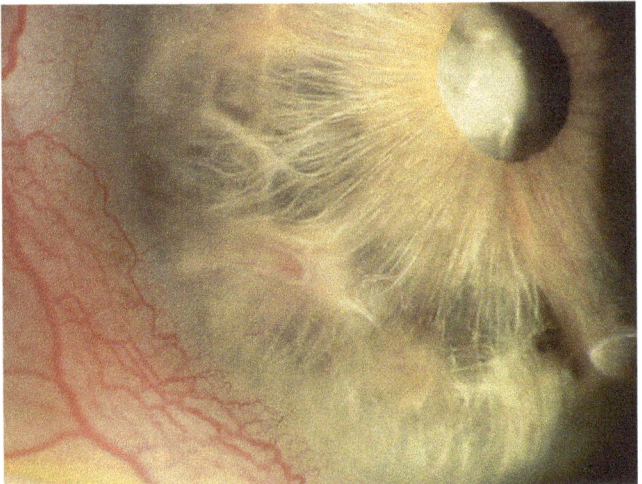

Fig. 7B.15: Slit-lamp photograph showing bundles of neovascularization at the surface of the iris.

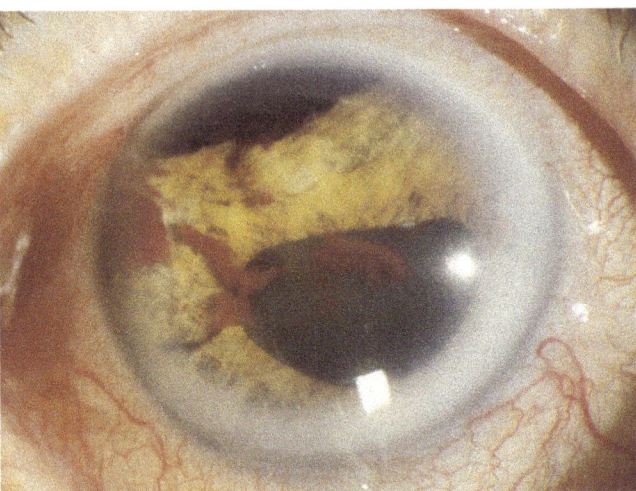

Fig. 7B.16: Slit-lamp photograph showing a large iridodialysis in the upper quadrant from 10 to 2 o'clock, with clots of blood in the anterior chamber.

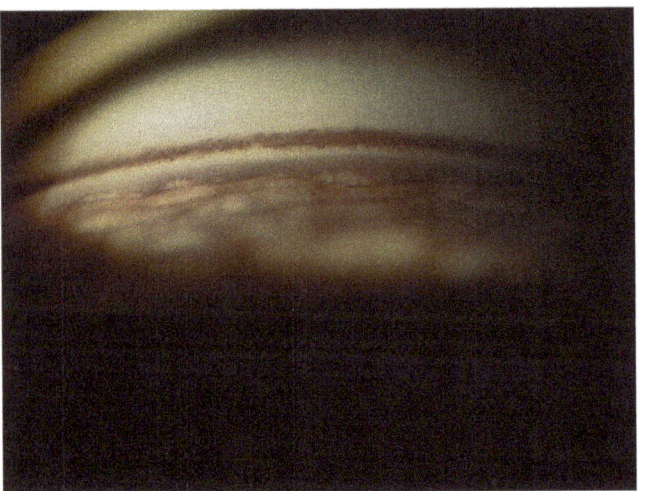

Fig. 7B.17: Gonioscopy view showing important pigment deposits at the level of Schwalbe line.

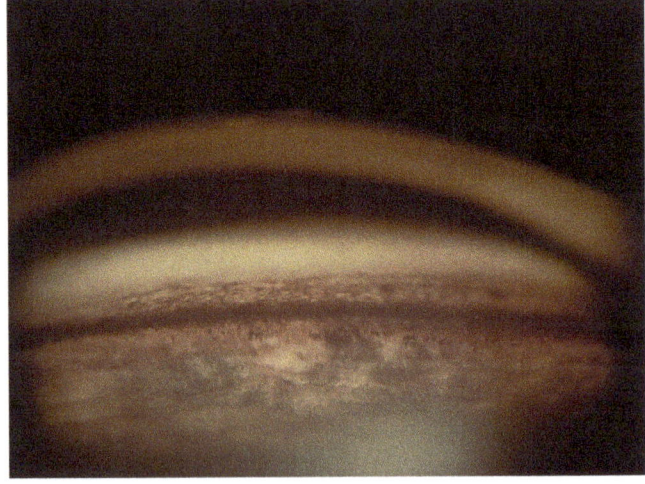

Fig. 7B.18: Gonioscopy view showing important pigment deposits in front of Schwalbe line and Sampaolesi line.

Case 7: Pigmentary glaucoma

Nonpenetrating deep sclerectomy is also efficient in pigmentary glaucoma where important deposits of iris pigmentation are present in the iridocorneal angle structures (Figs. 7B.17 and 7B.18). The creation of a large TDM allows for the aqueous humor to filter through that membrane, and the bypass of the dense grid of the trabeculum at the level of the juxtacanalicular meshwork contributes to a better control of the IOP. If necessary, an Nd:YAG goniopuncture can also be performed to enhance aqueous humor outflow in a late postoperative phase.

INVESTIGATIONS

Every glaucoma patient requiring an NPDS procedure should have the following comprehensive ophthalmology examination prior to surgery.

Mandatory tests include:

- Distance best corrected visual acuity and refraction

- *Tonometry (applanation):* Preoperative IOP under optimal or maximally tolerated medication
- *Pachymetry:* A central corneal thickness using a pachymeter (either ultrasound or noncontact) is required to correct for the corneal compensation of the applanation tonometry
- *Gonioscopy:* Images of the anatomy of the iridocorneal angle are necessary to exclude closed angle or neovascularization of the angle
- *Optic nerve assessment:* A dilated assessment of the ONH is essential together with a red-free evaluation of the peripapillary retinal nerve fiber layer (RNFL). The ONH can be documented using a hand drawn, labeled diagram (special emphasis on C:D ratio, notching, RNFL defects, and/or hemorrhage) and/or a clinical picture. A colored photo and a red-free photo of the ONH are essential for serial follow-up.
- *Visual field testing:* Reliable visual fields provide a baseline for future follow-up
- In addition, the following tests, if performed, help in managing the condition better, in case the facilities exist, and are affordable to the patient
- Stereo-optic disc photographs to confirm the optic nerve parameters and document baseline
- Imaging of the optic nerve with RNFL analysis (ocular coherence tomography, Heidelberg retinal tomography, or scanning laser polarimetry) provides a statistical comparison with the normative database, thereby providing additional information for subsequent management.
- Diurnal variation of IOP curve may provide additional information and influence timing of the surgery.

FOLLOW-UP PROTOCOL

Postoperative follow-up consists in regular clinical evaluation at days 1, 7, 14, 30, month 2, 3, 6, to ascertain the aspect of the filtering bleb, depth of the anterior chamber, flare level, IOP, and to document possible complications. Postoperative management consist in controlling the onset and growth of bleb fibrosis or encapsulation that can be treated with bleb needling associated with anti-metabolites. Increase in the outflow resistance through the TDM can be modulated by performing Nd:YAG laser goniopuncture.

BRIEF REVIEW OF LITERATURE

There is a consensus that complications related to over-filtration and infections are significantly lower than in trabeculectomy.[1-4] 10-year results indicate that NPDS remains a long-term successful procedure in stabilizing the IOP at around 12 mm Hg with low postoperative complication rates.[5] The success rate at 10 years was 44.6% and 77.6% for complete and qualified success, respectively. NPDS is also indicated for glaucoma secondary to uveitis and shows promising results in normal tension glaucoma (NTG).[6,7]

SUMMARY

Nonpenetrating deep sclerectomy lowers the resistance to aqueous humor egress by removing most of the resistance located at the level of the juxtacanalicular meshwork and inner wall of Schlemm's canal. Aqueous humor is essentially drained in the intrascleral and subchoroidal space in primary open-angle, pseudoexfoliative and NTG. Angle closure and neovascularization are contraindications for this procedure.

POINTS TO REMEMBER

1. Nonpenetrating deep sclerectomy is a safe and efficient glaucoma filtering procedure aimed at lowering the IOP while maintaining the structure of the anterior chamber.
2. Best results are obtained for the following glaucoma diagnosis:
   - Primary-open angle glaucoma
   - Pseudoexfoliation glaucoma
   - Pigmentary glaucoma
   - Glaucoma associated with myopia
   - Aphakic glaucoma
   - Pseudophakic glaucoma
   - Uveitic glaucoma
   - Normal tension glaucoma
   - Corticosteroid induced glaucoma
   - Traumatic glaucoma
3. Nonpenetrating deep sclerectomy lowers the number of complications and risks associated with penetrating surgery, that comprise:
   - Durable hypotony
   - Flat anterior chamber
   - Hyphema
   - Choroidal effusion, detachment or hemorrhage
   - Late endophthalmitis
   - Surgery-induced cataract development
4. Nonpenetrating deep sclerectomy lowers the IOP to a mean of about 12–14 mm Hg while removing the need for antiglaucoma medications, or reducing the burden of combined or multiple glaucoma therapy.

5. A gonioscopy must be performed to rule out angle closure, iridocorneal apposition, or congenital abnormalities of the angle that would prevent a functional filtration through the TDM. Neovascularization of the angle should also be excluded for the same reasons.

REFERENCES

1. Roy S, Mermoud A. How does nonpenetrating surgery work? J Fr Ophtalmol. 2006;29:1167-74.
2. Varga Z, Shaarawy T. Deep sclerectomy: safety and efficacy. Middle East Afr J Ophthalmol. 2009;16:123-6.
3. Roy S, Mermoud A. Deep sclerectomy. Dev Ophthalmol. 2012;50:29-36.
4. Roy S, Thi HD, Feusier M, Mermoud A. Crosslinked sodium hyaluronate implant in deep sclerectomy for the surgical treatment of glaucoma. Eur J Ophthalmol. 2012;22:70-6.
5. Bissig A, Roy S, Rivier Det al. Ten years follow-up after deep sclerectomy with collagen implant. J of Glaucoma. 2008; 17:680-6.
6. Anand N. Deep sclerectomy with mitomycin C for glaucoma secondary to uveitis. Eur J Ophthalmol. 2011;21:708-14.
7. Suominen S, Harju M, Kurvinen L et al. Deep sclerectomy in normal-tension glaucoma with and without Mitomycin-C. Acta Ophthalmol. 2014;92:701-6.

Transscleral Cyclophotocoagulation

Monica Gandhi, Suneeta Dubey, Julie Pegu, Nishtha Singh

INTRODUCTION

Refractory glaucoma is difficult to treat and several modalities like diathermy, cryotherapy, beta irradiation, therapeutic ultrasound and electrolysis have been used with limited success. Xenon arc lamps and ruby lasers were tried for transscleral destruction of the pars plicata of the ciliary body to decrease the aqueous production in order to decrease the intraocular pressure (IOP). This was replaced by neodymium:YAG and then by semiconductor diode lasers. This chapter will focus on transscleral cyclophotocoagulation (TSCPC) of the ciliary processes.

MECHANISM OF ACTION

The aqueous humor is produced by the pars plicata of the ciliary body. Histopathological studies in humans show that the diode laser leads to disruption of the pars plicata with focal damage and minimal inflammation.[1] There is nonspecific destruction of the pigmented and nonpigmented ciliary epithelium with pigment clumping and some associated destruction of muscle and vessels. There is less tissue disruption associated with endocyclophotocoagulation (ECP) than TSCPC. The loss of ciliary processes is not complete in most cases and this may be the cause of loss of IOP control over a period of time. Some regeneration of the epithelium takes place with time, however, may not be functional.

INDICATIONS

Transscleral cyclophotocoagulation is usually reserved for patients in whom the glaucoma is not controlled with medical and/or surgical means and who have limited visual potential. In some studies, it has been used as a primary procedure in patients with open-angle glaucoma and pseudoexfoliative glaucoma with no significant loss of visual acuity.[2] In these patients, however, one needs to evaluate the risk-benefit ratio in comparison to medical and other surgical modalities.

Indications include:

- Inadequate control of IOP despite maximal/tolerable medical therapy
- Painful blind eye with absolute glaucoma or minimal useful vision
- Primary treatment for glaucoma in patients where other modalities are not possible
  - Allergy or inability to tolerate antiglaucoma medication
  - Patients with poor systemic health which prevents invasive surgery
  - Patients unwilling for drainage surgery
- Refractory glaucoma:
  - After penetrating keratoplasty
  - Uveitic glaucoma
  - Pediatric glaucoma
  - Post-traumatic glaucoma
  - After failed trabeculectomy, tube shunts and other glaucoma surgeries
  - Glaucoma after intravitreal silicone oil
  - Postvitrectomy glaucoma
  - Neovascular glaucoma (NVG).

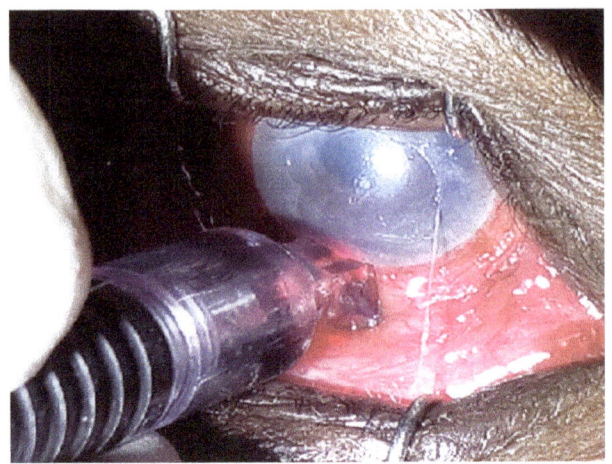

Fig. 7C.1: Transscleral cyclophotocoagulation using G-probe.

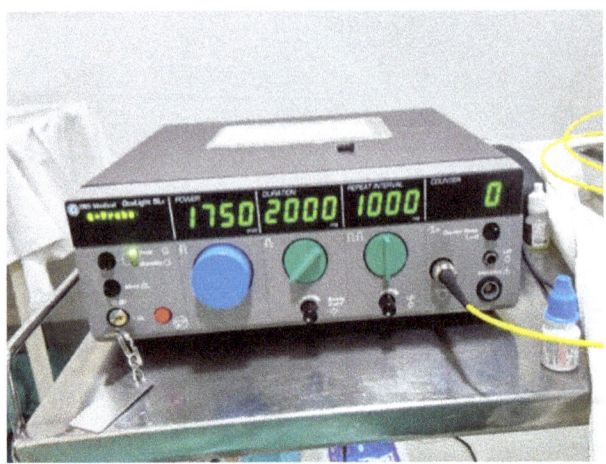

Fig. 7C.2: Laser console.

Case 1: TSCPC for NVG

A 61-year-old pseudophakic diabetic patient with lasered diabetic retinopathy of both eyes and NVG left eye presented with pain in the left eye. The best corrected visual acuity in the right eye was 6/12 and in the left eye was hand movements close to face (HMCF) with inaccurate projection of rays. Her IOP was 14 mm Hg in the right eye and 48 mm Hg in the left eye. Left eye had corneal edema, due to which fundus evaluation was difficult but previous records showed a 0.85:1 vertical cup-to-disc ratio (VCDR). Despite being on maximum tolerable antiglaucoma treatment, the patient was suffering from constant pain in the eye. She refused surgical options explained to her and thus she was planned for TSCPC.

A peribulbar block with 6 mL of a 50:50 mixture of 2% lidocaine and 0.75% bupivacaine was given. Laser safety glasses were worn by the surgeon. The anterior edge of the footplate of the G-probe was placed on the limbus so that the laser energy gets directed 1.2 mm posterior to the limbus, corresponding to the pars plicata of the ciliary body. The probe was kept parallel to the visual axis (Fig. 7C.1). Our initial settings were 1750 mW and no popping sound was heard so the power was increased in steps of 250 mW to 2,000 mW where popping sound was noted. The power was then decreased to 1750 mW (Fig. 7C.2). 270 degrees were treated sparing 3 o'clock and 9 o'clock positions (site of the long ciliary nerves and vessels). The superior temporal quadrant was avoided as to allow for a filtering surgery in the future if the need arose.

The treatment was started at 4 o'clock position and moved clockwise for each subsequent application. Applications were made by placing the side of the footplate

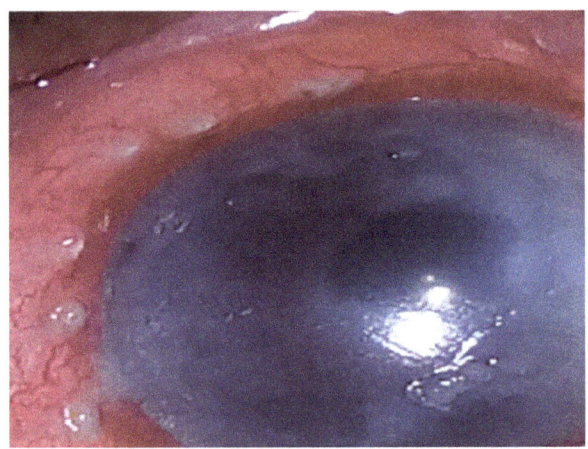

Fig. 7C.3: Case 1: Immediate post-transscleral cyclophotocoagulation.

slightly overlapping the indentation of the fiberoptic made by the prior application (Fig. 7C.3). The treatment was continued for a total of 21 applications. Pulse duration was fixed at 2000 ms at a repeat interval of 1000 ms.

Upon completion of the procedure, a subconjunctival injection of steroid and antibiotic combination was given and eye was patched after instillation of 1% atropine drop and an antibiotic eye drop.

Postoperatively, the patient was started on prednisolone acetate 1% eyedrop 8 times a day, atropine 1% eyedrop 3 times a day, an antibiotic eye drop 4 times a day for 7 days and tablet acetazolamide twice a day for 3 days to control the immediate postoperative spike that is noticed after the procedure due to inflammation. The prednisolone and atropine were tapered off as the inflammation and discomfort improved over the course of 1 month. The IOP-lowering drugs were tapered off gradually until safe IOPs were attained over the next 1 month. However, prostaglandin analog was stopped immediately after the procedure.

At the end of 6 months, left eye vision was HMCF and IOP was maintained at 16 mm Hg with no antiglaucoma medication.

Case 2: TSCPC for postkeratoplasty glaucoma

A 60-year-old female had undergone therapeutic penetrating keratoplasty (TPK) for fungal keratitis in the left eye a year ago. Subsequently the eye had graft failure and developed a membrane covering the pupillary area and very shallow anterior chamber (AC) for which a repeat TPK with extracapsular cataract extraction with anterior vitrectomy and pupilloplasty was done. Following the surgery, she complained of severe pain in the left eye with associated headache. On examination, her vision in the right eye was 6/9 and HMCF in the left eye. The left eye had scarred conjunctiva, corneal epithelial edema due to the high IOP, very shallow AC due to extensive PAS, aphakia with advanced glaucomatous damage with cup-to-disc (C:D) ratio of 0.9:1. IOP ranged from 48 mm Hg to 54 mm Hg in the left eye, despite maximal medical therapy. Gonioscopy revealed total synechial angle closure in the left eye. TSCPC was planned in view of the uncontrolled IOP and guarded visual prognosis.

A peribulbar block with 6 mL of a 50:50 mixture of 2% lidocaine and 0.75% bupivacaine was given. We used the semiconductor diode laser, which is portable, solid state, and requires no special electrical outlet or water for cooling. Our initial settings were 1350 mW and the power was increased

in steps of 250 mW up to 1850 mW till popping sound was heard, then it was decreased to 1500 mW. G-probe was placed as in the earlier case. The procedure was done in 270° sparing 3 o'clock and 9 o'clock positions and the superior temporal quadrant (Fig. 7C.4A). We started at 8 o'clock position and moved clockwise for each subsequent application. Lastly, the superonasal quadrant was done. The treatment was continued for a total of 24 applications. Pulse duration was fixed at 2000 ms at a repeat interval of 1000 ms.

Postoperative management was similar to the previous case. At the end of 6 months, left eye vision was counting finger close to face and IOP was maintained at 14 mm Hg (Fig. 7C.4B).

Most patients continue with their IOP-lowering drops for at least 15–30 days until the IOP-lowering effect of TSCPC is observed.

Case 3: TSCPC for failed glaucoma surgery

A 10-year-old male underwent congenital cataract surgery with intraocular lenses (IOL) implantation. He suffered a blunt trauma after 7 years of the surgery, leading to lens subluxation, which required IOL explantation. His visual acuity was FC 1 meter with accurate projection of rays and IOP of 38 mm Hg in that eye postoperatively. Optic disc showed a 0.8 VCDR and the IOP was not controlled with medications. He underwent Ahmed glaucoma valve surgery post which his IOP was controlled for about 2 months subsequent to which he developed hypertensive phase which did not resolve with maximal antiglaucoma medication and he was advised TSCPC. The IOP postoperatively was maintained with single antiglaucoma drug (Figs. 7C.5A and B).

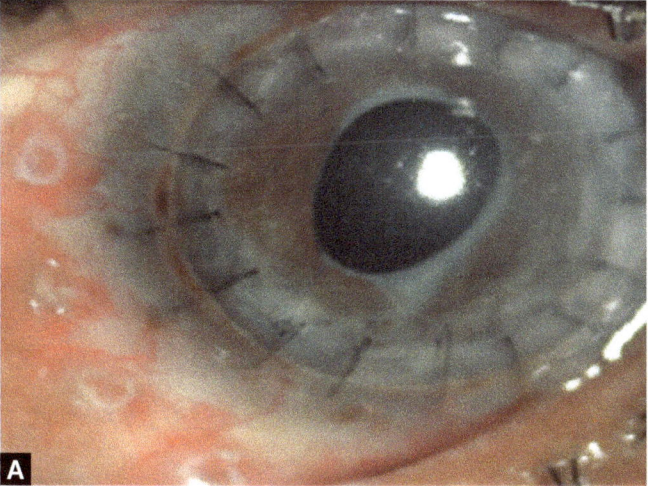
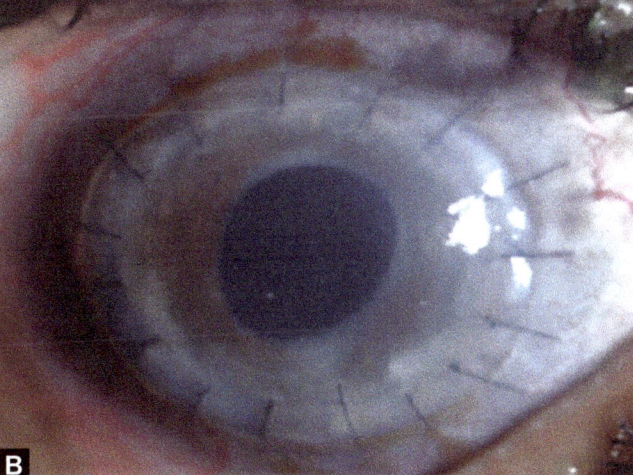

Figs. 7C.4A and B: (A) At the time of transscleral cyclophotocoagulation. (B) Six months post-transscleral cyclophotocoagulation.

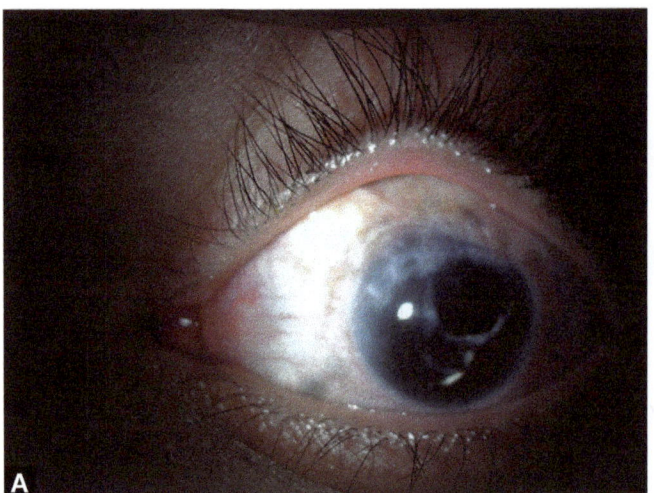
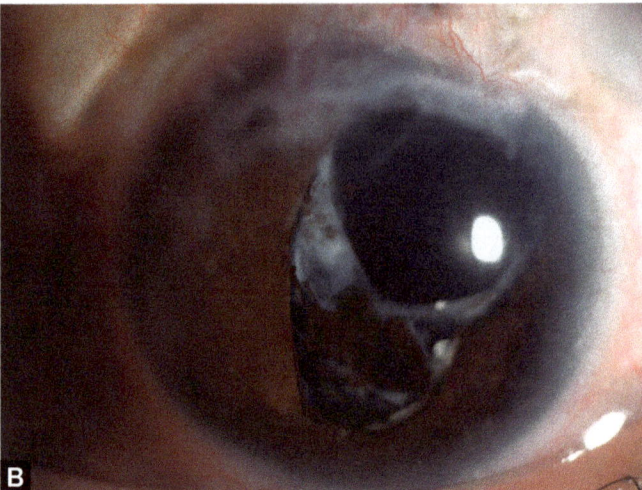

Figs. 7C.5A and B: (A) Left eye, Aphakia, Ahmed glaucoma valve implant; (B) After trans-scleral cyclophotocoagulation 180°.

Transscleral cyclophotocoagulation is a safe and effective therapy for the treatment of secondary pediatric glaucomas with uncontrolled IOP in the long-term.

HOW TO USE A G-PROBE?

The G-probe is designed for one-time use. However at our center, we clean it, sterilize it with ethylene oxide and use it for 2–3 times. We check the probe carefully, and if it causes charring or produces no evident result, we replace it. Also one needs to watch out for scleral burns. The probe tip should be kept free of charred debris as that can burn into or even through the sclera.

HOW MANY QUADRANTS TO TREAT?

The number of quadrants to be treated depends on the disease profile. However not more than 270 are treated in one sitting. The quadrant usually left is temporal when the first sitting is done and during the second sitting, if needed at a later stage, the upper temporal or lower temporal is omitted. We prefer to omit the superior quadrant such that trabeculectomy can be planned if needed.

The G-probe helps to identify the site to be lasered by its design but in cases where the anatomy is distorted or in congenital glaucoma eyes, transillumination has been used to identify the ciliary body position.[3]

COMPLICATIONS

Hypotony remains a risk in a certain subset of patients. Patients with NVG and those who have undergone a pars plana vitrectomy are predisposed to this complication. Vision loss post-TSCPC may be due to advancing cataracts, poor control of patients' IOP, cystoid macular edema and/ or chronic hypotony.[4]

CONCLUSION

Transscleral cyclophotocoagulation is a relatively safe and effective management option in glaucomas refractory to conventional treatment modalities. It helps to control the IOP and decrease the antiglaucoma medications along with symptomatic relief of associated symptoms. Proper patient selection and surgical technique help to minimize the procedure's known side effects and improve its long-term success.

REFERENCES

1. Mckelvie PA, Walland MJ. Pathology of cyclodiode laser: a series of nine enucleated eyes. Br J Ophthalmol. 2002; 86:381-6.
2. Grueb M, Rohrbach JM, Bartz-Schmidt KU, Schlote T. Transscleral diode laser cytophotocoagulation as primary and secondary surgical treatment in primary open angle and psuedoexfoliative glaucoma. Long-term clinical outcomes. Graefes Arch Clin Exp Ophthalmol. 2006;244:1293-9.
3. Kirwan JF, Shah P, Khaw PT. Diode laser cyclophotocoagulation: role in the management of refractory pediatric glaucomas. Ophthalmology. 2002;109:316-23.
4. Ansari E, Gandhewar J. Long-term efficacy and visual acuity following transscleral diode laser photocoagulation in cases of refractory and non-refractory glaucoma. Eye (Lond). 2007;21:936-40.

Endocyclophotocoagulation

Parul Ichhpujani, Shibal Bhartiya

INTRODUCTION

Reduction of aqueous production by ciliary body ablation is an important treatment modality for intractable glaucomas. The two modalities of laser cyclodestruction are ECP and TSCPC. In the former, the laser is applied under direct endoscopic view causing localized shrinkage of the ciliary processes due to thermal coagulation. This causes an initial reduction in blood supply to the ciliary processes, and a consequent reduction in aqueous production. Partial reperfusion of the ciliary body over 4–6 weeks means that the rates of hypotony and phthisis are lower than those associated with other methods of cyclodestruction.

The main advantages of this procedure include its excellent patient tolerability, short procedure duration and reasonable side effect profile. Another advantage is that it may be performed in conjunction with phacoemulsification and/or vitrectomy.

In comparison to other methods of cyclodestruction, ECP has some obvious drawbacks. It is an invasive procedure, and requires considerable surgeon expertise, especially in phakic patients. Given that it is an invasive procedure, it carries a risk of endophthalmitis, despite a reduced risk of vision loss due to hypotony or phthisis. Its efficacy may be limited in certain cases and the equipment is costly.

Typically, ECP only produces an IOP in the mid-teens but that is because of episcleral venous pressure, which limits how low we can get the IOP using this approach.

INDICATIONS

Transscleral cyclophotocoagulation is limited to refractory cases of glaucoma where vision is poor, but ECP can be considered in mild, moderate and advanced cases of glaucoma. It augments all therapeutic modalities that increase aqueous outflow; including trabeculectomy, tube surgery, nonpenetrating glaucoma surgery (NPGS) and angle shunt implants. It is usually reserved for pseudophakic eyes, and may be performed in conjunction with cataract surgery. The usual approach is via limbal incisions, the pars plana route being used rarely.

The main indications for ECP include:
- Intolerance to topical treatment
- To decrease the number of glaucoma medication in conjunction with planned cataract surgery
- Previous failed glaucoma surgery (trabeculectomy, aqueous shunt or NPGS)
- Patients with advanced disease who may not be good candidates for filtering surgeries or shunts due to their inability/unwillingness to comply with frequent postoperative visits and intensive postoperative drop and wound healing interventions required.
- Postpenetrating keratoplasty glaucoma.

Endocyclophotocoagulation is preferable to filtration surgery in eyes where an ocular fistula is problematic, such as cases of elevated episcleral venous pressure, intraocular tumor, contact lens wear or blepharitis.

Endocyclophotocoagulation involves fewer postoperative visits and additional treatments, such as laser suture lysis, bleb needling, 5-fluorouracil injections, etc. ECP may, therefore, be a good choice for patients who are unable to make frequent postoperative visits or who are unable to co-operate for manipulations of the bleb.[1]

CONTRAINDICATIONS

- It may be used with caution in postinflammatory glaucomas; uveitis, however, is not an absolute contraindication
- It may be used with caution in phakic patients due to the risk of lens trauma.

TECHNIQUE

Equipment

The ECP (Endo Optiks, Little Silver, NJ, USA) machine consists of an 810 nm continuous wave diode laser, a xenon light source, a helium neon aiming beam and a camera. These are transmitted via fiberoptics to an 18-gauge or 20-gauge probe. The endoscope provides a 70° field of view. The optimum focus for the laser is 0.75 mm from the tip (in practice, this translates into treatment of 4–6 ciliary processes).

Endocyclophotocoagulation is carried out under a sub-Tenon's or peribulbar block, rarely general anesthesia may be required. Under direct visualization, a temporal clear corneal incision is made. Viscoelastic is injected into the eye and into the ciliary sulcus, pushing the posterior peripheral iris forward and the lens capsule complex posteriorly. This ensures an easy visualization of, and access to, the ciliary processes.

A 360° treatment is usually carried out and requires 2 or 3 incisions of minimum 2.2 mm. The usual incisions include the phaco wound, a side port and a third fresh incision placed opposite the main phaco wound. The latter is usually inferonasal in case a temporal approach to cataract surgery has been used. The endo-probe is then inserted into the eye and activated. Under direct visualization, the ciliary processes are localized, and then treated with diode thermal laser.

The initial power is set at 0.35 W, with step ups up to 0.6 W; set to a continuous exposure for the duration of treatment, as controlled by the foot pedal. Laser energy is applied from the tip of the ciliary process to its base, and a blanching and shrinkage of each process is observed. As in the case of TSCPC, "pops" are a sign of supraoptimal energy. Therefore, if any pops are observed, the probe

should be withdrawn a little away from the ciliary processes. Usually, the position of the probe should enable a viewing angle of 4–6 processes.

When treatment has been applied through 360°, the probe is withdrawn and the viscoelastic is removed. This is followed by intracameral injection of unpreserved dexamethasone and antibiotic, followed by hydration and/or suturing of the ports.

Case 1: Endocyclophotocoagulation with phacoemulsification

Mr X, a 64-year-old gentleman, presented with moderate-to-severe ocular surface disease due to his antiglaucoma medication (travoprost-timolol fixed dose combination, brinzolamide). His baseline IOPs were oculus dexter (OD) 32 mm Hg and oculus sinister (OS) 38 mm Hg; and the target IOP of 16–18 mm Hg OU was achieved using the three eye drops. He had moderate glaucoma with a C:D ratio of 0.7–0.75 oculus uterque (OU), and biarcuate scotoma in visual field defects. His best-corrected visual acuity was 6/18 and 6/24 in the right and left eyes, respectively, due to an immature senile cataract on both eyes.

Since he was scheduled for phacoemulsification with posterior chamber intraocular lens implantation in the left and right eyes, consecutively, a combined procedure with approximately 220° of ECP (Fig. 7D.1) was planned.

Following the surgery, his vision was 6/6 OU (left eye with a correction of –0.75/+0.50@160); and both eyes had an IOP of 16 mm Hg, without any added antiglaucoma medication. This IOP drop has been maintained for the last 6 months.

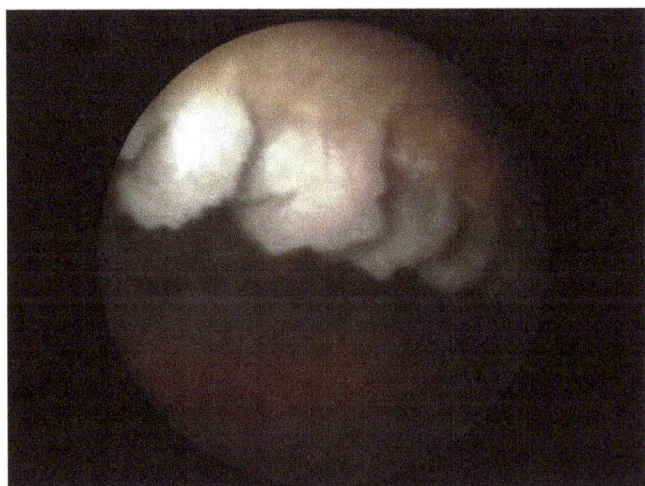

Fig. 7D.1: Shrinkage of ciliary processes.

Endocyclophotocoagulation is done after phacoemulsification but before insertion of the IOL as this provides an unrestrictive empty capsular bag. Some surgeons prefer a 360° ECP via two corneal incisions.

Case 2: Endocyclophotocoagulation in angle closure

Mr Y, 55-year-old hyperopic gentleman, had primary angle-closure glaucoma with 0.8–0.85 VCDR in both the eyes. He had IOPs of OD 28 and OS 30 mm Hg on brimonidine-timolol fixed drug combination. He was allergic to both bimatoprost and travoprost. He also had significant nuclear sclerosis. He was planned for a phacoemulsification along with an ECP (a supplement to the debulking effect of a primary lens removal).

In these individuals, ECP is effective not only for reducing aqueous production that lowers IOP, but also allows the surgeon to perform a posterior peripheral iris iridoplasty, shrinking the posterior tissue and opening up the narrow angle even more, thereby logically increasing outflow performance.

Endocyclophotocoagulation is especially useful in patients who have plateau iris, where the ciliary processes are riding very high up. Wherever the laser strikes, the tissue is coagulated, and the remaining tissue shrinks toward the coagulated area, thus opening the angle.[2]

Case 3: Endocyclophotocoagulation-plus

Mr A, a 58-year-old diabetic, underwent a pars plana vitrectomy for tractional retinal detachment; following which he developed refractory glaucoma. A glaucoma drainage device implantation was carried out to control IOP but after 2 months, despite 3 antiglaucoma medications, IOP ranged between late 30s and early 40s. An ECP-plus procedure was carried out. Before ECP-plus, a standard 2-port pars plana vitrectomy was performed and an AC maintainer was used. The ECP probe was then inserted into the posterior segment through a pars plana sclerotomy while another port was plugged and irrigation maintained. The probe was advanced toward the pars plana region and 180° of adjacent ciliary processes (anterior and posterior aspects of the ciliary processes) were treated. On the first postoperative day, patient had a fibrinous reaction in the AC. In the immediate postoperative period, patient was instructed to continue his prior glaucoma medical treatment regimen, in addition to starting Moxifloxacin drops 4 times daily, prednisolone acetate 1% every 1–2 hours, and a topical nonsteroidal anti-inflammatory 2–3 times a day. Fibrinous reaction resolved over 10 days and his IOP ranged from 16–19 mm Hg without any antiglaucoma medication.

It is believed that IOP reduction with ECP-plus is more with ECP. Possible explanations for the magnitude of IOP reduction with ECP-plus relate to treatment under direct visualization of: (a) the entire ciliary processes, (b) intervening regions between processes, (c) the pars plana, and (d) the extent of circumferential treatment. Pars plana treatment may have several effects. First, photocoagulation of any extension of the secretory ciliary epithelium from pars plicata onto pars plana results in more complete reduction of aqueous humor production. Second, a possible effect on the blood supply to the ciliary body would result in more profound aqueous suppression. Third, lasering the pars plana may increase uveoscleral outflow.[3]

Pars plana cannot be used for a phakic patient. Patients with severe anterior segment scarring are the best candidates for ECP-plus, which is appropriate for patients with any type of glaucoma but not for those with altered blood-aqueous barriers. Caution needs to be exercised in patients who have neovascular or uveitic glaucoma.

REFERENCES

1. Yang Y, Zhong J, Dun Z, et al. Comparison of efficacy between endoscopic cyclophotocoagulation and alternative surgeries in refractory glaucoma: a meta-analysis. Medicine (Baltimore). 2015;94:e1651.
2. Wang JC, Campos-Möller X, Shah M, et al. Effect of endocyclophotocoagulation on refractive outcomes in angle-closure eyes after phacoemulsification and posterior chamber intraocular lens implantation. J Cataract Refract Surg. 2016;42:132-7.
3. Tan JC, Francis BA, Noecker R, et al. Endoscopic Cyclophotocoagulation and Pars Plana Ablation (ECP-plus) to treat refractory glaucoma. J Glaucoma. 2016;25:e117-22.

CHAPTER 8

Complications after Trabeculectomy

Oana Stirbu, Jorge Vila Arteaga

INTRODUCTION

A trabeculectomy patient needs lifetime follow-up, very intensive in the first 2 months after surgery and every 6–9 months after clinical stabilization, depending on patient characteristics and glaucoma aggressiveness. Operated glaucoma patients can never be discharged from clinic and the patient with trabeculectomy deserves a special attention and postoperative care.

Early postoperative complications need quick management and effective resolution of the problem; nevertheless there is one specific late trabeculectomy complication, namely the bleb-related endophthalmitis that represents one of the few real ocular emergencies in which each hour of delay in diagnosing and starting the correct treatment can be fatal to the final outcome.[1]

Postoperative complications are classified according to the intraocular pressure (IOP), the bleb appearance, and the amplitude of the anterior chamber.

Case 1: Overfiltering bleb

A 74-year-old patient complained about fluctuating visual acuity with different gaze directions 3 weeks after trabeculectomy augmented with mitomycin C (MMC) (0.2 mg/mL for 2 minutes). The IOP was 4–6 mm Hg, patient's visual acuity ranged from 0.55 to 0.85 and automatic refractometer showed fluctuating astigmatism at different follow-up visits. The bleb was large, diffuse and extended circumferentially suggestive of an overdraining bleb (Fig. 8.1). Steroids were tapered and the patient gradually improved over 10 days.

Ocular hypotony can produce changes in corneal astigmatism in patients with thin sclera or thick eyelids. It is important to rule out hypotony maculopathy with macular folds when there is persistent visual discomfort. Management involves reducing the corticosteroid treatment to once or twice daily or discontinuing the steroids, this may facilitate faster episcleral scarring so you do not get as high a bleb; pressure eye patch; peri/intrableb autologous blood injection to promote fibrosis and/or surgical revision of the flap to place more sutures.[2] Compression sutures are not effective for dealing with circumferential blebs extending over 360°.

Case 2: Corneal dellen

A 65-year-old patient complained of foreign body sensation at 7-day follow-up visit after trabeculectomy. The bleb was diffuse from 10 hours to 2 hours and extended nasally

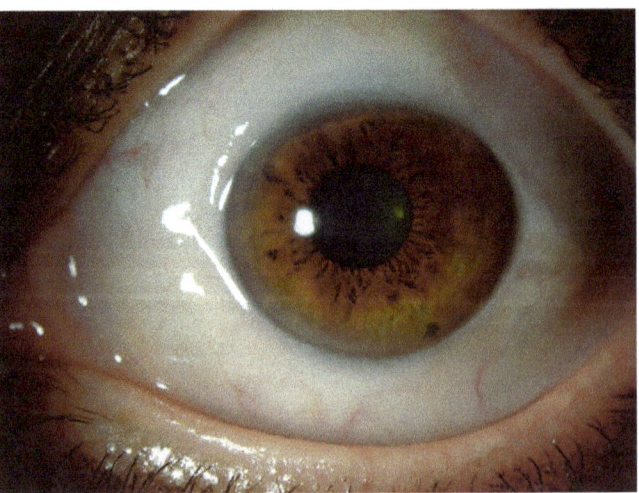

Fig. 8.1: Overfiltering bleb causing ocular hypotony.

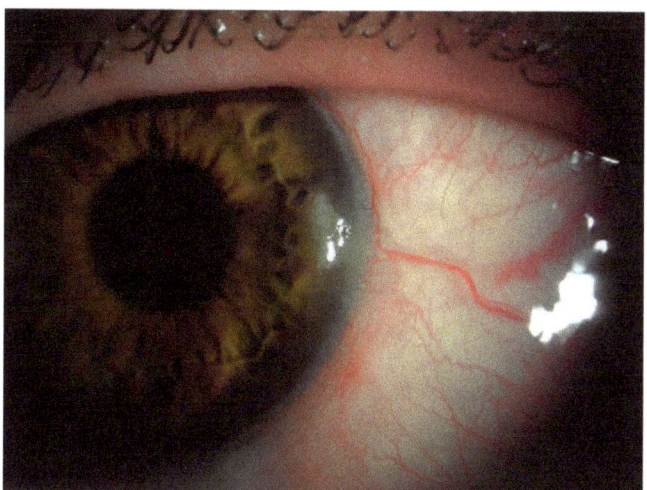

Fig. 8.2: Corneal dellen.

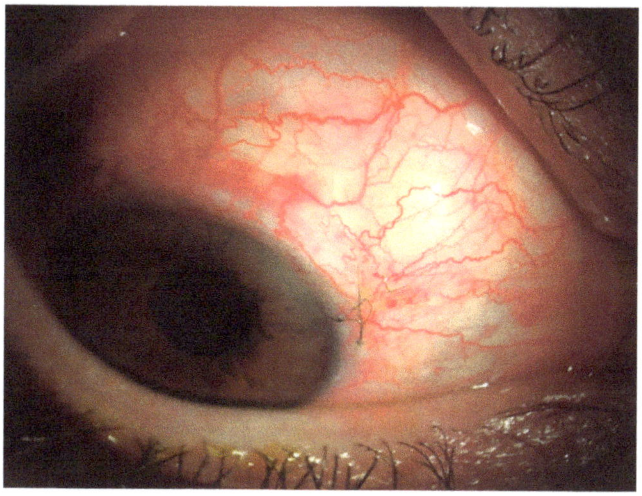

Fig. 8.3: Wound leak: suboptimal surgical suturing technique with loose nylon suture.

from 2 hours to 5 hours. A small area of corneal thinning, which stained with fluorescein, was seen in the peripheral cornea at 3 hours: Corneal dellen (Fig. 8.2). Patient was started on lubricating eyedrops QID and a lubricating gel BD; his symptoms improved and on subsequent visits, a reduction was noted in the area of corneal thinning.

Corneal dellen may develop in front of steep-walled nasally or temporally placed blebs, as the bulk of the bleb does not allow a correct contact between the tarsal conjunctiva of the upper lid and the peripheral cornea. Corneal lubrication is impaired as the tear film cannot reach and wet the epithelium producing local dehydration and thinning.[3] Dellen can be treated with intensive use of lubricants, gel-like tear supplements, ointments and bandage contact lens. When symptoms persist, a Palmberg compression mattress suture or a surgical revision should be considered.

Case 3: Wound leak

Mrs D was noted to have a very low height bleb and IOP 6 mm Hg on the second postoperative follow-up visit at 1 week after MMC-augmented fornix-based trabeculectomy. Pinpoint wound leaks (Fig. 8.3) were noted along the suture line at three points. A bandage contact lens was applied and after 3 days of its application, the leaking points had healed.

In cases with wound leak, look for retraction of the conjunctival flap caused by suboptimal suturing technique or hyper-reactive tissue scarring or leakage of aqueous through conjunctival tears and holes. Fluorescein stain always points the leaking spot, but sometimes patience is needed in order to see small conjunctival defects.

Ocular hypotony can be accompanied by shallow or flat anterior chamber and choroidal detachment. Choroidal effusion forms a vicious circle with ocular hypotony, reinforcing each other through a feedback loop. Complete rest and mydriatic or cycloplegic agents are used.[3]

In some cases of wound leak, application of one drop of tissue glue at the slit lamp, followed by bandage contact lens covering the area to reduce the foreign body sensation, eliminates the need of re-entering the operating room to place new sutures.

Ciliary body shutdown is a very rare circumstance in patients with uveitis, juvenile open-angle glaucoma or due to toxic levels of intraoperative antifibrotic agents. When you hear hoof beats, think horses not zebras. In early postoperative hypotony, think wound leak or overdraining bleb.

A fearsome and unpredictable consequence of intraoperative or postoperative ocular hypotony in patients with severe glaucoma is the wipe-out syndrome, which implies the irreversible loss of the remaining vision field.[4]

- Remember that most hypotony in the early postoperative period resolves with conservative measures
- Hypotony with lens-corneal touch and hypotony maculopathy with persistent foveal folds require anterior chamber reformation with BB, gas or high-density viscoelastic material
- Kissing choroidals need surgical intervention with *L*-shaped or *I*-shaped deep scleral incisions.

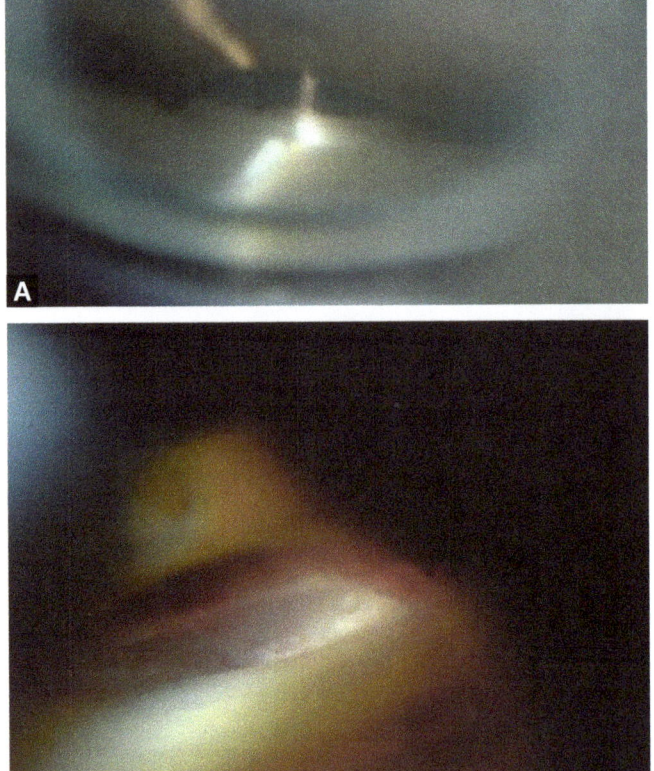

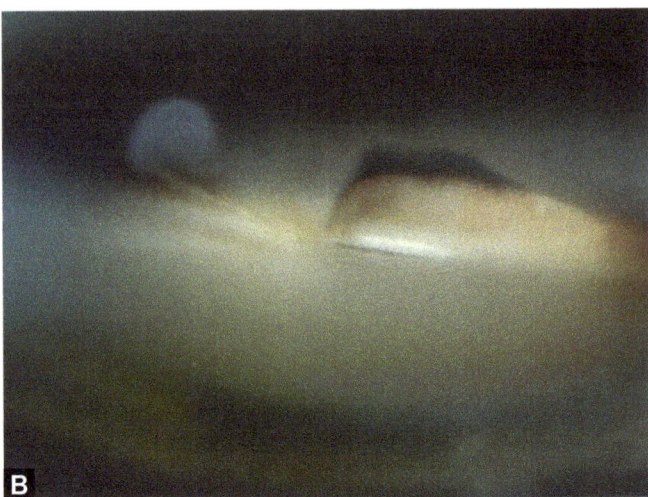

Figs. 8.4A to C: Gonioscopy after trabeculectomy: (A) Normal appearance of internal scleral ostium with large basal iridectomy; (B) Partial iris incarceration in the sclerostomy, which does not impede trabeculectomy function; (C) Blood-stained vitreous plugs the internal aspect of the sclerostomy, as a result of vitreous loss during surgery.
Photos courtesy: Dr Susana Duch, ICO Barcelona, Spain.

Case 4: Fistula obstruction

Mrs X, a 58-year-old patient with pseudoexfoliation glaucoma had IOP of 24 mm Hg on day 4 after a trabeculectomy complicated with intraoperative vitreous loss. The peripheral iridectomy was performed too posteriorly and the vitreous emerged through the traumatized zonule causing ab-interno obstruction of the scleral window. The iridectomy was accompanied by moderate bleeding, which stained the vitreous and made easier the identification of the vitreous filament (Fig. 8.4C).

Fistula obstruction is the most frequent cause of raised IOP in the early postoperative period. Look for too tight or too many scleral flap sutures, fibrin or blood at the level of the flap, iris or vitreous or blood incarceration at the sclerostomy or an inadequately excised corneoscleral block (Figs. 8.4A to C). Always perform gonioscopy to rule out internal obstruction.

Case 5: Postoperative hyphema

Mr A, a 61-year-old patient, had hyphema on postoperative day 1 after a fornix-based trabeculectomy with a small iridectomy and no intraoperative anterior chamber bleeding (Fig. 8.5). The IOP was 3 mm Hg and anterior segment examination showed a blood clot in anterior chamber along the vertical axis, which possibly originated at the site of superior iridectomy and a 1 mm high horizontal hyphema. When the patient was interviewed regarding any drug use, which he might have forgotten to mention preoperatively, he mentioned taking an ayurvedic preparation that acted as a blood thinner. Topical steroids were instilled hourly and patient was advised not to do any strenuous activity and keep head end of his bed elevated.

It is important to know that many times patients do not inform the doctor that they are on naturopathy, homeopathy or any other alternative medicine; as some of these

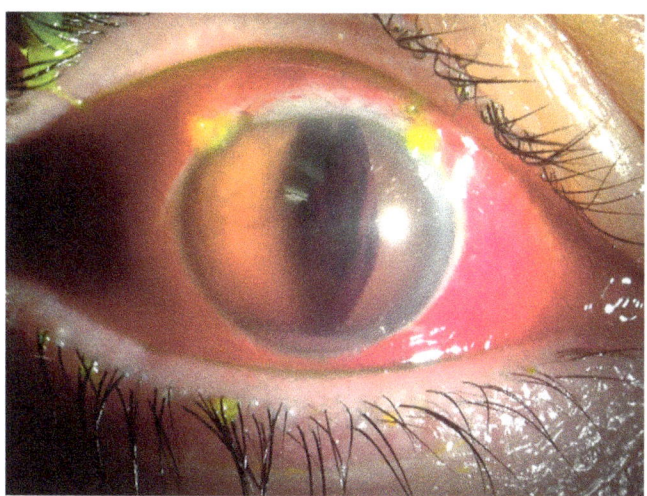

Fig. 8.5: Early postoperative hyphema.

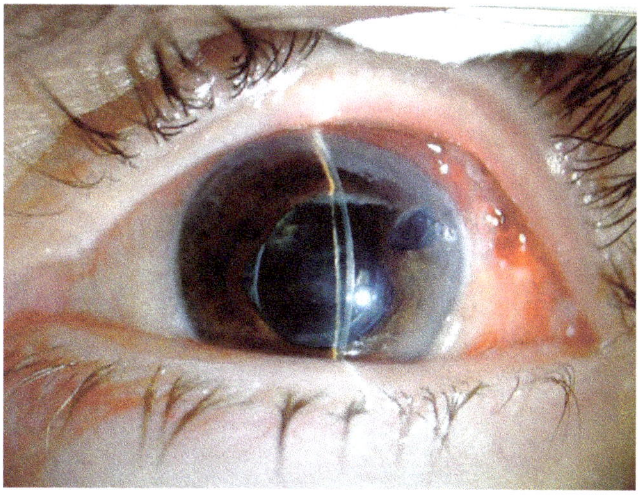

Fig. 8.6: Malignant glaucoma.

drugs (such as nettle, garlic, *Ginkgo biloba*, etc.) can affect blood coagulation and increase the risk of anterior chamber, bleb and suprachoroidal hemorrhage.[5] The hyphema resolved with conservative treatment with atropine, rest and cortisone eyedrops 5 times per day. Intraocular bleeding tends to occur when the IOP is low. In special cases using high-density viscoelastic material in the anterior chamber can increase the IOP and arrest the hemorrhage.

Case 6: Malignant glaucoma

Mr D, a 65-year-old pseudophake with short-axial length (19 mm), was referred to glaucoma clinic with 360° closed angle and an IOP of 46 mm Hg on maximal treatment. A superior trabeculectomy with iridectomy plus hyaloidotomy with anterior vitrectomy were performed. Despite all these prophylactic measures, on the first postoperative day 1, the patient presented IOP of 30 mm Hg and a shallow central anterior chamber suggestive of malignant glaucoma (Fig. 8.6). He was started on topical steroids qid and atropine ointment tid. On day 3, laser-assisted hyaloidotomy was done.

In eyes predisposed for developing choroidal detachment, inadequate response to vasoconstriction and vasodilatation and impermeable anterior hyaloid, the vitreous pushes forward the lens-zonule complex, leading to flat anterior chamber and high IOP. If atropine, hyaloidectomy and complete supine rest do not improve the condition, vitrectomy is recommended.[6]

Suprachoroidal hemorrhage: Ultrasound imaging is diagnostic, but the intense pain spontaneously reported by the patient should arouse your suspicion. Systemic risk factors include anticoagulant therapy, hypertension, arteriosclerosis and bleeding disorders.

Case 7: Blebitis and bleb-related endophthalmitis

Mr E, a 56-year-old patient with a trabeculectomy (performed 2 years back) and IOP ranging between 8 mm Hg and 12 mm Hg at follow-up visits, came to the emergency department complaining of foreign body sensation and photophobia. On examination, IOP was 26 mm Hg; chronic blepharitis and the *white on red* sign were present. A diagnosis of incipient blebitis was made (Fig. 8.7). Hourly preservative free moxifloxacin eye-drops were started and on the second day-fluorometholone twice a day was added with complete resolution of the signs and symptoms in 8 days.

At every follow-up visit, look for blepharitis and, if present, treat it. Patient should be reminded not to rub their eyes and to present urgently if any mucopurulent or purulent discharge is noticed. The chronic use of topical corticosteroids in eyes that have undergone trabeculectomy can lead to the thinning of conjunctiva, and later become susceptible to highly virulent bacterial strains like *Staphylococcus aureus*.

Blebitis and bleb-related endophthalmitis are potentially devastating complications that can occur months to years after trabeculectomy. Symptoms include redness, pain, tearing or discharge, photophobia and decreased vision and the sign *white on red* is clearly visible. The presence of hypopyon or vitritis is indicative of endophthalmitis.

Blebitis is treated with hourly topical antibiotic and systemic antibiotics for 5–7 days. Bleb-related endophthalmitis management includes oral and topical blebitis treatment plus intravitreal antibiotics and/or vitrectomy. Blebitis risk factors include use of antimetabolites intra- or postoperatively, bacterial conjunctivitis, blepharitis and diabetes mellitus.[7]

Case 8: Ischemic bleb

A 55-year-old patient presented with conjunctival scarring and bleb failure after deep sclerectomy at 12 hours performed 3 months before. A series of five subconjunctival temporal injections with 5 FU is performed, but the IOP rises to 24 mm Hg and trabeculectomy is planned as rescue surgery using the previous scleral flap. At the beginning of the surgery, a hole in the conjunctiva was noted and suture with Ologen implant patch and 10.0 nylon circular atraumatic needle was performed. Instead of using the same scleral flap, MMC-augmented trabeculectomy was performed at 2 hours, temporally to the prior surgery. In the immediate postoperative period, the IOP was 14 mm Hg and an ischemic bleb was present (Fig. 8.8). Thin avascular or ischemic blebs, especially after antimetabolites (in this case, MMC and 5 FU), are at risk for late leaks.

Sometimes, a melted flap is seen in a patient with an autoimmune disease, such as rheumatoid arthritis or even prior MMC exposure. In that situation, you need to put a scleral patch graft where the flap reinforces it with sutures and then put conjunctiva over it.

In younger patients, an autologous Tenon's capsule can also be used as a patch graft.[8]

Case 9: Tenon cyst

A 62-year-old patient presented with an IOP 30 mm Hg at 5 weeks follow-up visit after a trabeculectomy. Examination showed encapsulated, elevated and tense bleb, impermeable to the passage of aqueous humor, a Tenon cyst (Fig. 8.9). After failure of conservative treatment, we opted for slit lamp bleb needling revision. Despite needling, the Tenon cyst persisted even 4 months after the trabeculectomy and then we undertook surgical bleb revision with excision of the Tenon cyst walls.

The initial approach in case of Tenon fibrous cyst consists of aqueous suppressants, digital massage and serial

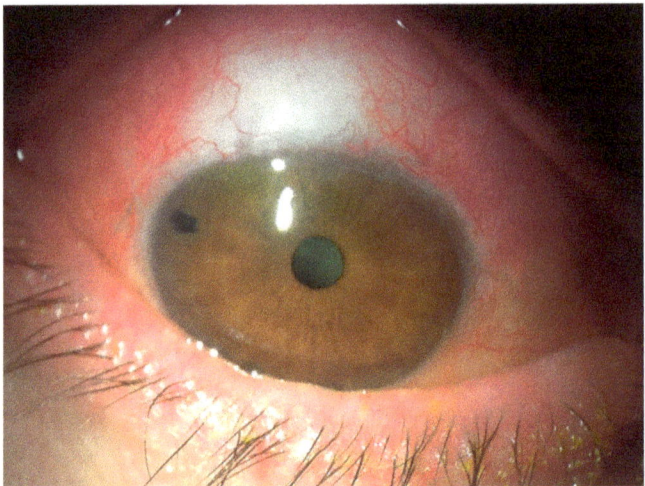

Fig. 8.7: White on red sign. The characteristic *white on red* appearance of acute blebitis.

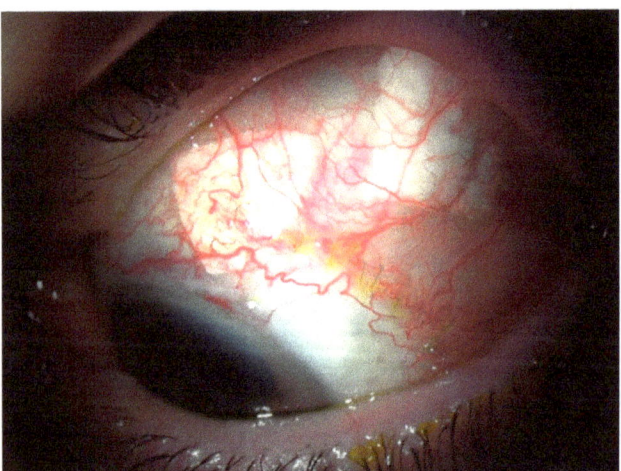

Fig. 8.8: Avascular blebs can develop late bleb leak: the surface epithelium necrosis results in transconjunctival percolation of aqueous humor (sweating or oozing).

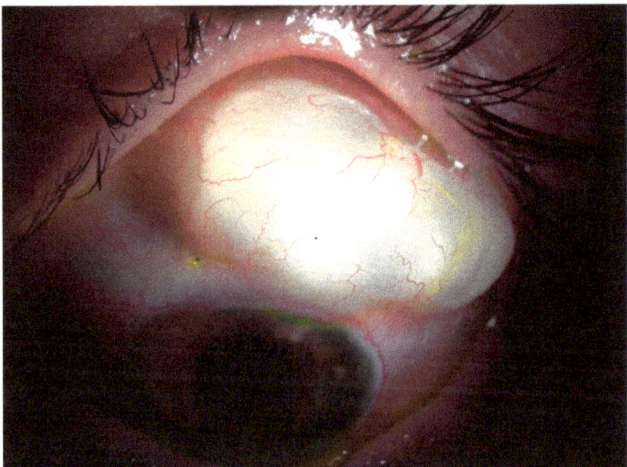

Fig. 8.9: Tenon cyst with thick walls.

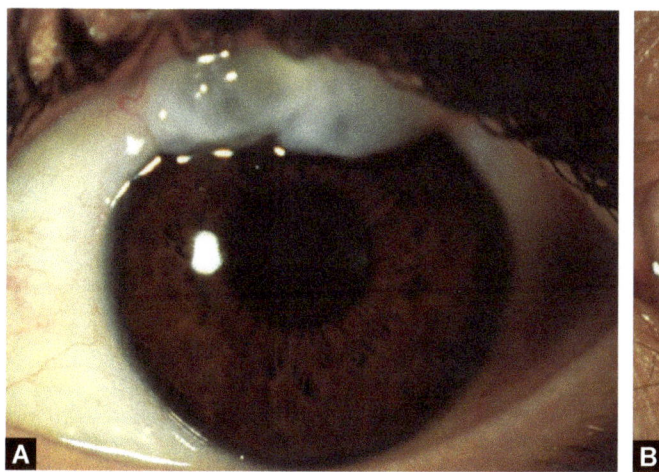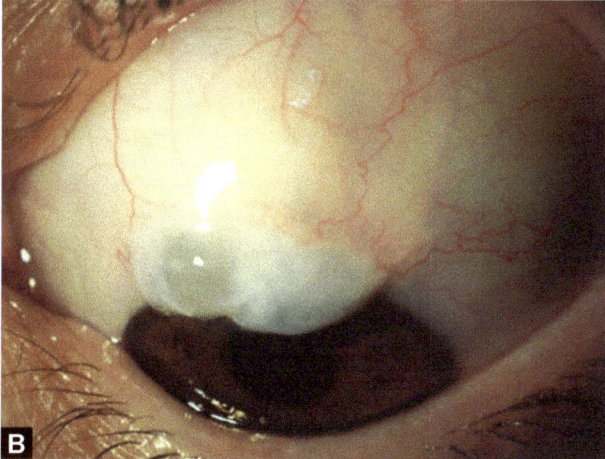

Figs. 8.10A and B: Steep-walled elevated bleb, at risk for blebitis, with corneal involvement, related to numerous complaints of foreign body sensation, pain, discomfort and stinging in trabeculectomy patients.

5 FU/MMC/antivascular endothelial growth factor peribleb injection. The next therapeutic step is slit lamp bleb needling revision or surgical bleb revision with excision of the Tenon cyst walls in the operating room. Postoperative protocols including orally taken (nonsteroidal anti-inflammatory drugs) NSAIDs may be an option.

Case 10: Dysesthetic bleb

A 67-year-old patient complained about stinging and *ripple sound* when blinking at 1-year follow-up visit after 0.2 mg/mL MMC for 2-minute-augmented trabeculectomy. Examination showed IOP 14 mm Hg with thin avascular elevated bleb, extended over the cornea not oozing but clearly interfering with the tear film impeding proper ocular surface lubrication: dysesthetic bleb (Figs. 8.10A and B). Cornea-dissecting blebs, forming a white, nonvascularized, spongy tissue that interferes with blinking, cause bubble formation and slowly remodulates in time. Surgical excision and bleb reformation with conjunctival advancement were done for this patient.

CONCLUSION

The success and failure of glaucoma surgery depend not only on the surgeon's skill and experience, but also on patient's idiosyncratic healing characteristics. The management of the bleb in the early postoperative period is fundamental for the long-term IOP control. The time window to act against conjunctival fibrosis is approximately 2 months and early complications, even diligently managed, can compromise surgery effectiveness. Adjustable sutures,

use of antimetabolites adapted to each case, careful manipulation of the conjunctiva and frequent follow-up visits in the early postoperative period decrease the likelihood of severe trabeculectomy complications.

REFERENCES

1. Khaw PT, Shah P, Sii F, Abbot J. Trabeculectomy. In: Shaarawy TM, Dada T and Bhartiya S (Eds). ISGS Textbook of Glaucoma Surgery, 1st edition. New Delhi: Jaypee Brother Medical Publishers (P) Ltd; 2014.
2. Leung DY, Tham CC. Management of bleb complications after trabeculectomy. Semin Ophthalmol. 2013;28(3):144-56.
3. Radhakrishnan S, Iwach AG. Complications of glaucoma surgery and their management. In: Ichhpujani P, Spaeth GL, Yanoff M (Eds). Expert Techniques in Ophthalmic Surgery, 1st edition. New Delhi: Jaypee Brothers Medical Publishers (P) Ltd; 2015. pp. 96-103.
4. Moster MR, Moster ML. Wipe-out: a complication of glaucoma surgery or just a blast from the past? Am J Ophthalmol. 2005;140(4):705-6.
5. Law SK, Song BJ, Kurbamnyan K, et al. Hemorrhagic complications from glaucoma surgery in patients on anticoagulation therapy or antiplatelet therapy. Am J Ophthalmol. 2008;145(4):736-46.
6. Wu ZH, Wang YH, Liu Y. Management strategies in malignant glaucoma secondary to antiglaucoma surgery. Int J Ophthalmol. 2016;9(1):63-8.
7. Yamamoto T, Sawada A, Mayama C, et al. The 5-year incidence of bleb-related infection and its risk factors after filtering surgeries with adjunctive mitomycin C: collaborative bleb-related infection incidence and treatment study 2. Ophthalmology. 2014;121(5):1001-6.
8. Kawai M, Nakabayashi S, Shimizu K, et al. Autologous transplantation of a free tenon's graft for repairing excessive bleb leakage after trabeculectomy: a case report. Case reports in ophthalmology. 2014;5(3):297-301.

CHAPTER 9

Tube Complications

Nadia Ríos-Acosta, Oscar Albis-Donado

INTRODUCTION

Glaucoma drainage implants can be valved or nonvalved devices. Most of the complications are observed on non-valved implants, but adverse events may occur after any kind of implant.

Early postoperative hypotony, suprachoroidal hemorrhage and choroidal effusions are among the most common complications, specially with nonvalved implants, but regardless of the device, we can find obstruction of the tube by debris, fibrin, iris, vitreous, blood, tube retraction or erosion, motility disturbances, corneal decompensation, endophthalmitis and retinal detachment.[1]

Case 1: Hypotony resolved without treatment

Mr Z, a 54-year-old gentleman, was found to have a shallow chamber with posterior synechiae on his left eye after his first day of the postsurgical period of a Baerveldt implant, intraocular pressure (IOP) 4 mm Hg visual acuity (VA) 20/200 (Fig. 9.1). At the posterior segment exploration, no abnormality was found and this was corroborated by A and B mode ultrasound. Observation with restriction of patient activities, an eye-shield and a cycloplegic was started. After 2 weeks of follow-up, IOP was 10 mm Hg and the anterior chamber was fully formed.

Case 2: Hypotony that requires treatment

Ten years later, Mr Z, now a 64-year-old gentleman (same patient as in Case 1), was found to have a flat chamber on his right eye after his second day of the postsurgical period of an Ahmed Valve implant, IOP 2 mm Hg VA 20/400,

corneal edema was found specially at the tube site, which had endothelial touch; the posterior segment was hard to evaluate clinically.

An A-B ultrasound showed medium-sized choroidal effusions. It was decided to inflate the anterior chamber with a high-density viscoelastic and increasing topical steroids and cycloplegics (Figs. 9.2A to C).

At 1-week follow-up, another ultrasound was performed demonstrating larger *kissing* choroidal effusions. Surgical drainage of the effusions was performed.

Case 3: Tube exposure

Mrs S, a 78-year-old lady with a severe primary angle-closure glaucoma and a failed phacotrabeculectomy performed

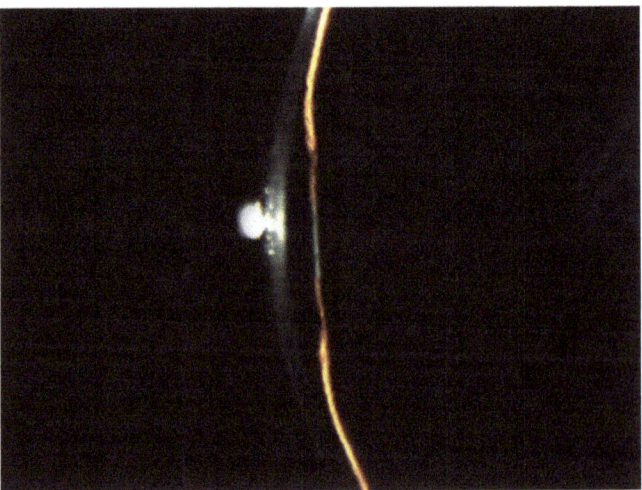

Fig. 9.1: A grade 2 flat anterior chamber with posterior synechiae and hypotony.

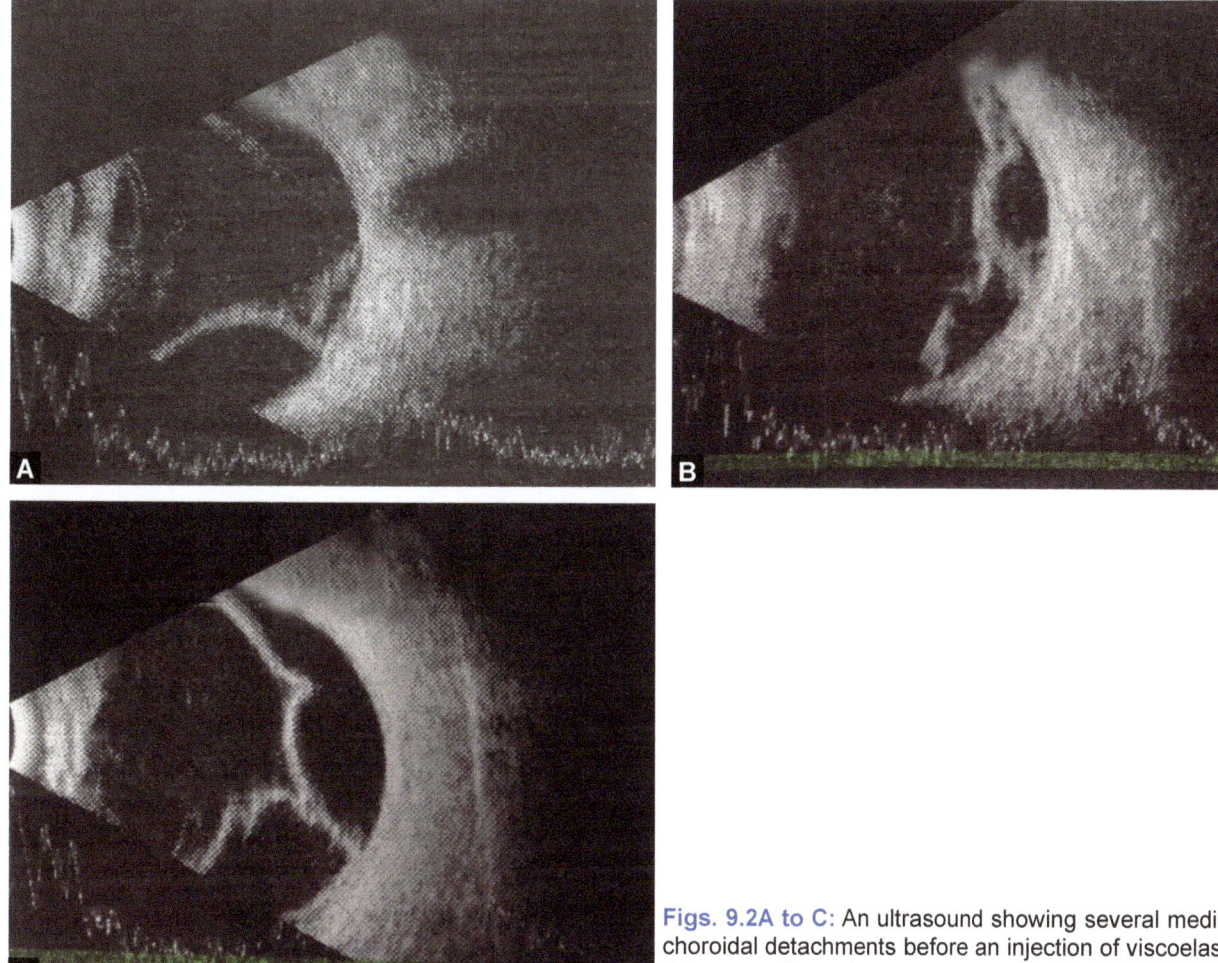

Figs. 9.2A to C: An ultrasound showing several medium-sized choroidal detachments before an injection of viscoelastic material was performed.

2 years ago, on triple hypotensive therapy since then, had an Ahmed valve implant a year ago.

During the first month of the postsurgical period, her IOP remained stable on 12 mm Hg without the need of hypotensive drugs. A year later, she returns with foreign body sensation and discharge. On examination a portion of the tube is seen exposed, the scleral patch has been completely reabsorbed (Fig. 9.3A). In surgery, the conjunctival defect is moved away from a new subepiscleral needle-created tunnel that is now covered with more healthy adjacent conjunctiva (Figs. 9.3B and C).

Case 4: Aqueous misdirection

Mr M, a 65-year-old patient, who had a failed previous phacotrabeculectomy 2 years before, had an Ahmed valve implant on his left eye 10 days ago. Three days ago he presents into the clinic with mild discomfort. At the examination

we find a shallow anterior chamber, IOP is 55 mm Hg, VA 20/100. Cycloplegia, corticosteroids and aqueous suppressant therapy was started. At the next day, IOP was 45 mm Hg and still a grade 2 athalamia was present. Posterior capsulotomy and hyaloidotomy were performed with neodymium-doped:yttrium aluminium garnet (ND:YAG) laser through an old iridectomy (Figs. 9.4A to D).

Case 5: Corneal decompensation

Mr J, aged 87 years, had an Ahmed implant surgery a few years ago. However, he has been presenting decreasing VA over the following years. At his ophthalmological examination, he is found to have IOP 13 mm Hg, loss of corneal transparency secondary to chronic corneal edema. The tube is in a good position. However, when reinterrogated, the patient has been sleeping on his right side, causing intermittent endothelial contact of the tube during those

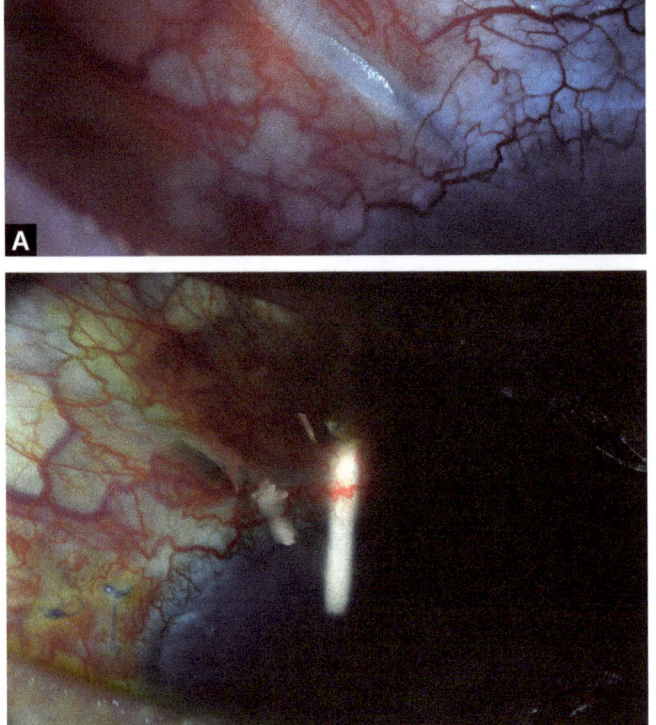

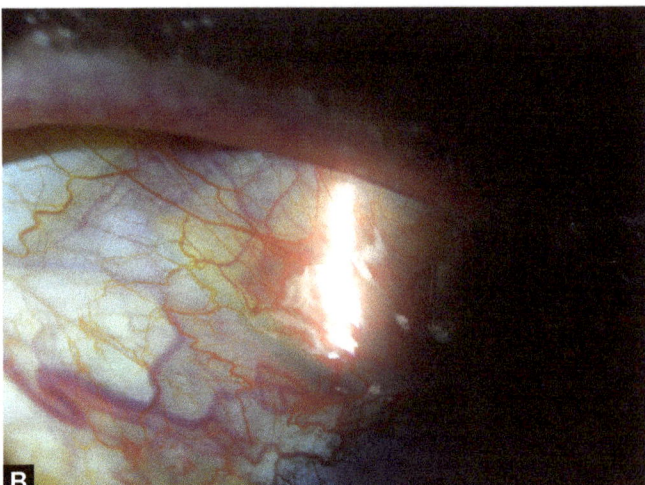

Figs. 9.3A to C: (A) A portion of the tube from an Ahmed valve implant is exposed, causing a small amount of discharge and foreign body sensation; (B and C) Two weeks later, the tube can be seen covered by healthy conjunctiva inside a needle-generated episcleral tunnel; the portion with the previous exposure has been moved toward the temporal side after removing the previously exposed borders and revitalizing the wound.

periods of time. He was planned for a Descemet stripping endothelial keratoplasty with repositioning and shortening of the tube (Figs. 9.5A and B).

Case 6: Tube blockage

Ms A, a 66-year-old female, had an Ahmed valve implant for neovascular glaucoma 3 days ago. However, her IOP remains on 35 mm Hg and there is no filtration bleb formed over the valve body.

At the anterior segment exploration, she has a 10% hyphema and there is a clot blocking the inner silicon tube. Tissue plasminogen activator (tPA) is administered directly on the anterior chamber. However the next day, the hyphema was 20%, IOP was 38 mm Hg and the clot was still blocking the tube. Nd:YAG laser was indicated to release the clot with adequate results lowering IOP to 16 mm Hg (Figs. 9.6A and B).

FOLLOW-UP PROTOCOL

Characteristics of the device implantation, corneal transparency, anterior chamber depth, IOP and posterior segment should be thoroughly assessed during the follow-up of patients who have undergone glaucoma drainage implant.

BRIEF REVIEW OF LITERATURE

The most descriptive study about long-term complications of tube implants is the tube versus trabeculectomy (TVT) study. TVT study reported that 21% of the tube patients had early postoperative complications.[2]

Results of the ABC and the AVB study suggest that although using a Baerveldt glaucoma implant may lead to better IOP outcomes, but with a significantly increased risk of postoperative complications and need for reintervention.[3,4] The occurrence of severe complications that

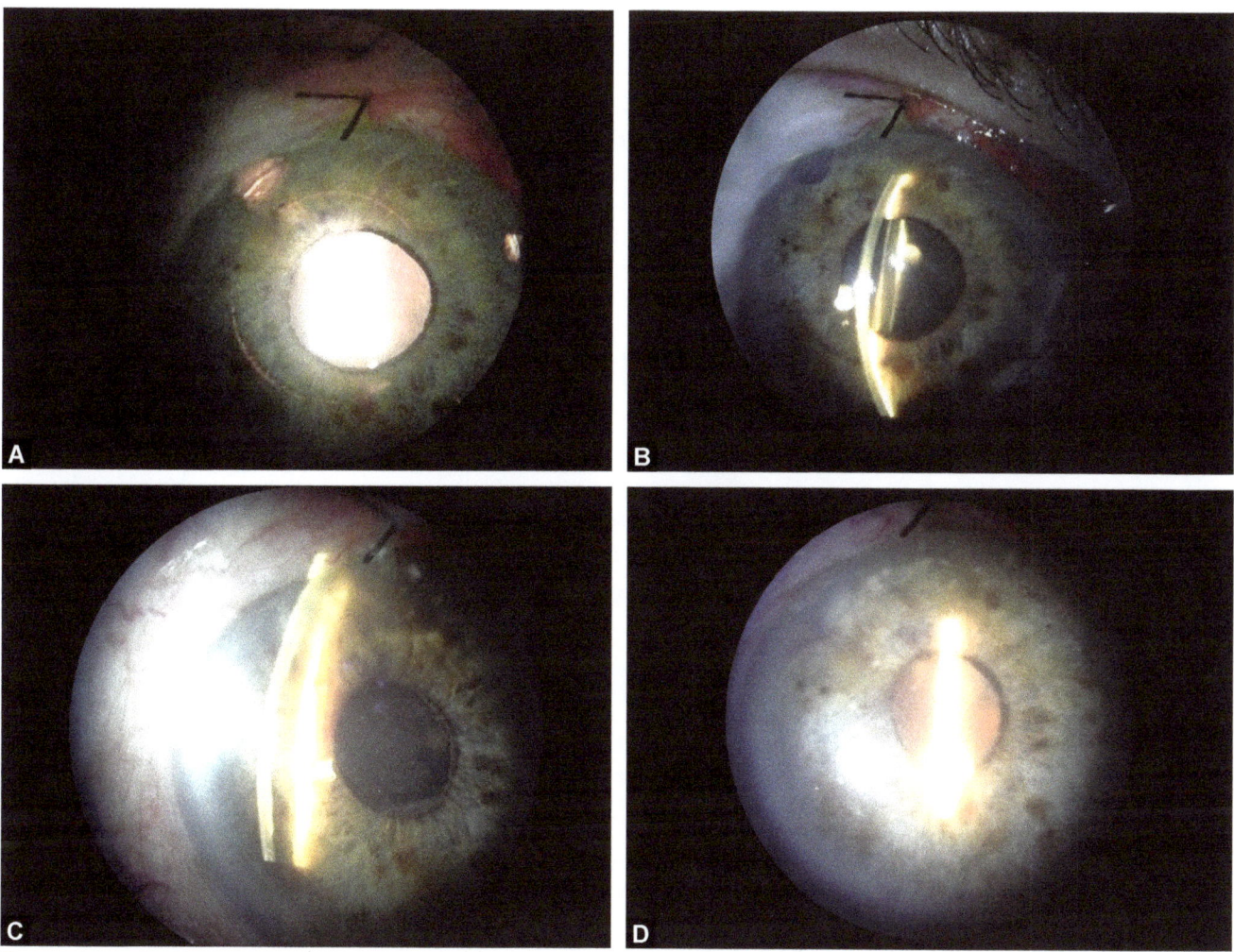

Figs. 9.4A to D: (A) On retroillumination, both the surgical and the laser iridectomies can be easily seen, but the border of the intraocular lens (IOL) is also bright, due to the forward pushing action of the aqueous humor trapped in the vitreous cavity; (B) The anterior chamber is shallow grade 2 with a small amount of space between the endothelium and the IOL. If it had been the natural lens (more protruding and not as rigid as the IOL), this would have been a grade 3 shallow anterior chamber; (C) Immediately after performing YAG laser capsulotomy and hyaloidotomy through the surgical iridectomy, the anterior chamber deepens as aqueous flows into it with some pigment. The IOL no longer draws its shape on the iris; (D) On retroillumination, the peripheral iridectomy remains visible, but the border of the IOL is no longer causing the perfectly round pigmentary defect.

could cause vision loss have also been described to be less frequent with Ahmed valve compared to Baerveldt (Table 9.1).

Similar complication rates have been described on neovascular glaucoma and non-neovascular glaucoma cases of Ahmed valve implant.[5]

On a recent report, the complications postoperatively of Ex-PRESS versus trabeculectomy (CPETS) study comparing trabeculectomy versus Ex-PRESS implant, reported similar postoperative complications to those described on the TVT study, except for a significant less frequency of hyphema on the Ex-PRESS group and a more frequent iris contact of this implant.[6]

SHALLOW OR FLAT ANTERIOR CHAMBER

One of the earliest postoperative complications is transient hypotony. It has been suggested to be due to leak around the tube in limbal tissues or failure of resistance from the valve.[1] By 1–2 weeks following the tube shunt surgery, a fibrous capsule has usually started to form around the plate to maintain an adequate IOP and formed anterior chamber.

On the TVT study, 21 patients reported a shallow anterior chamber. Among them, 10 patients had associated choroidal effusions, four had aqueous misdirection and

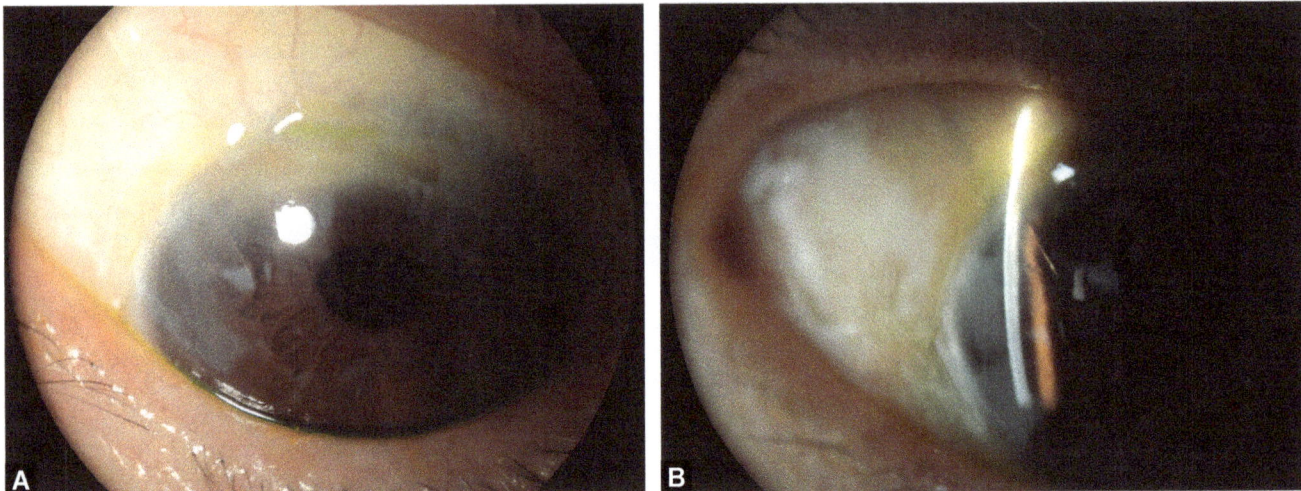

Figs. 9.5A and B: (A) The tube can be seen on an intermediate position between the iris and the corneal endothelium, but a small area of peripheral edema can be seen; (B) The slit lamp light shows an adequate distance between the tube and both the iris and the corneal endothelium, but a whitish zone of fibrous Descemet's membrane is seen at the place where intermittent contact happens.

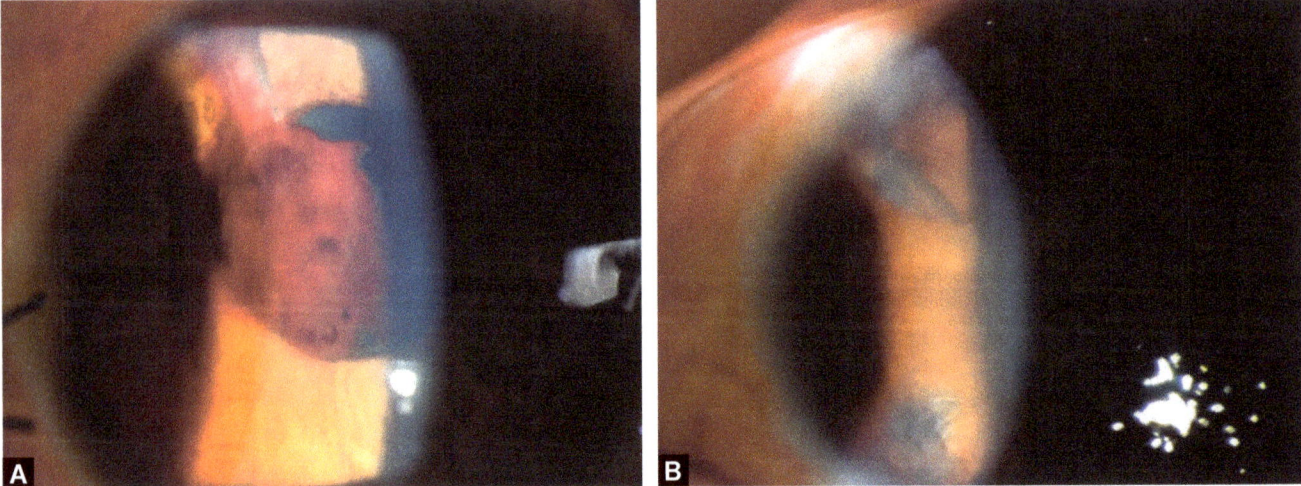

Figs. 9.6A and B: (A) A mid-sized clot is covering the tip of the tube. The anterior chamber is fully formed, but the intraocular pressure (IOP) is elevated; (B) Immediately after a failed tissue plasminogen activator injection and a successful yttrium aluminum garnet laser clot-removal, a diffuse hyphema can be seen, with the tip of the tube clearly visible achieving a lower IOP.

three patients had suprachoroidal hemorrhages.[2] Depending on the literature, a choroidal detachment after a valve implantation may develop in 8–22% of cases.[7-9] Hypotension due to choroidal effusions may lead to loss of vision.[7]

HYPERTENSIVE PHASE

Reports have described a postsurgical hypertensive phase, probably due to inflammation induced by flow of aqueous humor around the explants. Clinical failure can present due to excessive fibrosis and impermeability of the capsule around the explant.[1]

According to different authors, the incidence of encapsulated filtering bleb formation varies from 5% to 30%. It has been postulated that this complication depends on the properties of an implant, namely its size, shape, surface of the biomaterial, which leads to adhesion and proliferation of fibroblasts.[7]

The Ahmed valve has been associated with higher incidence of the hypertensive phase, which usually peaks at the first month and then is stabilized by 6 months after surgery.[10,11]

CORNEAL DECOMPENSATION

The main long-term complication of anterior chamber aqueous shunts is corneal endothelial decompensation.[1] In the TVT study, the most common late postoperative complication of this device was persistent corneal edema on 16% of the patients. The loss rate of endothelial cells after Ahmed glaucoma valve (AGV) implantation is reported to be 5.8% within 1 month, 11.5% after 6 months, 15.3% after 12 months, 16.6% after 18 months and 18.6% after 24 months. The greatest loss of endothelial cells has been observed in the area of the valve's tube, while in the central area of the cornea, the loss was only 15.4%, even 24 months after the surgery.[12]

MOTILITY DISORDERS

It has been described that up to 6% of the patients have diplopia or motility disorders, but only some of them have required extraction of the implant, while some others have undergone strabismus surgery to treat this condition.[7]

TUBE EXPOSURE

Meenakshi et al. reported an increased risk of tube exposure related to younger age and inflammation state.[13] Pakravan et al. compared the effectiveness of the AGV implantation in the upper and lower sectors, reporting that complications (cosmetic discomfort, tube erosion, endophthalmitis, diplopia) were more marked when implanted on the lower sector.[7,14]

Chances of tube erosion through the conjunctiva can be reduced by coating the tube with either of the graft materials *sclera*, fascia, pericardium and autologous sclera.[7] A needle-generated tunnel for the tube implant has been used and reports have shown possibly even lower chances of exposure than patches.[15-17]

ENDOPHTHALMITIS

This is a rare complication and occurs in 0.8–6.3% of cases. Mostly it has been related to tube extrusion. Explantation of the graft, vitrectomy and intravitreal injection of antibiotics resulted in inflammation relief in most cases.[15,16]

COMPLICATIONS OF AHMED VALVE IMPLANT ON CHILDREN

Hazem et al. reported on primary congenital glaucoma the main complication hyphema, which spontaneously resolved within 5–7 days without additional treatment, flat anterior chamber, encapsulated bleb and choroidal effusion presented with the same frequency of 6%, the cases of choroidal effusion resolved spontaneously with topic atropine and steroids and systemic steroid treatment.[20-24]

Postoperative interventions for common complications are enlisted in Table 9.2.

Table 9.1: Early and late postoperative complications of tube implant by decreasing frequency as described on the Tube Versus Trabeculectomy Study.[2]

Early postoperative complications	Late postoperative complications
Choroidal effusion	Persistent corneal edema
Shallow or flat anterior chamber	Persistent diplopia
Aqueous misdirection	Tube erosion
Hyphema	Cystoid macular edema
Suprachoroidal hemorrhage	Tube obstruction
Wound leak	Encapsulated bleb
Vitreous hemorrhage	Chronic or recurrent iritis
	Choroidal effusion
	Dysesthesia
	Endophthalmitis
	Flat or shallow anterior chamber
	Hypotony maculopathy
	Retinal detachment

Table 9.2: Postoperative interventions and reoperations for complications by decreasing frequency as described on the Tube Versus Trabeculectomy Study.[2]

Postoperative interventions	Reoperations for complications
Removal of rip chord	Penetrating keratoplasty
Laser suture lysis	Pars plana vitrectomy
Anterior chamber reformation	Tube shunt revision with patch graft
Needling	Drainage of choroidal effusion
5-FU injection	DSAEK
Injection of intracameral tPA	Tube repositioning or revision
	Cataract extraction
	Removal of implant

(DSAEK: Descemet's stripping automated endothelial keratoplasty; tPA: Tissue plasminogen activator).

REFERENCES

1. Minckler DS, Vedula SS, Li TJ, et al. Aqueous Shunts for Glaucoma. Cochrane Database Syst Rev. 2006;2:CD004918.
2. Gedde SJ, Herndon LW, Brandt JD, et al. Postoperative complications in the Tube Versus Trabeculectomy (TVT) study during five years of follow-up. Am J Ophthalmol. 2012;153(5):804-14.
3. Barton K, Feuer WJ, Budenz DL, et al. Three-year treatment outcomes in the Ahmed Baerveldt comparison study. Ophthalmology. 2014;121(8):1547-57.e1.
4. Aminlari AE, Scott IU, Aref AA. Glaucoma drainage implant surgery—an evidence-based update with relevance to sub-Saharan Africa. Middle East Afr J Ophthalmol. 2013;20(2):126-30.
5. Li Z, Zhou M, Wang W, et al. A prospective comparative study on neovascular glaucoma and non-neovascular refractory glaucoma following Ahmed glaucoma valve implantation. Chin Med J. 2014;127(8):1417-22.
6. Arimura S, Takihara Y, Miyake S, et al. Randomized Clinical Trial for Early Postoperative Complications of Ex-PRESS Implantation versus Trabeculectomy: Complications Postoperatively of Ex-PRESS versus Trabeculectomy Study (CPETS). Sci Rep. 2016;6:26080.
7. Bikbov MM, Khusnitdinov II. The results of the use of Ahmed Valve in refractory glaucoma surgery. J Curr Glaucoma Pract. 2015;9(3):86-91.
8. Al-Aswad LA, Netland PA, Bellows AR, et al. Clinical experience with the double-plate Ahmed glaucoma valve. Am J Ophthalmol. 2006;141(2):390-1.
9. Coleman AL, Hill R, Wilson MR, et al. Initial clinical experience with the Ahmed glaucoma valve implant. Am J Ophthalmol. 1995;120(1):23-31.
10. Zarei R, Amini H, Daneshvar R, et al. Long-term outcomes of Ahmed Glaucoma Valve implantation in refractory glaucoma at Farabi Eye Hospital, Tehran, Iran. Middle East Afr J Ophthalmol. 2016;23(1):104-9.
11. Gessesse GW. The Ahmed Glaucoma Valve in refractory glaucoma: experiences in Southwest Ethiopia. Ethiop J Health Sci. 2015;25(3):267-72.
12. Lee EK, Yun YJ, Lee JE, et al. Changes in corneal endothelial cells after Ahmed glaucoma valve implantation: 2-year follow-up. Am J Ophthalmol. 2009;148(3):361-7.
13. Chaku M, Netland PA, Ishida K, et al. Risk factors for tube exposure as a late complication of glaucoma drainage implant surgery. Clin Ophthalmol. 2016;10:547-53.
14. Pakravan M, Yazdani S, Shahabi C, et al. Superior versus inferior Ahmed glaucoma valve implantation. Ophthalmol. 2009;116(2):208-13.
15. Ozdamar A, Aras C, Ustundag C, Tamcelik N, Ozkan S. Scleral tunnel for the implantation of glaucoma seton devices. Ophthalmic Surg Lasers. 2001;32(5):432-5.
16. Leong JK, McCluskey P, Lightman S, Towler HM. Outcome of graft free Molteno tube insertion. Br J Ophthalmol. 2006;90:501-5.
17. Albis-Donado O, Gil-Carrasco F, Romero-Quijada R, Thomas R. Evaluation of Ahmed glaucoma valve implantation through a needle-generated scleral tunnel in Mexican children with glaucoma. Indian J Ophthalmol. 2010;58(5):365-73.
18. Gedde SJ, Scott IU, Tabandeh H, et al. Late endophthalmitis associated with glaucoma drainage implants. Ophthalmology. 2001;108(7):1323-7.
19. Morad Y, Donaldson CE, Kim YM, et al. The Ahmed drainage implant in the treatment of pediatric glaucoma. Am J Ophthalmol. 2003;135(6):821-9.
20. Helmy H. Combined trabeculotomy-trabeculectomy versus Ahmed valve implantation for refractory primary congenital glaucoma in Egyptian patients: a long-term follow-up. Electronic Physician. 2016;8(2):1884-91.
21. Wang YW, Wang PB, Zeng C, et al. Comparison of the Ahmed glaucoma valve with the baerveldt glaucoma implant: a meta-analysis. BMC Ophthalmol. 2015;15:132.
22. HaiBo T, Xin K, ShiHeng L, et al. Comparison of Ahmed glaucoma valve implantation and trabeculectomy for glaucoma: a systematic review and meta-analysis. PLoS One. 2015;10(2):e0118142.
23. Budenz DL, Barton K, Gedde SJ, et al. Five-year treatment outcomes in the Ahmed Baerveldt comparison study. Ophthalmology. 2015;122(2):308-16.
24. Shaarawy T, Sherwood M, Hitchings R, et al. Chapters 115. Glaucoma, 2nd edition. Amsterdam: Elsevier; 2014. pp. 1086-102.

CHAPTER 10

Complications of Nonpenetrating Deep Sclerectomy

Sylvain Roy, André Mermoud

INTRODUCTION

Nonpenetrating deep sclerectomy (NPDS) aims at lowering the intraocular pressure (IOP) while reducing the complications prevailing during penetrating surgery. Nonetheless some specific complications pertaining to this technique may occur and a sound knowledge of the difficulties and limitations of this surgery is requested to prevent or control these mishaps from endangering the results of this modern filtering procedure.

Case 1: Rupture of the thin trabeculo-Descemet's membrane

Rupture of the thin trabeculo-Descemet's membrane (TDM) can occur during NPDS or in the postoperative period (Fig. 10.1). A good knowledge of the anatomy of the anterior segment, a precise dissection of the deep scleral flap into clear cornea, a reduction of the intraoperative IOP by performing a paracentesis and gentle severing of the scleral flap avoiding excessive pressure to the globe help in preventing this complication from happening (Fig. 10.2). Should a perforation of the TDM occur, the procedure is modified the following: for a small perforation of the TDM, with rapid egress of aqueous but without incarceration of the iris, buffering of the rupture can be achieved using viscoelastics in the anterior chamber to separate the cornea from the iris (Fig. 10.3). These ophthalmic viscosurgical devices help in limiting the outflow of aqueous and reducing the incidence of postoperative hypotony. Should the perforation be large enough to result in permanent iris

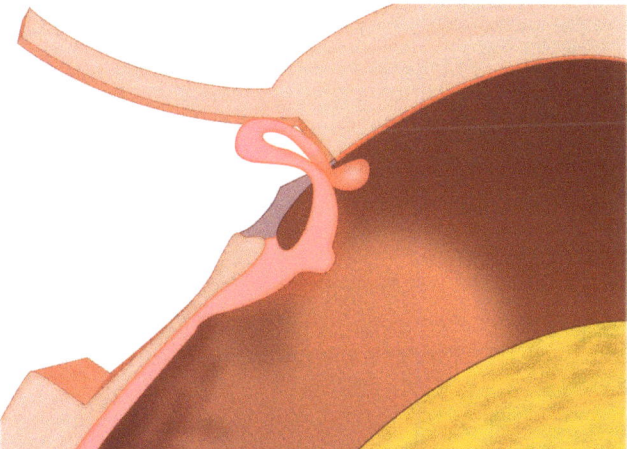

Fig. 10.1: Schematic drawing of iris incarceration in the trabeculo-Descemet's membrane.

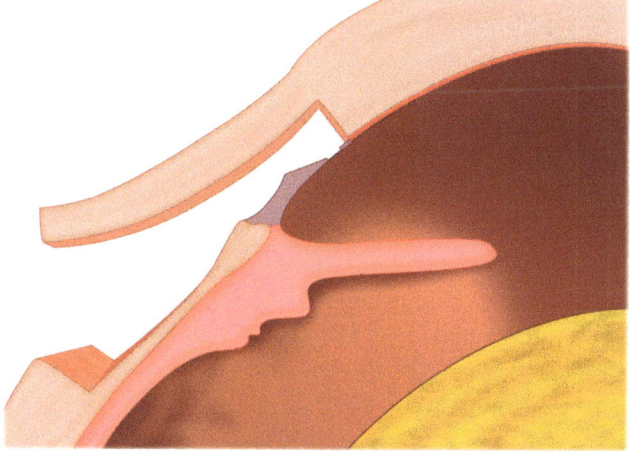

Fig. 10.2: Schematic drawing of a rupture of the trabeculo-Descemet's membrane without iris incarceration.

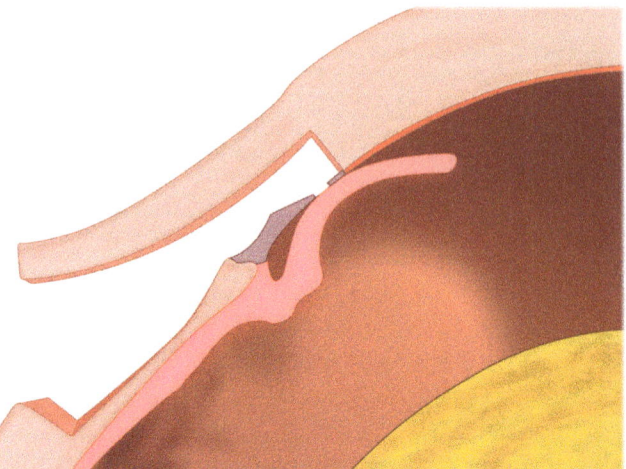

Fig. 10.3: Schematic drawing of iris apposition against the trabeculo-Descemet's membrane.

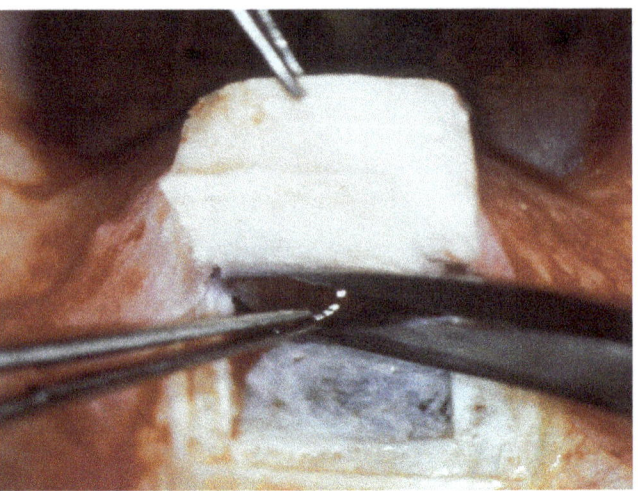

Fig. 10.4: Iris incarceration requiring peripheral iridectomy and conversion to trabeculectomy.

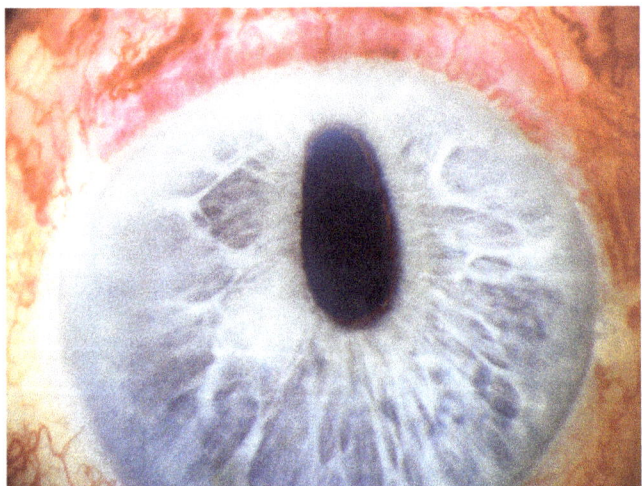

Fig. 10.5: An oval pupil resulting from iris incarceration after Nd:YAG goniopuncture.

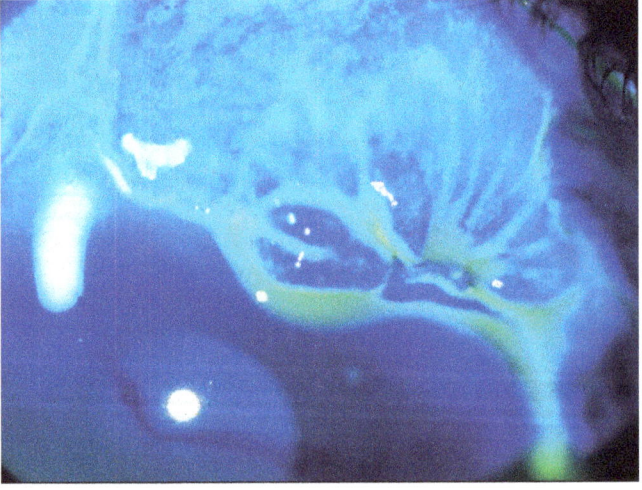

Fig. 10.6: Positive Seidel's sign of the filtering bleb using fluorescein and cobalt blue light.

incarceration in the breach, a peripheral iridectomy should be performed and the procedure converted to conventional trabeculectomy (Fig. 10.4). In this situation, the superficial scleral flap should be closed with multiple sutures and viscoelastics should be injected under the flap.

Late-onset of TDM rupture can occur after blunt ocular trauma, or after extensive neodymium-doped:yttrium aluminium garnet (Nd:YAG) goniopuncture that lead to iris incarceration in the punctured membrane, resulting in oval pupil (Fig. 10.5). In simple, stable cases with good IOP reaching the target values, there is no need for further action. If IOP is elevated, iris incarceration can be released using Nd:YAG laser and pilocarpine medication.

Conversely, surgical revision is required when the IOP is not correctly controlled despite Nd:YAG procedure intended to remove the iris incarceration. The surgery should clear the filtration site of any obstacle to aqueous humor outflow.

Case 2: Leak of the filtering bleb (Seidel's sign)

At the end of the surgery, the conjunctiva needs to be carefully closed to ensure a watertight filtering bleb. Wound dehiscence or insufficient closure of the conjunctiva can result in leak of the filtering bleb, which is indicated by a positive Seidel sign (Fig. 10.6). The postoperative examination should always include a proper assessment of the filtering bleb, and in any doubt, a fluorescein test should

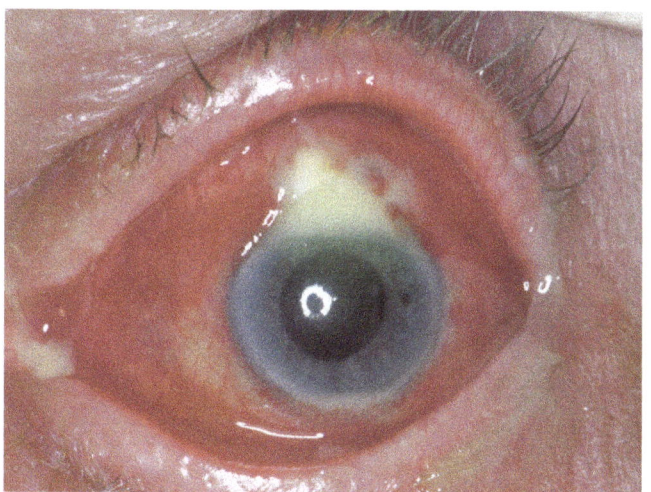

Fig. 10.7: Blebitis and endophthalmitis with hypopyon in ocular infection following glaucoma surgery.

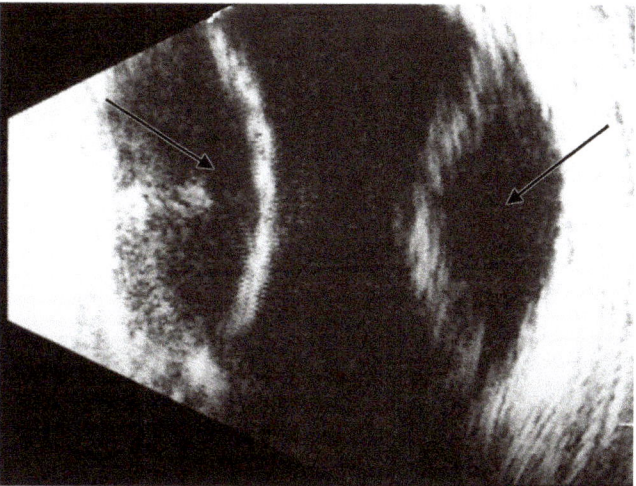

Fig. 10.8: Ultrasound biomicroscopy showing bilateral choroidal detachment (arrows).

be performed to rule out any leak of the bleb. If the IOP remains in acceptable range, i.e. higher than 5 mm Hg, moderate leak of the bleb can heal in a few days. Usually, corticosteroids administration should be stopped for some time to help healing process. In less benign cases, a therapeutic contact lens can be inserted to protect the conjunctiva from rubbing against the lids to help in promoting proper scarring and closure of the wound. In the most severe cases, a surgical revision of the wound is mandatory to prevent extreme hypotony, bleb (blebitis) and ocular (endophthalmitis) infections (Fig. 10.7).

Case 3: Hypotony

Overfiltration results in excessive IOP reduction and durable low-pressure situation below 5 mm Hg will lead to ocular hypotony with the related complications. After successful NPDS it is not uncommon to achieve a temporarily low-pressure condition, e.g. IOP around 4–5 mm Hg, 1 day after surgery. This condition will generally improve to achieve a target IOP at around 8–12 mm Hg the following weeks. Should the IOP remain lower than 5 mm Hg for more than 2 weeks with accompanying maculopathy, macular fold and choroidal detachment (Figs. 10.8 and 10.9), the causes for such hypotony should be investigated. Leak of the filtering bleb (*see* above), a chronic choroidal or ciliary body detachment can lead to hypotony. Surgical revision to close the bleb, drain the subchoroidal fluid, viscoelastics injected in the anterior chamber and extensive pharmacological cycloplegia are the remedies for such a complication.

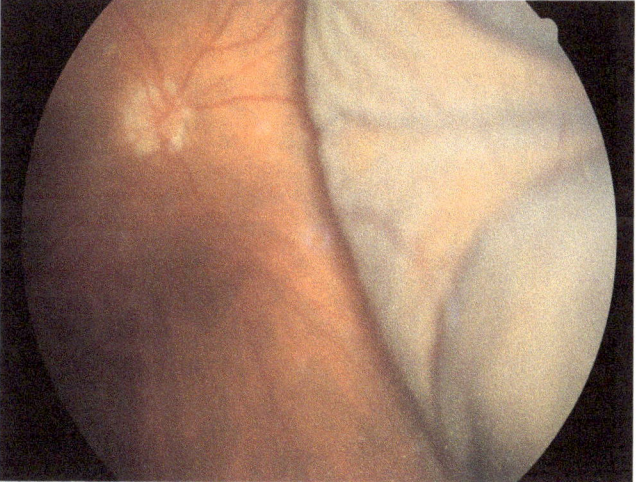

Fig. 10.9: Fundus photograph showing an important choroidal detachment.

Case 4: Bleb fibrosis and encystment of the bleb

In the weeks following NPDS fibrosis and/or encystment of the filtering bleb can occur that limit the aqueous humor outflow resulting in secondary rise in the IOP (Fig. 10.10). Excessive scarring responses and tissue remodelling are responsible for these fibrotic reactions. The use of antimetabolites, such as mitomycin C (MMC) during surgery, helps in preventing the outcome of such complications. Nonetheless, bleb fibrosis can develop in the early months after surgery. The treatment consists in injecting MMC under the conjunctiva in an area next to the filtering bleb to stop and reduce scarring of the bleb

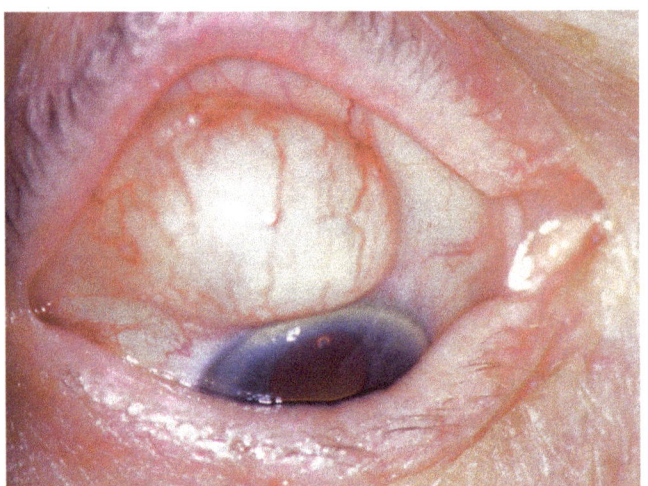

Fig. 10.10: Depicting an encystment of the filtering bleb.

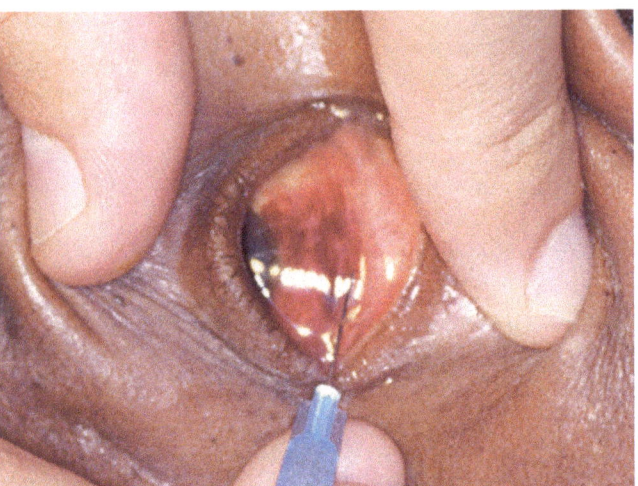

Fig. 10.11: Bleb needling to prevent scarring of the filtering bleb.

(Fig. 10.11). Alternatively, the filtering bleb can show encystment of the conjunctiva layers that severely reduce the egress of aqueous humor. This encystment of the bleb can be treated using a needling method that ruptures and severs the wall of the cysts. A combination of bleb needling and MMC injection can also be advocated in severe cases.

Case 5: Secondary rise in the intraocular pressure

If the IOP achieved a target range in the days following NPDS, but departs from that range in the weeks or early months after surgery, several causes might be responsible for that drift. First of all, a corticosteroids response should be rule out by tapering with the postoperative treatment. Alternatively, nonsteroids anti-inflammatory drops can be administered instead. A thickening of the TDM can lead to progressive increase in the resistance to aqueous humor egress. In that situation, Nd:YAG goniopuncture will create minute holes in the TDM and enhance aqueous humor outflow (Fig. 10.12). Finally, scarring of the scleral bleb, the subconjunctival space or the filtering bleb can equally prevent a sufficient drainage of the aqueous humor, all resulting in secondary rise in the IOP. As mentioned earlier, injection of MMC in the subconjunctival space and/or needling of the encysted bleb are therapeutics approaches to prevent departure from initially a good target IOP.

▎ INVESTIGATIONS

Every glaucoma patient, experiencing complications during or after NPDS, should be carefully and thoroughly

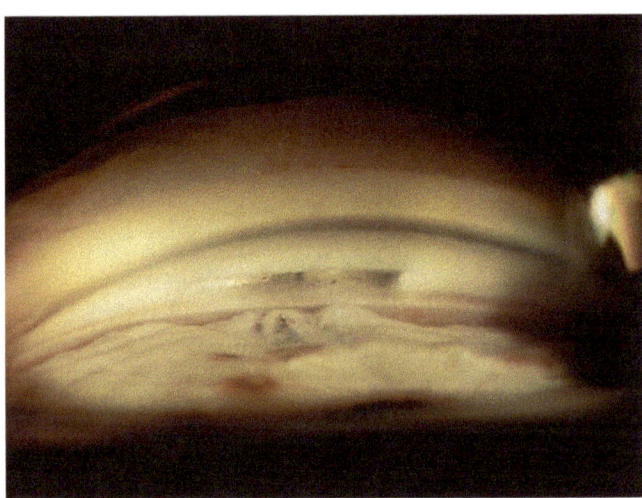

Fig. 10.12: Gonioscopic view of Nd:YAG goniopuncture performed in the TDM to enhance aqueous humor outflow.

examined to clearly identify the exact nature and cause of the complication for a proper management and treatment of such complication.

Clinical evaluation includes:

- Best-corrected visual acuity to assess change in vision
- Detailed slit-lamp biomicroscopy. A thorough examination of the conjunctiva, the filtering bleb, the cornea, the anterior chamber including the iris, the pupillary region and the lens is required for the handling of complications of NPDS
- *Tonometry (applanation):* Accurate IOP measurement to exclude or confirm hypotony or elevated IOP

- *Gonioscopy:* Precise and detailed images of the anatomy of the iridocorneal angle are necessary to assess the postoperative structures of the angle
- *Anterior segment imaging:* Ultrasound biomicroscopy or optical coherence tomography imaging help in visualizing the anatomical landmarks of the eye structures and the changes induced by the surgery, and can provide useful information about the cause of the complication
- Detailed fundus examination including the periphery to rule out choroidal hemorrhage or detachment of the choroid for instance.

FOLLOW-UP PROCEDURE

The etiology of the complication must be clearly identified before proper actions are taken. Depending on the kind of complications rapid measures have to be initiated, conversely a more conservative observational attitude can be taken. Some complications may resolve by themselves, whereas more sight-threatening situations will require immediate action, e.g. surgical revision. Late complications, such as bleb fibrosis or encapsulation of the bleb, can be treated with bleb needling associated with antimetabolites. Similarly, onset of ocular hypertension can be modulated by performing Nd:YAG laser goniopuncture to perforate the thin TDM.

BRIEF REVIEW OF LITERATURE

Nonpenetrating deep sclerectomy complications are a relatively rare event, but proper understanding of the precise cause is mandatory.[1] Goniopuncture is associated with a low-complication rate and demonstrates minimal inflammation, hemorrhage and hypotony when performed correctly.[2] Nonetheless, there are potentially serious complications associated with the procedure, such as peripheral anterior synechiae, IOP variation and occlusion of the goniopuncture by the iris.[3,4] Postlaser IOP was significantly lower than prelaser IOP at every time point.[5] Needle revision with subconjunctival MMC may successfully lower the IOP in eyes with a failing deep sclerectomy bleb in the long-term.[6]

SUMMARY

Complications of NPDS can occur during NPDS (rupture of the TDM) or after surgery (trauma), and the IOP can be low due to leaks on the conjunctiva, or elevated due to fibrosis or encystment of the bleb. Laser goniopuncture, antimetabolites and bleb needling can help in restoring a proper drainage of the aqueous humor outflow.

POINTS TO REMEMBER

- Rupture of the thin trabeculo-Descemet's membrane can occur during NPDS.
- If such rupture is small, viscoelastics material can be used to tamper the breach in the membrane.
- Else conversion to conventional trabeculectomy including peripheral iridectomy shall be performed.
- The filtering bleb can leak resulting in hypotony and elevated risk of blebitis (inflammation/infection of the bleb) and eventually endophthalmitis.
- Bleb revision is required to prevent onset of these complications.
- Conversely, injection of viscoelastics material in the anterior chamber helps in restoring the intraocular pressure.
- Late-onset of ocular hypertension can be treated by needling of the bleb and performing a Nd:YAG laser goniopuncture.
- Spontaneous iris incarceration in ruptured trabeculo-Descemet's membrane can be seen. In severe cases a surgical revision is required.

REFERENCES

1. Roy S, Mermoud A. Complications of deep nonpenetrating sclerectomy. J Fr Ophtalmol. 2006;29(10):1180-97.
2. Tam DY, Barnebey HS, Ahmed II. Nd: YAG laser goniopuncture: indications and procedure. J Glaucoma. 2013; 22(2):620-5.
3. Anand N, Pilling R. Nd:YAG laser goniopuncture after deep sclerectomy: outcomes. Acta Ophthalmol. 2010;88(1): 110-5.
4. Martín-Moro JG, Miguel YF. Management of post-goniopuncture iris herniation: a two-step procedure. Int Ophthalmol. 2014;34(3):603-6.
5. Di Matteo F, Bettin P, Fiori M, Ciampi C, Rabiolo A, Bandello F. Nd:Yag laser goniopuncture for deep sclerectomy: efficacy and outcomes. Graefes Arch Clin Exp Ophthalmol. 2016; 254(3):535-9.
6. Koukkoulli A, Musa F, Anand N. Long-term outcomes of needle revision of failing deep sclerectomy blebs. Graefes Arch Clin Exp Ophthalmol. 2015;253(1):99-110.

CHAPTER 11

Complications of Newer Surgeries

Youssef Abdelmassih, Sylvain el-Khoury, Ziad Khoueir, Tarek Shaarawy

INTRODUCTION

Trabeculectomy was introduced in the 1960s and quickly became the standard of care for filtering procedures.[1,2] However, despite numerous advances and modifications, reproducibility of trabeculectomy outcomes remained unsatisfactory when it came to lowering intraocular pressure (IOP). Furthermore, sudden decompression of the eye occurs upon penetration of the anterior chamber (AC) yielding to a relatively high risk of early postoperative complications such as overfiltration, hypotony, maculopathy and choroidal detachment.[3] The need for safer and more reliable surgical techniques as alternatives to traditional incisional surgeries led to the development of less-invasive procedures comprising surgical techniques with implants. Grouped under the acronym of minimally invasive glaucoma surgery (MIGS) they aim to necessitate, as the name suggests, less tissue manipulation while effectively reducing IOP with a better safety profile. The minimal invasive approach implies less postoperative scarring and thus reduced failure and complication rates. At the present stage these techniques are performed in selective mild-to-moderate glaucoma cases in combination with phacoemulsification or as a standalone procedure.

CLASSIFICATION

Minimally invasive glaucoma surgery and other implants can be subcategorized according to their anatomical outflow pathway as well as the surgical approach that is used to implant them:

- Subconjunctival space filtration
    - *Ab-interno implantation*: XEN Gel Stent (AqueSys, Inc., Aliso Viejo, California, USA)
    - *Ab-externo implantation*: EX-PRESS glaucoma filtration device (Alcon Inc, Forth Worth, Texas, USA); InnFocus Microshunt (InnFocus, Miami, Florida, USA). EX-PRESS and InnFocus shunts are not considered as MIGS
- Decreasing resistance of the Schlemm's canal
    - *Trabecular bypass*: iStent (Glaukos Corporation, Laguna Hills, California, USA)
    - *Schlemm's canal expander*: Hydrus Micro-stent (Ivantis, Irvine California, USA)
- Suprachoroidal space drainage
    - *Ab interno*: CyPass Micro stent (Transcend Medical Inc.).

COMPLICATIONS

The rate and type of complications with MIGS and other implants vary according to different techniques, implants, anatomical regions of action and surgeon experience.[4-6] In general most common complications are:
- Hypotony due to overfiltration
- Hyphema due to blood reflux either from the Schlemm's canal or from the suprachoroidal space
- Hypertony usually due to remaining viscoelastic in the AC or stent occlusion either from stent malpositioning or inflammatory fibrinous reaction.

Complications of MIGS and other implants as well as their anatomical sites are summarized in Figures 11.1A to F.

Suprachoroidal implants usually risk leading to hypotony and hyphema in the early postoperative period as well as implant obstruction with subsequent transient IOP increase[5,7-10] (Fig. 11.1A).

Implants acting on the Schlemm's canal carry a risk of occlusion. The one acting as a canal expander can be obstructed with peripheral anterior synechiae[4,11] (Fig. 11.1B) and the one acting as a trabecular bypass can be obstructed because of malpositioning or fibrosis[12,13] (Fig. 11.1C). Hyphema is reported to be more common in the trabecular bypass then in the canal expander.[11,12]

Devices implanted into the subconjunctival space have a high risk of scarring with secondary failure[14] as well as early postoperative hypotony[15,16] (Figs. 11.1D to F).

Case 1: Medical management of shallow anterior chamber after EX-PRESS glaucoma filtration device

A 64-year-old male patient presented to our clinic with a diagnosis of primary open-angle glaucoma in both eyes. Visual field in the left eye showed a superior arcuate defect in the Bjerrum area with a documented progression over the last 3 years. IOP in the left eye was 18 mm Hg at presentation with a central corneal thickness (CCT) of 525 μm. A 24-hour IOP measurement was performed and peaked up to 21 mm Hg under full topical treatment. The patient had a history of heart surgery with cardiac stent implantation in the last year and was on strict anticoagulation. An intervention to reach a lower target IOP was indicated and in order to avoid hemorrhage after iridectomy, the decision was taken to implant an EX-PRESS device into the subconjunctival space. The surgery was uncomplicated and straightforward, but on the first postoperative day, the AC was shallow with peripheral iris touch (AC depth grade 1) and bleb was elevated. A small choroidal effusion was detected on fundus examination and verified by B-scan. IOP was at 5 mm Hg. The patient was put on atropine 1% b.i.d. along with his regular postoperative treatment consisting of topical steroid and antibiotic and asked to return to clinic on the following day, at which the situation was stable with low IOP and shallow AC. Medication was continued and 1 week later the patient returned to clinic presenting with a slightly deeper chamber with no peripheral iris touch and an IOP of 8 mm Hg. Choroidal effusion had disappeared. Atropine was tapered to once daily. Two weeks later, AC had regained its preoperative depth, IOP was at 11 mm Hg and atropine was ceased.

Learning Points

- If a shallow AC is present, check IOP and rule out the presence of a choroidal effusion using a B-scan
- Medical treatment with Atropine 1% and steroid drops is the first-line therapy for a flat AC with low IOP
- A surgical reformation of the chamber using viscoelastic is indicated in case of no improvement over time or in case of AC depth grade 3 to avoid corneal decompensation and synechiae
- In majority of cases, a postoperative shallow AC associated with low IOP regains depth progressively without additional intervention, but has to be closely observed.

Case 2: XEN Gel-stent implant combined with cataract surgery

A 66-year-old gentleman known to have moderate glaucoma in both eyes presented to our clinic with reincreased IOP of 22 mm Hg and CCT of 540 μm in the left eye under full medical treatment. His best corrected visual acuity (BCVA) was 20/50 in that eye due to a nuclear cataract. Gonioscopy showed open angles (Shaffer 3) and fundus examination revealed bilateral moderate optic disc cupping [cup-to-disc (C:D) ratio 0.6]. The patient was scheduled for a cataract surgery combined with XEN Gel Stent implantation without the use of mitomycin C. Surgical intervention was uncomplicated and IOP in the first month postoperatively did not exceed 12 mm Hg. Subsequently, however, IOP progressively rose to close to preoperative levels and bleb flattened. The patient was scheduled for needling of the bleb, under which IOP dropped to levels below 13 mm Hg. The patient received prednisolone 1% eyedrops q.i.d. tapered, 3 injections of 5-flurouracil at the 2nd, 3rd and 5th, postoperative day after needling and was instructed to do a careful massage of the globe. Following these measures, the bleb became diffuse and quiet. IOP remained stable.

Learning Points

- Bleb-related complications are present even in case of an intraoperative application of mitomycin C
- Postoperative bleb care is essential for surgical success and comprises massage of the globe, antifibrotics and steroids.

Case 3: CyPass Micro-stent implantation with postoperative hyphema

A 72-year-old male patient presented to our clinic for blurred vision, redness and foreign body sensation. He had

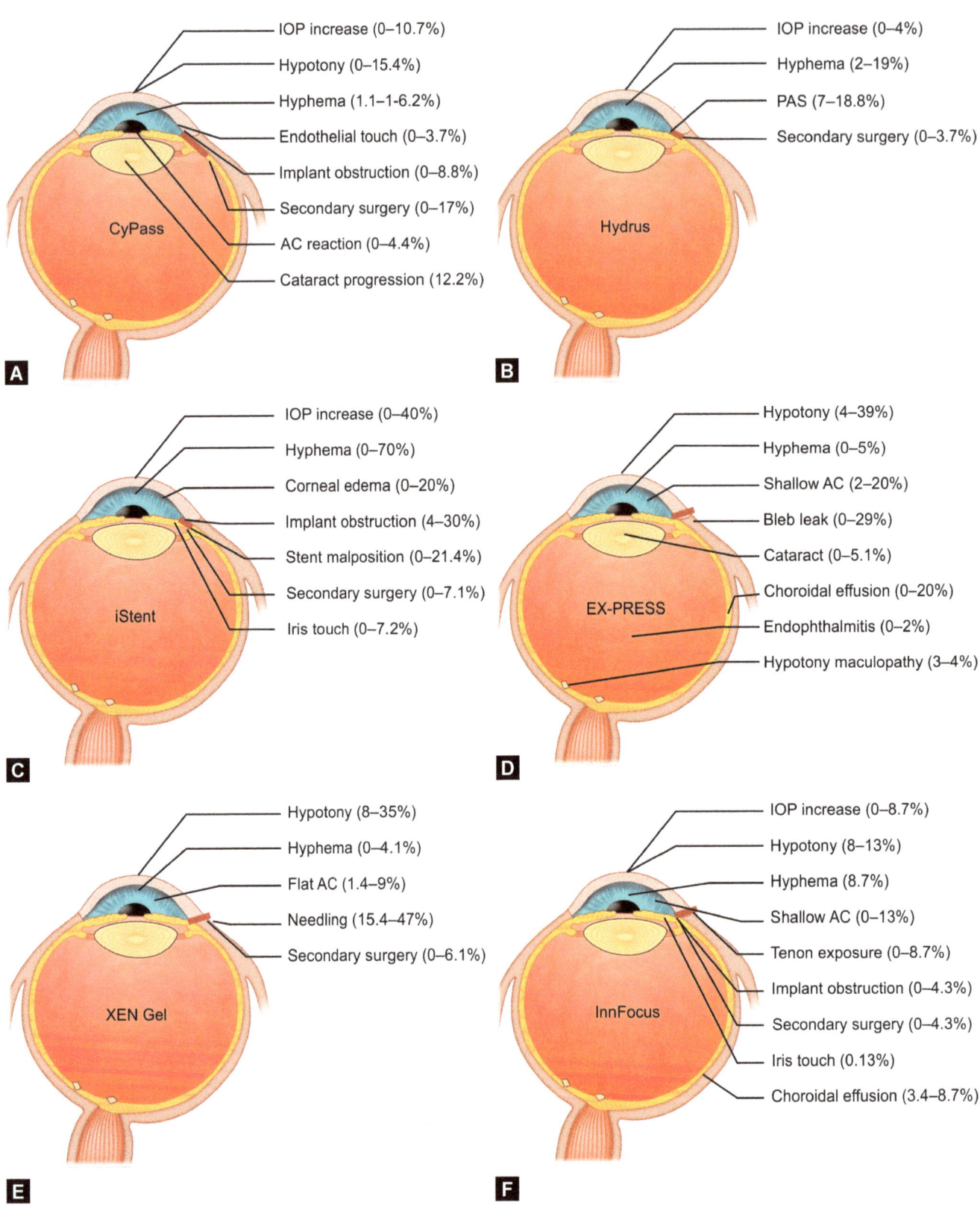

Figs. 11.1A to F: Complications of newer surgeries.
(AC: Anterior chamber; IOP: Intraocular pressure; PAS: Peripheral anterior synechiae).

been followed for glaucoma elsewhere and was on tri-therapy (bimatoprost, timolol and dorzolamide). On examination, BCVA was 20/40, anterior segment examination showed follicular conjunctivitis with hyperemia, eyelash hypertrichosis and inferior superficial punctate keratitis. IOP was 21 mm Hg in both eyes with a CCT of 540 μm and 535 μm. Anterior segment examination showed bilateral nuclear cataract. Gonioscopy showed opened angles (Shaffer 3) and fundus examination revealed bilateral moderate optic disc cupping (C:D ratio 0.7).

We decided to perform a combined cataract and CyPass Micro-stent implantation surgery for both eyes. The first surgery of the right eye went smoothly, except for a perioperative hyphema that was washed out at the end of the surgery. On the first postoperative day, anterior segment examination revealed a hyphema of 4 mm. IOP was 17 mm Hg. AC was well formed. The shunt was patent on gonioscopy with a minimal iris touch and no suprachoroidal hemorrhage or effusion was noted. We decided to continuously observe the patient with an interval of 3 days to increase prednisone eye drops to six times daily and to add a cycloplegic drug. By the first week postoperatively, the hyphema had completely resolved. IOP was at 16 mm Hg. Cycloplegic eye drops were ceased and prednisone eye drops slowly tapered.

Learning Points

- Hyphema can be caused by a reflux bleeding from the cyclodissection during CyPass implantation and does not per se constitute a complication
- The risk rate for hyphema in the first month postoperatively is 1–6%.[7,9] It is treated with steroids and cycloplegic topical medication and usually resolves without complications
- Great attention should be paid to the IOP in case of hyphema. If IOP subsequently increases, topical aqueous suppressants (first β-blocker then α-2 agonists) should be used as a first-line therapy. Be cautious using topical carbonic anhydrase inhibitors in sickle cell disease patients. In theory, prostaglandin analogs and miotics should be avoided postoperatively since they may increase inflammation
- Hyphema should be removed via paracentesis or surgical wash out in case[17,18]
  - Staining of cornea becomes visible
  - Hyphema fills more than 50% of AC and remains for a period of 8–9 days (in order to prevent peripheral anterior synechiae)

- Of total hyphema with IOP of more than 25 mm Hg for a period of 6 days (in order to decrease risk of corneal staining)
- Of high IOP more than 50 mm Hg for a period of 2 days (risk of optic nerve atrophy).

Case 4: Hypertony following iStent implantation

A 72-year-old lady presented to the clinic for a routine follow-up due to known open-angle glaucoma that was more advanced in the right eye. She was on full medical treatment (brimonidine, timolol, dorzolamide, latanoprost), but unable to take oral carboanhydrase-inhibitors due to renal problems. She had a history of bilateral cataract surgery. At presentation, BCVA was 10/10 in both eyes. Several visual field examinations of the right eye done in the last 2 years showed a superior arcuate scotoma with questionable progression.

On examination, IOP in the right eye was measured to be 24 mm Hg with a CCT of 530 μm and slit-lamp examination revealed some mild follicular reaction. Gonioscopy showed an open angle with a visible trabecular meshwork. Fundus examination exposed a cupped optic disc more pronounced in the inferotemporal rim and a C:D ratio of 0.8. The superotemporal notch was consistent with the visual field findings. A decision was made to implant a Glaukos iStent. At the first day postoperatively, IOP was 18 mm Hg without glaucoma medication. The implant was partially occluded by the iris. At that point no intervention was performed and we decided to closely observe the patient. At the 2 weeks follow-up visit, IOP increased to reach 23 mm Hg and implant was still obstructed by a fibrin membrane. An argon laser gonioplasty was performed to reopen the implant lumen. On the day following laser, IOP dropped to 13 mm Hg and remained stable henceforth.

Learning Points

- Stent occlusion is a frequent complication in the early postoperative period and is usually caused either by vitreous, fibrous overgrowth, fibrin, blood or implant malposition causing an iris or endothelial touch
- Gonioscopy along with IOP measurements are crucial to determine therapy in iStent patients suspected of having a stent occlusion
- If IOP is within normal limits, most complications related to stent malposition resolve spontaneously over time. If this is not the case secondary procedures, including neodymium-doped:yttrium aluminium garnet (Nd:YAG) laser, argon laser gonioplasty, recombinant

tissue plasminogen activator, stent repositioning, stent replacement or a new stent implantation can be considered as well as a return to medical treatment.

MANAGEMENT OF COMPLICATIONS

Intraocular Pressure Increase

Intraocular pressure increases after MIGS occurs most frequently in the early postoperative period.[5] There are multiple causes, including residual viscoelastic in the AC, steroid response (most MIGS are combined with cataract surgeries and need aggressive postoperative steroid treatment), stent occlusion or malpositioning, insufficient IOP control by the stent, failure of the bleb or failure of the surgery.

Most IOP elevations post-MIGS are transient in nature and should be treated with topical antiglaucoma medication until IOP decreases again to reach the desired target IOP with or without treatment. In case ocular hypertension persists, evaluate a stepwise approach consisting of resuming full medical treatment and moving forward with an incisional glaucoma surgery.

If IOP increase occurs in the first few days postoperatively, paracentesis using the side port of the surgery should be attempted to remove the remaining viscoelastic in the AC.[19] Gonioscopy is recommended in all cases of postoperative ocular hypertension. Bleb aspect and position of stent should be evaluated to check for any malpositioning, obstruction or kinking of the implant (especially in XEN Gel Stent) and depending on examination outcome, adequate measures have to be taken.

If IOP does not level after removal of viscoelastic and examination is normal, steroids should be tapered and medical glaucoma treatment started. If IOP remains uncontrolled then surgery is considered a failure.

Hyphema

Hyphema is a frequent complication in all MIGS. In most cases, however, it is minimal and resolves spontaneously. It is usually caused by a blood reflux from Schlemm's canal or the supraciliary space. It is recommended to wash out perioperative hyphema at the end of the surgery. Mild hyphema with no increase in IOP can be observed until it resolves spontaneously. More severe hyphema or any hyphema with increased IOP should be managed similarly to posttraumatic hyphema. Gonioscopy examination is mandatory, since a blood clot can obstruct the implant.[12] The application of tissue plasminogen activator (0.1–0.2 mL

of 5–20 µg),[13] iridoplasty with argon laser or YAG laser may be beneficial to dissolve or dispatch the blood clot as it was previously described and performed for other glaucoma drainage devices.[20,21]

Hypotony/Shallow Anterior Chamber

Hypotony occurs more frequently and is more severe in stents inserted into the subconjunctival space (XEN Gel, InnFocus, EX-PRESS) then in stents inserted into the supraciliary space (CyPass). No hypotony was reported in stents acting on Schlemm's canal.

Being the most described complication after CyPass insertion, hypotony commonly occurs and resolves in the first postoperative month without any treatment.[8] Only one case of hypotony associated shallow AC was reported, which resolved spontaneously without secondary AC refill.[9]

Hypotony is also the most frequent complication for stents inserted into the subconjunctival space. But contrary to CyPass, associated shallow AC is more frequent and sometimes require viscoelastic refill into the AC.[14] In these cases, associated choroidal effusion may be present and needs to be ruled out, but usually resolves after IOP stabilizes.

Additionally, treatment of hypotony consists of pressure bandage, treatment of bleb leak (*see* below) or medical application of atropine 1% and/or topical steroids.

Stent Occlusion

Stent occlusion has different causative mechanisms and the treatment varies according to the pathogenesis. If there is no increase in IOP, the condition may be observed and a spontaneous resolution may be awaited. If stent occlusion is due to a blood clot or iris, iridoplasty with argon laser constitutes an effective and safe therapy. Peripheral anterior synechiae can similarly cause stent occlusions (especially in Hydrus stents). Localized synechiae with well-controlled IOP is observed. If IOP is not well controlled, a goniopuncture using YAG laser may be applied for a synechiolysis.[4,7] Occlusion due to a fibrin film covering the lumen can be removed with a small paracentesis.

A stent occlusion may be caused by its malpositioning, often with an endothelial touch. If the malpositioning is causing complications, a surgical repositioning should be considered. Otherwise the patient should be closely observed since minor malposition often does not affect the outcome.[8,10]

Bleb Leak

Usually, bleb leak is only observed in the EX-PRESS glaucoma filtration device. Its treatment consists of observation, patching, bandage contact lens, direct suturing, compression stitches, conjunctival advancement or conjunctival autografts.[22-27]

CONCLUSION

Minimally invasive glaucoma surgery and other implants constitute a relatively safe and promising alternative to incisional glaucoma surgery. They are mainly used in cases of early-to-moderate glaucoma as a standalone procedure or in combination with cataract surgery.

REFERENCES

1. Cairns JE. Trabeculectomy: preliminary report of a new method. Am J Ophthalmol. 1968;66(4):673-9.
2. Sugar HS. Experimental trabeculectomy in glaucoma. Am J Ophthalmol. 1961;51(4):623-7.
3. Olayanju JA, Hassan MB, Hodge DO, Khanna CL. Trabeculectomy-related complications in Olmsted County, Minnesota, 1985 through 2010. JAMA Ophthalmology. 2015;133(5):574-80.
4. Gandolfi SA, Ungaro N, Ghirardini S, Tardini MG, Mora P. Comparison of surgical outcomes between canaloplasty and Schlemm's canal scaffold at 24 months' follow-up. J Ophthalmol. 2016;2016:3410469.
5. Hoeh H, Ahmed IIK, Grisanti S, et al. Early postoperative safety and surgical outcomes after implantation of a suprachoroidal micro-stent for the treatment of open-angle glaucoma concomitant with cataract surgery. J Cataract Refract Surg. 2013;39(3):431-7.
6. Seider MI, Rofagha S, Lin SC, Stamper RL. Resident-performed EX-PRESS shunt implantation versus trabeculectomy. J Glaucoma. 2012;21(7):469-74.
7. García-Feijoo J, Rau M, Grisanti S, Grisanti S, Höh H, Erb C, et al. Supraciliary micro-stent implantation for open-angle glaucoma failing topical therapy: 1-year results of a multicenter study. Am J Ophthalmol. 2015;159(6):1075-81.
8. Hoeh H, Vold SD, Ahmed IK, et al. Initial clinical experience with the CyPass Micro-Stent: safety and surgical outcomes of a novel supraciliary microstent. J Glaucoma. 2016;25(1):106-12.
9. Ianchulev T, Ahmed K, Hoeh HR, Rau M, DeJuan E. Minimally invasive ab interno suprachoroidal device (CyPass) for IOP control in open-angle glaucoma. AAO. 2010.
10. Höh H, Grisanti S, Grisanti S, Rau M, Ianchulev S. Two-year clinical experience with the CyPass Micro-stent: safety' and surgical outcomes of a novel supraciliary micro-stent. Klin Monatsbl Augenheilkd. 2014;231:377-81.
11. Pfeiffer N, Garcia-Feijoo J, Martinez-de-la-Casa JM, et al. A randomized trial of a Schlemm's canal microstent with phacoemulsification for reducing intraocular pressure in open-angle glaucoma. Ophthalmology. 2015;122(7):1283-93.
12. Buchacra O, Duch S, Milla E, Stirbu O. One-year analysis of the iStent trabecular microbypass in secondary glaucoma. Clin Ophthalmol. 2011;5:321-6.
13. Spiegel D, García-Feijoó J, García-Sánchez J, Lamielle H. Coexistent primary open-angle glaucoma and cataract: preliminary analysis of treatment by cataract surgery and the iStent trabecular micro-bypass stent. Adv Ther. 2008;25(5):453-64.
14. Sheybani A, Lenzhofer M, Hohensinn M, Reitsamer H, Ahmed IIK. Phacoemulsification combined with a new ab interno gel stent to treat open-angle glaucoma: pilot study. J Cataract Refract Surg. 2015;41(9):1905-9.
15. Riss I, Batlle J, Pinchuk L, Kato YP, Weber BA, Parel JM. One-year results on the safety and efficacy of the InnFocus MicroShunt™ depending on placement and concentration of mitomycin C. J Fr Ophtalmol. 2015;38(9):855-60.
16. Wagschal LD, Trope GE, Jinapriya D, Jin Y-P, Buys YM. prospective randomized study comparing Ex-PRESS to trabeculectomy: 1-year results. J Glaucoma. 2015;24(8):624-9.
17. Crouch ER, Frenkel M. Aminocaproic acid in the treatment of traumatic hyphema. Am J Ophthalmol. 1976;81(3):355-60.
18. Read J. Traumatic hyphema: surgical vs medical management. Ann Ophthalmol. 1975;7(5):659-62, 664-6, 668-70.
19. Samuelson TW, Katz LJ, Wells JM, Duh Y-J, Giamporcaro JE, Group USiS. Randomized evaluation of the trabecular micro-bypass stent with phacoemulsification in patients with glaucoma and cataract. Ophthalmology. 2011;118(3):459-67.
20. Netland PA, Schuman S. Management of glaucoma drainage implant tube kink and obstruction with pars plana clip. Ophthalmic Surg Lasers Imaging. 2005;36(2):167-8.
21. Tessler Z, Jluchoded S, Rosenthal G. Nd: YAG laser for Ahmed tube shunt occlusion by the posterior capsule. Ophthalmic Surg Lasers Imaging. 1997;28(1):69-70.
22. Ritch R, Schuman JS, Belcher CD III. Management of the leaking filtration bleb. J Glaucoma. 1993;2(2):114-8.
23. Azuara-Blanco A, Katz LJ. Dysfunctional filtering blebs. Surv Ophthalmol. 1998;43(2):93-126.
24. Palmberg P, BJ Leader, JC Calkwood. "Late complications after glaucoma filtering surgery." Proceedings of the 45th Annual Symposium of the New Orleans Academy of Ophthalmology. The Hague: Kugler Publications. 1996; pp. 183-94.
25. Blok MDW, Kok JHC, van Mil C, Greve EL, Kijlstra A. Use of the megasoft bandage lens for treatment of complications after trabeculectomy. Am J Ophthalmol. 1990;110(3):264-8.
26. Galin MA, Hung T. Surgical repair of leaking blebs. Am J Ophthalmol. 1977;83(3):328-33.
27. Buxton JN, Lavery KT, Liebmann JM, Buxton DF, Ritch R. Reconstruction of filtering blebs with free conjunctival autografts. Ophthalmology. 1994;101(4):635-9.

Glaucoma in Children

Alejandra Hernandez-Oteyza, Oscar Albis-Donado

INTRODUCTION

Glaucoma is a rare, but devastating condition in children. Its effect will literally last a lifetime, and the amount of years with vision or blindness will solely result from our decisions for its treatment at the earliest possible time. Childhood glaucomas pose a steep diagnostic and therapeutic challenge to all ophthalmologists, and adequate training often requires additional years of experience with afflicted children. Medical treatment for childhood glaucomas has a limited role and surgery remains the primary therapeutic approach for most congenital and secondary glaucomas.

DEFINITION

Childhood glaucoma is diagnosed if at least two of the following criteria are met in a patient less than 16 years of age:
- Intraocular pressure (IOP) greater than 21 mm Hg
- Optic disc cupping
- Corneal changes such as Haab's striae
- Corneal edema or an increase in its diameter
- Progressive myopia
- A reproducible glaucomatous visual field defect

In some countries childhood ends at 18 years of age.

Case 1: Primary congenital glaucoma

A 10-day-old boy born at 36 weeks of gestational age through a cesarean section was noted to have bilateral corneal edema at birth. The mother received several doses of systemic corticosteroids due to a threatened preterm delivery, starting at week 21. Betaxolol 0.25% every 12 hours was started on his first day of life, on the day of examination, IOP under treatment using an iCare tonometer was 21 mm Hg and 20 mm Hg, the optic nerve could not be seen. On his right eye, a superior trabeculotomy combined with trabeculectomy without mitomycin C (MMC), and on his left eye a superior trabeculotomy with nonpenetrating deep sclerectomy, also without MMC, was performed. IOP on day 1 was 8 mm Hg oculus dexter (OD) and 10 mm Hg oculus sinister (OS), the corneal edema persisted, but photophobia was reduced. The steroid drops were slowly tapered over the next 3 weeks. One year later, iCare IOP is 10 mm Hg in OU with no medications, no bleb is seen in any of the eyes, a patent iridectomy is seen in OD. Cycloplegic refraction is +2.00D/−1.00D Cyl × 180° OU, with symmetric fix, follow and maintain visual acuity. Cups are 0.5 OD and 0.3 OS (Figs. 12A.1A and B).

Case 2: Juvenile open-angle glaucoma

A 14-year-old girl was sent for evaluation due to suspect discs. On her first visit Goldmann tonometry was 18 mm Hg and dynamic contour tonometry was 22 mm Hg OU. Cup-to-disc ratio (C:D) was 0.8, and her left optic disc had a hyaloid artery remnant with active circulation. The angle was wide open with embryotoxon, but without iris processes or pigment. For her second visit visual fields had some mild defects that had a good correlation to mild defects of the optic nerve fibers, but her Pascal IOP was 18 mm Hg OD and 16 mm Hg OS. We decided to make an at-home nocturnal IOP monitoring using iCare tonometry measured by her sister after training her at the office and found fluctuations of 10 mm Hg and 9 mm Hg (Table 12A.1). Due to the marked fluctuations of IOP G. Travoprost QD was started (Figs. 12A.2A to D).

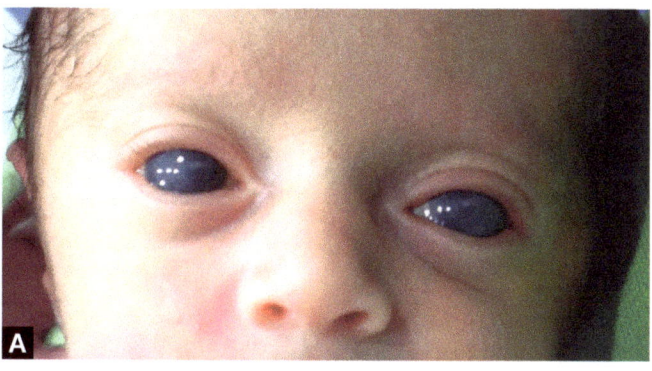
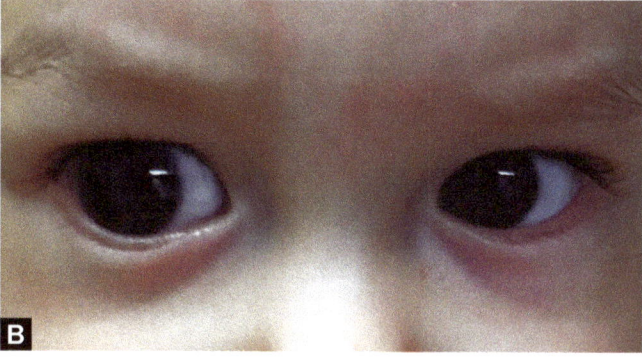

Figs. 12A.1A and B: (A) Buphthalmos, corneal edema and elevated intraocular pressure (IOP) despite betaxolol were observed. Horizontal corneal diameter was 14.5 mm OU. (B) One year later IOP is 10 mm Hg, the corneas are clear, and despite a seemingly larger right eye, cycloplegic refraction is symmetrical with low with-the-rule astigmatism.

Table 12A.1: Nocturnal intraocular pressure curve of case 2 done with iCare tonometry by training her older sister.		
Time	*OD iCare IOP (mm Hg)*	*OS iCare IOP (mm Hg)*
6:00 PM	14	14
7:20 PM	19	19
10:00 PM	15	15
12:12 AM	13	11
2:12 AM	9	10
4:20 AM	14	13
6:20 AM	15	13
8:20 AM	19	15

(IOP: Intraocular pressure).

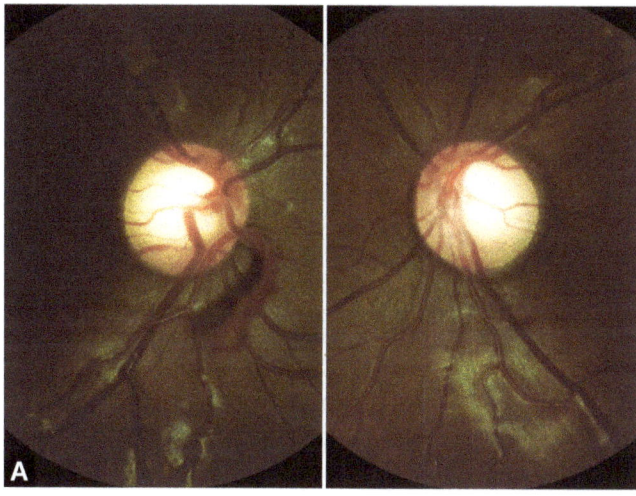

Fig. 12A.2A: Enlarged cups in a 14-year-old girl. Her right optic nerve has mild loss of superior fibers and a remnant of the hyaloid artery; her left optic disc has loss of some nasal fibers.

Case 3: Glaucoma associated with non-acquired ocular anomalies

A 4-month-old infant had been born prematurely and spent 40 days in the newborn intensive care unit, where they noted diminished red-reflex and possible cataracts. On first evaluation we found dilated pupils, no corneal edema and marked lens opacities. During the examination under anesthesia (EUA) her IOP was 10 mm Hg with Pascal tonometry OU, she had posterior embryotoxon with long iris processes that reached the embryotoxon and produced discoria, with a mostly dilated pupil, axial length was 19.23 OD and 19.5 OS. Bilateral cataract extraction was performed with anterior vitrectomy and both eyes received +30D lenses (a planned under correction of about 12D OU). She had an uneventful recovery and had residual nystagmus, despite the fact that she could fix her sight and make eye contact. Eight months later, the mother brought her to the emergency room with photophobia, tearing, corneal clouding and apparent pain. iCare IOP was 45 mm Hg OD and 50 mm Hg OS, the angle was found to be closed due to contraction

of the existing adherences from the iris to the embryotoxon. Bilateral FP7 Ahmed valve implants were placed in the superotemporal quadrants OU, and the larger-sized implants were chosen due to increased axial length of 20.3 mm OD and 20.5 mm OS (Figs. 12A.3A and B).

Case 4: Glaucoma associated with non-acquired systemic disease or syndrome

A 6-year-old boy with Sturge-Weber and secondary glaucoma in his right eye had a trabeculectomy with MMC 3 years before and an Ahmed valve implant in his superotemporal quadrant 2 years before. Using G. Timolol-brinzolamide bid and G. Bimatoprost QD his IOP was 22 mm Hg OD. On gonioscopy, his angle was

Central 24-2 Prueba de umbral

Monitor de fijación: APAGADO
Objetivo de fijación: Central
Pérdidas de fijación: 0/0
Errores falsos positivos: 4 %
Errores falsos negativos: 4 %
Duración de la prueba: 05:16

Foveal: 35 dB

Estímulo: III, Blanco
Fondo: 31.5 ASB
Estrategia: SITA-Standard

Diámetro de pupila:
Agudeza visual:
RX: -1.75 DS   DC X

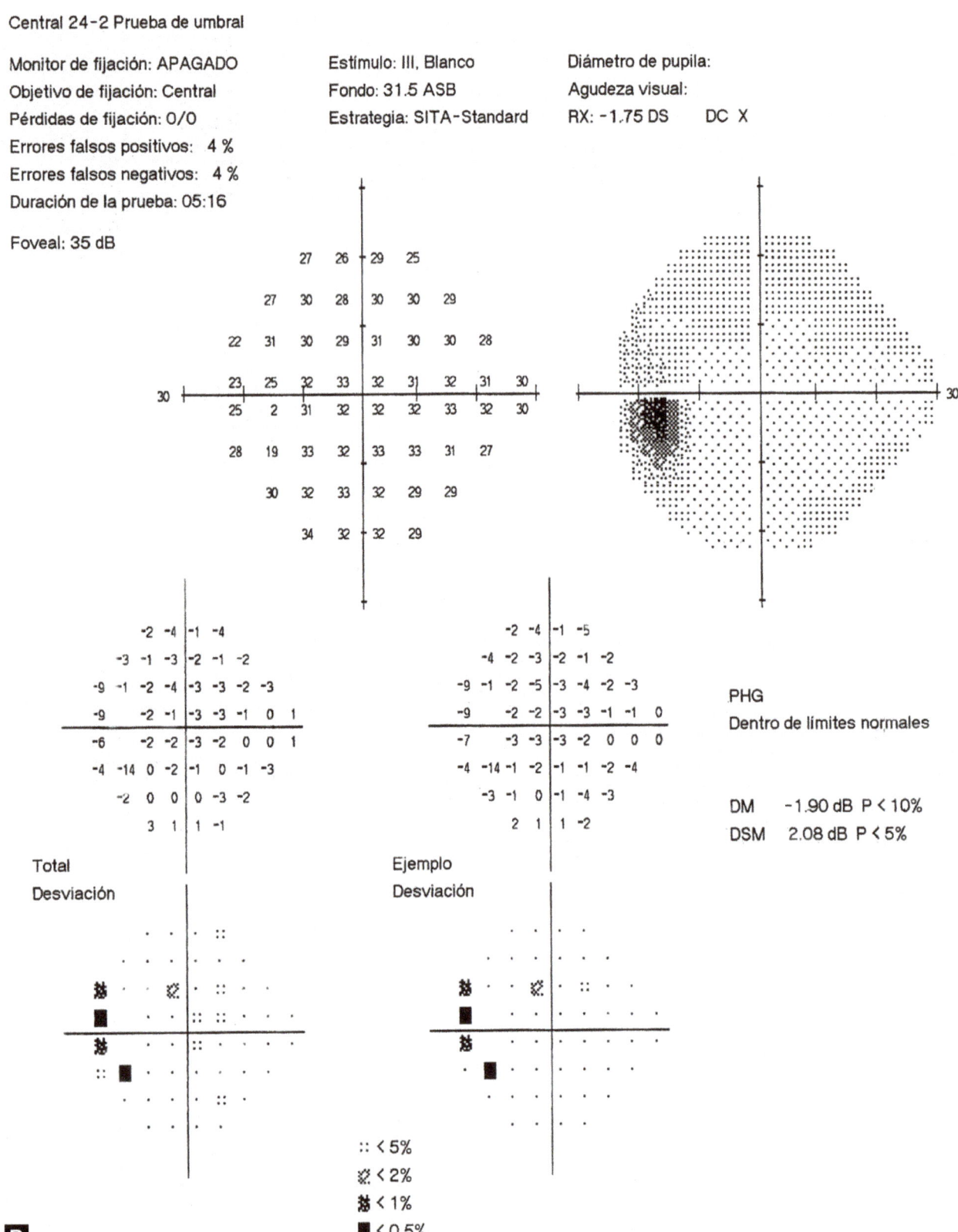

PHG
Dentro de límites normales

DM   -1.90 dB P < 10%
DSM   2.08 dB P < 5%

Total
Desviación

Ejemplo
Desviación

:: < 5%
▧ < 2%
▨ < 1%
■ < 0.5%

B

Fig. 12A.2B: Visual field of the left eye shows a temporal relative scotoma that correlates well with the lost fibers seen at the optic disc.

Central 24-2 Prueba de umbral

Monitor de fijación: Mirada/Punto ciego   Estímulo: III, Blanco   Diámetro de pupila: 4.8 mm
Objetivo de fijación: Central   Fondo: 31.5 ASB   Agudeza visual:
Pérdidas de fijación: 2/14   Estrategia: SITA-Standard   RX: -1.75 DS   DC X
Errores falsos positivos: 3 %
Errores falsos negativos: 2 %
Duración de la prueba: 05:17

Foveal: 36 dB

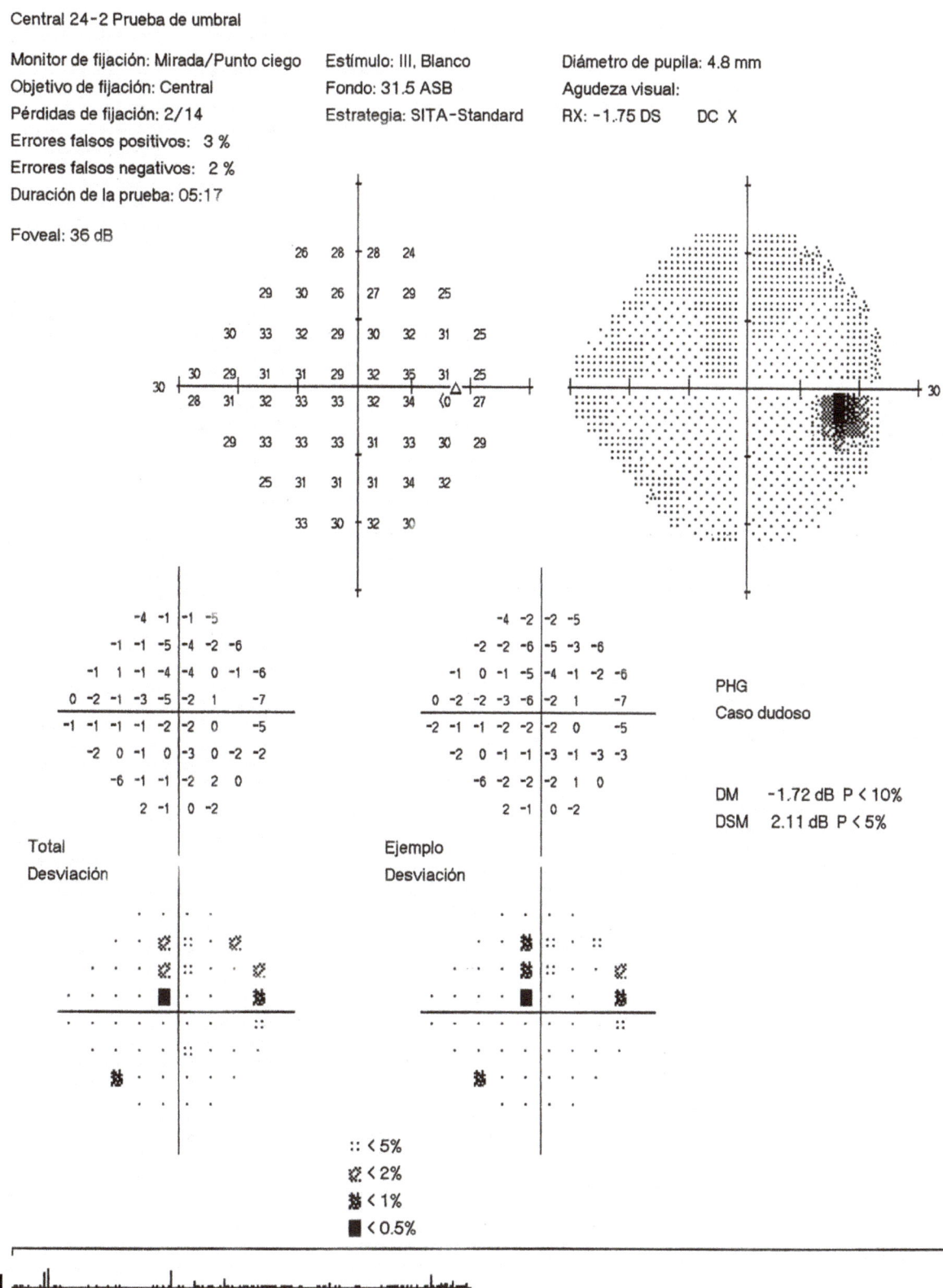

PHG
Caso dudoso

DM   -1.72 dB P < 10%
DSM   2.11 dB P < 5%

Total Desviación

Ejemplo Desviación

:: < 5%
⊠ < 2%
⊛ < 1%
■ < 0.5%

Fig. 12A.2C: The visual field of the right eye has relative superior scotomas that do not correlate well with either the optic disc or the optical coherence tomography (OCT) image.

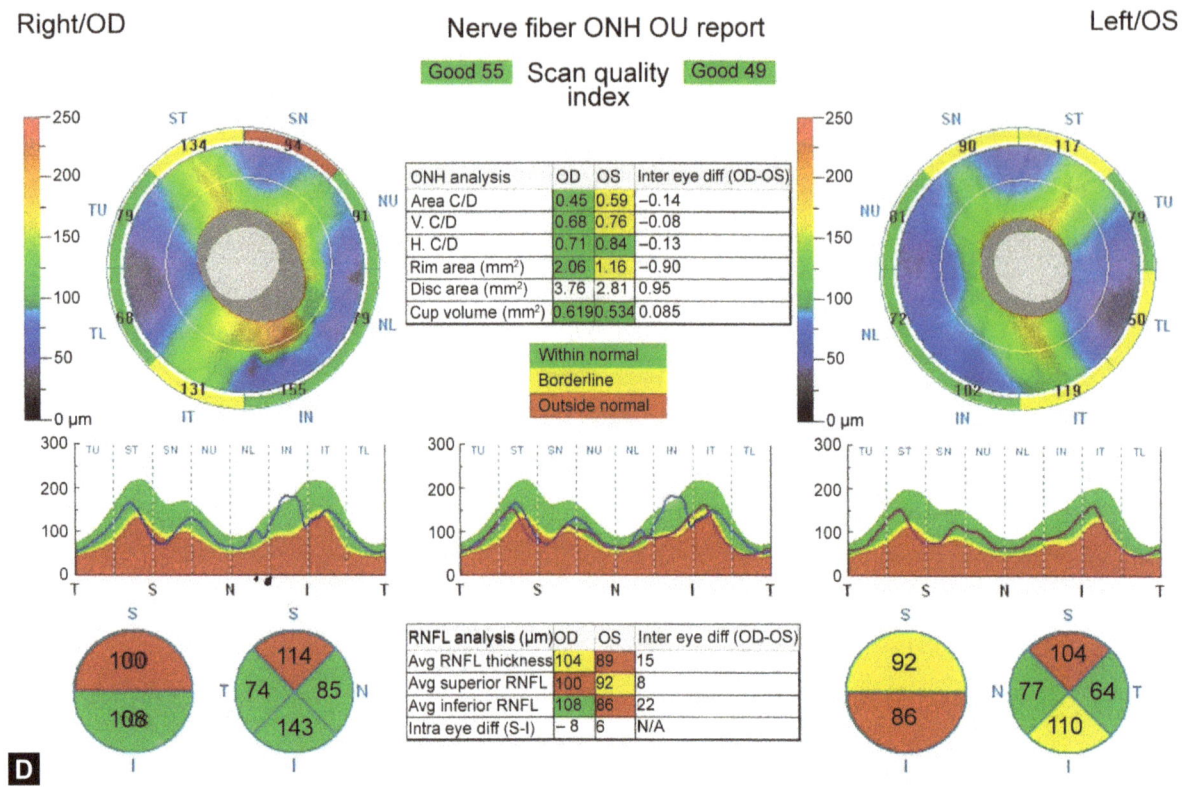

Fig. 12A.2D: OCT images show large discs with very mild defects of the optic nerve fiber layer. (OCT: Optical coherence tomography).

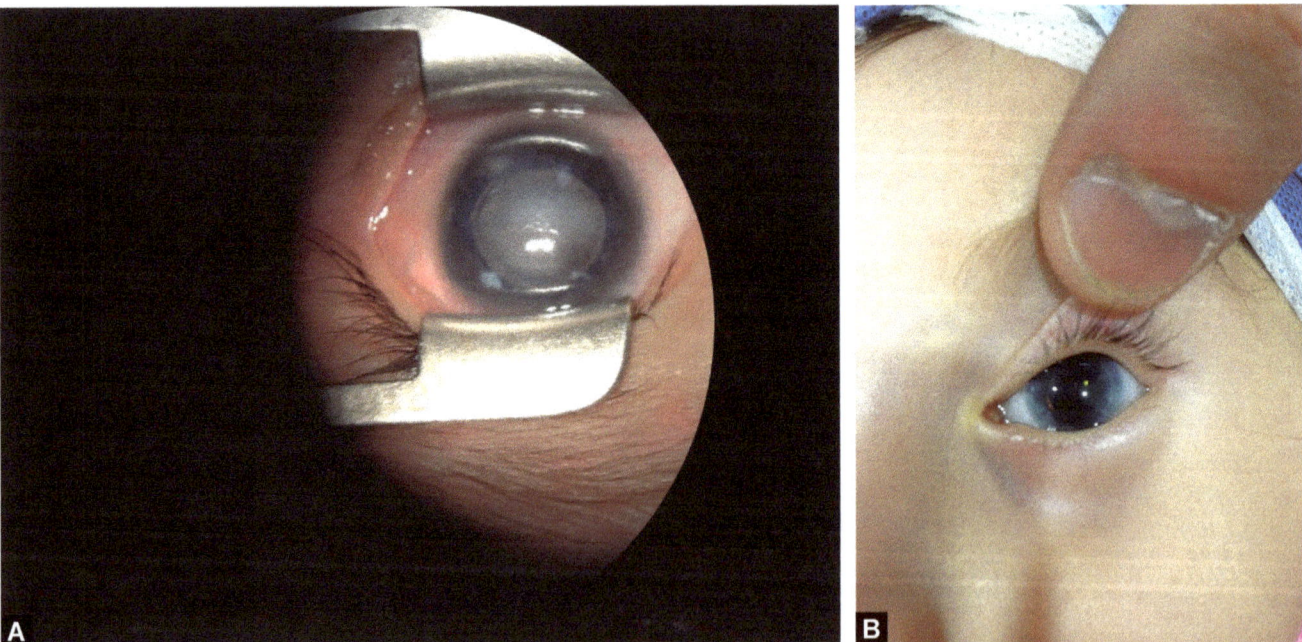

Figs. 12A.3A and B: (A) Apparent pupil dilation due to extensive adherences between the iris and the embryotoxon in this Axenfeld-Rieger syndrome left eye with an associated congenital cataract that was removed at the time of the picture. (B) The intraocular lens is well centered, the pupil remains dilated and the tube from the Ahmed valve implant has solved the corneal edema 1 month after implantation behind the iris and in front of the intraocular lens, intraocular pressure is 14 with no medications, cup-to-disc ratio is 0.3.

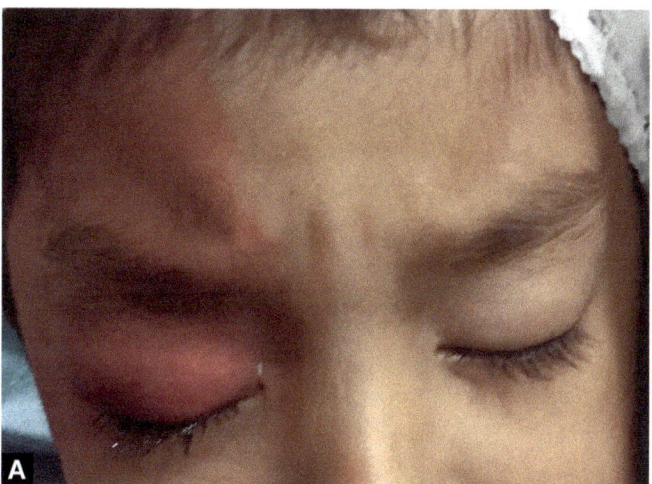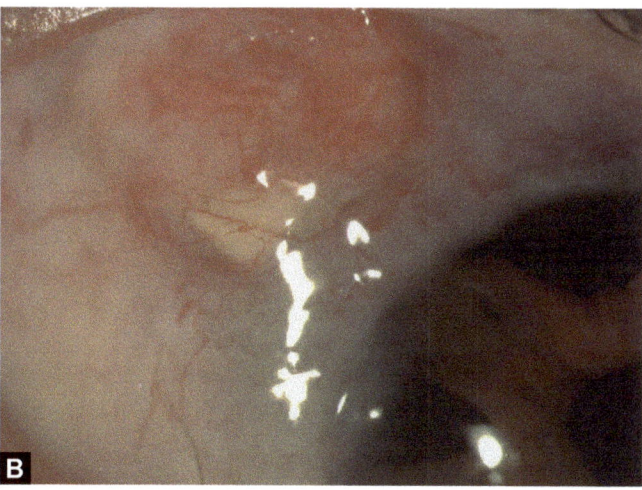

Figs. 12A.4A and B: (A) Sturge-Weber syndrome with associated secondary glaucoma. Mild photophobia, intraocular pressure (IOP) was 22 mm Hg with three medications; a filamentary trabeculotomy with an illuminated fiber-optic was planned. (B) The tube from the original Ahmed valve is in good position, no bleb is present temporal to the tube, despite it being the place of conjunctival dissection for filamentary trabeculotomy a year before. The cornea has no edema intraocular pressure is 11 mm Hg with no medications.

found to have a mild anterior iris insertion, resembling a congenital glaucoma angle, with blood reflux at the canal. On surgery Schlemm's canal was found and a filamentary trabeculotomy was performed starting at the superotemporal quadrant, next to the tube and ending in the superonasal quadrant next to the previous trabeculectomy, where a new linear incision was made to fish out the fiber-optic. One year later, IOP is 11 mm Hg without the use of medications (Figs. 12A.4A and B).

INVESTIGATIONS

All patients in whom childhood glaucoma is suspected require a thorough eye examination complemented by a physical examination to properly approach the disease and to classify it accordingly.

Mandatory tests include:

General Appearance/General Examination

A search for any systemic defects or malformations can be performed, since it will allows syndromes to be ruled out. Special attention to any systemic drug effects is mandatory, since some life-threatening signs can be observed in some children.

Visual Acuity and Refraction

Even though visual acuity may be challenging to measure in preverbal infants, an effort must be made to record it.

Teller's method may be used in infants under 2 years of age, Allen's pictures can be useful in young illiterate infants and in older children Snellen acuity charts must be used. Cycloplegic refraction must be performed in every EUA and when the child cooperates, in office visits too, to monitor refractive changes. Increasing myopia due to increasing axial length is a sign of glaucomatous progression in children.

Tonometry

In cooperative patients any method can be used (applanation tonometry, rebound tonometry, dynamic contour tonometry). Rebound tonometry is useful in awake babies and children. Schiötz indentation tonometry or Perkins applanation tonometry may be performed under general anesthesia, but IOP must be measured right after sedation has been achieved, to minimize the effect that the anesthetic agents have on IOP. It is important to note that normal IOP values in children are lower than those of adults with applanation tonometry.

Corneal Diameter Measurement

It may be measured on the slit lamp or using a caliper in patients undergoing EUA.

Gonioscopy

It is usually performed under general anesthesia using either a direct gonioscope, such as a Koeppe lens, or an indirect gonioscope, such as Zeiss, Goldmann or Posner goniolens. Gonioscopy must be attempted at the slit lamp in cooperative children.

Optic Nerve Assessment

Normal children have C:D of less than 0.3, so a C:D greater than 0.3 or C:D asymmetry must be considered suspicious. Whenever possible, it is desirable to have a photographic record of the optic disc appearance.

In addition some of the following tests, if available and affordable, may be performed:

Ultrasound

It is very important in children under 3 years of age to measure the eye's anterior-posterior (AP) diameter. Both eyes must be measured and compared to each other and to a nomogram according to the child's age. Follow-up ultrasounds to compare the AP diameter to the baseline measurements may be useful.

Anterior Segment Images

Intraocular surgeries may alter the anterior segment's anatomy and appearance; baseline photographs of the anterior segment are helpful for a retrospective accurate diagnosis and classification.

Automated Perimetry

It is useful for follow-up in cooperative children older than 7–8 years of age.

Ocular Coherence Tomography with Retinal Nerve Fiber Layer and Ganglion Cell Complex Analysis

Even when normative database are not available for children, it can provide an objective value to compare overtime.

FOLLOW-UP PROTOCOL

Follow-up examinations and studies must be individualized depending on the type of childhood glaucoma. Other factors to take into account for deciding the frequency and type of follow-up tests include: IOP control, number of surgeries and drugs required to obtain such IOP control, refraction, visual acuity, optic nerve photography and visual fields.

Most childhood glaucoma cases require surgical treatment as soon as possible. Follow-up visits after surgical management must be frequent initially and several EUA may be required; therefore, it is important to assess liver function prior to each EUA and to keep an open line of communication with the child's pediatrician.

Visual rehabilitation is an essential part of the management of childhood glaucoma; properly calculated spectacles are necessary to obtain the best possible visual performance, and therefore, the refraction must be constantly updated. Childhood glaucoma is a disease that requires a multidisciplinary approach; both the child and the parents require a support network and genetic counseling.

SUMMARY

Childhood glaucoma is the consequence of high IOP and causes optic disc cupping, corneal changes, progressive myopia and/or a glaucomatous visual field defect in children under 16 (or 18) years of age.

Its classification comprises seven groups: (1) primary congenital glaucoma (PCG), (2) juvenile open-angle glaucoma (JOAG), (3) glaucoma associated with nonacquired ocular anomalies, (4) glaucoma associated with nonacquired systemic disease or syndrome, (5) glaucoma associated with acquired condition, (6) glaucoma following cataract surgery, and (7) glaucoma suspect.

To properly identify, classify and manage children with childhood glaucoma several tests are needed, such as: general examination, visual acuity and cycloplegic refraction, tonometry, anterior segment evaluation (with special attention to the cornea and gonioscopy) and fundoscopy; auxiliary studies may include ultrasonography, anterior and posterior segment imaging, visual field testing and ocular coherence tomography.

Although the mainstay of management for most childhood glaucomas is surgery, glaucoma medication may be useful before surgery or as an adjuvant after it. Angle surgery (goniotomy or trabeculotomy) is the treatment of choice for congenital primary glaucoma. Multiple surgeries are often required to achieve IOP control.

There is a recognized genetic pathogenesis involved in many cases of childhood glaucoma, so an assessment by a geneticist is essential to understand the disease, dismiss systemic associations and provide genetic counsel to both the patient and the parents.

Childhood glaucoma management requires a multidisciplinary effort in which glaucoma specialists, ophthalmo-pediatric specialists, pediatricians, geneticists, optometrists, psychologists and the child's parents must work together to achieve the best possible visual rehabilitation and the best possible quality of life for the patient.

In 2013, the 9th Consensus Report of the World Glaucoma Association on Childhood Glaucoma was published. The reports' summary is described briefly in Box 12A.1.

Box 12A.1: Childhood glaucoma. The 9th Consensus Report of the World Glaucoma Association.

Objectives: To provide a foundation for diagnosing and treating childhood glaucoma and how it can be best done in clinical practice

Participants: Global experts on pediatric ophthalmology and on glaucoma

Summary:

Section 1: Definition, classification and differential diagnosis

- Childhood glaucoma is the damage to the eye caused by intraocular pressure (IOP)
- IOP measurement in infants can be affected by many factors, such as general anesthesia
- Childhood glaucoma is classified as primary vs. secondary. Secondary childhood glaucoma is classified as acquired or nonacquired (present at birth), which is divided depending if the signs are mostly ocular or systemic
- It is important to exclude other diseases and to be sure of the diagnosis before labeling or operating on a child

Section 2: Diagnosis and progression

- Early diagnosis and treatment can belittle visual compromise
- It is important to exclude other diseases and to be sure of the diagnosis before labeling or operating on a child
- Childhood glaucoma is characterized by high IOP and disc cupping; additional features such as buphthalmos can be found
- IOP measurement in infants can be affected by many factors, making it unreliable for the diagnosis and management
- IOP measurement can be altered by anesthetic agents
- A large corneal diameter is characteristic of childhood glaucoma
- Gonioscopy is essential for the diagnosis and surgical plan
- Optic disc cupping is important for the diagnosis and identification of progression in childhood glaucoma
- Changes in refraction (miopization) and axial length can help in the diagnosis and in assessing treatment response
- Visual field testing in children is useful but difficult to obtain

Section 3: Genetics

- In cases where there is a known genotype-phenotype correlation, genetic counseling is important
- Primary congenital glaucoma (PCG) has a known correlation with *CYP1B1* gene mutations
- There have been identified mutations in the *MYOC* gene in families with autosomal-dominant juvenile open-angle glaucoma (JOAG)
- Mutations with in *PITX2* and *FOXC1* are associated with Axenfeld-Rieger anomaly and syndrome
- *PAX6* mutations cause Aniridia, which has an autosomal-dominant inheritance with high penetration and variable expressivity
- Ectopia lentis, megalocornea (without high IOP), microspherophakia and associated secondary glaucoma have been related to *LTBP2* mutations
- An accurate clinical diagnosis is crucial to optimize genetic counseling
- General pediatric evaluation is important for the management and diagnosis, as it helps to identify systemic-associated conditions
- Genetics review is important

Section 4: Medications

- Medications alone are not efficient as a primary treatment for childhood glaucoma, especially in PCG
- Childhood glaucoma may have varied responses to glaucoma medications
- Pharmacokinetics for glaucoma medications differ in children as compared to adults
- Systemic adverse reactions that are potentially serious or fatal may be seen in children exposed to glaucoma medications
- Compliance and adherence are complex issues in children
- Target pressure must be assessed and adjusted according to all available information indicating glaucoma control
- Surgical treatment must be considered when medical treatment fails to control glaucoma

Section 5: Glaucoma surgery in children

- Surgical management is a crucial component of childhood glaucoma's management
- Surgical procedures must be performed by expert surgeons
- Glaucoma surgery in children has a higher failure and complications rate than in adult
- Angle surgery is the gold standard for PCG
- Trabeculotomy can have good outcomes in appropriate cases

Contd…

Contd...

- In refractory cases, glaucoma drainage devices may offer the most effective long-term IOP control
- Cyclophotocoagulation has limited success in the long-term and may require reinterventions and adjuvant medical treatment
- Other glaucoma procedures have not proven to be efficacious or safe in children
- Visual development must be encouraged with ametropic correction and amblyopia therapy
- Risks and benefits of each surgical intervention must be carefully assessed

Section 6: Primary congenital glaucoma and juvenile open-angle glaucoma

- The most common nonsyndromic glaucoma in infancy is PCG
- PCG inheritance pattern is usually autosomal recessive; family history is positive in 10–40% of cases and it is more common in consanguineous populations
- Pathogenesis of PCG is unknown; apparently it is due to the arrested maturation of tissues derived from cranial neural crest cells that form the angle
- PCG management requires angle surgery with high success rates reported in favorable cases and in repeated procedures
- If angle surgery fails, the subsequent procedure must be trabeculectomy or a glaucoma drainage device
- JOAG is rare and presents after the age of 4 years; angle appearance is normal and there are no signs of ocular or systemic diseases
- Glaucoma medications are the first-line of treatment, but surgical management is often required
- There is no consensus toward the first-line of surgery for JOAG

Section 7: Glaucoma associated with nonacquired ocular anomalies

- Infants with nonacquired ocular anomalies require pediatric evaluation to assess systemic conditions
- There is a genetic pathogenesis to most nonacquired ocular anomalies
- Nonacquired ocular anomalies may present with glaucoma at birth or glaucoma may develop afterwards, so regular evaluations are required
- High IOP associated to nonacquired ocular anomalies must be treated to prevent glaucoma from developing
- Children with nonacquired ocular anomalies that develop glaucoma have buphthalmos and may develop Haab's striae
- Even though medical treatment is given at first, surgical management is usually required in the treatment of congenital/infantile presentations and it must be performed promptly
- Infants with nonacquired ocular anomalies have genetic mutations that are associated to a variety of phenotypes
- Axenfeld-Rieger anomaly is a spectrum of disease that used to be referred to as Axenfeld anomaly and Rieger anomaly. Axenfeld-Rieger syndrome is the addition of Axenfeld-Rieger anomaly plus systemic abnormalities
- Peter's anomaly is an ocular disorder that when associated to systemic abnormalities of neural crest origin is then called Peters-Plus syndrome
- Aniridia can cause open-angle or closed-angle glaucoma
- Persistent fetal vasculature has a heterogeneity of clinical presentations, making its management challenging.

Section 8: Glaucoma associated with nonacquired systemic disease or syndrome

- Glaucoma can occur as a sign of syndromes with systemic anomalies or diseases present at birth
- Glaucoma is commonly found in Sturge-Weber syndrome
- Glaucoma is not commonly associated with neurofibromatosis
- Ectopia lentis can present either as an isolated ocular anomaly or as part of a syndrome
- Glaucoma signs may not be as evident at birth in infants with known or suspected congenital rubella, so close vigilance is recommended.

Section 9: Glaucoma associated with acquired conditions

- The management of uveitic glaucoma in children is difficult requiring intraocular inflammation control
- The pathogenesis of traumatic glaucoma is multifactorial
- Children receiving topical or systemic corticosteroids may develop severe steroid-induced high IOP
- Secondary glaucoma due to intraocular tumors in children is rare
- Glaucoma induced by retinopathy of prematurity is usually secondary to angle closure, but other factors may be involved.

Section 10: Glaucoma following cataract surgery

- Glaucoma secondary to cataract surgery may occur after cataract surgery of a congenital idiopathic or associated to ocular or systemic cataract, or an acquired cataract
- Both aphakic and pseudophakic eyes may have glaucoma
- Risk factors for glaucoma are young age at the time of the surgery and microcornea
- Usually this type of glaucoma is associated to open angles, but closed angle may be found
- Glaucoma may develop at any point following cataract surgery in children, so regular examinations are necessary
- Medical management is the first-line of treatment, but if it fails, surgical therapy may be required with no consensus as to which one to perform

POINTS TO REMEMBER

1. Childhood glaucoma is a challenging spectrum of diseases that require a multidisciplinary approach
2. Intraocular pressure is difficult to measure in children and it is often nonreliable, so other ocular signs, such as axial length and corneal edema, must be evaluated both in the diagnosis phase and to assess progression
3. Gonioscopy is essential for a proper classification and to plan a surgical approach
4. Surgical management is usually required and multiple procedures are often needed to obtain an appropriate IOP control
5. Medical treatment is sometimes necessary but must be used with caution as adverse effects may present more severely in children
6. Visual rehabilitation is essential.

SUGGESTED READING

1. Grajewski A, Papadopoulos M, Grigg J, Feedman S, Robert N, Weinreb. Childhood Glaucoma. The 9th Consensus Report of the World Glaucoma Association, 1st edition. Amsterdam, Netherlands: Kugler Publications; 2013.
2. Shaarawy TM, Sherwood MB, Hitchings RA, Crowston JG. Glaucoma. Medical diagnosis and treatment, 1st edition. China: Saunders Elsevier; 2009.

Postrefractive Surgery Glaucoma

Mona Khurana, Aditya Neog

▌ INTRODUCTION

Refractive surgery has impressive outcomes in terms of vision with the constantly improving cutting-edge technology. However, postrefractive surgery glaucoma can defeat the purpose of the surgery and lead to irreversible blindness. This chapter focusses on different causes of glaucoma after refractive surgery, their prevention, early detection and management.

▌ INVESTIGATIONS

Prerefractive Surgery Screening

History

A detailed history regarding risk factors for glaucoma.

Clinical Evaluation

Clinical evaluation to rule out pre-existing glaucoma or glaucoma suspect:

- *Intraocular pressure:* Establish a good baseline with multiple prerefractive surgery intraocular pressure (IOP) measurements. IOP measurement with instruments apart from Goldmann applanation tonometer (GAT) like dynamic contour tonometer (DCT), which are less dependent on central corneal thickness (CCT) is preferred.
- *Gonioscopy:* It should be performed in all cases under standard conditions to rule out any pre-existing angle-closure disease [especially in case of phakic intraocular lens (PIOL) and hyperopic refractive surgery] and risk factors for secondary glaucomas, like pigment dispersion, angle recession.

- *Optic nerve head:* A thorough evaluation of the optic nerve head with baseline stereoscopic optic disc photograph is recommended in all cases.
- *Anterior segment imaging:* Appropriate measurements to determine the size of the phakic IOL with appropriate anterior segment imaging.

Patient Counseling

The patient should be clearly explained the risks and the need for periodic follow-up.

Postrefractive Surgery

Postoperative Medication

Judicious use of topical steroids is the key.
Monitoring: Close follow-up is must in case of prolonged topical corticosteroid use.
Steroid response: Rule-out steroid response and interface fluid syndrome in case of postoperative inflammation.

Clinical Examination

- *Intraocular pressure:* New baselines for IOP preferably with DCT should be obtained following refractive surgery.
- *Optic nerve head examination:* Stereoscopic optic nerve head photograph should be taken and a copy should be given to the patient.
- *Imaging:* In case of suspicious discs, baseline imaging by optical coherence tomography (OCT) or confocal scanning laser tomography, like Heidelberg retina tomography (HRT), may be useful for monitoring progression.

- *Visual fields:* A new baseline following refractive surgery in case of suspicious discs.
- *Following Phakic Intraocular lens implantation:*
  - Screening for increased IOP in both early-operative and late-postoperative period is quintessential
  - Regular gonioscopy to detect goniosynechiae must be done
  - Monitor pigment dispersion.

Follow-up

Periodic follow-up with a comprehensive eye examination is essential as these eyes have a higher risk of developing glaucoma.

Case 1: Steroid-induced glaucoma post-refractive surgery

A 25-year-old male reported with complaints of mild irritation and blurring of vision in the left eye two weeks following laser-assisted in-situ keratomileusis (LASIK). He was noted to have diffuse granular corneal haze in the interface. The best corrected visual acuity was 6/6 in the right eye and 6/12 in the left eye. Preoperative refraction was –4.0D in the right eye and –4.5D in the left eye. He was diagnosed as having diffuse lamellar keratitis (DLK) and started on topical fluorometholone 2 hourly. The granular haze increased progressively and the patient was switched to topical prednisolone acetate 2 hourly. There was no prior history of glaucoma. Preoperative IOP was noted to be 14 mm Hg with a vertical cup-to-disc ratio (C:D) of 0.3 in both the eyes. On subsequent examination IOP with GAT was 6 mm Hg and 8 mm Hg and with DCT was 12 mm Hg and 30 mm Hg. On slit-lamp examination, fluid was seen in the corneal flap stroma interface, which was confirmed with anterior segment optical coherence tomography (ASOCT). Topical steroids were tapered fast and aqueous suppressant was started. Following this the corneal edema cleared, IOP decreased and vision improved to 6/6. Visual field examination was normal. This case illustrates the development of pressure-induced interlamellar stromal keratitis (PISK) following LASIK, which can be mistaken as a nonresolving DLK.

Case 2: Primary open-angle glaucoma in the postrefractive surgery period

A 35-year-old male with history of LASIK for myopia, 4 years back, reported for a routine eye examination. On examination the best-corrected visual acuity was 6/6 in both the eyes, IOP with GAT was 6 mm Hg and 9 mm Hg,

gonioscopy revealed open angles. Both eyes had a vertical C:D of 0.7 with inferior rim thinning with corresponding defects on visual field examination. The CCT was 449 microns and 460 microns in the right eye and left eyes, respectively. IOP with DCT was 28 mm Hg in the right eye and 32 mm Hg in the left eye. ASOCT revealed no interface fluid. The patient was started on IOP-lowering medications in both the eyes with which the IOP was controlled for 4 months. He subsequently underwent selective laser trabeculoplasty (SLT) in both eyes, following which IOP was controlled. However, the right eye IOP started to increase after 2 months despite maximum IOP-lowering medications and the patient underwent trabeculectomy with mitomycin C. The GAT IOP was 2 mm Hg with signs of early hypotony maculopathy postoperatively. He subsequently underwent compression sutures with autologous blood injection in the bleb in the right eye for the management of post-trabeculectomy hypotony secondary to an overfiltering bleb, following which the hypotony maculopathy resolved. This case highlights the fact that myopes are predisposed to developing POAG which can go undetected in the post refractive surgery period. It also illustrates how these eyes are prone to develop hypotony and related complications following filtering surgery.

Case 3: Late detection of secondary glaucoma following laser-assisted in-situ keratomileusis

A 27-year-old male with history of LASIK, 4 years back, reported mild blurring of vision in the right eye. On examination visual acuity was 6/9 and 6/6, IOP was 12 mm Hg and 8 mm Hg in the right and left eye. Slit-lamp examination revealed polycoria in the right eye. High peripheral anterior synechiae were noted on gonioscopy in three quadrants in the right eye with open angles in the left eye. The vertical C:D was 0.2 in both the eyes. The visual fields were normal. Right eye was diagnosed to have secondary angle closure due to iridocorneal endothelial syndrome. DCT revealed an IOP of OD 27 mmm Hg and OS 13 mm Hg. The patient was prescribed timolol 0.5% eye drops twice a day in the right eye. Subsequently, prostaglandin analogs, brimonidine and brinzolamide were added. However, the IOP remained uncontrolled despite maximum medication. The patient underwent Ahmed glaucoma valve implantation in the right eye following which IOP was controlled (8 mm Hg GAT/12 mm Hg DCT in OD). This case shows that secondary glaucoma developing in eyes, which have undergone refractive surgery, may go undetected due to low measurement of IOP.

Case 4: Bilateral acute angle-closure glaucoma following hyperopic laser-assisted in-situ keratomileusis

A 31-year-old female presented with complaints of severe pain, headache, redness, photophobia and blurring of vision in both eyes about 6 hours following LASIK surgery done elsewhere. The best corrected visual acuity was 6/18 in the right eye and 6/24 in the left eye. Slit-lamp biomicroscopic examination revealed bilateral severe conjunctival congestion, corneal epithelial edema and shallow anterior chamber in both the eyes. The IOP was 38 mm Hg and 44 mm Hg in the right and left eye. Gonioscopy showed 360° of angle closure in both eyes. Optic nerve head status could not be assessed due to corneal edema. The preoperative refraction was +3.5D in the right eye and +4D in the left eye with normal IOP. The diagnosis of bilateral acute angle closure attack was made due to pre-existing occludable angles, precipitated by pupillary dilation during or after the procedure probably due to the stress of surgery. The patient was given oral acetazolamide 500 mg stat. Topical timolol 0.5%, brimonidine 0.15% and prednisolone acetate 1% drops were instilled in both the eyes following IOP reduction. Pilocarpine 2% drops were applied to both eyes and neodymium-doped:yttrium aluminum garnet (Nd:YAG) laser iridotomy was performed successfully. At follow-up, IOP was controlled without medication in both the eyes and gonioscopy revealed open angles with healthy optic nerve head in both eyes. This case highlights the importance of preoperative gonioscopy in patients undergoing hyperopic LASIK to rule out pre-existing angle-closure disease.

Case 5: Unilateral acute angle-closure glaucoma following phakic intraocular lens implantation

A 28-year-old myopic female with history of phakic IOL implantation, 6 months back, reported to the emergency with complaints of severe pain, headache nausea, redness, photophobia in the right eye since 1 day. Best corrected visual acuity in the right eye was 6/60 and left eye was 6/6. Slit-lamp examination showed conjunctival injection, microcytic corneal edema and a shallow anterior chamber. The posterior chamber phakic IOL was seen hazily and noted to be in position. The patient gave history of laser iridotomy done 1 week prior to the phakic IOL implantation. On slit-lamp examination the laser iridotomy was noted to be blocked the right eye and patent in the left eye.

After lowering the IOP with oral acetazolamide, syrup glycerol and topical aqueous suppressants, pilocarpine 2% eye drops were instilled and the iridotomy was enlarged with Nd:YAG laser. Following this the IOP decreased to 14 mm Hg in the right eye. Gonioscopy revealed open angles. This case highlights the importance of regular follow-up in patients following phakic IOL implantation (especially the older designs) and the possibility of acute angle closure with pupillary block due to blockage of the iridotomy. The newer design, however, does not require laser iridotomy due the presence of holes allowing aqueous flow in the lens precluding the need for iridotomy.

MANAGEMENT OF GLAUCOMA

The treatment of glaucoma or elevated IOP after refractive surgery is similar to that for primary open-angle glaucoma (POAG).

Medical Management

- Acute reduction of IOP can be achieved with oral carbonic anhydrase inhibitors, hyperosmotics, like oral glycerol or intravenous mannitol
- Aqueous humor suppressants (β-blockers, α-agonists and topical carbonic anhydrase inhibitors) and prostaglandin analogs can be used for long-term IOP control.

Laser

Selective laser trabeculoplasty can be done in case of:
- Uncontrolled IOP
- Progression of glaucoma despite maximum medication
- Poor adherence
- Patients intolerant to topical IOP-lowering medications.

Surgery

In case of glaucoma progression despite maximum tolerated medical therapy
- Trabeculectomy with antimetabolites/ologen implant
- Glaucoma drainage devices
- Judicious use of antimetabolites during trabeculectomy is advisable. Application of releasable sutures as these myopic eyes are more prone to develop hypotony and related complications, like hypotony maculopathy.

Follow-up

- Periodic and regular follow-up is important
- IOP measurement with DCT is preferable
- Important to look for progression of glaucoma or conversion to glaucoma [in case of ocular hypertension (OHT)] with imaging modalities, like stereoscopic disc photography, HRT, OCT and serial visual field examination.

REVIEW OF LITERATURE

Glaucoma is two-to-three times more prevalent among myopes, the patients most frequently undergoing refractive surgery.[1,2] The reported incidence of increased IOP-following refractive surgery ranges from 11% to 25%.[3]

Intraocular Pressure Measurement

Goldmann applanation tonometer, the gold standard for IOP measurement is based on the modified Imbert Fick law assuming a CCT of 520 microns.[4] Refractive surgery while reshaping the cornea to alter its refractive status additionally changes its biomechanical properties. There is a change in corneal hysteresis, flattening of the corneal curvature and a decrease in the CCT. This cause a false underestimation of the measured IOP by instruments based on the principle of applanation and indentation delaying the detection of OHT or glaucoma.

Studies have reported a decrease in the measured IOP measurements following LASIK (myopic and hyperopic)[5-12] and photorefractive keratoplasty (PRK).[13-16] The decrease in measured IOP following LASIK is due to thinning of the central cornea.[15] It is theorized that following PRK the decrease in IOP may be due to a decreased resistance in corneal indentation-following removal of Bowman's layer.[16]

Different studies have reported a variable postrefractive surgery, change in IOP and there are no corrective nomograms for estimating the true IOP from GAT or other tonometer readings. Studies have measured IOP in the unaltered corneal periphery, however, no conclusive guidelines are present for estimating the true IOP. The DCT is a nonapplanation contact tonometer that reflects the surface contour of a resting human cornea when intraocular and extraocular pressures are equal, thus removing the influences of the corneal properties.[17] Many studies evaluating IOP measurements with DCT after LASIK, PRK, and LASEK have found that of all the tonometric methods, DCT is the least affected by refractive surgery.[17-20] Dynamic contour tonometry is the preferred method for measurement for IOP due to its minimal dependence on corneal characteristics.

Steroid Response

Steroid-induced glaucoma is a secondary open-angle glaucoma due to topical or systemic corticosteroid use. It is a prevalent, early postoperative complication of refractive surgery as steroids are commonly used after refractive procedures. It is seen more often in patients with risk factors, like pre-existing chronic open-angle glaucoma, family history of glaucoma, high myopia, previous steroid response, African American ethnicity, age and history of connective tissue disease.

The incidence of DLK following refractive surgery ranges from 0.4% to 32%.[21] It is treated by increasing the frequency of topical steroids. Steroid-induced glaucoma has been reported in patients treated with corticosteroids for DLK. A prevalence of 7.9–12% has been reported following PRK.[22-24] Steroid-induced glaucoma has also been reported following phakic IOL implantation.

Interface fluid syndrome or PISK is an undetected steroid-induced increase in IOP in the early postoperative period following LASIK. It is associated with the presence of fluid between the flap and stroma subsequent to the failure of the endothelial pump. It can mimic DLK, an inflammatory condition leading to clinicians prescribing more topical steroids and starting a vicious cycle. Lyle first described it and subsequently similar cases were reported by other authors.[25-28] The treatment includes stopping steroids and starting the patient on IOP-lowering medication.

Acute Optic Neuropathy Postlaser-assisted in-situ Keratomileusis

There is marked elevation of IOP up to 60–80 mm Hg during the suction cup application and passage of microkeratome in LASIK. This can lead to ischemic or direct barotrauma to susceptible optic nerve heads. The risk factors include age more than 35 years, diabetes mellitus, cardiovascular disease. tilted disc, optic nerve head drusen and small optic disc. As a rare complication, patients can develop positive scotoma and profound loss of vision in the immediate postoperative period. The optic disc may appear normal or show edema. Retinal nerve fiber layer defects may be present. Altitudinal visual field defects have been reported in the immediate postoperative period, which persist but usually do not progress.[29]

Acute Angle-Closure Glaucoma

Acute angle-closure glaucoma, although rare but has been reported following hyperopic LASIK. It has been postulated that the suction ring, steroid drops, emotional stress, dark room and mechanical deformity of anterior segment structure may precipitate an acute angle closure attack in predisposed eyes.[30,31]

Acute angle-closure glaucoma after phakic posterior chamber IOL implantation has been reported due to several mechanisms, like oversizing, vaulting, residual viscoelastic and blockage of peripheral iridotomy. Malignant glaucoma has been reported to occur following the older generation phakic IOLs.

Urrets-Zavalia syndrome has been reported following phakic IOL implantation with intermittent pupillary block with sudden IOP rise causing iris or pup sphincter ischemia and atonic pupil.[32]

CONCLUSION

Diagnosing and managing glaucoma is challenging following refractive surgery.

Challenges

- Eyes with myopia are at a greater risk of developing POAG
- There is a higher risk of developing steroid-induced OHT and steroid-induced glaucoma
- All keratorefractive procedures alter the biomechanical properties of the cornea
- Due to the change in corneal biomechanics and thickness, OHT/POAG are more like to be undetected due to deceptive low-to-normal IOP readings
- It is challenging to distinguish between a myopic and glaucomatous optic nerve head
- Whether to plan refractive surgery in a glaucoma suspect is an issue of debate.

REFERENCES

1. Mitchell P, Hourihan F, Sandbach J, Wang JJ. The relationship between glaucoma and myopia: the Blue Mountains Eye Study. Ophthalmology. 1999;106(10):2010-5.
2. Perkins ES, Phelps CD. Open angle glaucoma, ocular hypertension, low-tension glaucoma and refraction. Arch Ophthalmol. 1991;100(9):1464-7.
3. Rapuano CJ. 2008-2009 Basic and Clinical Science Course (BCSC) Section 13 Refractive Surgery. California: American Academy of Ophthalmology; 2008.
4. Goldmann H. Applanation tonometry. In: Newell FW (Eds). Glaucoma Transactions of the Second Conference. New York: Josiah Macy Jr. Foundation; 1957. pp. 167-220.
5. Agudelo LM, Molina CA, Alvarez DL. Changes in intraocular pressure after laser in situ keratomileusis for myopia, hyperopia, and astigmatism. J Refract Surg. 2002;18(4):472-4.
6. Alonso-Muñoz L, Lleó-Pérez A, Rahhal MS, Sanchis-Gimeno JA. Assessment of applanation tonometry after hyperopic laser in situ keratomileusis. Cornea. 2002;21(2):156-60.
7. Arimoto A, Shimizu K, Shoji N, Enomoto K, Kohara M. Underestimation of intraocular pressure in eyes after laser in situ keratomileusis. Jpn J Ophthalmol. 2002;46(6):645-9.
8. El Danasoury MA, El Maghraby A, Coorpender SJ. Change in intraocular pressure in myopic eyes measured with contact and non-contact tonometers after laser in situ keratomileusis. J Refract Surg. 2001;17(2):97-104.
9. Fournier AV, Podtetenev M, Lemire J, et al. Intraocular pressure change measured by Goldmann tonometry after laser in situ keratomileusis. J Cataract Refract Surg. 1998;24(7):905-10.
10. Wang X, Shen J, McCulley JP, et al. Intraocular pressure measurement after hyperopic LASIK. CLAO J. 2002;28(3):136-9.
11. Zadok D, Raifkup F, Landao D, et al. Intraocular pressure after LASIK for hyperopia. Ophthalmology. 2002;109(9):1659-61.
12. Faucher A, Grégoire J, Blondeau P. Accuracy of Goldmann tonometry after refractive surgery. J Cataract Refract Surg. 1997;23(6):832-8.
13. Montés-Micó R, Charman WN. Intraocular pressure after excimer laser myopic refractive surgery. Ophthalmic Physiol Opt. 2001;21(3):228-35.
14. Chatterjee A, Shah S, Bessant DA, et al. Reduction in intraocular pressure after excimer laser photorefractive keratectomy. Correlation with pretreatment myopia. Ophthalmology. 1997;104(3):355-9.
15. Recep OF, Cagil N, Hasiripi H. Correlation between intraocular pressure and corneal stromal thickness after laser in situ keratomileusis. J Cataract Refract Surg. 2000;26(10):1480-3.
16. Mardelli PG, Piebenga LW, Whitacre MM, et al. The effect of excimer laser photorefractive keratectomy on intraocular pressure measurements using the Goldmann applanation tonometer. Ophthalmology. 1997;104(6):945-8.
17. Kaufmann C, Bachmann LM, Thiel MA. Intraocular pressure measurements using dynamic contour tonometry after laser in situ keratomileusis. Invest Ophthalmol Vis Sci. 2003;44(9):3790-4.
18. Sadigh AL, Fouladi RJ, Hashemi H, et al. A comparison between Goldmann applanation tonometry and dynamic contour tonometry after photorefractive keratectomy. Graefes Arch Clin Exp Ophthalmol. 2013;251(1):603-8.
19. Shemesh G, Soiberman U, Kurtz S. Intraocular pressure measurements with Goldmann applanation tonometry and dynamic contour tonometry in eyes after IntraLASIK or LASEK. Clin Ophthalmol. 2012;6:1967-70.

20. Han KE, Kim H, Kim NR, et al. Comparison of intraocular pressures after myopic laser-assisted subepithelial keratectomy: tonometry-pachymetry, Goldmann applanation tonometry, dynamic contour tonometry, and noncontact tonometry. J Cataract Refract Surg. 2013;39(6):888-97.

21. Choe CH, Guss C, Musch DC, et al. Incidence of diffuse lamellar keratitis after LASIK with 15 KHz, 30 KHz and 60 KHz femtosecond laser flap creation. J Cataract Refract Surg. 2010;36(11):1912-8.

22. Machat JJ, Tayfour F. Photorefractive keratectomy for myopia: preliminary results in 147 eyes. J Refract Corneal Surg. 1993;9(2 Suppl):S16-9.

23. Shimizu K, Amano S, Tanaka S. Photorefractive keratectomy for myopia: One-year follow-up in 97 eyes. J Refract Corneal Surg. 1994;10(2 Suppl):S178-87.

24. Gartry DS, Kerr Muir MG, Marshall J. Excimer laser photorefractive keratectomy. 18-month follow-up. Ophthalmology. 1992;99(8):1209-19.

25. Lyle WA, Jin GJ. Interface fluid associated with diffuse lamellar keratitis and epithelial ingrowth after laser in situ keratomileusis. J Cataract Refract Surg. 1999;25(7):1009-12.

26. Fogla R, Rao SK, Padmanabhan P. Interface fluid after laser in situ keratomileusis. J Cataract Refract Surg. 2001;27(9):1526-8.

27. Hamilton DR, Manche EE, Rich LF, Maloney RK. Steroid-induced glaucoma after laser in situ keratomileusis associated with interface fluid. Ophthalmology. 2002;109(4):659-65.

28. Brashford KP, Shafranov G, Tauber S, Shields MB. Considerations of glaucoma in patients undergoing corneal refractive surgery. Surv Ophthalmol. 2005;50(3):245-51.

29. Lee AG, Kohnen T, Ebner R, Bennett JL, Miller NR, Carlow TJ, et al. Optic neuropathy associated with laser in situ keratomileusis. J Cataract Refract Surg. 2000;26(11):1581-4.

30. Osman EA, Al Turki T, Alsaleh AA, Al Obeidan SA. Bilateral acute angle closure glaucoma after hyperopic LASIK correction. Saudi J Ophthalmol. 2009;(3-4):215-7.

31. Paciuc M, Velasco CF, Naranjo R. Acute angle-closure glaucoma after hyperopic laser in situ keratomileusis. J Cataract Refract Surg. 2000;26(4):620-3.

32. Yuzbasioglu E, Helvacioglu F, Sencan S. Fixed, dilated pupil after phakic intraocular lens implantation. J Cataract Refract Surg. 2006;32(1):174-6.

Glaucoma after Vitreoretinal Surgery

Gowri J Murthy, Praveen R Murthy

INTRODUCTION

Post-vitreoretinal (VR) surgery glaucoma is a postoperative acute or chronic rise of intraocular pressure (IOP) after VR surgery, which could cause glaucomatous optic nerve damage if untreated.

The various vitreous substitutes used, namely expanding gases, silicone oil and perfluorocarbon liquids, each because of its chemical composition and physics in the eye can contribute toward raised IOP. Use of encircling elements and buckles also can cause decreased outflow by altering the anterior chamber (AC) angle. Intravitreal pharmacological agents, like steroids, also contribute. Pre-existing angle abnormalities or neovascularization of the iris and angle as part of the VR pathology can play a role in the IOP rise. The challenge of managing this entity in eyes with retinal and other ocular comorbidities lies in early detection and understanding the mechanism of IOP rise.[1,2]

CLASSIFICATION

Classification can be based on following:
- Time after VR surgery:
  - Early/immediate postoperative secondary glaucoma
  - Late postoperative secondary glaucoma
- Mechanism of raised IOP:
  - Closed-angle mechanism
  - Open-angle mechanism

RISK FACTORS FOR POSTVITREORETINAL SURGERY GLAUCOMA

- Pre-existing primary open-angle glaucoma/primary angle-closure glaucoma[3]
- High myopia[4]
- Diabetes mellitus
- Pre-existing angle pathology due to inflammation/neovascularization[5]
- Intraoperative factors, such as high buckle, nondrainage buckle surgery, extensive endolaser, lens removal, fibrinous reaction, rubeosis, oil in AC[6-8]
- Failed retinal detachment repair, Schwartz syndrome.[9]

Case 1: Postsilicone oil-removal glaucoma

A 67-year-old lady presented to us with complaints of decreased vision. She had undergone pars plana vitrectomy with silicone oil injection and endolaser for a retinal detachment in her only seeing right eye, 2 years back. Three months back, she underwent silicone oil removal. Subsequent to the silicone oil removal, she developed raised IOP, which ranged between 24 mm Hg and 28 mm Hg despite maximal medication (Brimonidine, timolol, Dorzolamide, travoprost). She had undergone cataract surgery in the same eye 5 years back. She was a diabetic and hypertensive on treatment. On examination best-corrected visual acuity (BCVA) was 6/24, and anterior segment examination showed pseudophakic status with emulsified silicone oil globules on the iris and AC (Fig. 12C.1). Gonioscopy showed open angles with emulsified silicone oil globules in the superior angle. IOP was

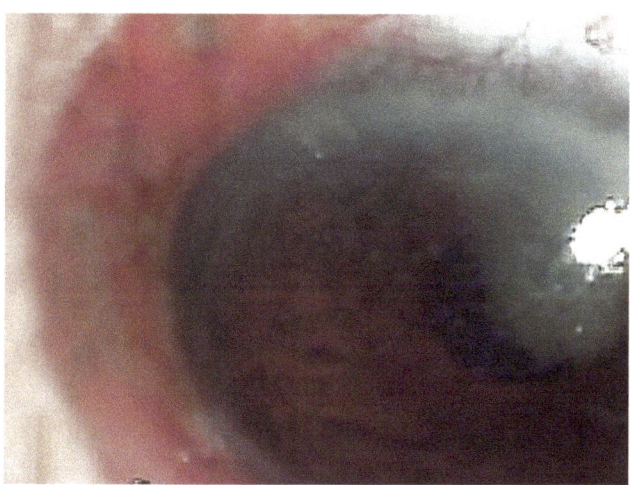

Fig. 12C.1: Anterior segment photo: Right eye showing emulsified silicone oil globules in anterior chamber.

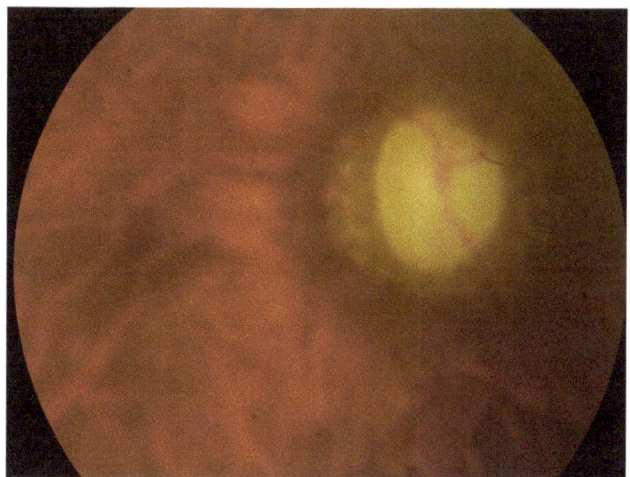

Fig. 12C.2: Optic disc right eye showing advanced glaucomatous damage.

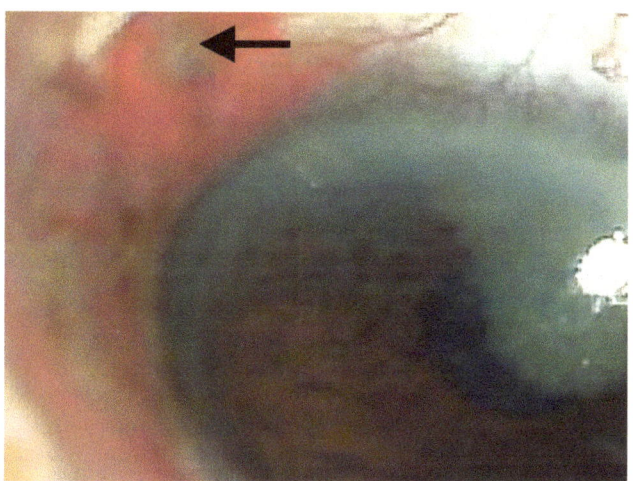

Fig. 12C.3: Tube exposure withconjunctival erosion (arrow) 1.5 mm posterior to limbus.

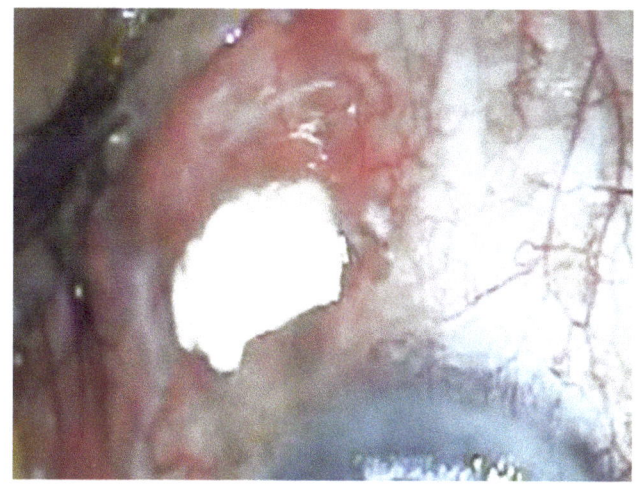

Fig. 12C.4: Conjunctival erosion and exposure of scleral patch graft.

26 mm Hg by applanation and retina was on with optic nerve head (ONH) showing significant pallor and shallow cupping of 0.9 (Fig. 12C.2). Due to the presence of scarred conjunctiva, and lower chances of success with trabeculectomy in an only seeing eye, a decision was taken to surgically manage with Ahmed glaucoma valve (AGV) implant with scleral patch graft. The patient was counseled regarding the risks and benefits of the procedure and she underwent the same uneventfully. Postoperatively, she achieved good IOP control (8 mm Hg) without medications.

However, at 3 months postoperative, she presented to us with complaints of irritation and watering of the eye, and

was found to have tube exposure 1 mm from the limbus (Fig. 12C.3). A repeat scleral patch graft with amniotic membrane graft with fibrin glue was performed. After initial resolution, after 1 month, again the scleral patch graft was exposed (Fig. 12C.4). A second conjunctival pedicle graft was then done with injection of botulinum toxin to the lid to decrease lid movements and promote conjunctival healing. The exposure resolved initially, but after 2 months, once the lid movement recovered, again the scleral graft exposure recurred. Taking into consideration of a myopic eye ball with increased axial length with a pseudoproptosis appearance, and the presence of tight

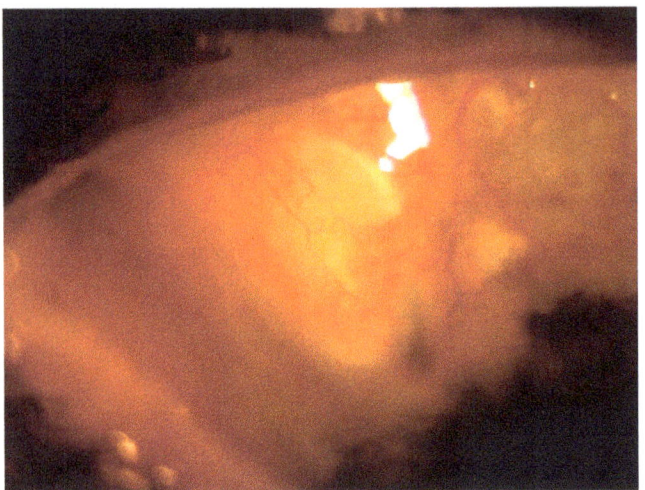

Fig. 12C.5: Healed conjunctiva after pars plana relocation of tube.

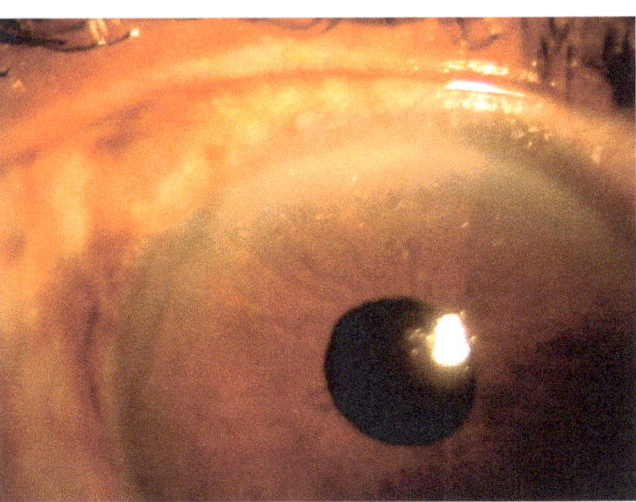

Fig. 12C.6: Anterior segment after pars plana relocation.

lids causing friction at the limbus as the probable cause of the repeated exposure at the limbus, a decision was taken to shift the entry of the tube into the eye, posteriorly to the pars plana region. The tube was trimmed and inserted into the pars plana region. Scleral patch graft was trimmed and conjunctiva sutured. The conjunctiva healed uneventfully, and the patient has a well-functioning tube with good IOP control for the last 1.5 years (Figs. 12C.5 and 12C.6).

Learning Points

- In many instances, IOP rise occurs after silicone oil removal as it is impossible to completely remove the emulsified oil droplets. The droplets clog the trabecular meshwork and cause secondary glaucoma
- In a prominent myopic eye with tight lids, repeated lid, conjunctival friction may be the cause for a tube/ scleral graft exposure. In such a situation, planned posterior/pars plana entry of the tube can relieve this repeated friction and lead to successful outcomes.

Case 2: Postoperative steroid-induced glaucoma-managed medically

A 73-year-old lady, known diabetic and hypertensive for the last 20 years, with history of bronchial asthma, presented to the retina clinic with sudden decrease in vision right eye. She had undergone cataract surgery 10 years back. On examination, she had a BCVA of 1/60, OD, and 6/9, N6 left eye. Anterior segment examination showed pseudophakia OU. IOP was 16 mm Hg OU, dilated fundus examination showed OD—vitreous hemorrhage,

OS—nonproliferative diabetic retinopathy. Ultrasound B-scan showed attached retina OD. She underwent micro-incision vitrectomy surgery (25 gauge) with endolaser OD, uneventfully (Fig. 12C.8). Postoperatively, the patient was on topical prednisolone acetate eye drops 2 hourly, along with antibiotic eye drops and homatropine eye drops (Fig. 12C.9). Four days postoperatively, the patient presented with pain and headache, which was right-sided. Examination showed, OD, BCVA 6/24, cornea-stromal and epithelial edema and deep AC with pharmacologically dilated pupil, IOP 33 mm Hg, fundus showed attached retina status post-pan-retinal photocoagulation. Gonioscopy with aseptic precautions with 4-mirror lens showed open angles. Patient was started on tablet Acetazolamide 250 mg twice a day and Brimonidine 0.15% eye drops thrice a day. Patient returned again the same evening with severe pain in the right eye and complained of inability to take tablet Acetazolamide due to abdominal discomfort. IOP in the right eye was 40 mm Hg. Patient was admitted and started on intravenous (IV) mannitol 20% 100 mL stat, and topical Brimonidine was continued. Also a decision was taken to shift the patient to a lower potency steroid (dexamethasone 0.1%), and reduce the frequency to 4 times a day. Next day the IOP reduced to 20 mm Hg and patient was comfortable. Patient was advised a tapering schedule of dexamethasone 0.1% over 4 weeks and asked to continue Brimonidine 0.15% eye drops thrice a day. Patient's IOP remained between 14 mm Hg and 17 mm Hg over the 4-week period, and once the topical dexamethasone was stopped, it came down to 10 mm Hg. Topical Brimonidine was stopped and at final postoperative visit. Her BCVA was 6/9 and pseudophakic status with retina stable.

Learning Points

- Steroid-induced IOP rise can present as early as few days after starting topical steroids in some patients[10]
- Shifting the patient to a lower potency steroid and adjunctive medical management helped in resolution of the IOP rise[10,11]
- Patients after retinal surgery need to be warned of symptoms of IOP rise and asked to review as necessary for IOP check.

Case 3: Multiple mechanisms for raised intraocular pressure requiring surgical management

A 55-year-old lady with history of Bilateral granulomatous uveitis, known steroid responder, presented with history of decreased vision in OD. She had been treated for tuberculosis in the past.

She was on brimonidine with timolol maleate eye drops twice a day, and dorzolamide eye drops twice a day to both eyes. Examination revealed BCVA 6/12, N8 OD, and 6/6, N6 OS. OD had a significant posterior subcapsular cataract (Fig. 12C.7). Dilated fundus examination showed vitreous opacities, as well as disc pallor, with vertical cup-to-disc ratio (C:D) of 0.7, inferior rim thinning with an epiretinal membrane (ERM) (Fig. 12C.10). Threshold visual fields central 30° showed generalized depression of retinal sensitivity with superior arcuate scotoma, OD, and only generalized loss in OS. Optical coherence tomography (OCT) of the macula OD showed ERM with no distortion of the macula.

Patient underwent OD, phacoemulsification + foldable hydrophobic acrylic intraocular lens (IOL) implant + 25 gauge vitrectomy with injection of dexamethasone sustained release implant intravitreally under local anesthesia. She had a bleed from the sclerotomy site at the end of the surgery when the trocar was removed. The blood tracked into the vitreous cavity-obscuring fundus view (Fig. 12C.11).

On the first postoperative day, BCVA was PL+ PR accurate, hand movements close to face and anterior segment showed IOL in position with minimal inflammation. View of retina was not possible due to vitreous hemorrhage. IOP

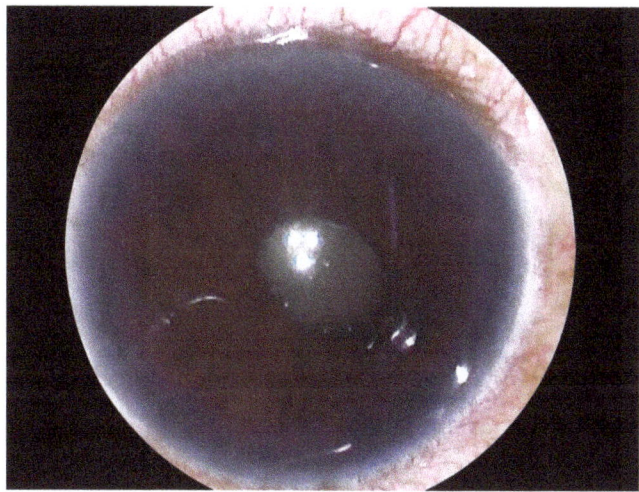

Fig. 12C.7: Preoperative photograph showing cataract right eye.

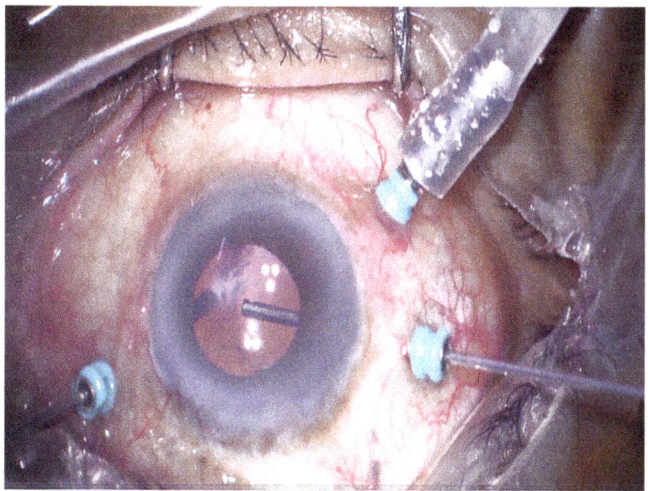

Fig. 12C.8: Twenty-five gauge vitrectomy in progress.

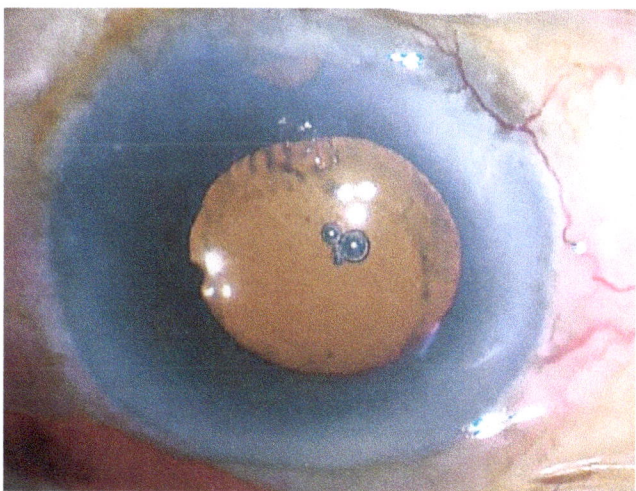

Fig. 12C.9: Postoperative photograph after vitrectomy with endolaser.

was 10 mm Hg and patient continued to use topical Brimonidine and timolol eye drops along with Dorzolamide with topical prednisolone acetate and antibiotic eye drops hourly. One week postoperatively, on review, OD had BCVA of hand movement close to face, anterior segment showed pseudophakic with resolving inflammation (Fig. 12C.12), IOP was 50 mm Hg and fundus showed hazy view due to vitreous hemorrhage.

At this stage the following factors were considered as probable reasons for the rise in IOP:

- Patient is a known steroid responder, and intravitreal dexamethasone implant coupled with topical prednisolone acetate could be contributing
- *Vitreous hemorrhage*—Red blood cells possibly clogging the trabecular meshwork
- Trabeculitis due to inflammation postoperatively in a uveitic eye.

Initial medical management with IV mannitol, tablet Acetazolamide and topical Brimonidine + timolol failed to achieve control of IOP. After discussing risks and benefits with the patient, OD vitreous lavage with trabeculectomy was done.

Post-trabeculectomy + vitreous lavage, initially IOP came down to the high teens (Fig. 12C.13), but started going up again within few weeks, and was at 36 mm Hg with tablet Acetazolamide, and topical Brimonidine with timolol at 4 weeks postsurgery. At this stage the patient's topical steroid had been reduced to dexamethasone 0.1%, four times per day. Gonioscopy showed open angles with pigmentation of the trabecular meshwork. BCVA had improved to 6/12, N6. Fundus examination showed

dexamethasone implant in the vitreous cavity with disc and fundus status stable.

The cause of IOP rise was now narrowed down to:

- Steroid-induced IOP response due to intravitreal dexamethasone implant, status-post failed trabeculectomy, in an eye with chronic uveitis.

After discussing the risks and benefits with the patient, OD, AGV implant with corneal patch graft over the tube was done. Post-AGV IOP stabilized at 12–16 mm Hg with no topical antiglaucoma medications. At last visit, 3 months postoperation OD had BCVA 6/9, N6, quiet anterior segment, pseudophakic (on tapering schedule of fluorometholone eye drops) IOP was 14 mm Hg and fundus was stable (Fig. 12C.14).

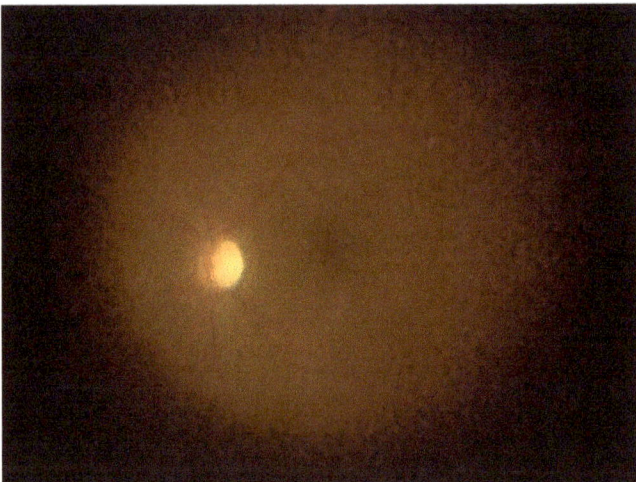

Fig. 12C.10: Fundus view during vitrectomy (inverted view).

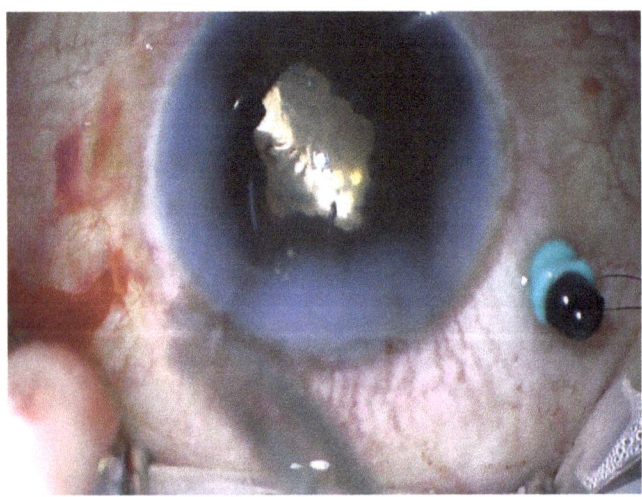

Fig. 12C.11: Bleeding from the vitrectomy port seen tracking into the vitreous cavity at end of surgery.

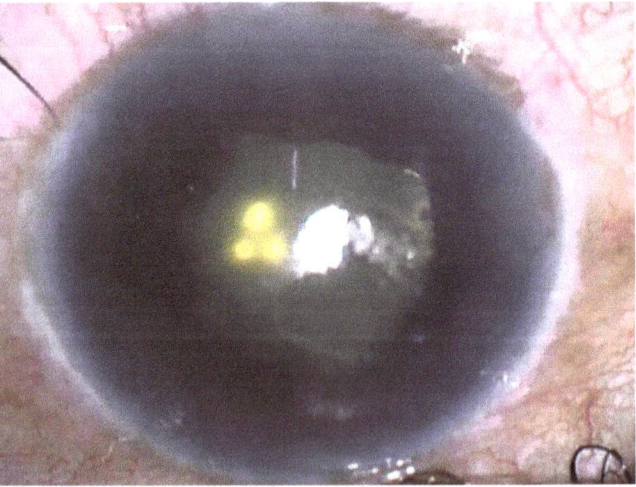

Fig. 12C.12: Postoperative photo showing corneal edema due to raised intraocular pressure.

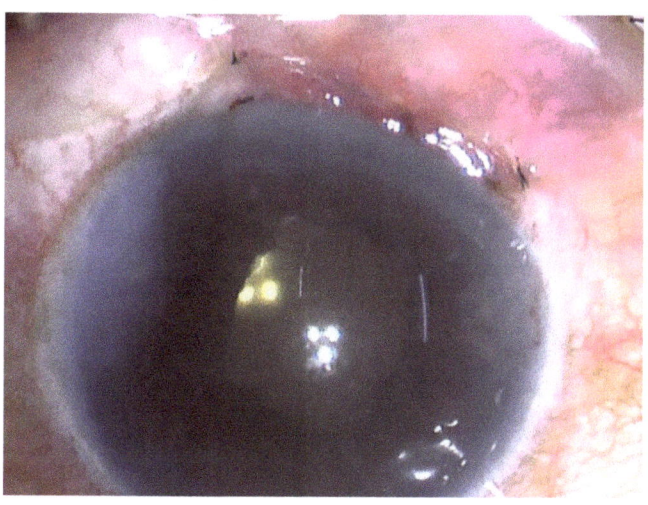

Fig. 12C.13: Anterior segment photograph status post trabeculectomy and vitreous lavage.

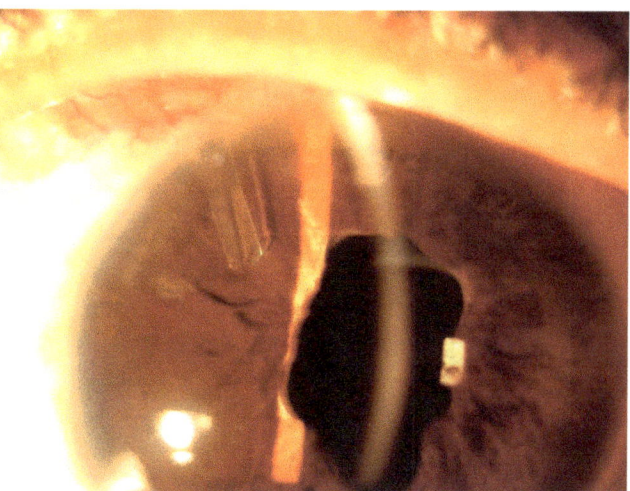

Fig. 12C.14: Anterior segment photo status post Ahmed glaucoma valve implant.

Learning Points

- More than one cause could be contributing to the IOP elevation postvitrectomy surgery
- Frequent post operative follow-ups and checking of IOP are required to detect the IOP spikes and to assess the efficacy of glaucoma management
- Trabeculectomy can fail in postoperative eye, do not procrastinate and proceed to the next option when one option fails
- Discuss with patients risks and benefits preoperatively and keep him/her informed about the situation throughout.

Case 4: Iris bombe causing secondary angle closure and silicone oil overfill

A 75-year-old lady was diagnosed with OD, rhegmatogenous retinal detachment with immature cataract. She had a previous history of being treated for anterior uveitis with topical steroids in the past. She was diabetic and hypertensive on treatment.

She underwent OD, phacoemulsification with foldable hydrophobic acrylic IOL implant with vitrectomy with fluid gas exchange, endolaser and silicone oil injection under local anesthesia.

As her first postoperative day, IOP was 26 mm Hg. She was started on Dorzolamide and timolol eye drops twice a day and Brimonidine eye drops thrice a day to OD along with topical steroids.

In the third postoperative week, patient presented with pain and redness OD. On examination OD, BCVA was counting of fingers close to face, and anterior segment showed iris bombe configuration with 360° posterior synechiae to the IOL. IOP was 50 mm Hg. B-scan showed attached retina with silicone oil in situ.

A diagnosis of pupil block leading to secondary angle closure was made and patient underwent laser peripheral iridotomy (Fig. 12C.15). Postiridotomy, her IOP reduced to low 20s. Medical management of IOP was continued along with topical steroids and atropine 1% eye drops. Patient returned, 1 week later, again with recurrence of iris bombe and IOP of 50 mm Hg, and the peripheral iridotomy (PI) was found to be blocked with fibrin. The PI was enlarged with yttrium aluminum garnet (YAG) laser, and patient was also started on a course of systemic steroids in addition to the topical steroid and mydriatic-cycloplegic. However, the IOP stabilized to between 34 mm Hg and 40 mm Hg. Anterior segment showed resolving fibrin and inflammation, pseudophakia and resolution of iris bombe (Fig. 12C.16). Fundus examination showed attached retina with silicone oil in situ. After discussion with the VR surgeon, it was decided to tap the silicone oil. Under aseptic precaution, 1 mL of silicone oil was removed (Fig. 12C.17). Post-tapping of silicone oil, the IOP reduced to 15–18 mm Hg, and the antiglaucoma medications and the steroids were gradually tapered off.

Learning Points

- On the first postoperative day, a moderate IOP elevation was managed medically
- 360° posterior synechiae due to inflammation caused pupil block and further raised IOP

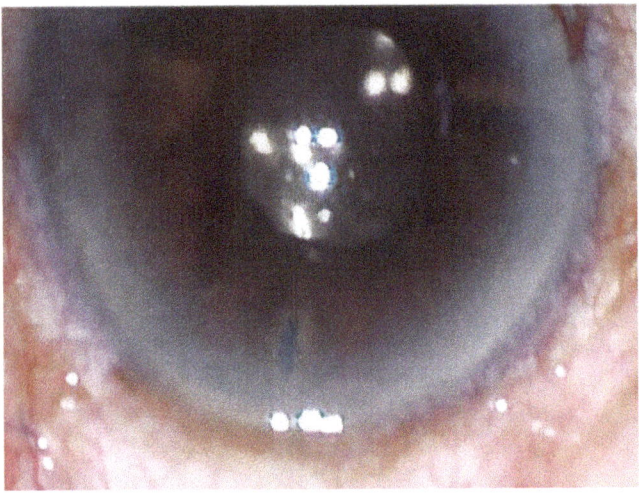

Fig. 12C.15: Inferior yttrium aluminium garnet laser iridotomy done for iris bombe.

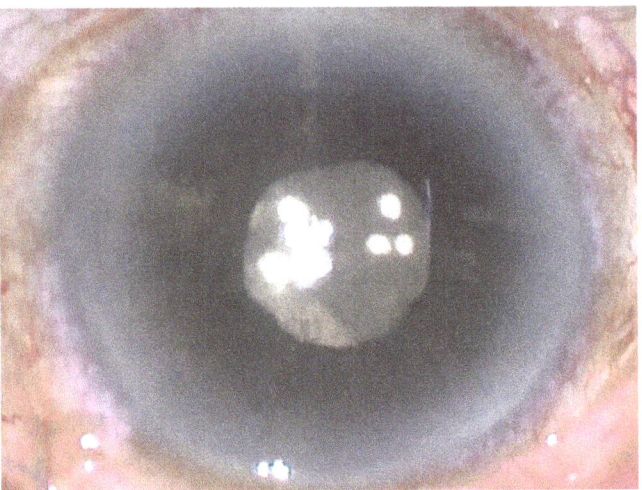

Fig. 12C.16: Postiridectomy picture with corneal edema due to raised intraocular pressure.

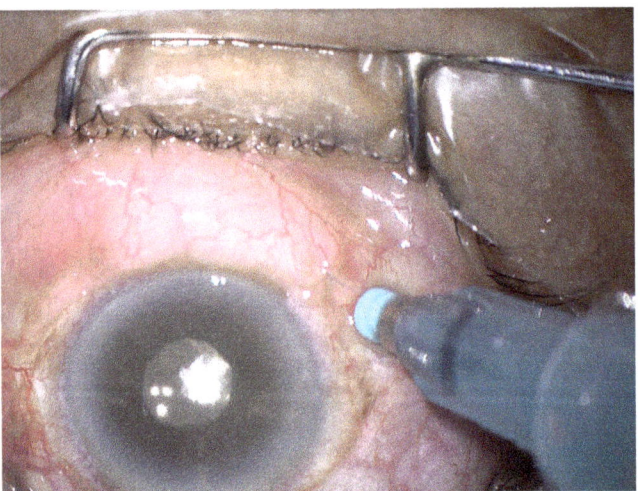

Fig. 12C.17: Single 25 gauge port being used for tapping silicone oil.

- Yttrium aluminum garnet PI in eyes with inflammation can get blocked due to fibrin and needs to be enlarged/ large iridotomy needs to be done. Postlaser intensive steroids and cycloplegic mydriatics are necessary
- In this eye, the angle damage following the pupil block and secondary angle closure might have compromised the aqueous outflow and resulted in persistent high IOP
- Partial tapping of the silicone oil resulted in re-establishing the homeostasis and control of IOP
- There might have been a slight overfill to start with as the first postoperative day IOPs were moderately high.

Case 5: Silicone oil-induced glaucoma in a high myope managed with silicone oil removal with endoscopic cyclophotocoagulation

A 35-year-old lady, a high myope, presented to us with OD rhegmatogenous retinal detachment with choroidal detachment. She underwent OD, vitrectomy + encircling band + fluid gas exchange + endolaser + silicone oil injection uneventfully (Fig. 12C.18). Postoperatively retina was attached (Fig. 12C.19).

During the third week following surgery, the IOP was found to be high (26 mm Hg) and medical management of glaucoma was started, Brimonidine + timolol eye drops. The IOP elevation initially responded, but after a couple of weeks was again elevated and IOP was 44 mm Hg at the seventh postoperative week (Fig. 12C.20). Retina was attached.

As the IOP was not responding to maximal medical management, she was taken up for phacoemulsification + IOL + silicone oil removal + endoscopic cyclophotocoagulation (ECP) (Fig. 12C.21). Postsurgery after 6 weeks, she has a BCVA of 6/18, N10, and IOP 16 mm Hg (on Brimonidine + timolol) and attached retina with myopic fundus (Fig. 12C.22).

Learning Points

- Patients with high myopia are at risk for developing glaucoma
- A VR surgery in these eyes can cause raised IOP due to various mechanisms

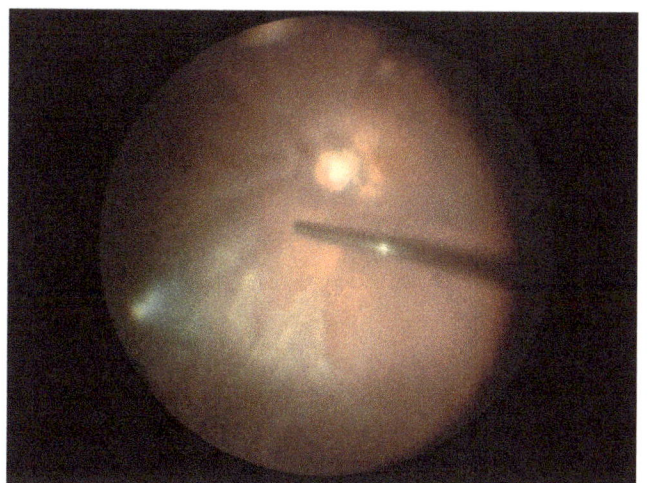

Fig. 12C.18: Retinal detachment vitrectomy in progress (inverted image).

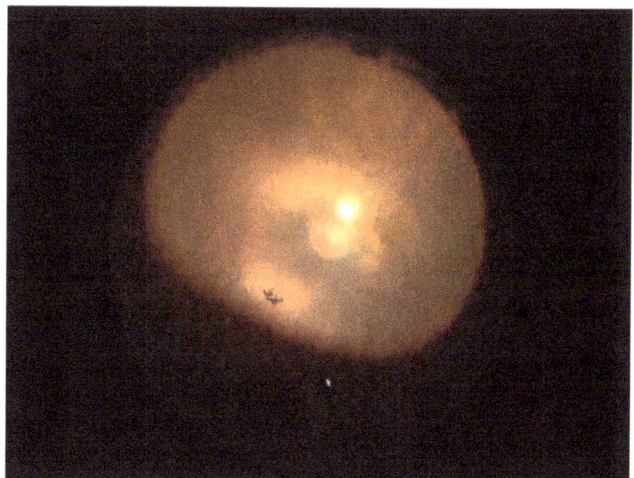

Fig. 12C.19: Retina attached at the end of surgery (inverted image).

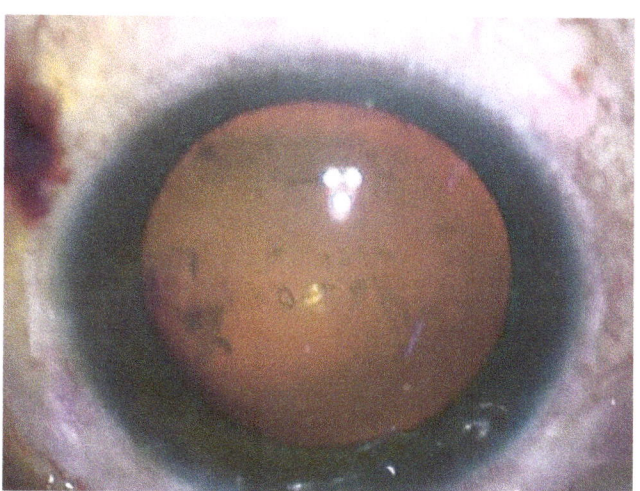

Fig. 12C.20: Postoperative anterior segment photo with raised intraocular pressure.

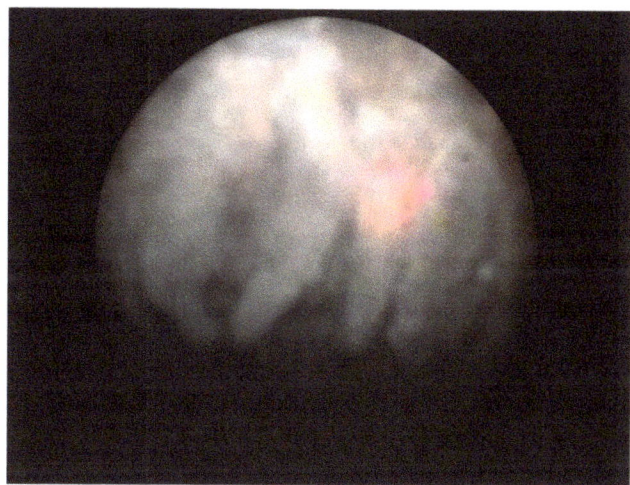

Fig. 12C.21: Pars plana endoscopic cyclophotocoagulation in progress.

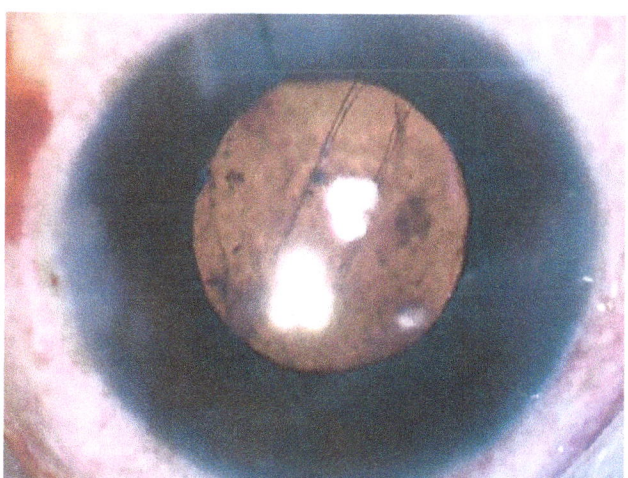

Fig. 12C.22: Anterior segment photo after phacoemulsification + intraocular lens + SOR + endoscopic cyclophotocoagulation. (SOR: Silicon oil removal).

- As the retina attached and IOP did not respond to medical management early removal of the silicone oil was considered
- Endoscopic cyclophotocoagulation can be combined with VR procedures to manage raised IOP
- Phacoemulsification with IOL was combined to enable ECP by the pars plana route.

INVESTIGATIONS

Patients with raised IOP-following VR surgery should be examined in a systematic way and all efforts should be made to identify the mechanism of the IOP rise. A step-by-step approach taking into the account the operative details and thorough slit-lamp examination, including gonioscopy, and fundus examination is the key to identifying the mechanism of IOP rise.

Corneal Findings or Considerations

Raised IOP causes corneal edema, both stromal and epithelial edema, if the IOP rise is significant and occurs over a short period of time. A slow rise in IOP like that which occurs in steroid-induced glaucoma may produce no/minimal corneal edema.[10] In the immediate postoperative period, if the corneal epithelium has been debrided for operative viewing purposes, it may not be possible to check applanation IOP in the presence of an epithelial defect. In such eyes, a tono-pen can be used to check IOP over a bandage contact lens.[12] Presence of air/gas in the AC may cause inaccuracies in applanation IOP.[12] Also in the presence of silicone oil/air/gas in the AC in the immediate postoperative period, the IOP rise may not cause corneal edema. The presence of a clear cornea may lull one into thinking that the IOP is normal.

Anterior Segment

The depth of the AC can provide a clue to the cause of IOP rise. A uniformly shallow AC indicates either a pupil block mechanism or forward movement of the iris lens diaphragm due to pushing pressure from the vitreous cavity. The anterior movement of the iris lens diaphragm could be caused by overfill of vitreous substitutes and also by aqueous misdirection, which could occur especially in eyes with pre-existing angle-closure glaucoma.[6]

An iris bombe configuration implies pupillary block due to posterior synechiae to lens/IOL without a patent iridectomy. Use of atropine in the postoperative period-following vitrectomy may result in the posterior synechiae

being formed peripherally with a dilated pupil and the typical iris bombe configuration may not be seen in these eyes. One has to specifically look at the iris contour and the angle in such eyes.

Iris

Findings in the iris include areas of atrophy and new blood vessels on the iris and ectropion uveae in neovascular glaucoma. Fine globules of emulsified silicone oil can also be seen over the iris in eyes with emulsified silicone oil causing raised IOP. Inferior iridectomies are usually performed in eyes, which have undergone silicone oil injection during VR surgery. The inferior PI serves as a route for passage of aqueous humor from the posterior to AC as silicone oil tends to float up and occlude the pupil and a superior PI.[13,14] Sometimes inflammation in the postoperative period can cause a thin layer of fibrin to form over the PI and this may cause pupil block leading to raised IOP. YAG laser to the fibrin results in resolution of this block. If heavy silicone oil is used, a superior PI is indicated.[15] Intraocular gas after vitrectomy can also be a cause for pupil block and can escape into the AC in pseudophakic/aphakic eyes (Fig. 12C.23). Proper postoperative positioning of the patient can relieve pupil block in such eyes.

Angles

Gonioscopy is an important examination in all eyes with secondary glaucoma. The status of the angle, either open or closed, helps to determine the mechanism of IOP rise. A 4-mirror gonioscope of the Zeiss/Susmann type is preferred. In addition, other angle findings, such as new blood vessels, silicone oil globules and peripheral anterior synechiae help to correctly identify the mechanism of glaucoma.[6]

Lens

The lens status of the eye, either phakic or pseudophakic, if so the type of lens—in the bag/sulcus fixated/AC/iris clip lens should be factored in deciding the mechanism and also in planning management of the raised IOP. Prostaglandin (PG) analogs are relatively contraindicated in aphakic single chamber eyes with raised IOP, as the occurrence of cystoid macular edema is a possibility.[16]

Fundus Examination

Assessment of the ONH may pose challenges in eyes with post-VR surgery secondary glaucomas. Presence of retinal

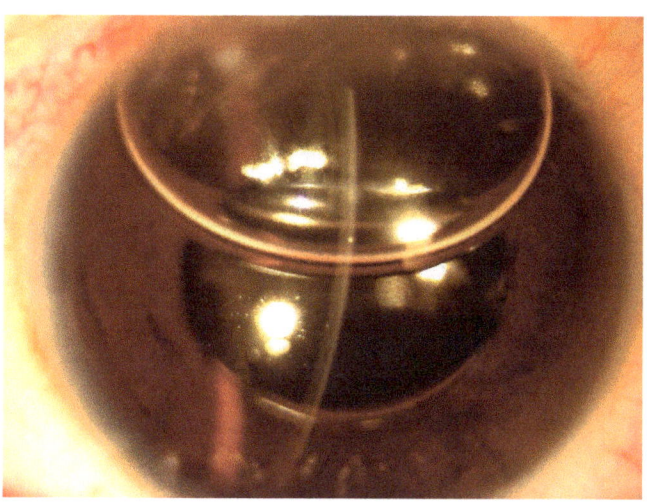

Fig. 12C.23: Anterior migration of gas bubble status post vitrectomy.

comorbidities, like proliferative diabetic retinopathy and laser to the retina/branch retinal vein occlusions/nonarteritic anterior ischemic optic neuropathies, can cause pallor of the ONH.[17] Also an acute episode of raised IOP for a variable period of time causes a very shallow cupping and more marked pallor of the optic disc and may not result in the typical glaucomatous cupping seen in eyes with primary glaucomas. Myopes have discs, which are atypical in size and shape, and the border of the disc is not made out well due to peripapillary atrophy. Detection of glaucomatous change in these discs can be very challenging.[18] A thorough examination of the rest of the retina including the periphery should also be done. Thinning of the sclerotomy sites can be present in eyes with raised IOP for a long period of time.

In addition, the following tests, if performed, help in managing the condition better in case the facilities exist and are affordable to the patient:

Ultrasound B-scan

When the view of the posterior pole is not clear due to media opacity/vitreous hemorrhage, an ultrasound B-scan can provide a wealth of information about the posterior segment. In addition to confirming the retinal status, it can also help in detecting advanced optic disc cupping. Small supraciliary accumulations of fluid and choroidal detachments pushing the iris forward and causing angle closure can be detected.[19] In eyes, where the operative details are not available and the presence of silicone oil in the vitreous cavity may be confirmed by a B-scan. B-scan

ultrasound may not be very useful in gas-filled eyes. Silicone oil-filled eyes look extremely long on ultrasound B-scan and the posterior pole details may not be made out clearly.

Ultrasound Biomicroscopy

Ultrasound biomicroscopy (UBM) is an investigation, which significantly helps in the identification on angle closure and the mechanism of angle closure, and detection of angle pathology in the presence of a nontransparent cornea. Small supraciliary choroidal detachments, which cause anterior rotation of the ciliary body and angle closure can only be picked-up by UBM.[19,20] Lens zonular integrity can be assessed. The position of the IOL haptics in a pseudophakic eye can be ascertained. Presence of anterior hyaloid proliferation, especially in relation to the sclerotomy sites and mass lesions in the ciliary body area can also be detected.[21]

Iris or Fundus Fluorescein Angiography

Iris angiography is indicated to detect subtle neovascularization of the iris. When the cause for neovascularization of the iris is not clearly apparent on fundus examination, and fluorescein angiogram can help in detecting retinal ischemia.[22,23]

Optical Coherence Tomography Scans of the Macula and the Optic Nerve Head

Optical coherence tomography scan of the macula can help in detecting subtle vitreomacular traction/subretinal fluid, which may be contributing to the vision loss in eyes with coexisting secondary glaucoma. The ONH scans are not very useful in eyes with large myopic discs. The additional macular/retinal pathology can confound the findings of the retinal nerve fiber layer/ONH scans and cannot be taken at face value.[24]

Visual Fields

Documenting the visual field status is an often forgotten investigation when one is managing post-VR secondary glaucoma. In eyes with chronically elevated IOP, wherever, possible one should consider documenting the function of the optic nerve by a visual field. However, interpretation should take into account the contribution of the retinal pathology to the same. Use of central 10–2 programs/size 5 targets may be of help in patients with low vision. The fields can help to determine progression of glaucomatous damage over time. Flowchart 12 C.1 summarises the entire diagnosis.

Flowchart 12C.1: Diagnosis of glaucoma after vitreoretinal surgery.

```
                    ┌─────────────────────┐
                    │ Raised IOP after    │
                    │ vitreoretinal surgery│
                    └──────────┬──────────┘
                               ▼
                    ┌─────────────────────┐
                    │ Primary or          │
                    │ secondary?          │
                    └──────────┬──────────┘
                               ▼
                    ┌─────────────────────┐
                    │ Other eye           │
                    │ findings—IOP/angle/ │
                    │ disc/VFT            │
                    └──────────┬──────────┘
```

| Primary glaucoma | Secondary glaucoma |

| Open angle | Closed angle |

| Early/intermediate "postoperative" | Late postoperative | Pupil block mechanism | Nonpupil block mechanism |

| Silicone oil/Gas overfill/expansion | Latent POAG unmasked | | UBM |

| Steroid-induced IOP rise | Structural angle damage due to pathology and surgery | | Supraciliary fluid or anterior rotation of ciliary body |

| Anterior segment ischemia | Silicone oil/emulsified oil blocking the angle | | Synechial angle closure |

| | Ghost cell glaucoma | | |

(IOP: Intraocular pressure; POAG: Primary open-angle glaucoma; UMB: Ultrasound biomicroscopy; VFT: Visual field testing).

MANAGEMENT

Early recognition of IOP rise is the first key to tackling the entity of post-VR surgery secondary glaucoma. The treatment is tailored to the cause.

Medical Management

In the immediate postoperative IOP rise, medical management needs to be instituted promptly. Systemic Acetazolamide and, if necessary, hyperosmotics, such as IV mannitol, and oral glycerol may be needed. However, hyperosmotics may be of limited value in gas-filled/silicone oil-filled eyes. Generally, aqueous suppressants form the mainstay, timolol maleate 0.5%, and Dorzolamide 2% or Brinzolamide 1%, Brimonidine 0.15% can also be used as adjuncts. Generally, PG analogs are relatively contraindicated in the immediate postoperative period, and also in eyes with neovascularization. In the long-term management, however, PG analogs can be used and can be effective. One should always keep in mind the potential for IOP rise with the use of topical/intravitreal steroids. In the situation of a steroid-induced IOP elevation, switching to a lower potency steroid can be of help. Intravitreal steroids can also cause intractable IOP rise. Medical management is the initial choice, and if it does not resolve then surgical management will be required.[25,26]

Laser Iridotomy

Yttrium aluminum garnet laser iridotomy is used specifically in the context of a pupillary block leading to iris bombe and secondary glaucoma. Iridotomy relieves the pupil block and restores the circulation of aqueous humor. In silicone oil-filled eyes, an inferior iridotomy is done. YAG laser can also be used to disrupt fibrinous membranes, which may be blocking the PI or the pupil.[13-15]

Surgical Management

Surgical management involves glaucoma surgery, either to increase outflow of aqueous humor or to decrease its production, or involve retinal surgeries, which address the underlying pathology or a combined approach.

Vitreous Tap

In the context of an expanding gas bubble in surgeries, like pneumatic retinopexy, a vitreous tap to reduce the amount of gas in the vitreous cavity may result in resolution of the IOP rise (C3F8 triples its volume in 72 hours and SF6 doubles in 24 hours). In some vitrectomy surgeries, a nonexpansile gas mixture is injected at the end of surgery. The calculation is done based on rule of thumb, i.e. 14% C3F8 and 20% SF6 is considered nonexpansile. However, this depends on the purity of the source gas, and sometimes errors could occur causing further expansion of the gas-air mixture in the vitreous cavity. A patient having a general anesthesia, after a VR surgery, can also have expansion of the gas bubble in the eye due to influx of anesthetic gas. In such situations, a predetermined amount of gas can be withdrawn from the vitreous cavity, while ensuring adequate amount of gas remains in the eye, to achieve the required tamponade effect.[25-27]

In silicone oil over fill it is not possible to remove adequate amount of oil through a fine needle. It is better to make a 23/25-gauge trocar opening into the vitreous cavity and actively withdraw a small amount of the oil using the silicone oil-removal mode of the vitrectomy machine.[26]

After tapping gas/silicone oil, it is imperative to continue to monitor the IOP.

Vitreous Lavage

Residual heme/bleeding into the vitreous cavity post-VR surgery can later result in ghost-cell glaucoma. Vitreous lavage and washing out the deformed red blood cells can result in resolution of the glaucoma.

Trabeculectomy with Mitomycin C

Trabeculectomy carries lower success rates due to scarring of the conjunctiva and presence of encircling elements and buckles. However, it is a modality, which can effectively reduce IOP in the medium-term and long-term for some eyes. Certain surgical considerations:

- Choose a quadrant where conjunctiva is freely mobile, check on the slit lamp with a Q tip/move the conjunctiva through the upper lid
- Use of mitomycin C. Antimetabolites prevent scarring and are indicated in these eyes
- In the setting of neovascularization of the iris/angle, preoperative injection of anti- vascular endothelial growth factor (VEGF) antibodies, e.g. bevacizumab/ranibizumab/aflibercept, will cause regression of the new vessels and prevent intraoperative bleeding and improves the success rates of trabeculectomy due to its antiangiogenesis action[28,29]
- Consider the use of releasable sutures to titrate the IOP in the postoperative period.

Glaucoma Drainage Devices

The Ahmed glaucoma valve (AGV) and the Baerveldt glaucoma drainage implant or the Arvind aqueous drainage device are useful devices in the management of these secondary glaucomas.[25-30]

Considerations for drainage device implantation in eye post-VR/buckle surgery:

- Position the plate of the drainage device away from segmental buckles but, tube can be passed over encircling bands
- Presence of 360° encircling buckles may present a difficult proposition
- Under the buckle, sclera tends to be thin and one should be careful while dissecting in this area
- Avoid opening the fibrous capsule around the buckle, rather, pass the valve over the band area
- Avoid passing tube over large buckles.
- Avoid exposing the buckle suture as far as possible, as this may precipitate buckle or tube exposure
- Anterior chamber/pars plana tube placement, the position of placement of the tube can be in the pars plana, if the space in the AC is less due to extensive peripheral anterior synechiae, or if the corneal endothelium is borderline decompensated or in a postkeratoplasty context
- If silicone oil needs to be retained in the eye, the drainage device should be placed inferiorly. When the tube

is inserted into the AC and the IOP reduced, silicone oil bubbles may move forward into the AC. Do not attempt to remove this, as more oil will keep coming anteriorly.

Cyclodestructive Procedures

Reduction of inflow of aqueous humor by destruction of the ciliary body is a management modality, which could be considered in eyes with post-VR surgery glaucoma nonresponsive to traditional surgical methods. Irrespective of the method used, destruction of the ciliary body is irreversible. The dose-response curve or the amount of IOP reduction per degree/extent of cyclodestruction is unpredictable. Hypotony and phthisis bulbi, therefore, are possibilities. There is always associated inflammation, which is incited by the destructive procedure. Loss of visual acuity may result due to inflammatory and other changes due to cyclodestruction.[31-34]

Endoscopic cyclophotocoagulation: Endoscopic delivery offers precision in terms of location and energy delivery. The development of the 20 gauge and 23 gauge ECP probe with combined functions of an 810 nm red diode laser, video endoscope and illumination in a single probe, enabled ECP. It offers a better safety profile, better preservation of BCVA and has similar success rates as compared to trans-scleral cyclophotocoagulation (TSCPC). ECP can be performed by either limbal or pars plana route. The advantage of the procedure is that it can be combined with VR procedures and can be performed in the presence of scarred conjunctiva in eyes with scleral buckles. Laser photocoagulation of the peripheral retina can also be done with the ECP probe in eyes with neovascular glaucoma.[34]

Trans-scleral cyclophotocoagulation: TSCPC with the 810 nm diode laser using the G probe is a noninvasive method of destroying the ciliary processes.[31-33]

Considerations during TSCPC in post-VR surgery eyes:
• Avoid areas of scleral thinning
• Postoperatively one can expect intraocular inflammation due to breakdown of blood-ocular barrier
• Vision loss in up to 40% of patients has been reported, could be avoided in eyes with good visual acuity.[31-33]

FOLLOW-UP PROTOCOL

Follow-up protocol is to be customized to the individual patient depending on extent of IOP rise, retinal pathology and the cause. In the immediate postoperative period, one should be vigilant and check the IOP frequently. In the late postoperative period, follow-up is tailored to the individual patient. IOP/disc and other variables need to be periodically assessed.

BRIEF REVIEW OF LITERATURE

The incidence of IOP elevation after VR surgery has been defined in different ways and at different time points after surgery in literature. The incidence of early postoperative IOP rise is seen in up to 52% of eyes,[35] and late postoperative up to 50%.[36] The rates vary with type of surgery performed and type of vitreous substitute used.

Vitrectomy alone has been shown to increase the IOP to 30 mm Hg or greater in 40% of operated eyes.[2] Early postoperative elevation of IOP is common with use of intraocular gas,[37-40] and silicone oil injection is associated with both short-term and long-term IOP elevation.[41-43] IOP elevation can be caused by both nonemulsified and emulsified silicone oil.

Reporting of outcomes of secondary glaucoma following VR surgery in literature: In majority of the eyes post surgical IOP elevation is transient.[35] The use of antiglaucoma medication is sufficient for resolution in most eyes requiring treatment.[25,30,35,44] Supplemental VR procedures or modification of the VR surgery can help in resolution.[44] A small percentage requires glaucoma surgery, which is largely successful, but can be associated with complications including hypotony.[25,27,30,44] Trabeculectomy with antimetabolites, glaucoma drainage implants and cyclodestruction are well-described surgical procedures in literature for this subset of secondary glaucomas.

SUMMARY

Raised IOP is a distinct possibility following VR surgery. The elevated IOP can cause glaucomatous disc damage and decrease vision in an eye with retinal comorbidities. Thorough evaluation, understanding the mechanism of IOP elevation and prompt management helps in successful resolution of the condition. The patient should be an informed partner at all stages in the care process.

REFERENCES

1. Costarides A, Alabata P, Bergstrom C. Elevated intraocular pressure following vitreoretinal surgery. Ophthalmol Clin North Am. 2004;17(4):507-12.
2. Desai UR, Alhalel AA, Schiffman RM, Campen TJ, Sundar G, Muhich A. Intraocular pressure elevation after simple pars Plana Vitrectomy. Ophthalmology. 1997;104(5):781-6.

3. Phelps CD, Burton TC. Glaucoma and retinal detachment. Arch Ophthalmol. 1977;95(3):418-22.
4. Podos SM, Becker B, Ross Morton W. High myopia and primary open-angle glaucoma. Am J Ophthalmol. 1966; 62(6):1038-43.
5. Sebestyen JG. Retinal detachment and glaucoma. Arch Ophthalmol. 1962;67(6):736.
6. Han DP, Lewis H, Lambrou FH, et al. Mechanisms of intraocular pressure elevation after pars plana vitrectomy. Ophthalmology. 1989;96(9):1357-62.
7. Wu L, Berrocal MH, Rodriguez FJ, et al. Intraocular pressure elevation after uncomplicated pars plana vitrectomy. Retina. 2014;34(10):1985-9.
8. Chang S. LXII Edward Jackson lecture: open angle glaucoma after vitrectomy. Am J Ophthalmol. 2006;141(6):1033-43.
9. Schwartz A. Chronic open-angle glaucoma secondary to rhegmatogenous retinal detachment. Am J Ophthalmol. 1973;75(2):205-11.
10. Armaly MF. Effect of corticosteroids on intraocular pressure and fluid dynamics. Arch Ophthalmol. 1963;70(4):482-91.
11. Shammas HF, Halasa AH, Faris BM. Intraocular pressure, cup-disc ratio, and steroid responsiveness in retinal detachment. Arch Ophthalmol. 1976;94(7):1108-9.
12. Fogelman KL, Hines MW, Jost BF. Oculab tono-pen, Goldmann applanation tonometry, and pneumatic tonometry for intraocular pressure assessment in gas-filled eyes. Am J Ophthalmol. 1988;106(2):174-9.
13. Ichhpujani P, Jindal A, Jay Katz L. Silicone oil induced glaucoma: a review. Graefes Arch Clin Exp Ophthalmol. 2009;247(12):1585-93.
14. Ando F. Usefulness and limit of silicone in management of complicated retinal detachment. Jpn J Ophthalmol. 1987;31(1):138-46.
15. Cheung BT, Lai TY, Yuen CY, Lai WW, Tsang CW, Lam DS. Results of high-density silicone oil as a tamponade agent in macular hole retinal detachment in patients with high myopia. Br J Ophthalmol. 2007;91(6):719-21.
16. Halpern DL, Pasquale LR. Cystoid macular edema in aphakia and pseudophakia after use of prostaglandin analogs. Semin Ophthalmol. 2003;17(3-4):181-6.
17. Lim MC, Tanimoto SA, Furlani BA, Lum B, Pinto LM, Eliason D, et al. Effect of diabetic retinopathy and panretinal photocoagulation on retinal nerve fiber layer and optic nerve appearance. Arch Ophthalmol. 2009;127(7):857-62.
18. Jonas J, Dichtl A. Optic disc morphology in myopic primary open-angle glaucoma. Graefes Arch Clin Exp Ophthalmol. 1997;235(10):627-33.
19. Liebmann JM, Weinreb RN, Ritch R. Angle-closure glaucoma associated with occult annular ciliary body detachment. Arch Ophthalmol. 1998;116(6):731-5.
20. Liu W, Wu Q, Huang S, Wang N, Cheng X. Application of ultrasound biomicroscopy in diagnosis of anterior segment vitreoretinal disorders. Yan Ke Xue Bao. 1997;13(4):192-6.
21. Bhende M, Agraharam SG, Gopal L, Sumasri K, Sukumar B, George J, et al. Ultrasound biomicroscopy of sclerotomy sites after pars plana vitrectomy for diabetic vitreous hemorrhage. Ophthalmology. 2000;107(9):1729-36.
22. Oya Y, Sugiyama W, Ando N. Anterior segment fluorescein angiography for evaluating the effect of vitrectomy for neovascular glaucoma. Nippon Ganka Gakkai zasshi. 2005;109(11):741-7.
23. Ino-ue M, Azumi A, Shirabe H, et al. Iridopathy in eyes with proliferative diabetic retinopathy: detection of early stage of rubeosis iridis. Ophthalmologica. 1998;212(1):15-8.
24. Kim KE, Jeoung JW, Park KH, Kim DM, Kim SH. Diagnostic classification of macular ganglion cell and retinal nerve fiber layer analysis: differentiation of false-positives from glaucoma. Ophthalmology. 2014;122(3):502-10.
25. Tranos P, Asaria R, Aylward W, Sullivan P, Franks W. Long term outcome of secondary glaucoma following vitreoretinal surgery. Br J Ophthalmol. 2004;88(3):341-3.
26. Gedde SJ. Management of glaucoma after retinal detachment surgery. Curr Opin Ophthalmol. 2002;13(2):103-9.
27. Budenz DL, Taba KE, Feuer WJ, Eliezer R, Cousins S, Henderer J, et al. Surgical management of secondary glaucoma after pars plana vitrectomy and silicone oil injection for complex retinal detachment. Ophthalmology. 2001; 108(9):1628-32.
28. Kobayashi S, Inoue M, Yamane S, et al. Long-term outcomes after preoperative intravitreal injection of bevacizumab before trabeculectomy for neovascular glaucoma. J Glaucoma. 2016;25(3):281-4.
29. Shen C, Salim S, Du H, Netland P. Trabeculectomy versus Ahmed glaucoma valve implantation in neovascular glaucoma. Clin Ophthalmol. 2011;5:281-6.
30. Al-Jazzaf AM, Netland PA, Charles S. Incidence and management of elevated intraocular pressure after silicone oil injection. J Glaucoma. 2005;14(1):40-6.
31. Han SK, Park KH, Kim DM, Chang BL. Effect of diode laser trans-scleral cyclophotocoagulation in the management of glaucoma after intravitreal silicone oil injection for complicated retinal detachments. Br J Ophthalmol. 1999;83(6):713-7.
32. Ghazi-Nouri SMS, Vakalis AN, Bloom PA, et al. Long-term results of the management of silicone oil-induced raised intraocular pressure by diode laser cycloablation. Eye. 2004;19(7):765-9.
33. Sivagnanavel V, Ortiz-Hurtado A, Williamson TH. Diode laser trans-scleral cyclophotocoagulation in the management of glaucoma in patients with long-term intravitreal silicone oil. Eye. 2004;19(3):253-7.
34. Murthy GJ, Murthy PR, Murthy KR, Kulkarni VV, Murthy KR. A study of the efficacy of endoscopic cyclophotocoagulation for the treatment of refractory glaucomas. Indian J Ophthalmol. 2009;57(2):127-32.
35. Chen CJ. Glaucoma after macular hole surgery. Ophthalmology. 1998;105(1):94-100.
36. Hussain RN, Banerjee S. Densiron® 68 as an intraocular tamponade for complex inferior retinal detachments. Clin Ophthalmol. 2011;5:603-7.
37. Silicone Study Report 2. Vitrectomy with silicone oil or perfluoropropane gas in eyes with severe proliferative vitreoretinopathy: results of a randomized clinical trial. Arch Ophthalmol. 1992;110(6):780-92.

38. Silicone Study Report 1. Vitrectomy with silicone oil or sulfur hexafluoride gas in eyes with severe proliferative vitreoretinopathy: results of a randomized clinical trial. Arch Ophthalmol. 1992;110(6):770-9.

39. Abrams GW, Swanson DE, Sabates WI, Goldman AI. The results of sulfur hexafluoride gas in vitreous surgery. Am J Ophthalmol. 1982;94(2):165-71.

40. Chang S, Lincoff HA, Coleman DJ, Fuchs W, Farber ME. Perfluorocarbon gases in vitreous surgery. Ophthalmology. 1985;92(5):651-6.

41. Burk LL, Shields MB, Proia AD, McCuen BW 2nd. Intraocular pressure following intravitreal silicone oil injection. Ophthalmic Surg. 1988;19(8):565-9.

42. Lucke KH, Foerster MH, Laqua H. Long-term results of vitrectomy and silicone oil in 500 cases of complicated retinal detachments. Am J Ophthalmol. 1987;104(6): 624-33.

43. Nguyen QH, Lloyd MA, Heuer DK, et al. Incidence and management of glaucoma after intravitreal silicone oil injection for complicated retinal detachments. Ophthalmology. 1992;99(10):1520-6.

44. Mittra RA, Pollack JS, Dev S, et al. The use of topical aqueous suppressants in the prevention of postoperative intraocular pressure elevation after pars plana vitrectomy with long-acting gas tamponade. Ophthalmology. 2000;107(3):588-92.

CHAPTER 12D

Neovascular Glaucoma

Jasleen Dhillon

INTRODUCTION

Neovascular glaucoma (NVG) is a potentially blinding secondary glaucoma, which is therapeutically challenging to manage and is often associated with a poor prognosis. It is a sequela of ocular ischemic conditions, most commonly in 97% of cases caused by central retinal vein occlusion (CRVO) and proliferative diabetic retinopathy (PDR).

ETIOPATHOGENESIS

Diabetes

- Two percent in diabetes mellitus; 21% in PDR; 80% after pars plana vitrectomy (PPV)
- Neovascularization of iris (NVI) can be as high as 65% in PDR
- Incidence higher in case the posterior capsule integrity is compromised.

Ischemic Central Retinal Vein Occlusion

- Twenty-three to sixty percent (as high as 80% over 12–18 months)
- Eighty percent present in the first 6 months of CRVO
- Fifteen percent of nonischemic CRVO can convert to ischemic CRVO in 4 months and a total of 34% after 3 years.

Carotid Artery Obstructive Disease

This is the third most common cause accounting for 12% of cases. Severe hypoxia of ciliary body with resultant decreased aqueous production in this subset can cause eyes to be normotensive or hypotensive despite synechial closure.

Less common etiologies include:
- Branch retinal vein occlusion
- Intraocular tumors
- Chronic ocular inflammation
- Central retinal artery occlusion
- Chronic retinal detachment
- Anterior segment ischemia, e.g. postsquint surgery
- Ocular ischemic syndrome
- Sickle cell retinopathy.

The retinal hypoxia releases vasoproliferative factors, which induce neovascularization of the anterior segment with subsequent fibrovascular closure of the angle leading to a rapidly developing severe glaucoma.

CLINICAL FEATURES

The best management of NVG lies in its prevention and early detection. It is important to evaluate high-risk patients undilated on the slit lamp under high magnification to look for iris neovascularization and with gonioscopy to evaluate neovascularization of the angle.

Early iris neovascularization is seen as small tufts of blood vessels at the pupillary ruff, which can be easily missed unless looked for. These can also begin at the edges of an yttrium aluminum garnet iridotomy. The vessels then follow over the iris surface toward the angle in an irregular radial meandering fashion. At the angle, fine new vessels are seen to cross the scleral spur and ramify over the trabecular meshwork. The fibrosis of these vessels leads to development of ectropion uveae and synechial angle closure.

MANAGEMENT

The two-key aspects of managing the disease are: (1) managing the underlying ischemic pathology and (2) lowering the intraocular pressure (IOP). For the purpose of management, the following classification has been proposed.

Grades of Neovascular Glaucoma

- *Stage 1*: Early NVI or neovascularization of the angle (NVA) with open angles and normal IOP
- *Stage 2*: Clinically evident NVI or NVA with open angle and IOP between 20 mm Hg and 30 mm Hg
- *Stage 3*: Prominent NVI/NVA with angle closure, ectropion uvea and IOP over 30 mm Hg.

Stage 1: Neovascularization of iris+/Neovascularization of the Angle–Intraocular Pressure within Normal Limits
- *Target cause:* pan-retinal photocoagulation (PRP)
- Anti-vascular endothelial growth factor (VEGF)
- Pars plana vitrectomy + Endolaser/cataract surgery and PRP

Stage 2: Neovascularization of the Angle, Open Angles, High Intraocular Pressure
- *Address ischemic drive:* PRP
- ±Anti-VEGF
- Medical management
- Surgery if needed

Stage 3: Closed Angles and High Intraocular Pressure
- Panretinal photocoagulation, anti-VEGF
- Medication
- Surgery depending on visual potential, metabolite-augmented trabeculectomy/glaucoma drainage device (GDD)/cyclodestructive procedure
- Start multipronged treatment early.

Majority of patients present with stage 3 NVG with pain, photophobia, redness and decreased vision. Ocular examination reveals circumcorneal congestion, corneal edema, aqueous flare, iris and angle neovascularization, ectropion uveae and a markedly raised IOP. They may even have hyphema (Fig. 12D.1) and vitreous hemorrhage.

Management depends upon the grade of the disease, the visual potential, media clarity and underlying etiology.

Panretinal Photocoagulation

The definitive treatment is directed at the cause of ischemia and thus the mainstay of therapy is panretinal photocoagulation. PRP destroys ischemic retinal cells, thereby

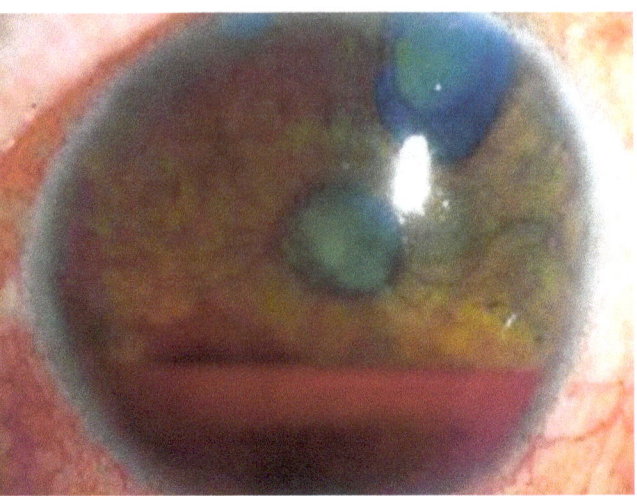

Fig. 12D.1: Hyphema in an eye with florid neovascularization of iris.

decreasing the stimulus for NV. PRP remains the treatment modality that affects the course of NVG in terms of decreasing the need for surgery to control IOP, reduce the metabolic needs of the hypoxic retina by reducing the total amount of functional retina, so remaining retinal circulation is sufficient to prevent further production of vessel growth factors by the nonablated retinal tissue. It takes 3–4 weeks for effect and has to be done extensively. If due to media haze or nondilating pupil, it is not possible to laser the periphery, one may need to couple it with endophotocoagulation or cryotherapy.

In established cases of PDR, PRP with or without intravitreal anti-VEGF is the procedure of choice to prevent NVG. Such patients deserve careful monitoring of iris and angle, even after standard course of PRP, so that further retinal ablation can be done if new vessels develop or progress in the anterior segment.

However, in patients with CRVO with no evidence of neovascularization, prophylactic PRP showed no significant difference in the incidence of NVG as compared to eyes without PRP. The Central Retinal Vein Occlusion Study (CVOS) essentially recommended careful follow-up of patients with ischemic CRVO and PRP was indicated for fundus fluorescein angiography (FFA) confirmed ischemic CRVO who developed 2 o'clock hours of NVI or NVA.

Antivascular Endothelial Growth Factor

Anti-VEGF injections provide a rapid regression of new vessels and are a useful adjunct for glaucoma surgery and PRP. They provide a temporizing measure while the effect of PRP comes and in glaucoma surgery reduce intra- and postoperative complications, like hyphema.

The main cause of proliferative anterior segment neovascularization is posterior segment ischemia. Due to the posterior location—as well as the potential for the vitreous body to serve as a reservoir for the anti-VEGF medication and ensure a prolonged effect—intravitreal injections are a preferred location for injections in NVG. When anatomic landmarks are unclear, or the clinician is more comfortable with anterior segment surgery, intracameral injections are also effective at decreasing NVI and NVA.

Close monitoring is essential as recurrence of neovascularization or synechial closure due to fibrosis of ghost vessels remains a risk.

Medical Management of Neovascular Glaucoma

The IOP is medically managed temporarily with topical β-blockers and carbonic anhydrase inhibitors. Prostaglandins may be added to the armamentarium, wherever needed, although not as first choice since they increase inflammation and with synechial closure they are not effective enough. Systemic hypo-osmotics and carbonic anhydrase inhibitors are used where indicated after ruling out systemic contraindications.

Symptomatic relief is brought about by anti-inflammatory agents and atropine.

Surgical Management of Glaucoma

There is no consensus on which glaucoma incisional surgery works best for NVG. Because of its complicated nature, NVG was an exclusion criterion for the tube versus trabeculectomy study. Both trabeculectomy with adjunctive antimetabolite and GDD surgery is advocated for NVG depending upon the clinical picture, age, previous ocular surgery, presence of scarring and surgeons expertise. It is best to control inflammation and neovascularization as far as is possible before glaucoma surgery for better clinical outcome. It is usually timed 3–4 weeks after PRP and within a week of anti-VEGF. A higher risk of complications and failure is expected due to the inflammation, hyphema, choroidal detachment, shallow anterior chamber (AC) and postoperative hypotony. The antimetabolite is applied for longer duration and may be applied both subconjunctival and subscleral, avoid sudden hypotony and use preplaced sutures. The tube may be placed via the pars plana route where the anterior segment has excessive scarring.

The surgery may be combined with phacoemulsification where the media haze is precluding adequate laser and with vitrectomy in case of vitreous hemorrhage.

The success rate is reasonable in the short-term (62–86% at 1 year) coming down to about 10% at 5 years. A significant number had no light perception (31–48%).

Management options are elucidated in the following clinical scenarios.

Case 1: NVG in a diabetic with PDR

A 65-year-old male presented to the clinic with blurring of vision in right eye for the past 1 month. He had a history of long-standing diabetes moderately controlled for 20 years. On examination he was found to have a best-corrected visual acuity (BCVA) of 6/9 in the right eye and 6/60 in the left eye. The applanation tonometry revealed an IOP of was 18 mm Hg in the right eye and 26 mm Hg in the left eye. Slit-lamp examination revealed neovascularization of the iris at the pupillary ruff over 3-clock hours and early cortical cataract in left eye. The angles were open with no evidence of neovascularization. Fundus examination revealed moderate non-PDR in the right eye and PDR with clinically significant macular edema in the left eye. The optic disc was perfused with no evidence of glaucomatous changes.

The IOPs were brought down by topical brimonidine and timolol combination BD. Following FFA, early PRP was performed over three sittings. The NVI was seen to regress at 2 weeks follow-up and the glaucoma medications were tapered over 2 months. The IOPs were normal on single glaucoma medication and the retina was stable at last follow-up.

Careful high magnification undilated slit-lamp examination is mandatory in all high-risk patients to pick-up early neovascularization even in the absence of high IOP.

It is also to be noted that neovascularization angle may in rare instances be present in the absence of NVI (noted in 6–12% of CRVO patients), so gonioscopy should also be routinely done in this category of patients.

Case 2: NVG in vascular occlusion

A 58-year-old female patient presented with pain and blurring of vision in right eye since 1 week. She had a history of hypertension for over 12 years and had undergone angioplasty few months back. She was diagnosed with CRVO with NVG in her right eye. The IOP was oculus dexter (OD) 42 mm Hg/oculus sinister (OS) 16 mm Hg and the right eye had corneal stromal edema, aqueous flare, NVI with the gonioscopic examination showing open angles with NVA over nearly 270°. The BCVA was OD FC 4 meters and OS 6/12.

Medical lowering of IOP was achieved with systemic acetazolamide and topical dorzolamide and brimonidine-timolol combination. The cornea cleared to allow early completion of PRP. The NVI regressed over 2 weeks and the angle showed fine peripheral anterior synechiae over 2 clock hours. At 8 weeks, IOP was maintained between 14 mm Hg and 17 mm Hg with brimonidine TID and the optic had regressed NVD with shallow cupping of about 0.5. The patient was advised to follow-up every 6 weeks.

At 4 months follow-up, IOP was found to be 28 mm Hg and the angle had synechial closure over 180°. There was no active neovascularization and the patient was advised to undergo trabeculectomy with mitomycin C (MMC). The postoperative period was uneventful and the patient was maintained at 6 months follow-up on no antiglaucoma medications.

Careful frequent follow-up is important in patients of NVG since the ghost-regressed vessels over the iris can cause scarring and zipping-up of the angle even after a thorough extensive PRP.

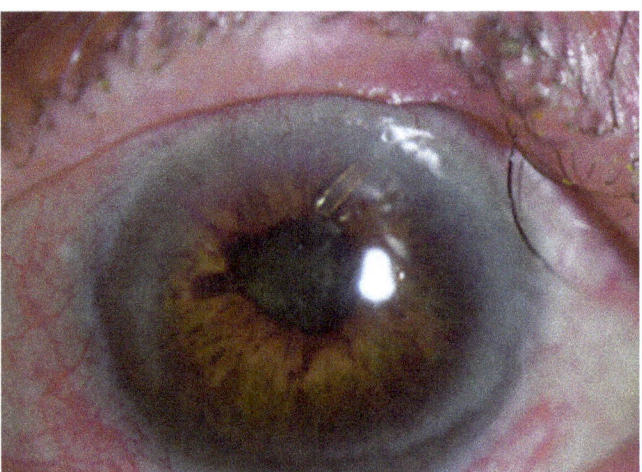

Fig. 12D.2: Ahmed glaucoma valve in an eye with partially regressed neovascularization of iris.

Case 3: Anti VEGF for NVG

A 71-year-old male with systemic history of diabetes and kidney disease came with painful red eye to the clinic of 1 week duration. He was found to have extensive NVI and NVA with synechial closure 270°. Fundus examination revealed PDR. The applanation IOP of affected eye was 50 mm Hg and since there was relative contraindication of systemic hypotensive agents, he was started on dorzolamide TID, brimonidine-timolol combination and prostaglandin analog HS. Intravitreal anti-VEGF was given along with controlled paracentesis following which an Ahmed glaucoma valve surgery was performed 2 days later (Fig. 12D.2). On the day of surgery, the NVI was regressing, the anterior chamber was quieter, IOP was 28 mm Hg and the visual acuity had improved from finger count close to face and the visual acuity had improved from finger count close to face to finger count at 3 meters. The PRP was started on postoperative day 2 with laser indirect ophthalmoscope and completed over more frequent sittings where fewer lower energy laser shots were applied to reduce risk of choroidal detachment. The IOP was controlled at 14–16 mm Hg at 2 months follow-up. The visual acuity was 6/60.

- In cases, where oral hypo-osmotics are contraindicated prostaglandins may be added
- Anti-VEGF can raise the IOP further and in cases with very high IOP should be done under systemic hypo-osmotics, wherever, not contraindicated and

with controlled paracentesis. Some surgeons advocate combining it with limited core vitrectomy

- Early intervention is paramount in preserving vision
- Under the cover of anti-VEGF glaucoma surgery can be performed within the week to decrease the neovascularization and to decrease complications, like hyphema.

Case 4: PRP for NVG

A 58-year-old woman came with diminished vision in right eye with redness. On examination, the visual acuity in OD was FC 3 meter with relative afferent pupillary defect and NVI extending across the iris surface. Gonioscopy revealed NVA with synechial closure over 270°. The applanation IOP was 56 mm Hg OD. The fundus details were poorly appreciated due to cataract, but a diagnosis of ischemic CRVO was established. Prompt medical management with systemic hypotensive agents, full regime of topical antiglaucoma drugs was started. PRP was only possible to a very limited extent due to the cataract and it was decided to proceed with combined phacoemulsification and tube shunt surgery after 3 days of intracameral and intravitreal anti-VEGF (Figs. 12D.3A and B). This was followed by PRP starting post day 2. The vision improved to 6/60 p and the IOP was controlled to 15–18 mm Hg.

- Preferably, wherever, possible avoid combining phacoemulsification with glaucoma surgery-increased inflammation and poorer success
- Panretinal photocoagulation and anti-VEGF improves the surgical success and decreases complications of glaucoma surgery

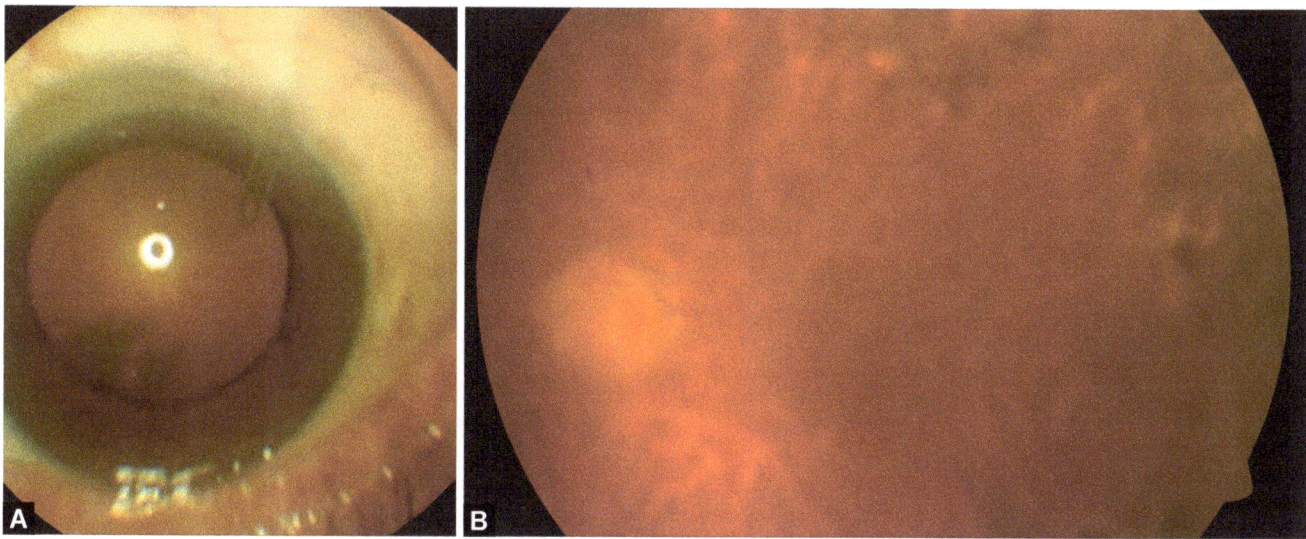

Figs. 12D.3A and B: (A) Ahmed glaucoma valve implanted following intravitreal bevacizumab in a case of neovascular glaucoma with central retinal vein occlusion; (B) central retinal vein occlusion as seen through hazy media.

- If media haze not allowing PRP then may need to go for combined procedure
- Glaucoma drainage devices preferred over trabeculectomy and in case of extensive synechiae a ciliary sulcus tube placement is a better option
- *Special precautions in glaucoma surgery:* avoid sudden hypotony (preplaced sutures, sodium hyaluronate); higher dose/longer duration of MMC, avoid pulling iris root during iridotomy; air tamponade. Postoperatively advise head end elevation and aggressive steroids and cycloplegics, closer follow-up, intervene early.

Case 5: PPV with GDD for NVG

A 63-year-old male presented with sudden blurring of vision in left eye. On examination, he was diagnosed with NVG with PDR with vitreous hemorrhage. After initiating medical treatment for glaucoma, intravitreal anti-VEGF was injected and PRP was attempted in, whatever, area was visible. By a week, there was only partial regression of neovascularization and IOP was 34 mm Hg on treatment. A PPV was done along with endolaser diode photocoagulation combined with a tube surgery. The IOPs were in the middle teens and the visual acuity was 6/36 at 2 months follow-up.

Case 6: TSCPC for NVG

A 75-year-old man with florid NVG, no PL and stony hard eye presented to the OPD. He had been diagnosed with CRVO 2 years ago and had incipient NVI then. He had undergone incomplete PRP and was lost to follow-up. He now presented with IOP of 72 mm Hg and had corneal edema, florid new vessels over the iris, angle and cornea with hyphen over the lower half. The patient was pseudophakic and posterior segment could not be evaluated due to vitreous hemorrhage. After discussing the treatment options and visual prognosis the patient opted for diode laser photocoagulation diode laser cyclophotocoagulation (DLCP) over 180°. At 1 month, the IOP was settled at 32 mm Hg on antiglaucoma medications and cycloplegics and the patient was comfortable. He was explained probable need for a second sitting in case of symptoms.

SUGGESTED READING

1. Castaneda-Díez, García-Aguirre, Vitrectomía en Pacientes Diabéticos con Glaucoma Neovascular, Highlights of vitreoretina, 2010.
2. Calugaru D, Calugaru M. Prevention of neovascular glaucoma. Ophthalmology. 2013;120(7):1507-8.
3. Chalam KV, Gupta SK, Grover S, et al. Intracameral Avastin dramatically resolves iris neovascularization and reverses neovascular glaucoma. Eur J Ophthalmol. 2008;18(2): 255-62.
4. Chatterjee S, Rao A. Intraocular pressure following combined routes of bevacizumab-augmented trabeculectomy for refractory neovascular glaucoma. Semin Ophthalmol. 2013;28(2):72-4.
5. Chen TC, Ahn Yuen SJ, Sangalang MA, et al. Retrobulbar chlorpromazine injections for the management of blind and seeing painful eyes. J Glaucoma. 2002;11(3):209-13.

6. Ehlers JP, Spirn MJ, Lam A, et al. Combination intravitreal bevacizumab/panretinal photocoagulation versus panretinal photocoagulation alone in the treatment of neovascular glaucoma. Retina. 2008;28(5):696-702.

7. Gedde SJ, Schiffman JC, Feuer WJ, et al. Treatment outcomes in the Tube Versus Trabeculectomy (TVT) Study after five years of follow-up. Am J Ophthalmol. 2012;153(5):789-803.

8. Horsley MB, Kahook MY. Anti-VEGF therapy for glaucoma. Curr Opin Ophthalmol. 2010;21(2):112-7.

9. Huddleston SM, Feldman RM, Budenz DL, et al. Aqueous shunt exposure: a retrospective review of repair outcome. J Glaucoma. 2013;22(6):433-8.

10. Lüke J, Nassar K, Lüke M, et al. Ranibizumab as adjuvant in the treatment of rubeosis iridis and neovascular glaucoma-results from a prospective interventional case series. Graefes Arch Clin Exp Ophthalmol. 2013;251(10):2403-13.

11. Ma KT, Yang JY, Kim JH, et al. Surgical results of Ahmed valve implantation with intraoperative bevacizumab injection in patients with neovascular glaucoma. J Glaucoma. 2012;21(5):331-6.

12. Mermoud A, Salmon JF, Alexander P, et al. Molteno tube implantation for neovascular glaucoma. Long-term results and factors influencing the outcome. Ophthalmology. 1993; 100(6):897-902.

13. Moraczewski AL, Lee RK, Palmberg PF, et al. Outcomes of treatment of neovascular glaucoma with intravitreal bevacizumab. Br J Ophthalmol. 2009;93(5):589-93.

14. Saito Y, Higashide T, Takeda H, et al. Beneficial effects of preoperative intravitreal bevacizumab on trabeculectomy outcomes in neovascular glaucoma. Acta Ophthalmol. 2010;88(1):96-102.

15. Sidoti PA, Dunphy TR, Baerveldt G, et al. Experience with the Baerveldt glaucoma implant in treating neovascular glaucoma. Ophthalmology. 1995;102(7):1107-18.

16. SooHoo JR, Seibold LK, Kahook MY. Recent advances in the management of neovascular glaucoma. Semin Ophthalmol. 2013;28(3):165-72.

17. Takihara Y, Inatani M, Fukushima M, et al. Trabeculectomy with mitomycin C for neovascular glaucoma: prognostic factors for surgical failure. Am J Ophthalmol. 2009; 147(5):912-8.

18. The Central Vein Occlusion Study Group N report. A randomized clinical trial of early panretinal photocoagulation for ischemic central vein occlusion. Ophthalmology. 1995; 102(10):1434-44.

19. Wakabayashi T, Oshima Y, Sakaguchi H, et al. Intravitreal bevacizumab to treat iris neovascularization and neovascular glaucoma secondary to ischemic retinal diseases in 41 consecutive cases. Ophthalmology. 2008;115(9): 1571-80.

20. Wand M, Dueker DK, Aiello LM, Grant WM. Effects of panretinal photocoagulation on rubeosis iridis, angle neovascularization, and neovascular glaucoma. Am J Ophthalmol. 1978;86(3):332-9.

21. Yildirim N, Yalvac IS, Sahin A, et al. A comparative study between diode laser cyclophotocoagulation and the Ahmed glaucoma valve implant in neovascular glaucoma: a long-term follow-up. J Glaucoma. 2009;18(3):192-6.

Cataract and Glaucoma

M Chockalingam

Cataract and glaucoma may coexist especially in elderly individuals. The management of either necessitates consideration of both conditions. Therefore, the decision for either cataract or glaucoma surgery or combined glaucoma and cataract surgery requires evaluation of need for visual rehabilitation and adequate intraocular pressure control.

Case 1: Cataract surgery alone in an eye with no prior glaucoma filtration surgery

Mr ABC, a 67-year-old gentleman, was found to have reduced visual acuity (6/36, N18) in the left eye. Slit-lamp evaluation revealed deep anterior chamber and immature cataract in both eyes (nuclear sclerosis Grade II in the right eye and nuclear sclerosis Grade III in the left eye). His intraocular pressure by applanation tonometry was 14 mm Hg and 13 mm Hg in the right eye and left eye, respectively. Gonioscopy showed open angles. The cup-to-disc (C:D) ratio was 0.30:1 and 0.40:1 in the right and left eye, respectively (Fig. 12E.1).

The visual fields showed early nasal step in the left eye and was normal in the right eye (Fig. 12E.2). The central corneal thickness by ultrasonic pachymetry was 543 microns and 534 microns in the right eye and left eye, respectively. He was on Brimonidine tartrate (0.15%) eye drops TID, both eyes. The status of condition, cataract and glaucoma (which was adequately controlled with one medication) was discussed with the patient, and he underwent phacoemulsification with foldable intraocular lens implantation through a clear corneal incision and was advised to continue with the glaucoma medication in the left eye.

Case 2: Cataract and glaucoma surgery

Mr XYZ, a 73-year-old gentleman, was found to have reduced visual acuity (6/60, N36) in the left eye. Slit-lamp evaluation revealed deep anterior chamber and immature cataract (nuclear sclerosis Grade III) in the left eye and early lens changes in the right eye. His intraocular pressure by applanation tonometry was 19 mm Hg and 21 mm Hg in

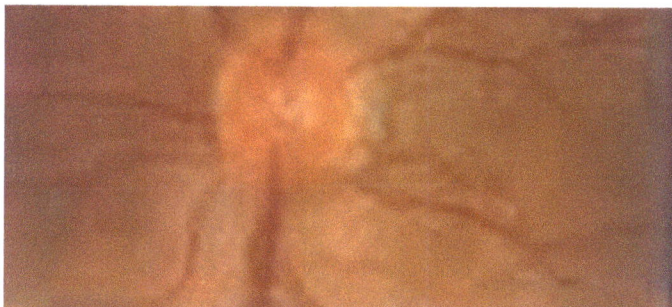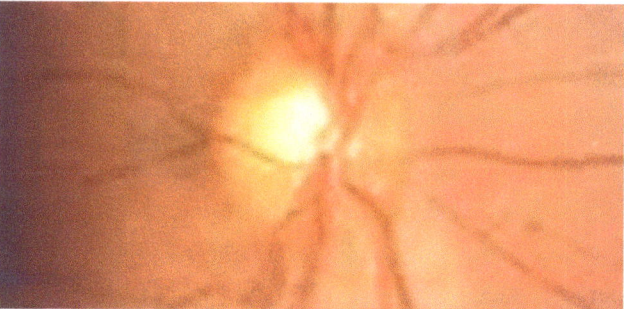

Fig. 12E.1: Optic nerve photograph showing early cupping in the left eye (Case 1).

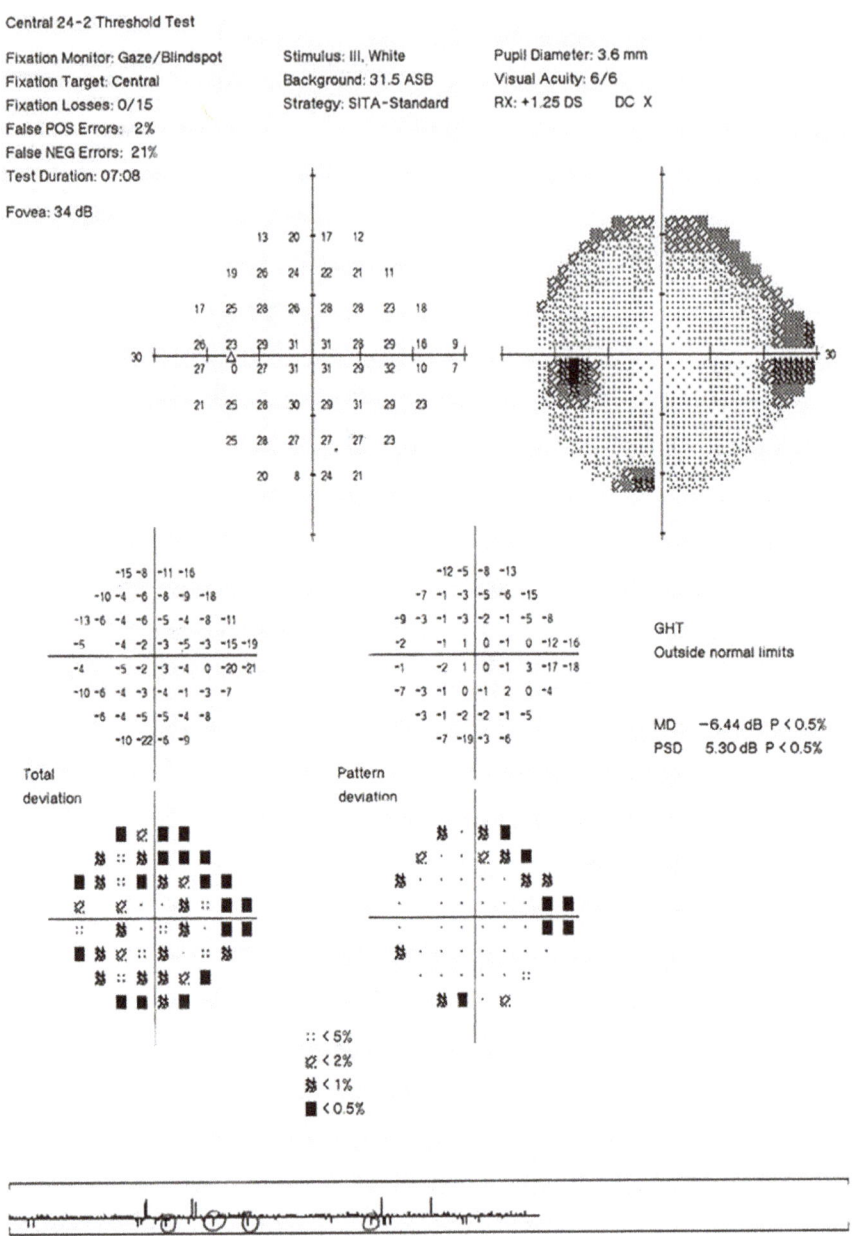

Fig. 12E.2: Visual fields showing nasal step in the left eye. (POS: Positive; NEG: Negative; SITA: Swedish interactive thresholding algorithm; GHT: Glaucoma hemifield test; MD: Mean deviation; PSD: Pattern standard deviation).

the right eye and left eye, respectively. Gonioscopy showed open angles. The C:D ratio was 0.65:1 and 0.80:1 in the right and left eye, respectively, with extensive neuroretinal rim loss, splinter hemorrhage in both eyes and bipolar notch in the left eye (Fig. 12E.3). The visual fields showed moderate field loss in the right eye and superior arcuate scotoma in the left eye (Fig. 12E.4). The central corneal thickness by ultrasonic pachymetry was 512 microns and 503 microns in the right and left eye, respectively. He was on brimonidine

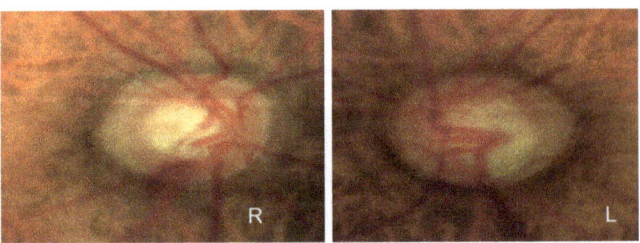

Fig. 12E.3: Optic disc photograph showing advanced glaucomatous cupping in the left eye (Case 2).

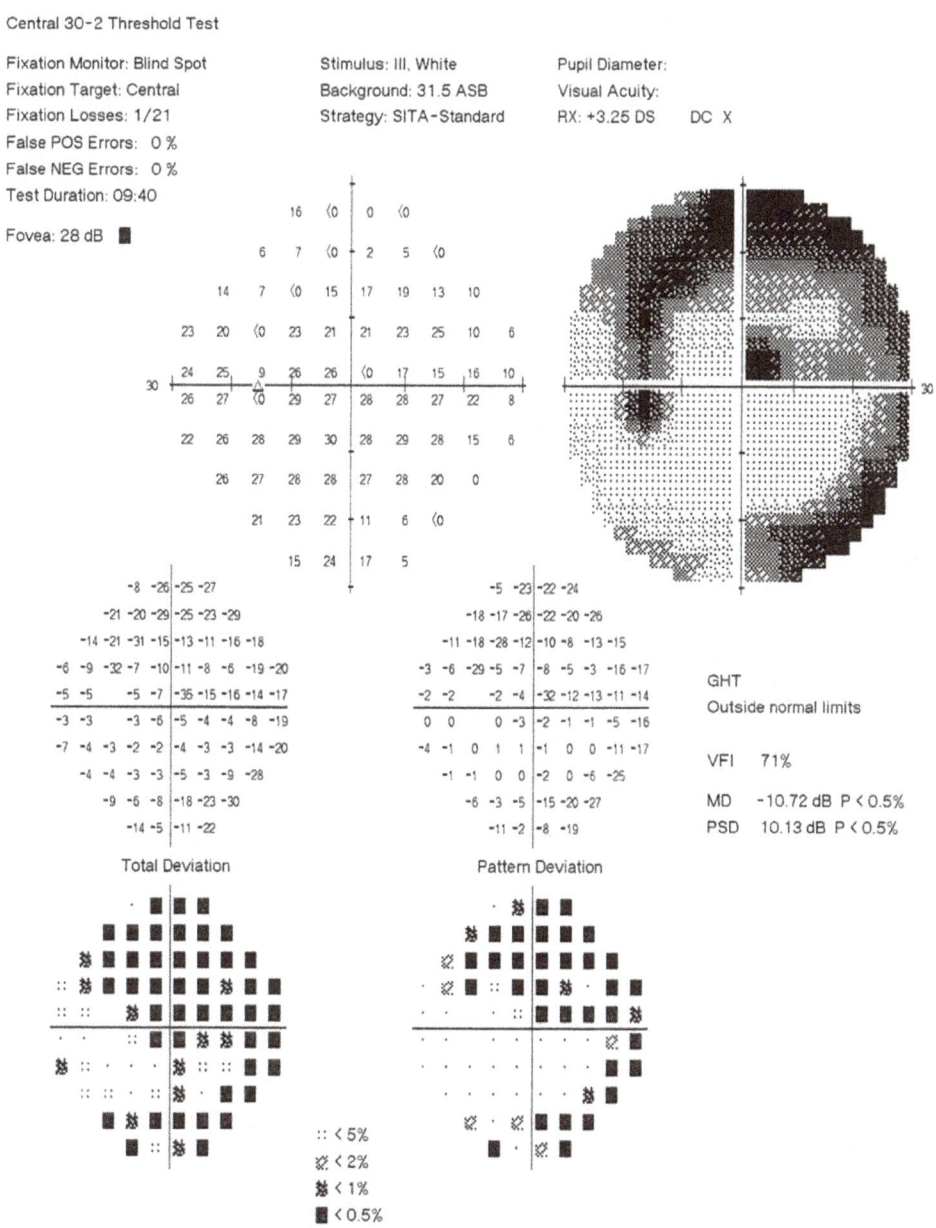

Fig. 12E.4: Visual fields showing double arcuate scotoma in the left eye in Case 2. (POS: Positive; NEG: Negative; SITA: Swedish interactive thresholding algorithm; GHT: Glaucoma hemifield test; MD: Mean deviation; PSD: Pattern standard deviation).

tartrate + timolol maleate 0.5% combination eye drops twice a day along with bimatoprost eye drops 0.1% to both eyes. The status of condition, cataract and glaucoma (which was not well-controlled with more one medication) was discussed with the patient, and he underwent phacoemulsification with foldable intraocular lens implantation through a clear corneal incision and trabeculectomy (separate site) in a single setting in the left eye.

Case 3: Sequential glaucoma and cataract (cataract surgery post-trabeculectomy)

Mr PQR, a 53-year-old gentleman, was found to have reduced visual acuity (6/60, N36) in the left eye. He gave a history of having undergone glaucoma filtration surgery in the left eye in the past and was on dorzolamide 2% + timolol maleate 0.5% eye drops in the right eye. Slit-lamp evaluation revealed deep anterior chamber and immature cataract (nuclear sclerosis Grade II–III) in both eyes. There was a filtering bleb in the superonasal quadrant of the left eye. His intraocular pressure by applanation tonometry was 21 mm Hg and 14 mm Hg in the right eye and left eye, respectively. Gonioscopy showed open angles in both eyes with patent internal ostium in the left eye (Fig. 12E.5). The C:D ratio was 0.70:1 and 0.80:1 with extensive neuroretinal rim loss in the right and left eye, respectively. The visual fields showed double arcuate scotoma in left eye (Fig. 12E.6). The central corneal thickness by ultrasonic pachymetry was 502 microns and 503 microns in the right and left eye, respectively. The status of condition, cataract and glaucoma (which was under control) was discussed with the patient, and he underwent phacoemulsification with foldable intraocular lens implantation through a clear corneal incision at a site away from in the left eye filtering bleb.

WORKUP OF A PATIENT BEFORE DECISION-MAKING AND SURGERY

Every patient, who presents with cataract and glaucoma, requires a careful and comprehensive eye examination to enable appropriate decision-making and management.

Workup the patient includes:

- *Details of glaucoma medications used*: number and type of medications, medication side effects, compliance, quality of life issues
- *History of prior trauma or inflammation*: which have a bearing on the performance and outcome of cataract and/or glaucoma surgery
- Visual acuity and refraction
- *Slit-lamp evaluation*: density and location of lenticular opacity, pseudoexfoliation, anterior chamber depth and asymmetry of depth between eyes (if any), presence of filtering bleb, peripheral iridotomy, presence of peripheral anterior and posterior synechiae, phacodonesis/iridodonesis/subluxation of lens, abnormal irido-lenticular gap, etc. pupil status and extent of pupil dilatation should be checked to enable needs for enhancing pupil dilatation during cataract surgery if needed by additional methods
- Tonometry with Goldmann applanation tonometer to record intraocular pressure
- Gonioscopy to look for status of angle, i.e. extent to which the angle is open, presence of ostium or internal opening of valve shunts, angle recession, etc.

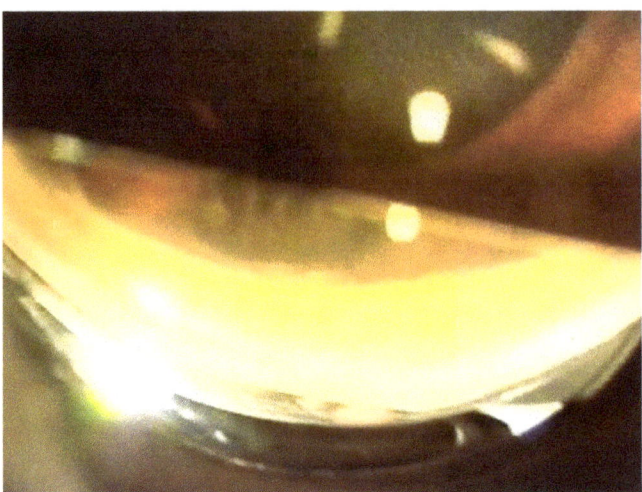

Fig. 12E.5: Trabeculectomy ostium.

- Ultrasonic pachymetry to measure the central corneal thickness
- *Optic nerve assessment*: A dilated fundus examination with assessment of the optic nerve head is a must with hand drawn, labeled diagram with emphasis on C:D ratio, notching, retinal nerve fiber layer defects and/or hemorrhage
- If feasible, a slit-lamp photograph in dilated state along with a color photo and red-free photo of the optic nerve head (subject to reasonable visualization of the fundus) may be done for documentation and serial follow-up
- Visual field testing to be done to establish extent of visual loss and can be followed-up after surgery to find changes in the same
- Imaging of the optic nerve with retinal nerve fiber analysis (ocular coherence tomography, Heidelberg retinal tomography or scanning laser polarimetry) may be done subject to appropriate visualization of the fundus and this provides a statistical comparison with the normative database.

FOLLOW-UP PROTOCOL

Monitoring of the intraocular pressure after cataract or combined surgery is essential and it is important to blunt any postoperative intraocular pressure spikes. In patients, who have undergone phacoemulsification only and were on glaucoma medications before surgery, the same may be continued after surgery. Following a combined surgery, glaucoma medications have to be summarily stopped from the day of surgery. We have to look out for

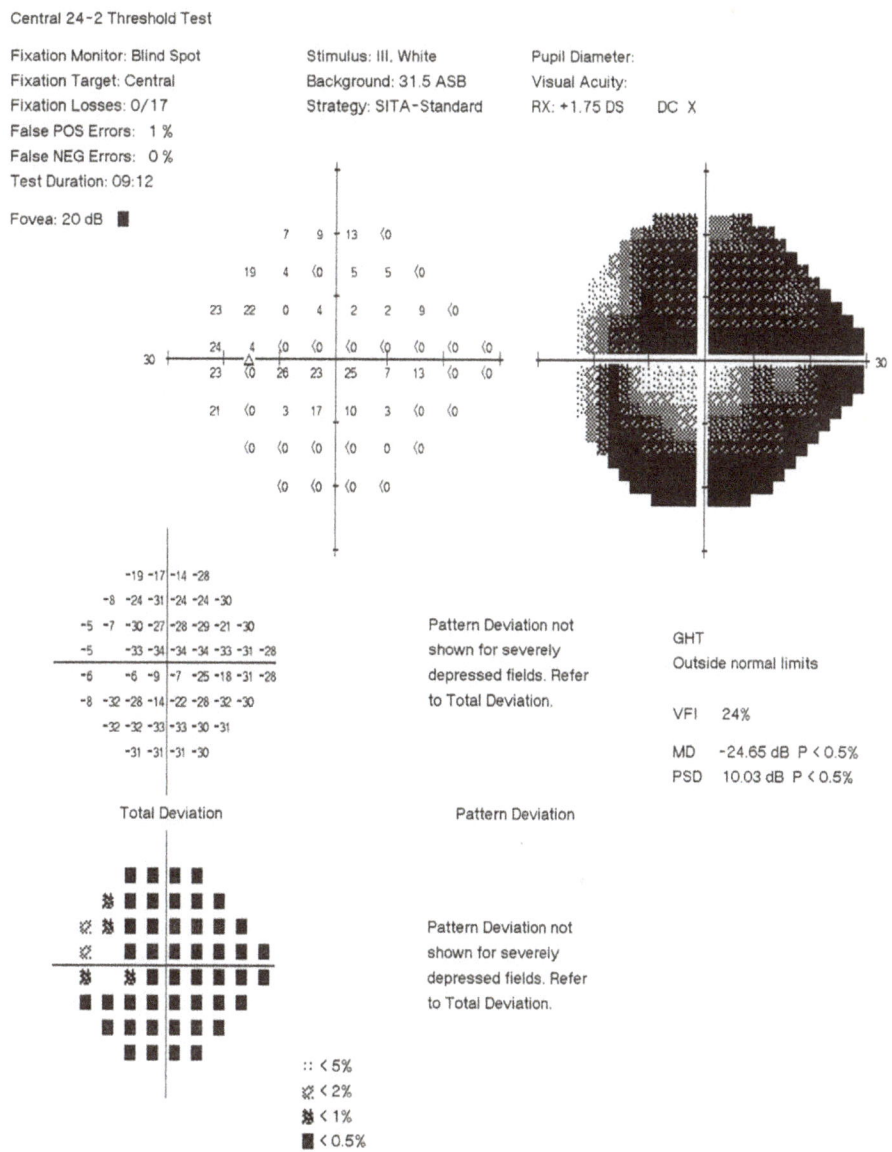

Fig. 12E.6: Visual fields showing dense double arcuate scotoma in the left eye.
(POS: Positive; NEG: Negative; GHT: Glaucoma hemifield test; MD: Mean deviation; SITA: Swedish interactive thresholding algorithm; PSD: Pattern standard deviation).

presence of inflammation, shallow anterior chamber and handle the same. Following a combined procedure, appropriate intervention, like suture removal or suture lysis, to achieve desired intraocular pressure should be done at an appropriate time. Aggressive management of bleb may be needed should there be bleb fibrosis or failure following cataract surgery in an eye with prior trabeculectomy.

Long-term follow-up is crucial as patients may return to preoperative or higher intraocular pressure at a later date necessitating reinstitution of medical therapy.

KEY POINTS TO BE CONSIDERED IN DECISION-MAKING

The following are the key points to be considered in decision-making as to whether a patient requires (A) Combined cataract and glaucoma surgery; (B) Cataract surgery alone or (C) Sequential cataract surgery followed by glaucoma filtration surgery:

- A small cataract may have a disproportionately large effect in the glaucomatous eye, especially in the presence of advanced visual field loss

Table 12E.1: Advantages and disadvantages of cataract surgery alone.

Advantages	Disadvantages
Restores vision	Early postoperative IOP elevation
Simple and short procedure	Continued dependence on medications and reduced long-term IOP control compared to combined surgery
Glaucoma filtration surgery may be done later if needed	Future filtration surgery is compromised if conjunctiva is compromised

(IOP: Intraocular pressure).

- Type of glaucoma, extent of intraocular pressure control, glaucoma medications used—number and type of medications, status of angle (closed or open), severity of optic nerve damage due to glaucoma, visual field loss, history of prior laser iridotomy, laser trabeculoplasty, incisional surgery—cataract, glaucoma or other surgery all influence the decision-making as to the surgical modality that is being planned.

Cataract Surgery Alone with No Previous Glaucoma Filtration Surgery

Indications

Glaucomatous eyes with:
- Visually significant cataract
- Intraocular pressure well controlled with one or two medications
- Good compliance and no major systemic side effects due to medications
- No significant glaucomatous visual field loss/cupping
- Anatomically narrow angles compromised by an enlarging cataractous lens
- A dense cataract that prevents adequate evaluation of the optic disc and visual fields in one eye but whose visual complaints are minimal due to normal vision in the other eye.

Advantages and Disadvantages of Cataract Surgery Alone

The advantages and disadvantages of cataract surgery alone are described in Table 12E.1.

Pearls in Surgical Technique

These are as follows:
- Use preoperative nonsteroidal anti-inflammatory drops to decrease risk of postoperative cystoid macular edema
- Do not discontinue antiglaucoma medications
- Perform surgery under topical anesthesia if feasible

- Perform surgery in a temporal aspect to preserve superior conjunctiva if filtration surgery is needed in the future
- Be prepared to manage special situations like:
  - Small pupil intracameral medications (epinephrine + lignocaine), viscoelastic pupil dilatation, release of posterior synechiae with an iris sweep, pupil manipulation manually by multiple sphincterotomies using a Rappazzo scissors, pupillary stretching using Kuglen's iris hooks and by using pupil expansion devices, like iris hooks and pupil expansion rings like the Malyugin ring
  - Intraoperative floppy iris syndrome in patients on α-1-blocking agents, like tamsulosin presents with poor pupil dilation, floppy iris, iris prolapse and progressive intraoperative miosis. The clear corneal tunnel should be long with a relative anterior entry to avoid iris prolapse, use high-density viscoelastic, like Healon 5 (Alcon Laboratories, Fort Worth, TX), keep low-flow parameters, avoid infusion directed at the iris plane and if the iris billows then use a Y-shaped retractor to move the iris back and up so that the billowing is stopped
  - *Zonular weakness*—very common in exfoliation syndrome and post-trauma. Do effective hydrodissection to achieve free rotation of the nucleus. Use capsule retractors, capsule tension rings or capsule-retaining segments to prevent zonule dehiscence during surgery
  - Crowded anterior chamber in high-hyperopic patients and in nanophthalmic eyes poses a challenge in performing phacoemulsification. The clear corneal tunnel should be long with a relative anterior entry to avoid iris prolapse, use high-density viscoelastic, like Healon 5 (Alcon Laboratories, Fort Worth, Texas) to maintain anterior chamber depth and flatten the iris/lens contour. If needed a pars plana vitrectomy or vitreous tap may be done to enable satisfactory anterior chamber depth to permit a reasonably sized and safe continuous curvilinear capsulorhexis, small pupil, if present, needs to be appropriately managed

– Vitreous loss during cataract surgery in patient with glaucoma with or without a functioning filtering bleb is a potentially serious complication. Dealing with this complication appropriately will minimize the possibility of a significant increase in the postoperative intraocular pressure. Complete and meticulous removal of vitreous from the anterior chamber will ensure success of subsequent filtering surgery if needed. If insufficient posterior capsule remains, residual anterior capsule allows sulcus fixation of a three-piece posterior chamber intraocular lens. An anterior chamber intraocular lens is best avoided. If an intraocular lens cannot be placed due to poor capsular support, the same may be deferred and done as a second stage procedure when a scleral-fixated intraocular lens may be placed, however; with a cost of loss of conjunctival integrity should a trabeculectomy be needed in the future.

Combined Cataract and Glaucoma Surgery

Indications

Glaucomatous eyes with:
- Visually significant cataract with uncontrolled intraocular pressure
- Visually significant cataract and controlled on multiple (more than two) medications or intolerant to medications
- Visually significant cataract and controlled intraocular pressure but with glaucomatous damage ranging from moderate-to-advanced (e.g. superior or inferior arcuate defect approaching fixation)

- Visually significant cataract and inadequate bleb function despite previous glaucoma filtration surgery necessitating reinstitution of medical therapy.

Advantages and Disadvantages of Combined Cataract and Trabeculectomy Surgery

The advantages and disadvantages of combined cataract and glaucoma surgery in comparison with cataract surgery alone or trabeculectomy alone is summarized in Table 12E.2.

Single-site versus Twin-site Combined Procedure

The salient difference between single-site and twin-site combined procedures is summarized in Table 12E.3.

Pearls in Surgical Technique

- Combined surgery necessitates the use of regional anesthesia
- In a single site combined surgery, superonasal or superotemporal quadrant is chosen leaving the other for future filtration surgery if needed; it is preferable to operate in a slightly superotemporal approach in combined surgery because it facilitates access to the surgical site
- In two site combined surgery, a temporal clear corneal phacoemulsification is combined with filtration surgery done in either the superonasal or superotemporal quadrant
- A fornix-based flap is preferred as it requires less manipulation of the conjunctiva during surgery, has less need for a surgical assistant, and provides better visualization of the limbus

Table 12E.2: Advantages and disadvantages of combined cataract and trabeculectomy surgery.

Advantages	Disadvantages
Immediate visual rehabilitation	Longer surgical time
Single procedure	Increased intraoperative and postoperative complications
Good short- and long-term intraocular pressure control	Intensive postoperative care needed unlike for simple cataract surgery

Table 12E.3: Differences between single-site and twin-site combined procedures.

Salient differences between single site and twin-site combined procedures	Twin-site surgery
Simple and less time-consuming	More time-consuming
Manipulation of the eye tissue at the filtering site during cataract surgery	Minimizes manipulation of conjunctiva and scleral flap intraoperatively
Surgically less comfortable to do the procedure	More comfortable to do the temporal site phacoemulsification
Increase in postoperative astigmatism	Lesser incidence of postoperative astigmatism

- Antiproliferative agents, like 5-fluorouracil or mitomycin may be used taking into account the potential risk factors like short-term or long-term hypotony, thin blebs, bleb leaks and endophthalmitis. Alternatively, Collagen Matrix may be used for enhancing filtration especially in myopic individuals with thinner sclera
- In twin-site combined surgery, either phacoemulsification is performed first via a temporal incision followed by trabeculectomy or the partial thickness scleral flap is created in the superonasal or superotemporal quadrant and stopped just short of entry into anterior chamber. Then a temporal clear corneal phacoemulsification is completed and a foldable intraocular lens is inserted; following this anterior chamber is entered from underneath the scleral flap, sclerectomy, iridectomy and flap closure are done
- A peripheral iridectomy should be done mandatorily after sclerostomy. It is also important to ensure the excised iris tissue is washed out of the anterior chamber to prevent any post operative pigment dispersion over the iol surface by the remanant iridectomy tissue
- In twin site incision, it is mandatory to place a 10–0 nylon suture at the cataract incision to maintain anterior chamber stability during trabeculectomy
- It is preferable to close the scleral flap with releasable sutures to enable titration of the intraocular pressure to the desired level after surgery.

Two-staged Cataract and Glaucoma Surgery

Indications

Glaucomatous eyes postfiltration surgery with:
- A well-functioning filtering bleb and adequate intraocular pressure control on no or minimal medical therapy with
- Progressive cataract.

Pearls in Surgical Technique

- With regards to the surgical approach, preservation of the bleb and remaining conjunctiva is the highest priority

- Ideally surgery should be done under topical anesthesia and should regional anesthesia be needed then digital massage or application of super pinky should be avoided to prevent damage to the pre-existing bleb
- Incision placement and wound configuration play an important role in ensuring successful outcome. Clear corneal phacoemulsification remains the surgery of choice in these patients as it aids in preserving conjunctiva in the event of bleb failure and the need for additional filtration surgery. Extensive iris manipulation and other maneuvers that might increase inflammation or decrease aqueous flow at the filtration site should be avoided. Bottle height should not be kept too high to avoid excessive anterior chamber deepening
- The chances of hypotony after surgery are eliminated by adequate wound closure with a 10-0 nylon suture if needed
- Following the surgery, subconjunctival injection of 5-fluorouracil (5-FU) on the table reduces the likelihood of bleb failure in patients with pre-existing blebs.

CONCLUSION

Decision making about the management of coexisting cataract and glaucoma involves consideration of multiple factors, careful decision-making individualized for each patient. Glaucoma is a lifetime disease and cataract surgery may alter the disease but not cure it.

SUGGESTED READING

1. Budenz DL, Gedde SJ. New options for combined cataract and glaucoma surgery. Curr Opin Ophthalmol. 2014;25(2):141-7.
2. Casson RJ, Salmon JF. Combined surgery in the treatment of patients with cataract and primary open angle glaucoma. J Cataract Refract Surg. 2001;27(110):1845-63.
3. Rehman Siddiqui MA, Khairy HA, Azuara-Blanco A. Effect of cataract extraction on SITA perimetery in patients with glaucoma. J Glaucoma. 2007;16:205-8.
4. Rosdahl JA, Chen TC. Combined cataract and glaucoma surgeries: Traditional and new combinations. Int Ophthalmol Clin. 2010;50(1):95-106.

CHAPTER 12F

Compliance

Shibal Bhartiya, Parul Ichhpujani, Suresh Kumar

INTRODUCTION

It is a well-accepted fact that a substantial proportion of patients with chronic glaucoma fails to comply with medical advice. Patient's collaboration in treatment is imperative if his/her intraocular pressures (IOPs) are to be kept under control to prevent visual field loss. It has been estimated that approximately 10% of all visual loss from glaucoma can be attributed to nonadherence to therapy.

- *Compliance* is defined as the degree of correspondence between the prescribed treatment regimen and the patient's actual dosing history[1,2]
- *Adherence* is used interchangeably and is the preferred term since it indicates the level to which active patients' behavior correspond with physician's recommendations
- *Medication persistency* is defined as the total time on therapy. Measures of persistency allow for some degree of patient noncompliance; for instance, a

patient who takes a daily prescribed medication every other day is persistent with therapy, although his level of compliance is 50%. Persistency is an indication of the patient's satisfaction with an agent's tolerability and also the physician's satisfaction with the degree of IOP control.[3,4]

The main causes for noncompliance are varied and below are a few case studies to elaborate the same.

Case 1: White coat adherence

Mr X, a 71-year-old gentleman, had previously been diagnosed with moderate open-angle glaucoma and prescribed travoprost eye drops to be used at bedtime for both eyes. He had no significant comorbidities. The peak baseline IOP was recorded as 24 mm Hg and 26 mm Hg and pachymetry was 532 microns and 534 microns for right and left eye, respectively, both optic nerves showed a cupping of 0.6:1 with a mild inferior rim thinning (Fig. 12F.1). His

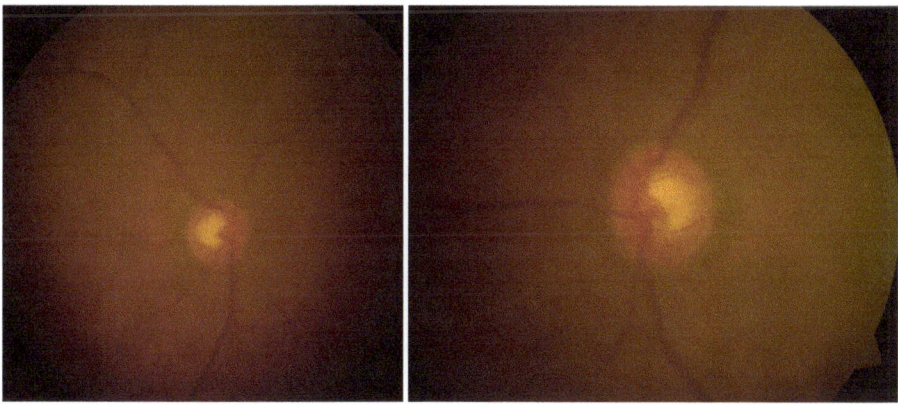

Fig. 12F.1: ONH OU shows C:D ratio of 0.6:1 with mild inferior rim thinning in OS.

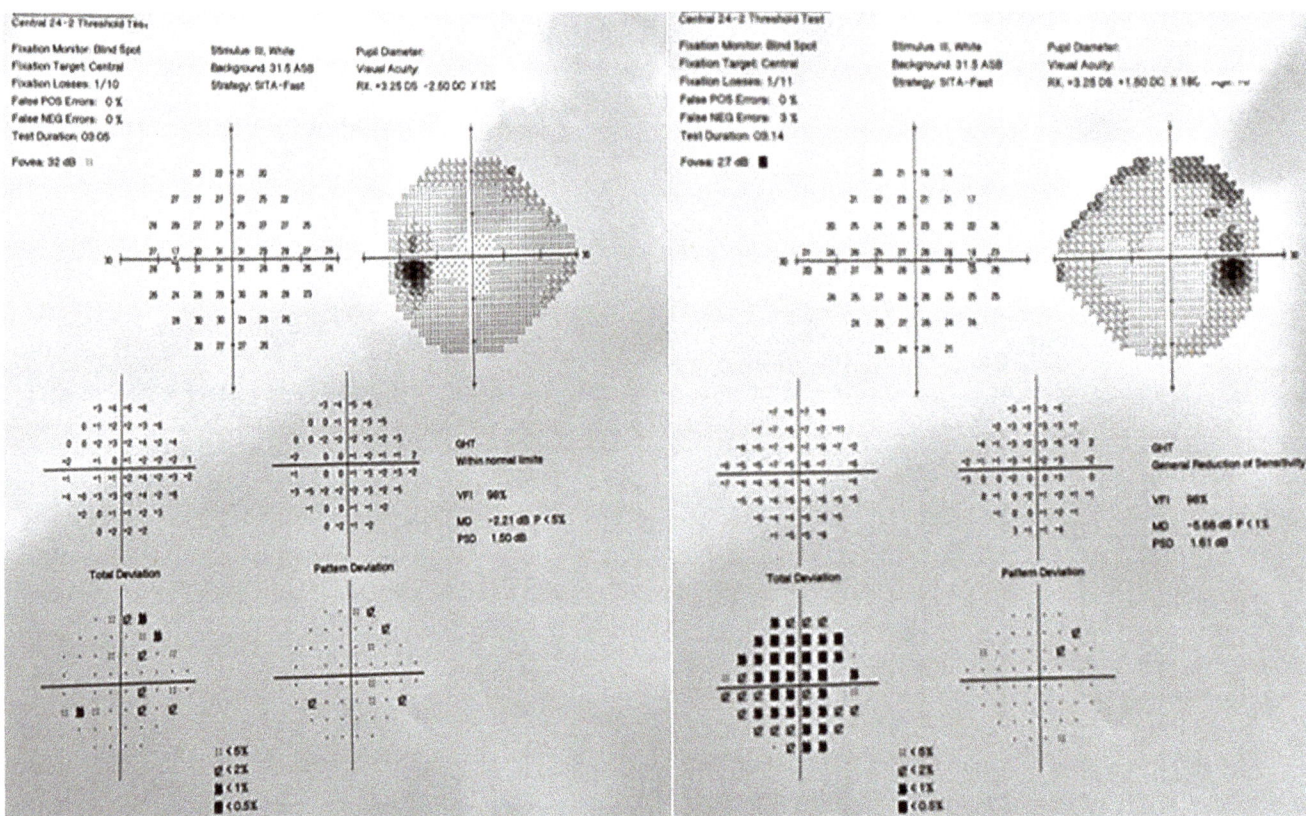

Fig. 12F.2: Humphrey SITA FAST 24-2 visual fields at presentation.

initial fields showed a mean deviation (MD) oculus dexter (OD) of –5.68 (Fig. 12F.2). The target IOP was, therefore, ascertained to be around the late teens with an acceptable fluctuation of around 5 mm of Hg. A diurnal control of IOP on travoprost, after 1 month of initiation of therapy, had shown that target IOP was achieved with peak IOP being 14 mm Hg and 15 mm Hg for right and left eye, respectively, with a fluctuation of 6 mm Hg.

Repeat fields carried out after 1 year of follow-up showed signs of progression on visual fields (Fig. 12F.3) despite good IOP control. A water drinking test (WDT) with 10 mL/kg body weight was then ordered to check for IOP fluctuation.

The WDT revealed peak IOP of 18 mm of Hg with a minimum IOP recorded 13 mm of Hg (fluctuation 5 mm Hg). All IOP recordings were found to be well within the target for both peak and fluctuation.

A repeat visual field was performed to confirm the visual field changes and the repeat fields confirmed progression.

A cursory conversation with the patient about adherence to prescribed medication revealed that she was very regular with her medication.

The glaucomatologist was then concerned enough to consider nocturnal dips in blood pressure (BP) as a plausible cause of progression and the need for a 24-hour BP recording was discussed with the patient. A detailed conversation about progression despite adequate IOP control as measured by the WDT was explained to her. She was also told that a 24-hour IOP monitoring at a government hospital (since Shibal Bhartiya's facility does not offer inpatient IOP monitoring) may be essential for better monitoring her condition. The possibility of adding another drug, brinzolamide/dorzolamide (for possible positive effect on optic nerve blood flow autoregulation), to be used thrice a day was also discussed with the patient since the progression rate seemed unacceptable.

After considerable time was spent in discussing the future course of action, Mr X revealed that he had stopped his eye drops after his last visit to the ophthalmologist, since his pressures were *normal*. He had only resumed his medication 3 weeks before his current visit because a chance IOP check as part of a routine screening camp in his residential area had revealed high IOPs.

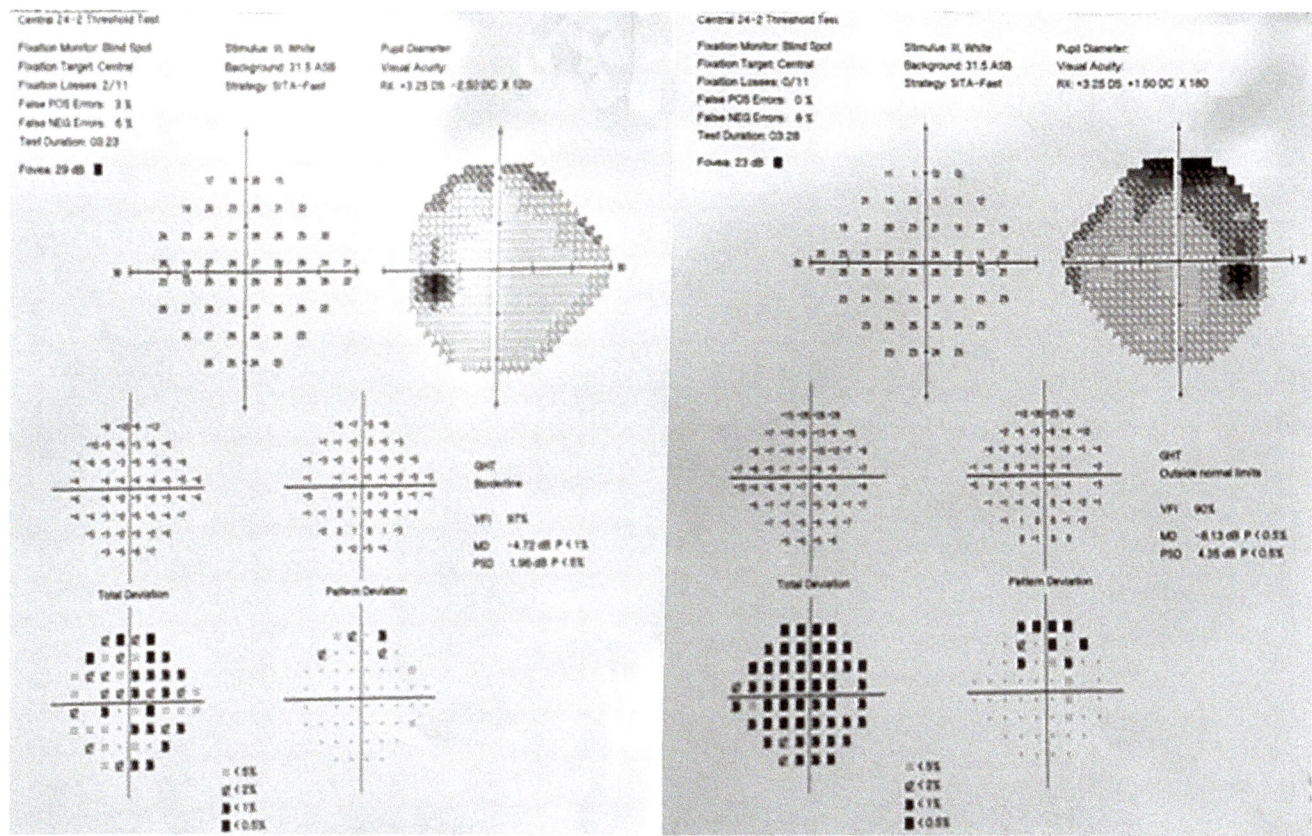

Fig. 12F.3: 1 year follow-up visual fields showing progression.

Comment

White-coat adherence is common in which patient adherence rises sharply 1 week before the appointment with the physician then declines rapidly following the appointment. White-coat adherence may make it difficult to assess IOP control over the longer term; cycling behavior with medication use is well-documented. Adherence and persistence rates differ by class of drug with higher rates associated with prostaglandin use. However, even with prostaglandins, it is important to consider the possibility of nonadherence when a progression of disease is noted despite good IOP control.[2]

Case 2: Drug induced nocturnal hypotension

Mrs ABC had previously been diagnosed with moderate-to-advanced open-angle glaucoma and prescribed bimatoprost eye drops to be used at bedtime and brinzolamide eye drops to be used thrice daily for both eyes. She was a diabetic and hypertensive, and also was on treatment for obstructive airway disease as well as coronary artery disease. The peak baseline IOP was recorded as 26 mm Hg and 27 mm Hg; and pachymetry was 521 microns and 514 microns for right and left eye, respectively, both optic nerves showed a cupping of 0.7:1 with a significant inferior rim thinning (Fig. 12F.4). Her left eye initial fields showed a MD of –4.92 dB. The target IOP was, therefore, ascertained to be around the mid-teens with an acceptable fluctuation of around 5 mm of Hg. A diurnal control of IOP on travoprost and brizolamide after 1 month of initiation of therapy had shown that target IOP was achieved with peak IOP being 14 mm Hg and 19 mm Hg for right and left eye, respectively, with a fluctuation of 5 mm Hg.

Repeat left eye fields carried out after 2 years of follow-up showed signs of progression on visual fields (Fig. 12F. 5) despite good IOP control. A WDT with 10 mL/kg body weight was then ordered to check for IOP fluctuation (a diurnal variation/phasing can also be done in place of WDT, if the facility is available). The WDT revealed peak IOP of 17 mm Hg and 21 mm of Hg for right and left eye, respectively, with a minimum IOP recorded 13 mm of Hg (fluctuation 4 mm Hg and 7 mm Hg, respectively, for right and left eye). All IOP recordings were found to be well within the target for both peak and fluctuation.

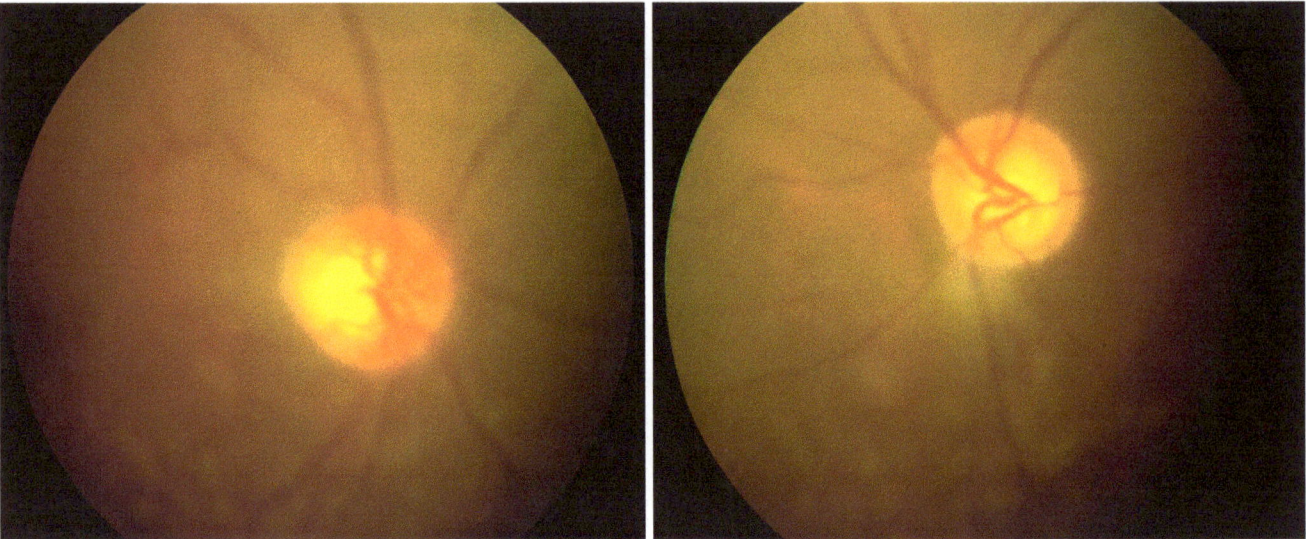

Fig. 12F.4: ONH OU shows C:D ratio of 0.7:1 with significant inferior rim thinning and broken ISNT rule.

A detailed conversation with the patient and her primary caregiver revealed strict adherence to prescribed medication with only one dose missed (which was documented in the patient diary over 4 months).

The glaucomatologist was then concerned enough to consider nocturnal dips in BP as a plausible cause of progression and the need for a 24-hour BP recording was discussed with the patient. The 24-hour ambulatory BP recording revealed nocturnal dips in BP (Fig. 12F.6). A discussion with the cardiologist resulted in a dose readjustment for her antihypertensive medication, and the visual fields have since been shown to be stable.

Case 3: Drug induced ocular surface disease

Mr X instead of Mr Y, a 73-year-old gentleman, had been diagnosed with moderate primary angle-closure glaucoma and had bilateral laser peripheral iridotomy (LPI) elsewhere. The peak baseline IOP, 1 month post-LPI was recorded as 30 mm Hg and 28 mm Hg; and pachymetry was 542 microns and 533 microns for right and left eye, respectively, both optic nerves showed a cupping of 0.8:1 with an inferior rim thinning. His initial fields showed a MD of –8.92 dB in right eye and –6.98 dB in left eye. He also had bilateral epibulbar dermoids (Fig. 12F.7). He had no significant comorbidities. He was prescribed latanoprost and timolol-fixed dose combination at bedtime; and brimonidine eye drops thrice a day for both eyes. He had been using the same drugs for over a year and had been brought for a second opinion by his son. Mr X was of the view that he should, rather, take a risk of going blind, rather than endure the extreme side effects of his glaucoma treatment.

A preliminary examination revealed both, his compliance and adherence to glaucoma therapy, as well as his obvious discomfort (Fig. 12F.8). Brimonidine eye drops were stopped and he was advised lubricatings eye drops 2 hourly initially for a week, the frequency decreasing to thrice a day thereafter.

He was asked to follow-up after 4 weeks and a visibly happier patient promised lifelong compliance to glaucoma medication.

The target IOP was ascertained to be around the early mid-teens with an acceptable fluctuation of around 5 mm Hg. A diurnal control of IOP on latanoprost and timolol-fixed dose combination at bedtime, after 1 month of cessation of brimonidine showed that target IOP was achieved with peak IOP being 14 mm Hg and 15 mm Hg for right and left eye, respectively, with a fluctuation of 6 mm Hg.

Mr X is a satisfied and compliant patient with no evidence of progression, 2 years after his new treatment regimen was established.

Comment

It is important to remember that glaucoma is an asymptomatic disease, and the treatment results in side effects, which are often unacceptable to the patient despite recognizing the plausible threat of blindness.

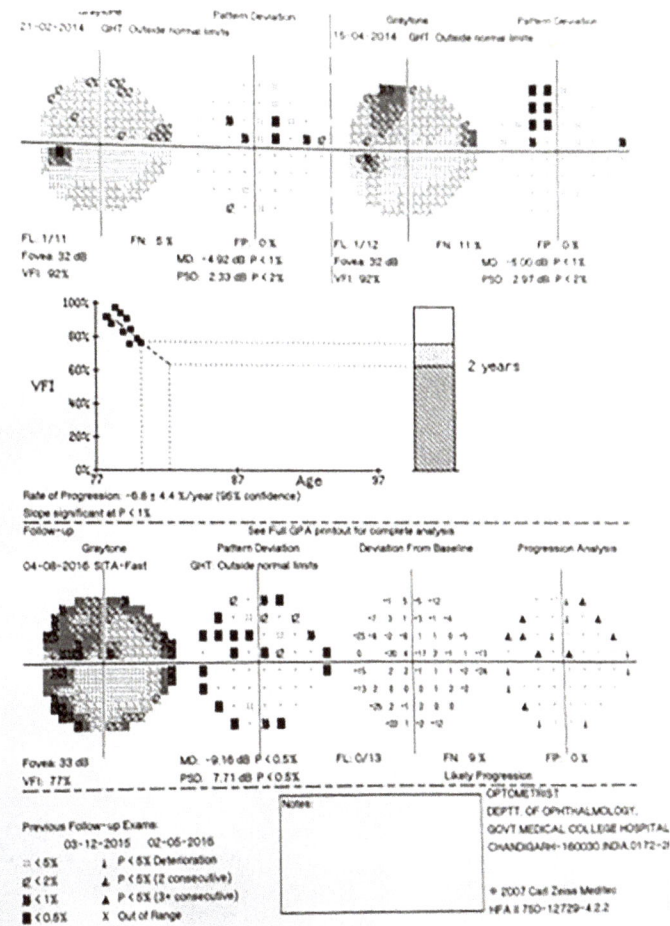

Fig. 12F.5: Follow-up visual fields showing likely progression.

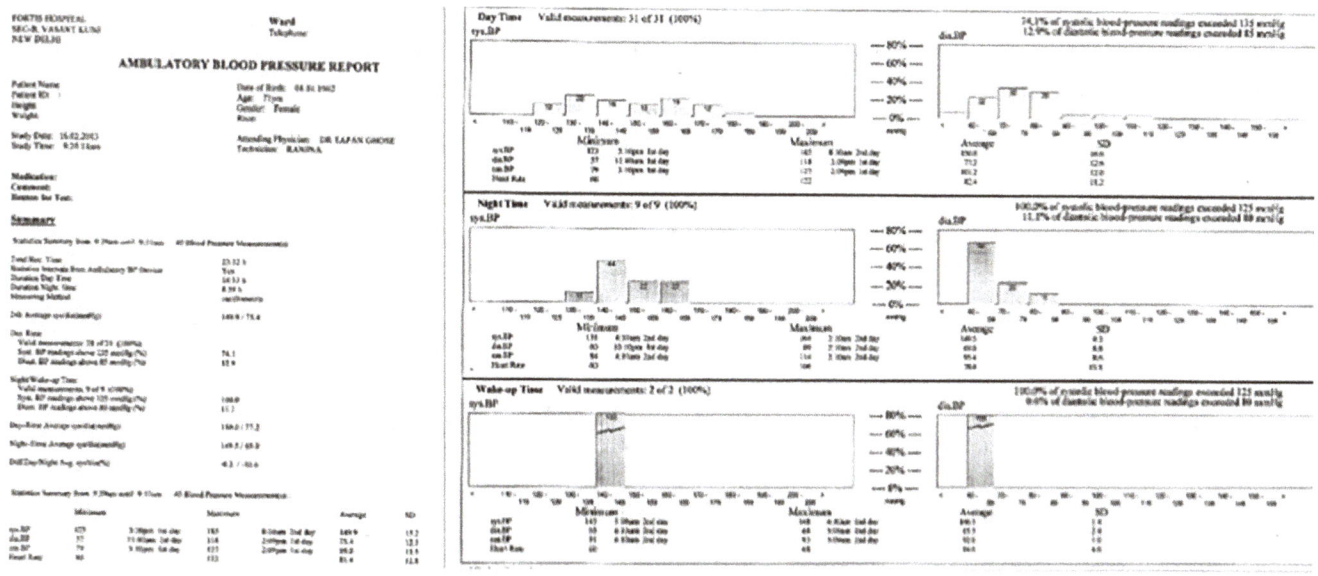

Fig. 12F.6: 24-hour ambulatory BP recording revealed nocturnal dips in BP.

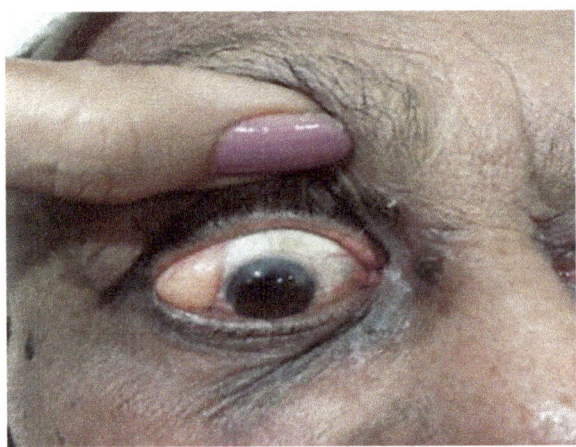

Fig. 12F.7: Epibulbar dermoid.

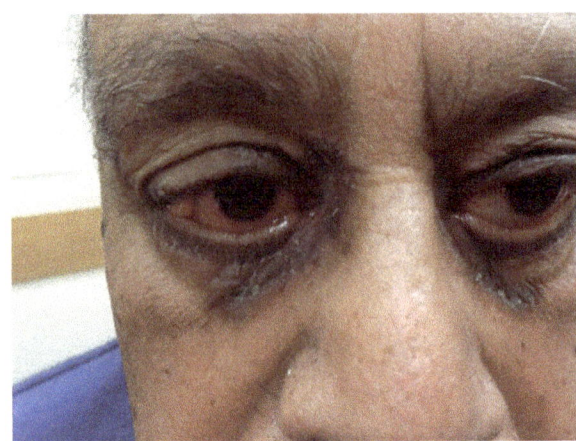

Fig. 12F.8: Compromised ocular surface secondary to anti glaucoma drugs.

The reasons for poor compliance can be broadly classified into:

- *Medical regimen*: These include side effects, complexity of the regimen in terms of the number of medicines and dosing schedules and medication costs
- *Situational and environmental reasons*: including lack of social support, difficulty in travelling to doctor/pharmacy
- *Patient factors*: including patient's beliefs about the severity of the disease and personal susceptibility, memory, comorbidities.[4]
- *Provider factors*: Patient physician relationship and the physician's ability to communicate.

REFERENCES

1. Schwartz GF, Quigley HA. Adherence and persistence with glaucoma therapy. Surv Ophthalmol. 2008;53(Suppl 1):S57-68.
2. Mohindroo C, Ichhpujani P, Kumar S. How 'Drug Aware' are our glaucoma patients? J Curr Glaucoma Pract. 2015;9(2):33-7.
3. Olthoff CM, Schouten JS, van de Borne BW, Webers CA. Noncompliance with ocular hypotensive treatment in patients with glaucoma or ocular hypertension: an evidence-based review. Ophthalmology. 2005;112(6):953-61.
4. Smith VA, DeVellis BM, Kalet A, Roberts JC, DeVellis RF. Encouraging patient adherence: primary care physicians' use of verbal compliance-gaining strategies in medical interviews. Patient Educ Couns. 2005;57(1):62-76.

CHAPTER 13

Informed Consents

Shibal Bhartiya, Parul Ichhpujani, Suresh Kumar

INTRODUCTION

Mutual trust is the foundation of a doctor-patient relationship. In this era of information overload, with a surplus of information available to each patient, it is imperative for the doctor to communicate with the patient about his/her treatment plan.

Consent may be defined as an instrument of mutual communication between doctor and patient with an expression of authorization/permission/choice by the latter for the doctor to act in a particular way.

Informed consent is a critical step in delivering quality care to our patients. A clear and open discussion between the caregiver and the patient and his/her family helps to discuss diagnosis, management and its implications. It also helps to ensure compliance and manages expectations of the patient. For a disease like glaucoma it becomes even more important since the chances of visual gain are poor and the risk of attendant complications, and multiple surgical interventions more than that, for say cataract surgery.

The process of consent should emphasize more on communication and managing expectation than on absolving the clinician of medicolegal liability alone, even though the latter is of importance given the litigious times we live in.

The basic tenets of the informed consent process are:

- *Full, free and voluntary consent*: document acceptance of risks of complications
- Document the patients complaints in his or her own words
- Discussion in the patients-preferred language, using a facilitator/interpreter, whenever, necessary
- Written, informed consent signed by the patient (or guardian) and witnessed by a third party. Document name, relationship and contact details of witness and interpreter
- Document and include description and cause of any functional impairment, especially if irreversible
- Treatment options and alternatives explained
- Risks and benefits of preferred treatment plan discussed
- Possible clinical outcomes
- Approximate cost and duration of surgery
- Expected follow-up schedule following the procedure
- Document comorbidities, which may influence treatment outcomes
- Document a list of possible common complications (by no means exhaustive)
- Document the eye to be operated first (right or left)
- Document the possible need for more than one surgical intervention, list common ancillary procedures
- Document possible impact on vision and possibility of vision fluctuation
- Discuss choice of anesthesia with patient, with anesthetist, and primary care physician in case of monitored anesthetic care or general anesthesia
- For simultaneous bilateral procedures, take a separate informed consent for each eye
- Provide the patient with a copy of the signed consent.

WHO CAN GIVE CONSENT?

Patient must be above the age of 18 years and should be of sound mind and competent to give consent. The patient must understand the implications of the treatment before being asked to sign the consent.

In case of children, the consent must be obtained from a parent, preferably both if possible. In case of incapacitated persons, close family members or legal guardians can give consent.

In case of a language barrier, an interpreter must explain in great detail the risks and benefits and treatment options to the patient and verify that the patient's questions have been answered to his/her satisfaction, before consent is sought.

This process may be recorded in the operating room for all major procedures:

- Identify the patient; verify the surgery and the site of surgery prior to administration of anesthesia. Mark the site of surgery at this stage. Crosscheck any implant specifications
- Immediately before starting surgery, verify same details verbally with operating theater technicians/anesthetists/patient.

ETHICS OF CONSENT

The concept of consent arises from the ethical principle of patient autonomy and basic human rights. It is the patients right to make an informed decision and to partner completely in his/her treatment plan. It is, therefore, incumbent upon the doctor to ensure that the patients' right to make an informed contribution to his/her own healthcare is honored.

Consent, however, is not only an ethical obligation, but also a legal compulsion. The level of disclosure has to be case-specific.

Important points to remember include:

- Ensure prompt and compassionate communication about the disease process and evolution
- Do not withhold any significant information about the disease severity and prognosis
- Do not withhold information about the alternatives to your preferred treatment plan. Discuss risks and benefits of each and explain why you prefer one
- Inform patients about any complications promptly
- Be truthful about your training and experience
- Advise the patient about the need for a second opinion/refer patient to a higher tertiary care center, when needed
- In case you are using an off-label drug, make sure the patient knows and signs a separate consent form for that.

Exemptions to Disclosure

Therapeutic Privilege

If the treating doctor is of the opinion that certain information can seriously harm a patient's health, physical, mental or emotional, he has the privilege to withhold such information. But, it should be shared with close relatives, and a written consent sought from the next of kin with complete disclosure.

Placebo

Use of placebos may be justified in certain conditions, as there are high chances of benefit to the patient with negligible risk. These include some self-limiting conditions in patients with a psychological overlay of symptoms, and those who insist for some form of medication.

SPECIAL CONSENTS

Special consents will be required in certain situations, outside of the operating room and these include:

- Participating in a research protocol
- Participating in a teaching process
- Change in operating surgeon
- Use of photos, in any forum, in which the patient may be recognized
- Use of patient data for analysis, even if anonymized.

There cannot be anything called a standard consent form, this chapter, however, provides consents, which may work as a generalized framework for the consent process, and may be customized to the individual patients.

Informed Consent for Trabeculectomy

Name:	Age/Sex:
(UID No: Unique identification number)	Date:

Glaucoma is a condition, where the pressure in the eye (intraocular pressure) leads to optic nerve damage and thus vision loss. The goal of glaucoma surgery is to lower the eye pressure to slow nerve loss and reduce the ongoing vision loss. It is important to realize that the purpose of glaucoma surgery is to lower eye pressure. It does not reverse the nerve damage that has occurred (it does not improve vision and does not reverse pre-existing vision loss).

If medications are not effective, laser and other surgical procedures may be of value in controlling the pressure and preventing further vision loss. Your doctor has informed you that a drainage operation called trabeculectomy is necessary to help control the pressure in your eye. If this pressure remains too high, your optic nerve can become damaged, leading to vision loss and eventual blindness.

This procedure allows your doctor to create a new drainage channel for the eye. A small hole is made in the eye to allow fluid to flow to a fluid pocket under the upper lid called a bleb. Usually, a medication called mitomycin C is used to prevent scarring so that the fluid drainage (and thus pressure lowering) will continue long-term. When successful, this procedure will lower the pressure in your eye, minimizing the risk of further vision loss from glaucoma.

The information presented is to educate you, so that your consent for an operation is an informed one. Your conversations with your ophthalmologist are also very important and you encouraged to ask as many questions as you think are necessary.

Risks of Trabeculectomy

The outcome of any surgical procedure cannot be guaranteed and there are certain risks associated with glaucoma drainage surgery. For instance, there is always the possibility that the surgery will not help to control eye pressure. Eye drops or more procedures may be needed. Not every conceivable complication can be covered in this form, but the following are examples of risks encountered with glaucoma drainage surgery. These complications can occur days, weeks, months or years after. They can result in loss of vision or blindness. Careful follow-up is required after surgery. After your eye heals you will still need regular eye examinations to monitor your pressure and to watch for other eye problems.

Complications from Surgery
- Eye pressure too high or too low
- Sudden permanent vision loss
- Infection (endophthalmitis)
- Retinal detachment or retinal swelling
- Corneal swelling, decompensation requiring corneal transplant
- Serious bleeding inside the eye
- Double vision
- Drooping of eyelid (ptosis)
- Need for further surgery
- Progression of glaucoma
- Worsening of cataract (if not already removed)
- Change in vision requiring new glasses

- Chronic discomfort, foreign body sensation or tearing problems with the bleb
- Abnormal pupil.

Most people undergo surgery with a local anesthetic. This significantly reduces the likelihood of, but does not eliminate, anesthetic complications, such as drug reactions or other problems that could lead to brain damage or even death. Complications of anesthesia injections around the eye include perforation of eyeball, needle damage to the optic nerve, which could destroy vision, double vision, interference with circulation of the retina, drooping of eyelid.

Consent for Operation

I declare that I understand the proposed surgery. The basic procedures involved in glaucoma surgery, its possible benefits and risks, and the alternative treatments have been explained to me by my doctor. I understand that it is impossible for every detail of the surgery and its possible complications to be explained to me. I have asked for and received answers to all my questions.

I have read this informed consent document or had it read to me and I fully understand it.

I wish to have a trabeculectomy with/without mitomycin C operation on my __ right __ left eye.

Name of Witness	Name of patient/guardian (in case of minor)
Sign	Sign
Date	Date

Informed Consent for Glaucoma Drainage Implant Surgery

Name:	Age/Sex:
UID No:	Date:

Glaucoma is a condition whereby the pressure in the eye (intraocular pressure) leads to optic nerve damage and thus vision loss. The goal of glaucoma surgery is to lower the eye pressure to slow nerve loss and reduce the ongoing vision loss. It is important to realize that the purpose of glaucoma surgery is to lower eye pressure. It does not reverse the nerve damage that has occurred (it does not improve vision and does not reverse pre-existing vision loss).

If medications are not effective, laser and other surgical procedures may be of value in controlling the pressure and preventing further vision loss. Medications, lasers and surgery are designed to lower eye pressure. Your doctor has informed you that a drainage operation called an Ahmed glaucoma valve/Baerveldt/Molteno tube shunt surgery is necessary to help control the pressure in your eye. If this pressure remains too high, your optic nerve can become damaged, leading to vision loss and eventual blindness. This procedure allows your ophthalmologist to create a new drainage channel for the eye. When successful, this procedure will lower the pressure in your eye, minimizing the risk of further vision loss from glaucoma.

The information presented is to educate you, so that your consent for an operation is an informed one. Your conversations with your ophthalmologist are also very important and you encouraged to ask as many questions as you think are necessary.

Risks of Glaucoma Drainage Implant Surgery

The outcome of any surgical procedure cannot be guaranteed and there are certain risks associated with glaucoma drainage surgery. For instance, there is always the possibility that the surgery you have will not help to control eye pressure. Eye drops or more procedures may be needed. Not every conceivable complication can be covered in this form but the following are examples of risk encountered with glaucoma drainage surgery. These complications can occur days, weeks, months or years after. They can result in loss of vision or blindness. Careful follow-up is required after surgery. After your eye heals you will still need regular eye examinations to monitor your pressure and to watch for other eye problems.

Complications from Glaucoma Drainage Implant Surgery

- Eye pressure too high or too low
- Sudden permanent vision loss
- Infection (endophthalmitis)
- Retinal detachment
- Choroidal detachment
- Corneal swelling, decompensation requiring corneal transplant
- Serious bleeding inside the eye
- Double vision
- Worsening of cataract
- Change in vision requiring new glasses
- Drooping of eyelid
- Need for further surgery related to initial surgery

- Progression of glaucoma
- Tube retraction
- Implant exposure/extrusion.

Most people undergo surgery with a local anesthetic. This significantly reduces the likelihood of, but does not eliminate, anesthetic complications, such as drug reactions or other problems, that could lead to brain damage or even death. Complications of anesthesia injections around the eye include perforation of eyeball, needle damage to the optic nerve, which could destroy vision, interference with circulation of the retina, drooping of eyelid.

Consent for Operation

I declare that I understand the proposed surgery. The basic procedures involved in glaucoma surgery, its possible benefits and risks and the alternative treatments have been explained to me by my doctor. I understand that it is impossible for every detail of the surgery and its possible complications to be explained to me. I have asked for and received answers to all my questions.

I have read this informed consent document or had it read to me and I fully understand it.

I wish to have an Ahmed glaucoma valve/Baerveldt/Molteno tube shunt surgery on my __ right __ left eye.

Name of Witness	Name of patient/guardian (in case of minor)
Sign:	Sign:
Date:	Date:

Informed Consent for Cataract Surgery

Name:	Age/Sex:
UID No:	Date:

Cataract surgery with intraocular lens implantation is a specialized microsurgical procedure in which the opacified crystalline lens is removed and an artificial lens is implanted in its place. _____(XYZ Hospital) is equipped with the latest machines and technology required for this procedure.

The modern techniques of cataract surgery are generally safe and the results are gratifying.

However, even in the best of hands there can be complications during surgery, like posterior capsular dehiscence, nucleus drop and damage to the corneal endothelium. Rarely intraocular bleed may occur.

Postoperatively, chances of infection are rare but not unknown. Retinal complications, such as cystoid macular edema, retinal detachment, causing decreased vision may occur. Delayed postoperative complications, such as corneal edema, posterior capsular opacification and glaucoma may occur.

In addition, there are risks of anesthesia (general/local) and of drug reactions, which are common to any surgery. These risks are higher in diabetics, hypertensives, asthmatics, obese patients, chronic smokers and heart patients. Since it is impossible to state here every complication that may occur as a result of surgery the list in this form is incomplete.

With the knowledge of the surgeon(s) and his/her/their facilities, the expected prognosis and the risks involved, I hereby authorize the consulting surgeon(s) of XYZ Hospital to carry out treatment and surgery/surgeries considered appropriate by them. I shall be satisfied as long as they have done their best.

Special comments regarding this particular case:

- I hereby declare that I have read and understood this informed consent or this informed consent has been read out and explained to me completely and I understand the risks involved in the procedure and give my full free and voluntary consent to Dr_____for performing_____surgery on my right/left eye
- It has been explained to me that during the course of the surgery unforeseen conditions may be encountered that necessitate surgical or other procedures in addition to or different from those planned and discussed. I thereby further request and authorize the above-mentioned physician/surgeon or his designates to perform such additional surgical or other procedure as he or they may deem necessary or desirable
- I consent to the administration of anesthesia and to the use of such anesthetics as may be deemed necessary
- I further consent to the administration of drugs or infusions deemed necessary in the judgment of the medical staff
- I consent to the observing, photographing or televising of the procedure to be performed for medical, scientific and educational purpose provided my identity is not revealed
- Any tissues or parts surgically removed may be disposed off by the institution in accordance with the appropriate practice designated by XYZ hospital

- The basic procedures of cataract surgery, the benefits, risks and alternatives have been explained to me. Although it is impossible for me to know of every possible complication that may occur, my questions have been answered to my satisfaction. In signing this informed consent for cataract operation, and/or implantation of intraocular lens, I am stating I have read this informed consent (or it has been read to me) and I fully understand it and the possible risks, complications and benefits that can result from the surgery.

Name of Witness	Name of patient/guardian (in case of minor)
Sign:	Sign:
Date:	Date:

Informed Consent Form for Neodymium-doped:Yttrium Aluminum Garnet Laser Capsulotomy

Name:	Age/Sex:
UID No:	Date:

Neodymium-doped:yttrium aluminum garnet capsulotomy is done for posterior capsular opacification that can develop after cataract surgery. LASER energy is used to disrupt the opacified posterior capsule.

The procedure itself is mostly very safe. There can be rare complications, such as transient rise in intraocular pressure, some post-LASER uveitis, etc. Most of these can be controlled by medication. Due to disruption of the posterior capsule yttrium aluminum garnet (YAG) does increase the risk of development of retinal detachment slightly (by about less than 1% as per international studies).

The procedure is done under topical (eye drop) anesthesia using paracaine 0.5% and/or xylocaine 4% eye drops. This form of anesthesia is very safe. Only rarely can it cause local allergy or superficial punctuate keratitis (mild corneal epithelial disturbance), which can usually be treated with medication.

The basic procedures of YAG LASER capsulotomy, the benefits, risks and alternatives have been explained to me. Although it is impossible for me to know of every possible complication that may occur, my questions have been answered to my satisfaction. In signing this informed consent, I am stating I have read this informed consent (or it has been read to me) and I fully understand it and the possible risks, complications and benefits that can result from the surgery.

I have read the above/been explained in the language I understand the procedure and give my full, free and voluntary consent to Dr_____for performing YAG capsulotomy in my right/left eye.

_____	_____
Name of Witness	Name of patient/guardian (in case of minor)
Sign:	Sign:
Date:	Date:

Neodymium-doped:Yttrium Aluminum Garnet Laser Iridotomy

Name:	Age/Sex:
UID No:	Date:

Neodymium-doped:Yttrium Aluminum Garnet iridotomy is done for pupillary block glaucoma. LASER energy is used to create a small opening in the peripheral iris to relieve the block. XYZ Hospital is equipped with the latest machines and technology required for this procedure.

The procedure itself is very safe. Most people notice some blurring in their vision after the laser. This clears within a few hours in most individuals. There can be rare complications, such as transient rise in intraocular pressure, post-LASER hyphema, uveitis, etc. Rarely local endothelial damage can occur. Most of these can be controlled by medication.

You will need to use drops after the laser to help the eye heal correctly. In most cases, you are asked to continue your other glaucoma medications after the laser procedure. The doctor will notify you, if there is any exception to continuing your medications. It will take several weeks to determine how well the laser has worked to lower your pressure. Sometimes the opening created in the iris may not be full thickness or may close down and may require a repeat procedure.

The procedure is done under topical (eye drop) anesthesia using paracaine 0.5% and/or xylocaine 4% eye drops. This form of anesthesia is very safe. Only rarely can it cause local allergy or superficial punctuate keratitis (mild corneal epithelial disturbance), which can usually be treated with medication.

The basic procedures of YAG LASER iridotomy, the benefits, risks and alternatives have been explained to me.

Although it is impossible for me to know of every possible complication that may occur, my questions have been answered to my satisfaction. In signing this informed consent, I am stating I have read this informed consent (or it has been read to me) and I fully understand it and the possible risks, complications and benefits that can result from the surgery.

I have read the above/been explained in the language I understand the procedure and give my full, free and voluntary consent to Dr_____ for performing YAG iridotomy in my right/left/both eye(s).

_____	_____
Name of Witness	Name of patient/guardian (in case of minor)
Sign:	Sign:
Date:	Date:

Informed Consent for Selective Laser Trabeculoplasty

Name:	Age/Sex:
UID No:	Date:

Selective laser trabeculoplasty (SLT) is used for patients with open angle types of glaucoma. The laser is utilized to treat the drainage system of the eye known as the trabecular meshwork. Treating this area of the natural internal draining system is designed to improve the outflow of fluid from the eye. This type of laser surgery will be effective in some patients but not others. Your response is determined by the type of glaucoma you have and the specific structures found in your drainage system. Your doctor cannot predict how well the laser will work before the laser surgery.

The procedure may be performed in one or two sittings. The laser machine is similar to the examination slit lamp that the ophthalmologist uses at each visit to look into your eyes. The laser itself makes little noise and flashes a light about as bright as the flash on a camera. Nearly all patients find the procedure comfortable and pain free. The procedure generally takes from 10 minutes to 20 minutes.

You may need to use drops both before and after the laser treatment. As the pressure in the eye may temporarily go up after the laser treatment, you will likely need to have your pressure measured after 1.5–1 hour following the laser surgery. If the pressure does elevate, you may need additional medicines to lower the pressure, which will be administered in the office. Rarely, the pressure in the eye could elevate to a level that might require surgery in the operating room to relieve the glaucoma. You will need to use drops after the laser to help the eye heal correctly. You will probably use the new drops for approximately 1 week. In most cases you will be asked to continue your other glaucoma medications after the laser surgery. The doctor will notify you if there are exceptions to continuing your medications.

Laser may be associated with a few complications. Some patients notice transient blurring of vision after SLT. This generally clears within 20–30 minutes following the procedure and is usually related to the gel that is used on the lens during the procedure. Although extremely rare and unusual, there may be bleeding within the eye, inflammation and increase in the pressure in the eye requiring different and more extensive treatment. It will take several weeks to determine how much of your eye pressure will be lowered with this treatment. You may require additional laser surgery to lower the pressure, if you have a response but one that is insufficient to control the pressure.

Not every conceivable complication could be covered in this form and I understand that no warranty or guarantee has been made to me regarding the result of the proposed laser surgery. I have read and understand the consent form, my questions have been answered and I authorize my surgeon to proceed with the operation on my _____ (state *right* or *left*) eye.

_____	_____
Name of Witness	Name of patient/guardian (in case of minor)
Sign:	Sign:
Date:	Date:

Informed Consent for Diode Laser Cyclophotocoagulation

Name:	Age/Sex:
UID No:	Date:

Your doctor has recommended that you undergo diode laser cyclophotocoagulation for managing your refractory glaucoma. If successful, it will lower your eye pressure by decreasing the eye's fluid production. A laser probe will be placed on the white wall of the eye, just outside the circle formed by the iris (the colored part of the eye) and the cornea (the clear window portion of the eye) to administer 15–25 laser treatment spots. The laser energy affects the fluid-forming cells in the eye and alters them in such a way that they produce less fluid, thus lowering the eye pressure.

Risks and Benefits of Laser Treatment

The benefit of this laser treatment is improved glaucoma control, often with a reduced need for medical treatment. In some instances, this laser treatment is done to lower the eye pressure to a level that will stop further visual loss from glaucoma. In other cases, the treatment may be done in an eye with low vision that has painful glaucoma to lower the pressure enough to make the eye comfortable. Like any procedure, complications can occur. These include a temporary or long-lasting decrease in vision, inflammation or bleeding inside the eye, swelling in the back of the eye, or, if performed in an eye with its own natural lens, development of a cataract. A single laser treatment may not achieve adequate control of the eye pressure, and repeat treatment may need to be considered. Occasionally, the treatment results in excessive lowering of the eye pressure, either immediately or some time afterwards. This can cause decreased vision, which may not be correctable.

Before the Laser Treatment

You will receive instructions regarding the laser surgery from your doctor and the staff. Usually no blood tests or other preoperative testing is required. As rather powerful laser energy is utilized for this treatment, local anesthesia in the form of an injection behind and/or around the eye is necessary. Because of this injection, blood thinners, aspirin-containing products may need to be discontinued usually a week prior to the surgery, if it is acceptable to your regular personal physician.

If you have diabetes, and particularly if you use insulin, you should receive special instructions from your doctor and the staff regarding your diet and the use of insulin on the day of the laser surgery.

During the Treatment

Once the local anesthesia is completed and the eye is numb, the untreated eye will be patched to protect it, and a small device to expose the treated eye, called a lid speculum, will be placed. You may feel some pressure from this, but there should be no pain during the procedure. You may hear some beeps and feel or hear some popping noises. These are normal and expected. The treatment should take no more then 10–15 minutes. When the procedure is completed, medications are placed in the eye, which will be covered with a patch.

After the Laser Treatment

Once you are felt to be stable after the treatment, you will be discharged home. You will be asked to keep the eye patched for a few hours to overnight. After that, no patching is required, and you may resume all usual activities. You will be given instructions regarding eye medications that you should begin once you remove the patch. In most instances, your doctor will see you the next day.

There is typically minimal postoperative pain, but sometimes the eye can be uncomfortable afterwards for several days. You will be prescribed painkillers in case of this, and you also will be on some eye drops to reduce inflammation. These will be tapered over the next few weeks as the inflammation subsides.

Depending on your eye's response to the laser treatment, the pressure immediately after the procedure may be high or low. You may need to continue some or all of your preoperative glaucoma medications, at least temporarily. As it may take up to a month for your eye to have its maximum response to the treatment, these medications may later be decreased or discontinued if the pressure begins dropping to an acceptable level. If the pressure does not drop to an acceptable level, or if the treatment was done for comfort and the eye remains painful, a repeat laser treatment may be recommended.

If you should have additional questions or concerns regarding your laser surgery, please feel free to speak with your doctor or a member of the staff.

I have read and understand the consent form, my questions have been answered and I authorize my surgeon to proceed with the laser cyclophotocoagulation on my _____ (state *right* or *left*) eye.

_____	_____
Name of Witness	Name of patient/guardian (in case of minor)
Sign:	Sign:
Date:	Date:

So to conclude, it is not enough for the doctor to list the risks, benefits and complications of a procedure as well as the available alternatives to the recommended procedure. The benefit of a surgical intervention may not always be noticeable in the immediate postoperative period, and, therefore, the patient should be made aware about the recovery time and the need for repeated follow-up visits. Educating patients about their disease as well as the mechanisms of the surgical or laser procedure would help them to understand the goal of the procedure and what to reasonably expect. The doctor must allow them time to consider the surgery and the healing process so that they can make the necessary preparations.

▌ SUGGESTED READING

1. Krishnamurti T. A patient-centered approach to informed consent: results from a survey and randomized trial. Med Decis Making. 2016;36(6):726-40.
2. O'Neill O. Some limits of informed consent. J Med Ethics. 2003;29(1):4-7.
3. Satyanarayana Rao KH. Informed consent: an ethical obligation or legal compulsion? J Cutan Aesthet Surg. 2008;1(1):33-5.

Chapter 14A

How to Overcome Imaging Artifacts and Prevent Misinterpretation of Imaging Results

Gábor Holló

INTRODUCTION

Optical coherence tomography (OCT) examination of the disc, the retinal nerve fiber layer and the inner macular retina thickness has become a part of the routine patient evaluation for glaucoma. However, the quality of the examination and the interpretation of the results and findings are frequently suboptimal, which has negative effect on the care of the glaucoma patient. This chapter presents the typical OCT artifacts and the most common reasons of misinterpretation of the findings, and gives easy-to-follow instructions how to avoid these pitfalls in routine glaucoma care.

BACKGROUND

Optical coherence tomography has been widely used to assist glaucoma diagnostics and detect structural progression during follow-up. However, in real life practice, the results of OCT examinations made for glaucoma detection are frequently misinterpreted. The three main reasons of misinterpretation are:

1. Lack of understanding of the technology and its limitation
2. Missed image quality control
3. Inadequate clinical examination and substitution of clinical examination with software-provided classification automatically given on the printed OCT report.[1-4]

This chapter shows how to avoid erroneous imaging practice in glaucoma diagnostics and follow-up.

TECHNICAL EVIDENCES

The principles of modern OCT technology are valid for all OCT instruments and software versions. However, it is important to know that the content of the similarly labeled software-provided parameters is different for the various OCT instruments, and therefore, the corresponding parameter values are not interchangeable. This is due to the different wavelengths, resolutions, segmentation algorithms, normal databases and analysis methods employed in the various OCT systems (Table 14A.1). Thus, for comparison and follow-up the same OCT instrument type and (as much as possible) the same software version are to be used. Software development and upgrading, which are faster than progression of glaucoma, may result in virtual alterations of the results when the current images are compared to those obtained with earlier software versions.[5] This may falsely influence clinical decision-making.

Optical coherence tomography measurements are based on image segmentation. In order to define the various layers, the software employs interpolation for filling in the space between the truly measured pixels. Interpolation, however, can be disturbed by abnormalities, which are not *expected* and not corrected for by the OCT's software. This results in incorrect segmentation, incorrect parameter values and as a consequence incorrect classification for glaucoma.[2-4,6-9]

Whenever, the illuminating light is blocked by an anatomical structure (shadow effect) the reflected light is reduced, which results in poor signal-to-noise ratio and incorrect classification. Therefore, image quality control

Table 14A.1: Some of the widely used optical coherence tomograph instruments and their most important parameters.

Manufacturer	Instrument	Axial resolution	Scanning speed (A scan/sec)
Optovue	RTVue Premier	5 μm (natív) 3 μm (digitális)	26,000
Optovue	Avanti	5 μm (natív) 3 μm (digitális)	70,000
Optovue	Angiovue	5 μm (natív) 3 μm (digitális)	70,000
Optovue	iVue	5 μm	26,000
Optovue	iFusion	5 μm	26,000
Optovue	iScan		
Optopol	Copernicus	5 μm	27,000
Optopol/Canon	Copernicus HR	3 μm	52,000
Bioptigen	EnvisuC-class	3.3 μm	32,000
Carl Zeiss Meditec	Cirrus	5 μm	27,000–68,000
Carl Zeiss Meditec	Cirrusphoto	5 μm	27,000–68,000
Heidelberg Technology	Spectralis HRA-OCT	3.8 μm	40,000
Topcon	3D OCT 2000	5–6 μm	50,000
Topcon	3D OCT 2000 FA plus	5–6 μm	50,000
Topcon	OCT-1 Maestro	5–6 μm	50,000
Topcon	DRI OCT Triton swept source OCT	2.6 μm (digitális)	100,000
Topcon	DRI OCT Triton plus swept source OCT	2.6 μm (digitális)	100,000
Optos	OCT SLO	4–6 μm	27,000
Haag Streit Surgical	iOCT		

(DRI: Digital retinal imaging; HR: High resolution; OCT: Optical coherence tomography; SLO: Scanning laser ophthalmoscope).

and replacement of poor-quality images and images containing artifacts with sufficiently high-quality images are essential prior to the evaluation of the results. Image quality control cannot be made on printed reports. OCT examinations comprise three-dimensional information pieces; information related to depth cannot be evaluated on the two-dimensional (2D) printouts. Exclusive use of printed reports leads to missed shadow effects due to vitreous floaters, undetected segmentation errors due to vitreoretinal abnormalities and unrecognized outer retinal abnormalities (e.g. drusens), which may modify segmentation in the inner retinal layers.[2-4,6-9]

INTERPRETATION EVIDENCES

For cross-sectional diagnostic purposes most OCT instruments provide *statistical classification* for each parameter, based on the parameter's relationship with the corresponding normal database.[1,4] The classification shows if the measured parameter value is within the statistically normal limits (green-color code); outside the statistically normal limits (red-color code); or between these categories (borderline, yellow-color code). One needs to understand that parameter values altered by measurement errors, diseases other than glaucoma or unusual but healthy anatomical variants all differ from the corresponding parameter ranges of the selected *supernormal* eyes in the normal database.

Therefore, ophthalmologists need to know that:

- The red-color code does not define true pathology/abnormality
- The green-color code does not define lack of pathology/abnormality
- When red-color code reflects a true pathological alteration it is not necessarily caused by glaucoma.

In clinical practice, unfortunately, misclassification of a healthy eye as glaucomatous simply because the color code of an OCT parameter is red is not uncommon (*red disease*).[2,3] Similarly, missing a true disease due to green OCT color code is not infrequent (*green disease*).[2,3]

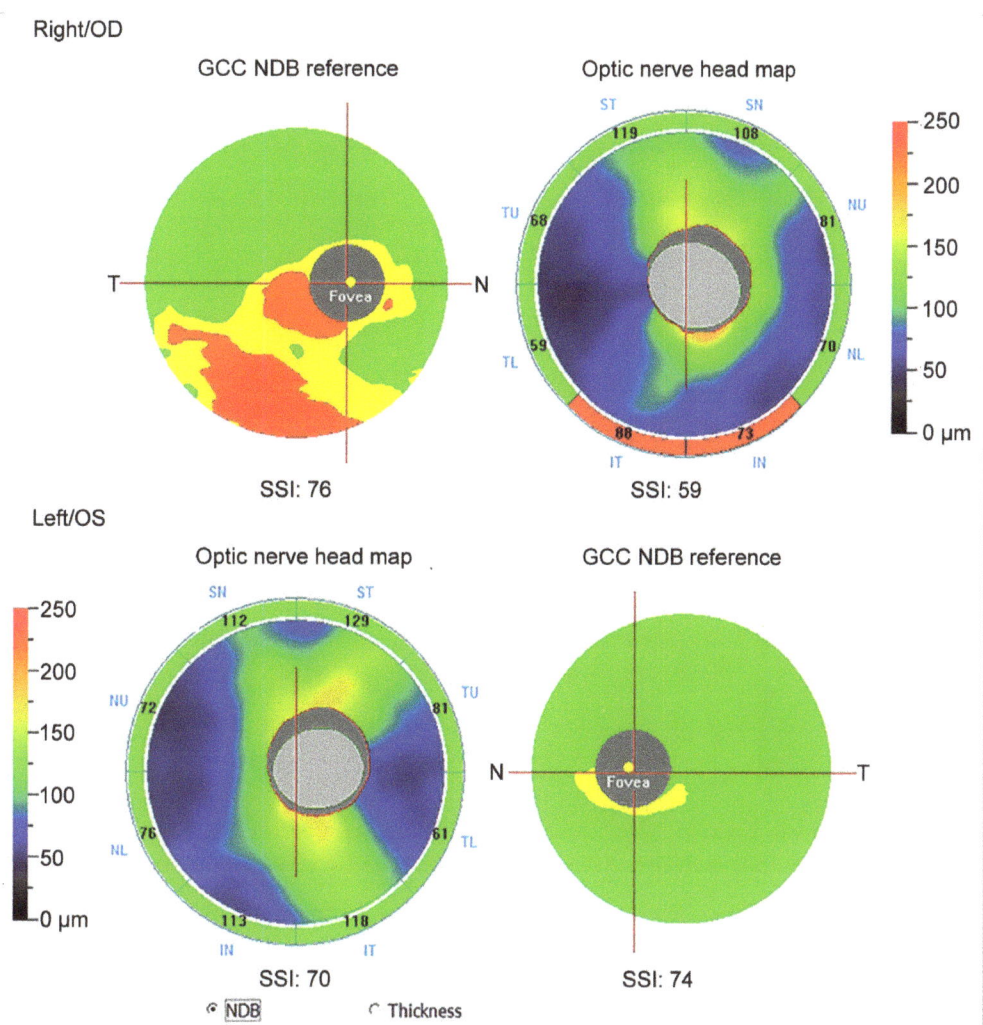

Fig. 14A.1: The true glaucomatous structural damage comprises spatially corresponding thinning of the inner macular retina (right eye, left image, red area) and the retinal nerve fiber layer (right eye, right image, red sectors). The left eye images show *within normal limits* thickness values for both the inner macular retina (right image) and the retinal nerve fiber layer (left image), thus the lack of structural damage is true.
(GCC: Ganglion-cell complex; NDB: Normal database; OD: Oculus dexter; OS: Oculus sinister).

Parameter Types and their Practical Clinical Value

The OCT instruments provide an *examination package* for glaucoma (*glaucoma protocol*). This comprises three parameter groups; each of them comprises several color-coded parameters. The three main parameter groups deal with:

1. The optic nerve head
2. The peripapillary retinal nerve fiber layer thickness (RNFLT)
3. The inner macular retina thickness.

Since the size of the optic nerve head shows a large interindividual variation[10] the optic nerve head parameters carry the least useful information for clinical decision-making.[1] In high myopia peripapillary RNFLT is decreased (independently from the presence or absence of glaucoma), thus this parameter group is less useful in high myopia than the inner macular thickness parameters.[11] It is important to understand that in glaucoma peripapillary RNFLT and inner macular retina thickness show spatially corresponding damages (Fig. 14A.1). This is due to the fact that they reflect the same pathology: the loss of ganglion cell bodies in the inner retina, and the loss of the ganglion cell axons

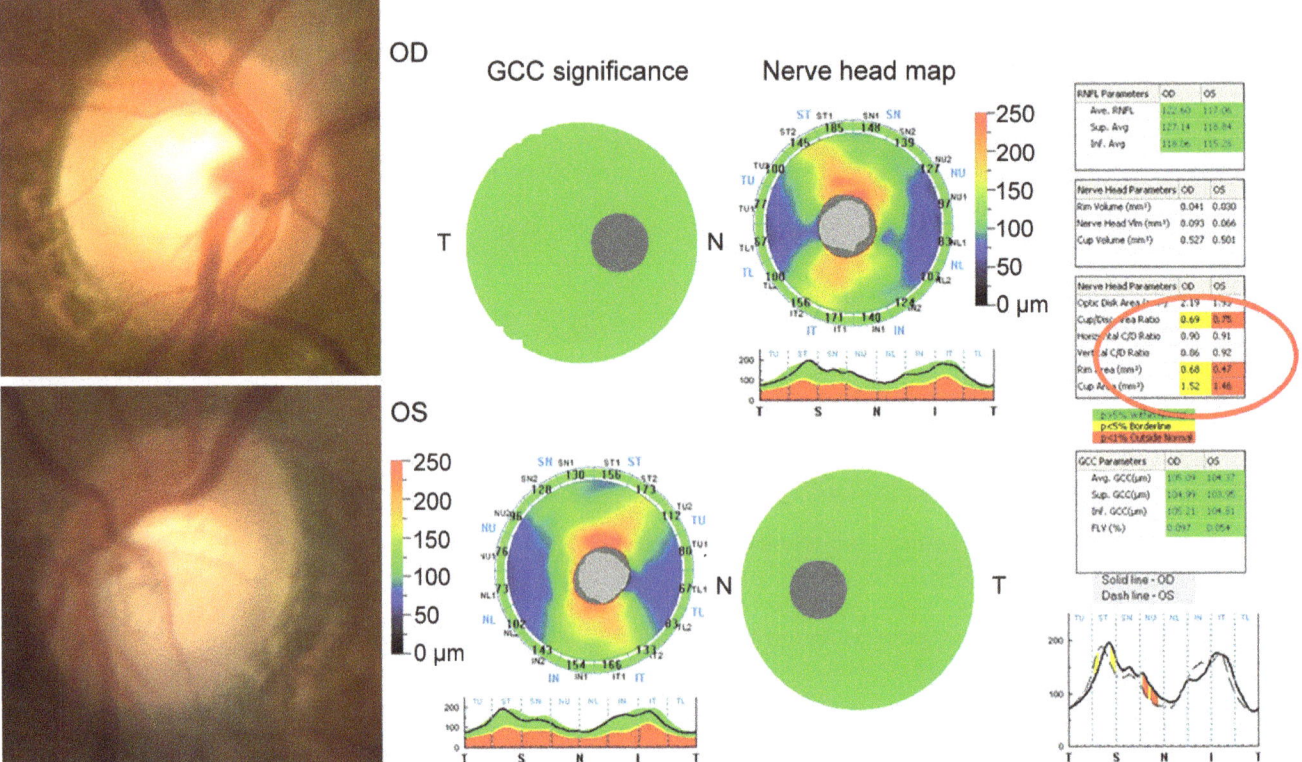

Fig. 14A.2: The congenital bilateral macrodiscs exceed the normal ranges of the disc parameters (encircled), but the retinal nerve fiber layer thickness and inner macular retina thickness parameter values are all *within normal limits*. (GCC: Ganglion-cell complex; OD: Oculus dexter; OS: Oculus sinister).

in the peripapillary retinal nerve fiber layer. When the spatial correspondence is missing or only one of the two parameter groups shows abnormalities the discrepancy is typically caused either by artifacts or a true pathology, which is not glaucoma.

Case 1: Red disease due to healthy macrodiscs

A 26-year-old gentleman presented on a routine eye examination. He had no visual complain and his best-corrected visual acuity was 1.0 on both eyes. His intraocular pressure was 24 mm Hg and 25 mm Hg, and his central corneal thickness measured was 586 microns and 590 microns on the right and left eye, respectively. The vertical cup-to-disc ratio was 0.75 in both the eyes (Fig. 14A.2). An OCT examination was made, which showed borderline (right eye) and outside normal limits (left eye) classifications for all optic nerve head parameters. The RNFLT and inner macular retina thickness parameters were all *within normal limits* in both eyes (Fig. 14A.2). The referring ophthalmologist set the diagnosis of *glaucoma OU*.

Explanation of the Case

The patient's intraocular pressure is explained with the relatively high-central corneal thickness. The discs are large and symmetric without any neuroretinal rim loss, thus the classification is macrodisc (macropapilla), which is a congenital normal variation. However, it results in parameter values outside the ranges of those in the OCT's database, thus the optic nerve head parameters are color-coded with red and yellow. The important information is that the RNFLT is normal and symmetric between the eyes, and the inner macular retina thickness parameters are all normal. The correct diagnosis is *macrodisc OU* with no acquired abnormality. The incorrect referral diagnosis was a typical *red disease*.

Case 2: Green disease due to macula edema

A 75-year-old female glaucoma patient, with advanced visual field defect on both eyes and decreased best-corrected visual acuity on the left eye, was referred for consultation. The referring ophthalmologist could not explain the

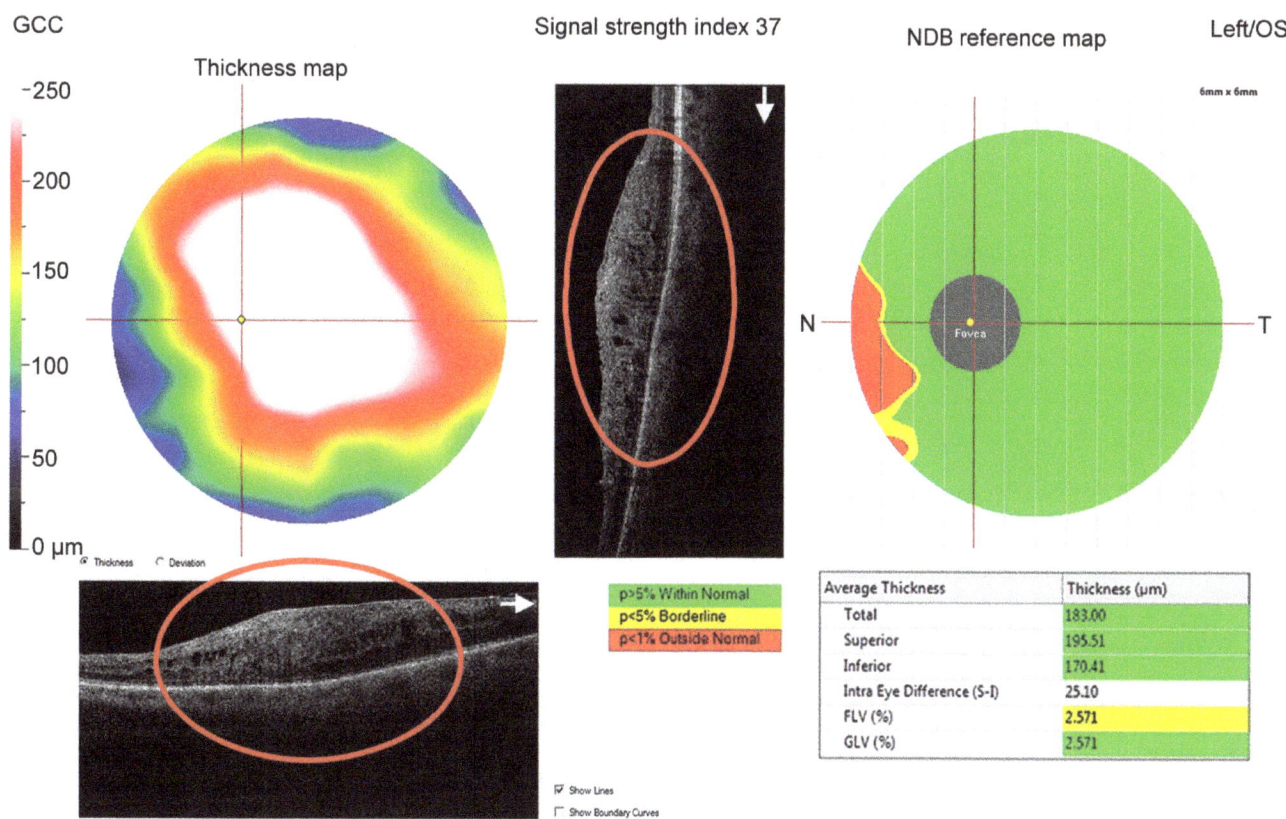

Fig. 14A.3: *Green disease*: The inner macular retina thickness is supernormal in severe glaucoma. This, however, reflects another disease: the severe edema of the macula is caused by an earlier retinal vein occlusion. If an ophthalmologist misses detailed image analysis on the screen and uses only the printed report, the glaucomatous inner macular retina damage remains undetected.
(GCC: Ganglion-cell complex; NDB: Normal database; OS: Oculus sinister).

coexistence of the severe RNFLT decrease and the *within normal limits* classification given to the inner macular retina thickness parameters on the left eye (Fig. 14A.3).

Explanation of the Case

The seemingly normal inner macular retina thickness of the left eye suffering from advanced glaucoma is due to thickened retinal layers (*green disease*, red circle). The thickening of the macular retina is caused by macula edema, which is a consequence of an earlier retinal vein occlusion.

Case 3: Blink artifact

This female patient was urgently referred to us for a very severe superior RNFLT damage of the right eye (Fig. 14A.4). The patient started her routine clinical assessment for

glaucoma a few days earlier, and OCT imaging was the first step of the examination.

Explanation of the Case

Based on the OCT image, we cannot tell if this patient has mild glaucoma or not, but we can tell that the reason of the urgent referral is an artifact. On the right eye, we see a complete loss of information and zero RNFLT superiorly (circles). Clinicians need to know that even when no retinal nerve fiber is preserved the RNFLT value provided by OCT instruments is different from zero: the measurement noise results in an approximately 50 microns RNFLT value.[12] In the current case, however, the value is 0 micron superiorly. This means that no information arrived back to the OCT instrument from the retina. This is caused by the upper eyelid (blink artifact), which

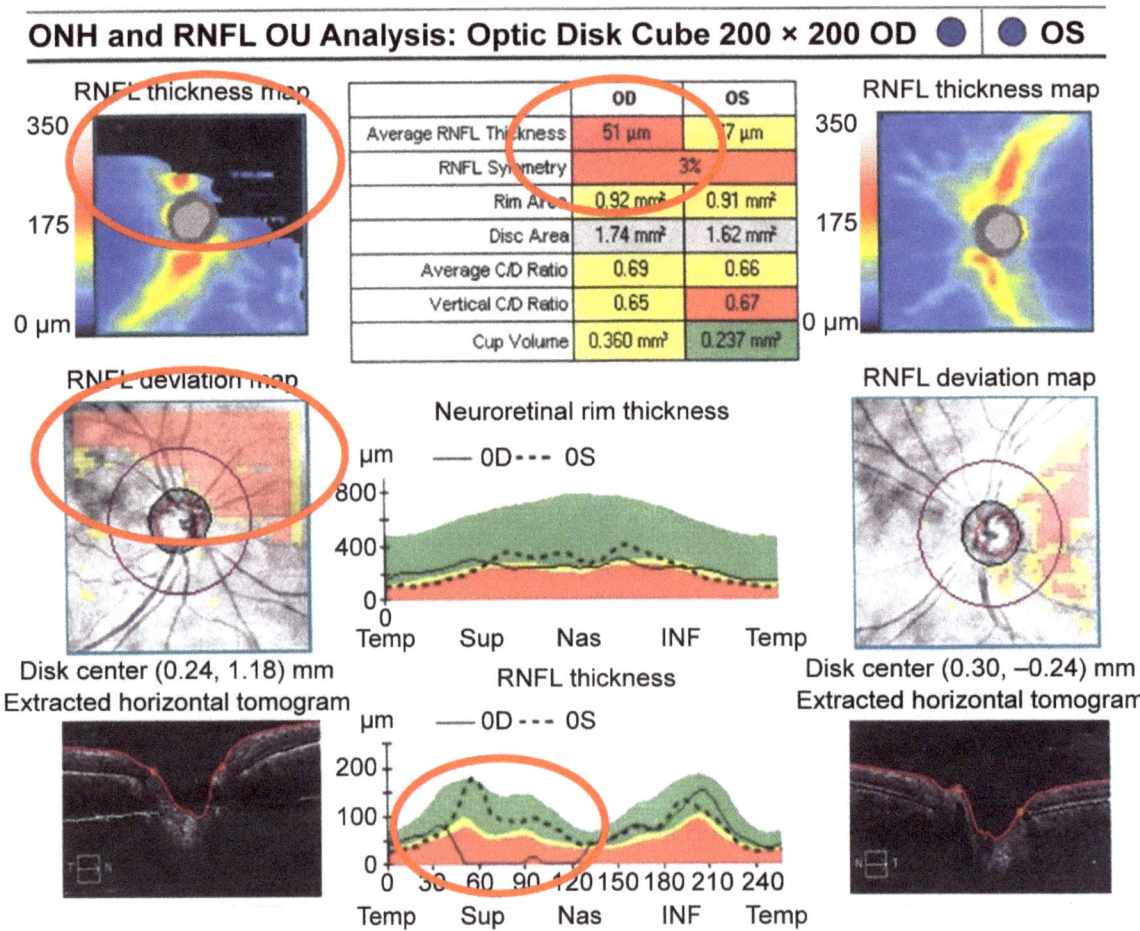

Fig. 14A.4: Blink artifact on the right eye image (encircled).
(OD: Oculus dexter; OS: Oculus sinister; ONH: Optic nerve head; RNFL: Retinal nerve fiber layer).

prevented the illumination light entering the eye. The image should have been deleted, and a new image should have been acquired to substitute the technically incorrect scan.

Case 4: Segmentation error due to a vitreoretinal surface abnormality

This 72-year-old female patient, with high myopia, had severely decreased RNFLT on both eyes (Fig. 14A.5). This can be due to pathological myopia with or without glaucoma, as discussed earlier in this chapter. Her referral was initiated to clarify a diagnostic problem: on the right eye the circumpapillary RNFLT was unexpectedly high (well within the normal range) superiorly and nasally, which did not fit to the findings of the clinical examination.

Explanation of the Case

The *within normal limits* classification of the superior and nasal RNFLT sectors of the right eye is caused by a segmentation error commonly seen in high myopia. It is due to an abnormality of the vitreoretinal surface. This type of segmentation error cannot be neutralized, thus it prevents using the RNFLT scans for clinical decision-making.

Case 5: Segmentation error caused by a vitreous floater

This case was a healthy nonglaucomatous control person who participated in a clinical research investigation. The inner macular retina thickness image shows no pathology, but a vitreous floater causes localized shadow effect

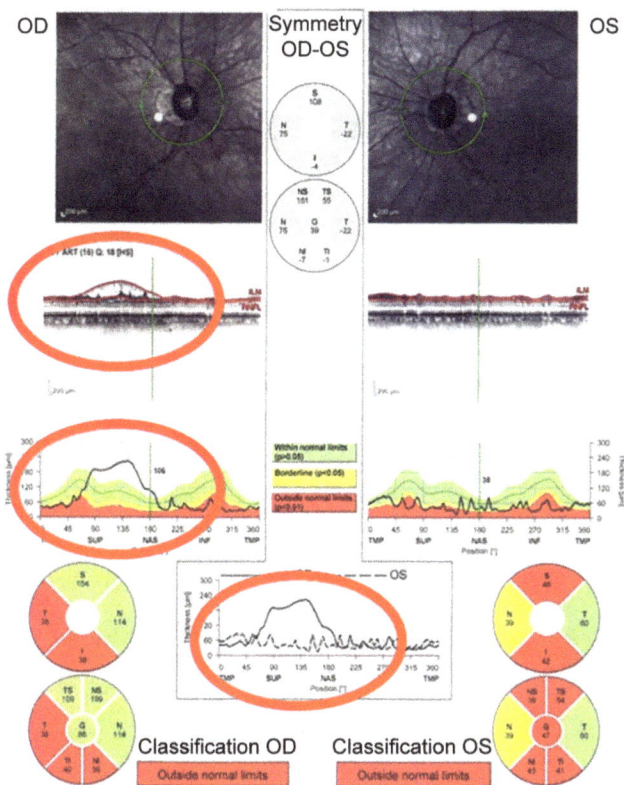

Fig. 14A.5: Segmentation error due to a vitreoretinal abnormality in high myopia (encircled). The segmentation error causes falsely high-retinal nerve fiber layer thickness values for the involved superior and nasal sectors.
(OD: Oculus dexter; OS: Oculus sinister; OCT: Optical coherence tomography).

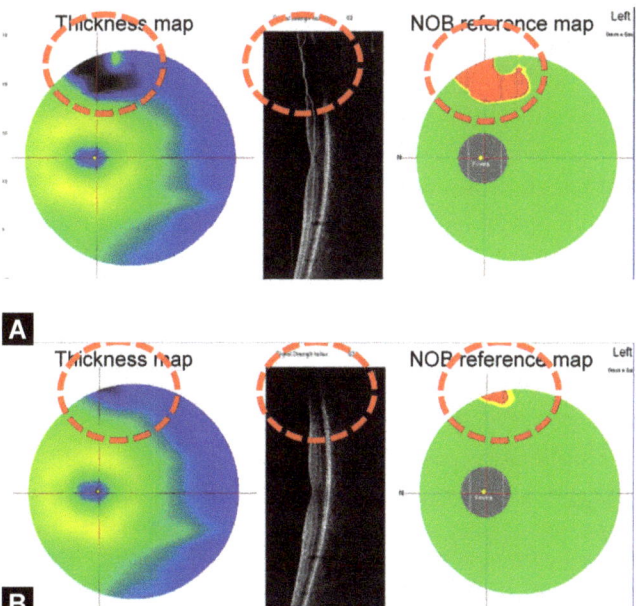

Figs. 14A.6A and B: Segmentation error caused by a vitreous floater on the inner macular retina thickness image: (A) The position of the vitreous floater is relatively central, thus the image is considerably influenced; (B) After some blinks the vitreous floater moves to a more peripheral location. The image is now less influenced and can be used for analysis. (NDB: Normal database).

superiorly (Fig. 14A.6A, circle). This reduces the signal and causes poor signal-to-noise ratio, which results in a segmentation error (circle). Such artifacts are common in glaucoma eyes, thus it is useful to know how to neutralize them.

Explanation of the Case

The operator asks the patient to blink a few times. Due to the forces during blinking the vitreous floater moves away from the image area (Fig. 14A.6B, circle). This reduces its influence on the measured values. With the OCT instrument employed in the actual case the periphery of the macular scan area is not used for the calculation of the inner macular retina thickness, thus the second image can be used for clinical purposes.

HOW TO AVOID MISINTERPRETATION OF RNFLT AND INNER MACULAR RETINA THICKNESS CHANGES DURING LONG-TERM FOLLOW-UP?

Progression analysis for detection and quantitative measurement of structural progression in glaucoma is a new and still developing application of OCT imaging. The software-provided progression analysis (linear regression analysis) is superior to the event analysis (comparison of two images obtained in different visits). Progression analysis provides information on thickness change per year (in microns/year), and indicates when the change is statistically significant.[13] However, it is mandatory to:

- Evaluate all images included in progression analysis for image quality
- Remove all images with artifacts and insufficient image quality from the analysis
- Identify progressing changes that are not related to glaucoma (e.g. increasing number of vitreous floaters,

progressing retinal damage due to progressive macular degeneration, decreasing image quality due to progressing cataract or progressing posterior capsule opacification after cataract surgery). In such cases, glaucoma progression analysis is misleading
- Carefully evaluate the various software versions used for image acquisition during follow-up, since software changes may result in unexpected changes, which can be misinterpreted for progression.

SUMMARY

Imaging cannot replace the detailed clinical evaluation of the optic nerve head and the ocular fundus. But information provided by modern OCT technology on RNFLT and inner macular retina thickness may usefully assist clinical decision-making and quantitative characterization of the structural parameters. Each ophthalmologist needs to be familiar with the technical and biological limitations of the imaging technique he/she uses, and needs to critically compare the images with the corresponding clinical findings. One should not replace clinical examination with reading the OCT report, but should use the possibilities offered by the OCT instrument's software for the evaluation of image segmentation, image quality and artifacts before an image is applied for clinical decision-making. Using only printed reports is a limitation since the layer-by-layer depth evaluation, which is essential to detect segmentation artifacts cannot be made on 2D printouts.

REFERENCES

1. European Glaucoma Society. (2011). 5th European Resident Glaucoma Course, Imaging technologies: hands on. [online] Available from http://www.eugs.org/eng/video_show2011.asp?id=2080. [Accessed July, 2016].
2. Asrani S, Essaid L, Alder BD, Santiago-Turla C. Artifacts in spectral-domain optical coherence tomography measurements in glaucoma. JAMA Ophthalmol. 2014;132(4):396-402.
3. Chong GT, Lee RK. Glaucoma versus red disease: imaging and glaucoma diagnosis. Curr Opin Ophthalmol. 2012;23(2):79-88.
4. Meier KL, Greenfield DS, Hilmantel G, et al. Special commentary: Food and Drug Administration and American Glaucoma Society co-sponsored workshop: the validity, reliability, and usability of glaucoma imaging devices. Ophthalmology. 2014;121(11):2116-23.
5. Naghizadeh F, Holló G. Influence of software upgrade on detection of localized nerve fiber defects with the RTVue optical coherence tomograph in glaucoma. Eur J Ophthalmol. 2013;23(3):423-6.
6. Holló G, Hsu SW, Naghizadeh F. Evaluation of a new software version of the RTVue optical coherence tomograph for image segmentation and detection of glaucoma in high myopia. J Glaucoma. 2016;25(6):e615-9.
7. Garas A, Papp A, Holló G. Influence of age-related macular degeneration on macular thickness measurement made with Fourier-domain optical coherence tomography. J Glaucoma. 2013;22(3):195-200.
8. Holló G, Naghizadeh F. Influence of a new software version of the RTVue-100 optical coherence tomograph on ganglion cell complex segmentation in various forms of age-related macular degeneration. J Glaucoma. 2015;24(3):245-50.
9. Nakanishi H, Akagi T, Hangai M, et al. Sensitivity and specificity for detecting early glaucoma in eyes with high myopia from normative database of macular ganglion cell complex thickness obtained from normal non-myopic or highly myopic Asian eyes. Graefes Arch Clin Exp Ophthalmol. 2015; 253(7):1143-52.
10. Holló G. The Optic Nerve in Glaucoma. In: Choplin NT, Traverso CE (Eds). The Atlas of Glaucoma, 3rd edition. London: Informa PLC; 2013. pp. 61-72.
11. Kim NR, Lee EK, Seong GJ, Kang SY, Kim JH, Hong S, et al. Comparing the ganglion cell complex and retinal nerve fibre layer measurements by Fourier domain OCT to detect glaucoma in high myopia. Br J Ophthalmol. 2011;95(8):1115-21.
12. Miki A, Endo T, Morimoto T, Matsushita K, Fujikado T, Nishida K. Retinal nerve fiber layer and ganglion cell complex thicknesses measured with spectral-domain optical coherence tomography in eyes with no light perception due to nonglaucomatous optic neuropathy. Jpn J Ophthalmol. 2015;59(4):230-5.
13. Holló G, Zhou Q. Evaluation of retinal nerve fiber layer thickness and ganglion cell complex progression rates in healthy, ocular hypertensive and glaucoma eyes with the Avanti RTvue-XR optical coherence tomograph based on 5-year follow-up. J Glaucoma. 2016. published online first, DOI: 10.1097/IJG.0000000000000410.

Sources of Errors While Interpreting Perimetry

Parul Ichhpujani, Sahil Thakur, Suresh Kumar

INTRODUCTION

Visual field testing is an important diagnostic test in the evaluation of conditions affecting the optic nerve such as glaucoma and other forms of neurological diseases. It is also helpful for retinal conditions and instances when visual field function needs to be measured. Given the subjective nature of the test, it is essential to differentiate true, disease-related defects and abnormalities from artifact and noise. In this chapter, we would discuss some scenarios, which highlight the need to evaluate visual field results cohesively linking all the data together.

Case 1: Error due to pupil size

A 64-year-old man was referred to the glaucoma clinic after routine Humphrey Swedish interactive thresholding algorithm (SITA) fast perimetry in both eyes, revealed a superior visual field defect in his left eye. The patient was asymptomatic and was visiting the hospital for a routine comprehensive annual check-up. There was no known family history of glaucoma. Past ocular history included a penetrating injury to the left eye with closure of an inferior limbal wound over 15 years ago. This had resulted in an inferiorly displaced pupil with loss of iris tissue inferiorly. On examination, best-corrected visual acuity (BCVA) was 6/6 in both eyes. Intraocular pressure (IOP) was 14 mm Hg oculus dexter (OD), and 12 mm Hg oculus sinister (OS). Examination of the anterior segment and gonioscopy of the right eye was unremarkable. Examination of the left eye revealed an inferior limbal scar with loss of iris tissue inferiorly and an inferiorly displaced pupil. Gonioscopy showed an abnormal angle over the inferior 90°, but the

remainder of the angle was normal. Fundus examination revealed healthy optic discs with a cup-to-disc (C:D) ratio of 0.2 and a healthy neuroretinal rim. Humphrey visual field perimetry using SITA standard algorithm in the left eye confirmed the superior field defect, as well as a more generalized depression more prominent in the left superior field. Visual field in the right eye was unremarkable. Repeat perimetry was performed 2 weeks later with the pupil dilated beforehand with 1% tropicamide. The visual field defect was no longer evident after pharmacological dilatation of the pupil. In view of the normal IOPs, normal optic disc appearances and normal visual fields post-dilatation, the patient was reassured and kept for routine follow-up, as there was no clinical evidence of glaucoma.

Inference

Pupil size is vital and an important parameter to consider when carrying out visual field examination, particularly where the patient is undergoing visual field monitoring. It is important to differentiate between true improvement and worsening of the visual field outcome from alterations in pupil size. Retinal illumination is determined by the pupil size and subsequently can influence visual field sensitivity. Deterioration in visual field sensitivity, resulting in a worsening of the visual field outcome, would be expected when the pupil size has decreased significantly, relative to the previous examination. Conversely, visual field improvement would be expected where the pupil size has increased over successive examinations. Pharmacological, surgical, traumatic or iatrogenic changes in the pupillary size can hence change the visual field outcome

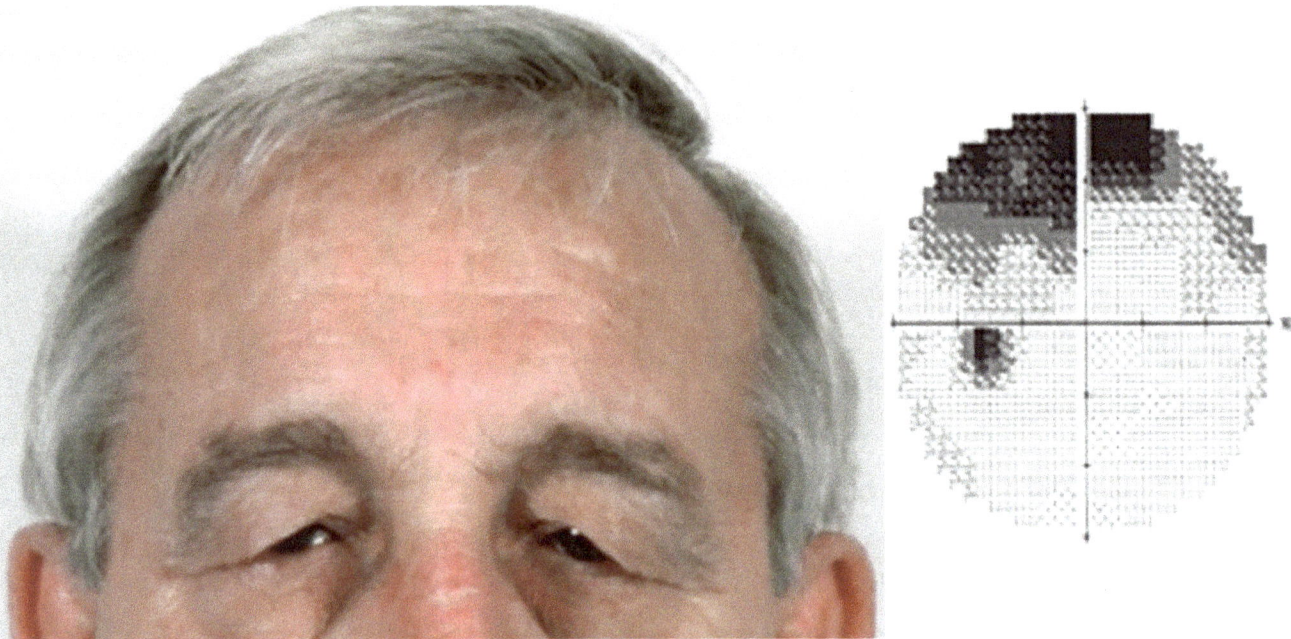

Fig. 14B.1: Dermatochalasis resulting in superior visual field defects.

of the patient. It is, therefore, good practice to measure and record the patient's pupil size under the illumination for the visual field examination so as to facilitate detection of artifacts due to pupillary size. Some perimeters have video-monitoring systems in addition to gaze tracking that are able to measure pupil diameter automatically and can account for changes in visual field outcome due to pupillary causes.

Case 2: Error due to drooping lid

A 70-year-old Asian-Indian man was referred to the glaucoma clinic as a disc suspect. His Humphrey SITA fast perimetry in both eyes revealed superior visual field defects. The patient was asymptomatic and there was no known family history of glaucoma. Past ocular history included uncomplicated cataract surgery for both eyes with good visual outcome. On examination, BCVA was 6/9 oculus utro (OU) and IOPs were 12 mm Hg OD, and 14 mm Hg OS. Anterior segment examination was unremarkable and gonioscopy showed open angles in both eyes. Fundus examination revealed symmetrical optic discs with a C:D ratio of 0.6 and a healthy neuroretinal rim. Repeat perimetry in both eyes also showed bilateral superior field defects, and more generalized depression prominent in the right superior field. On examination of ocular adnexa, dermatochalasis was noted and repeat perimetry was performed with the lids taped. The visual field defect was no longer

evident after taping of the lids. In view of the normal IOPs, symmetrical optic disc appearances suggestive of physiological cupping and normal visual fields postlid taping, the patient was reassured and referred to the oculoplasty clinic for opinion and subsequent uneventful blepharoplasties in both eyes that alleviated the visual field defects.

Inference

The normal extent of the superior visual field is approximately 55–60° at the 90° meridian. Impairment of the superior visual field can range from 20%, in mild ptosis to 64% in more severe cases where the eyelid crosses the middle of the pupil. Ptosis surgery is indicated when the superior visual field improves on taping by 12 degrees or more. Blepharoplasty is indicated, if there is 30% or more improvement after taping of superior visual field loss secondary to blepharochalasis, dermatochalasis (Fig. 14B.1) or pseudoptosis with upper field loss of atleast 20 degrees. It is important to record such interventions while visual field testing is done to make sure that the records are uniform and comparable.

Case 3: Error due to incorrect ocular aid

A 50-year-old male diagnosed with primary angle closure who had undergone bilateral laser iridotomy, elsewhere, was referred for further management to the glaucoma

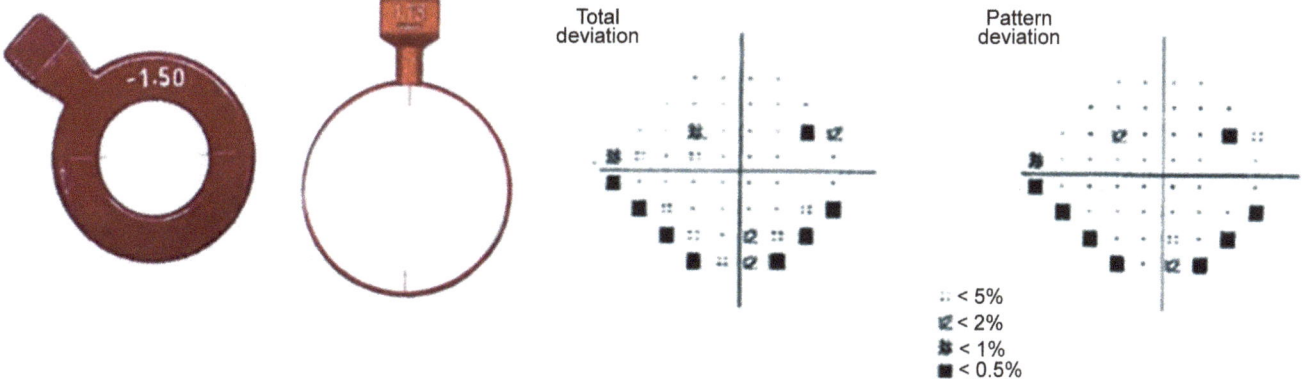

Fig. 14B.2: Thick-rimmed lenses induce rim artifact, which can be obviated by the use of thin-rimmed lenses.

clinic. His baseline Humphrey SITA fast perimetry in both eyes revealed inferior half ring defects in both eyes (Fig. 14B.2). On examination, his BCVA OU was 6/6. IOP was 14 mm Hg OD and 18 mm Hg OS; off drugs with patent iridotomies. Anterior segment examination was unremarkable. Fundus examination revealed healthy optic discs with a C:D ratio of 0.4 and a healthy neuroretinal rim. Humphrey visual field perimetry using SITA standard algorithm in both eyes confirmed the peripheral ring defect with low overall threshold values giving a total deviation error. It was, however, discovered that the thicker-corrective lenses were being used in the trial frame for testing on the Humphrey visual field analyzer. Examination was repeated with thin-rimmed lenses in the trial frame after proper centering and positioning of the lens. The visual field defect was no longer evident after testing with the trial frame. In view of the normal IOP, optic disc appearances and normal visual fields post use of correct trial frame, the patient was reassured and kept for routine follow-up, as there was no clinical evidence of glaucoma.

Inference

The choice of ocular aid while testing can cause significant artifacts and should always be checked, especially if the field defects do not correspond to the clinical findings. Spectacle rims, trial holder rims, position, nature, type and upkeep of the lenses used for providing correction can lead to visual field artifacts.

Case 4: Error due to fatigue

A 45-year-old female, ocular hypertensive patient, underwent Humphrey SITA fast perimetry in both eyes, which revealed a peripheral arcuate defect in the left eye. She had a positive family history of glaucoma and previous ocular history was unremarkable. On examination, visual acuity was 6/6 unaided in both eyes. IOP was 16 mm Hg OU. Anterior segment examination and gonioscopy of both eyes was unremarkable. Fundus examination revealed healthy optic discs with a C:D ratio of 0.45 and a healthy neuroretinal rim. Repeat Humphrey visual field perimetry in both eyes confirmed the peripheral arcuate defect in left eye with progressive worsening on repeat testing. She was advised to come after 2 weeks and examination repeated with the left eye being tested first. The peripheral visual field defect now manifested in the right eye and had classical *clover-leaf* pattern. The patient was reassured and on subsequent follow-ups the field became progressively better. In view of the normal IOPs, normal optic disc appearances and normal visual fields on follow-up, the patient was reassured and kept for routine follow-up, as there was no clinical evidence of glaucoma.

Inference

Fatigue is an important cause of visual field artifacts. It classically manifests as a cloverleaf pattern as the peripheral positions are thresholded in the latter stages of the visual field examination with increased false-negatives (Fig. 14B.3). Fatigue is also attributed to the Troxler fading or Ganzfeld blackout observed due to the influence of binocular rivalry from the occluded eye during monocular testing. This fading effect, which is thought to be cortical in origin, can be reduced by encouraging fixation to move during the visual field examination. Some perimeters periodically move the fixation target during the examination and, hence, reduce fatigue. Psychological factors also tend to affect visual field outcome and thus adequate patient

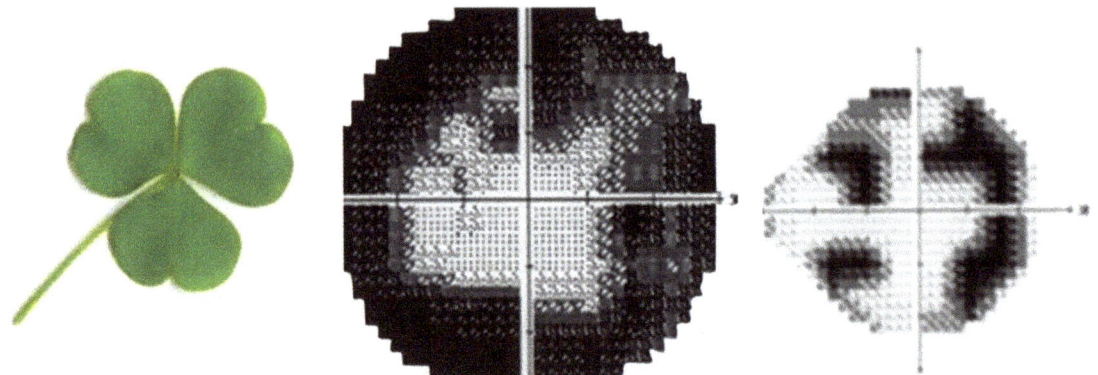

Fig. 14B.3: Central image shows the cloverleaf defect, and the extreme right image shows the inverse cloverleaf defect.

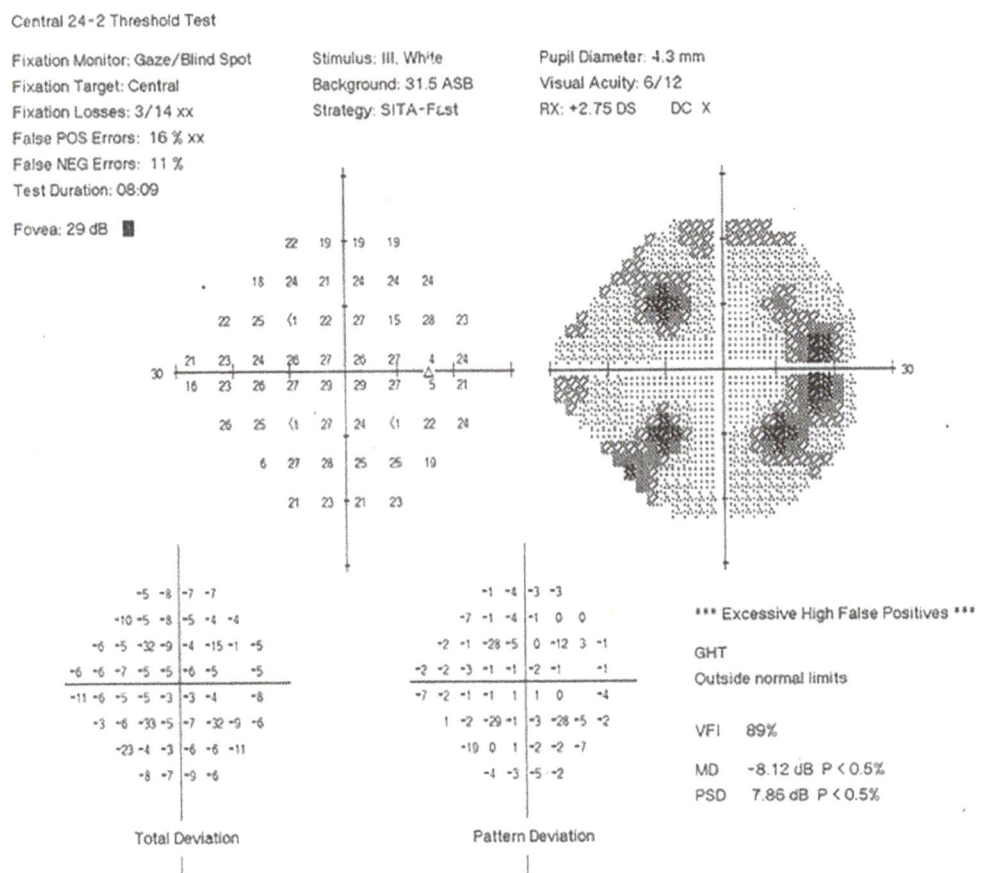

Fig. 14B.4: Unreliable test with an inverse cloverleaf pattern and high false-positive errors and a test duration of 8 minutes. (POS: Positive; NEG: Negative; SITA: Swedish interactive thresholding algorithm; GHT: Glaucoma hemifield test; VFI: Visual field index; MD: Mean deviation; PSD: Pattern standard deviation).

reassurance and encouragement can also aid to minimize such artifacts. By convention the right eye is tested first, but in cases like abovementioned one, the convention can be broken to aid correct diagnosis of the patient condition. Sometimes, cloverleaf pattern may also be seen if a patient is malingering. Inverse cloverleaf defect with high false-positives on the other hand suggests learning curve or functional loss.

One must also observe the time taken to perform the test. Long-test duration results in an unreliable test (Fig. 14B.4).

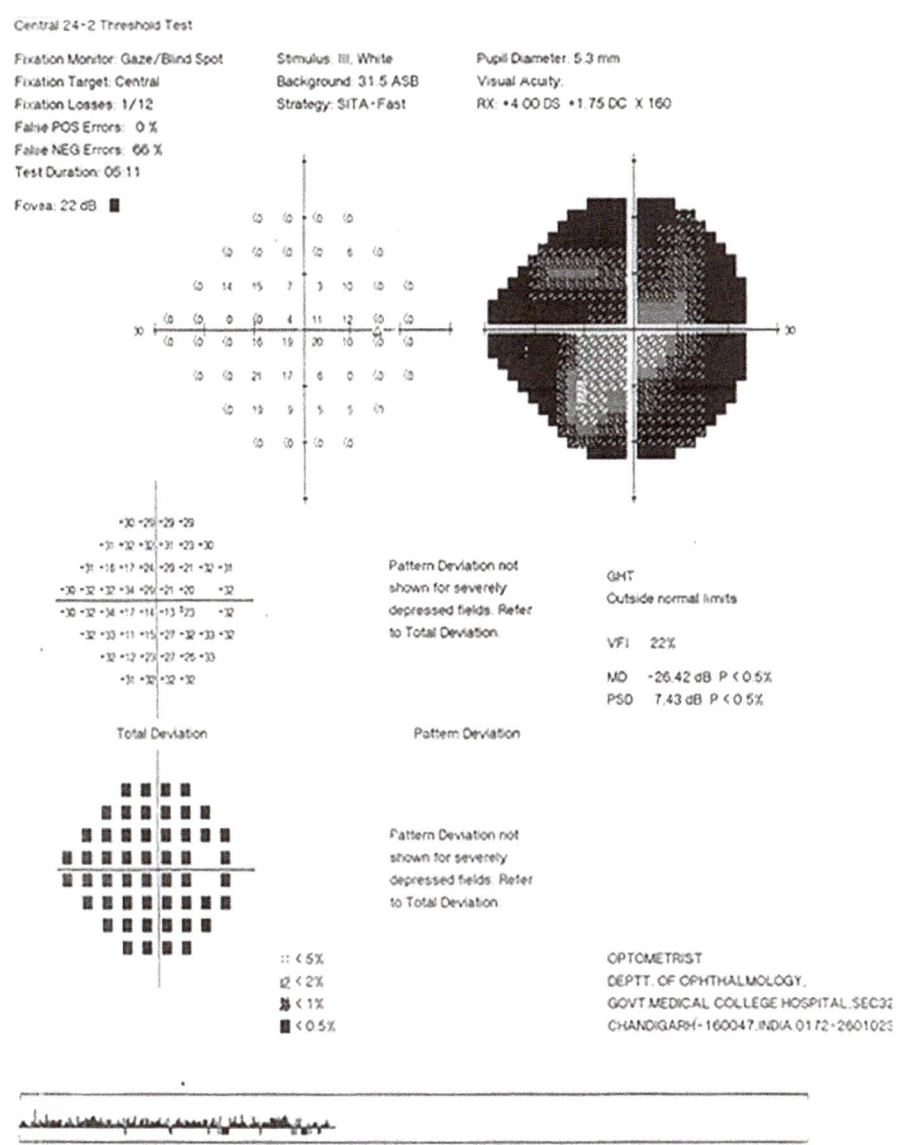

Fig. 14B.5: Very high false-negative errors in an inattentive patient.
(GHT: Glaucoma hemifield test; MD: Mean deviation; NEG: Negative; POS: Positive; PSD: Pattern standard deviation; SITA: Swedish interactive thresholding algorithm; VFI: Visual field index).

Some patients fail to understand the test and forget to press the button while performing. It is important that the test be fully explained and that the patient understands the purpose and process of the examination. A demonstration program can provide the practice to better understand the test and lessen learning effects (Fig. 14B.5).

POINTS TO REMEMBER

- It is a good idea for the physicians interpreting the visual field tests, to undergo the test themselves, so that they can better understand the difficulties faced by the patients while performing the test
- Eyelids that interfere with the visual field are taped open; then use artificial tears during the test to prevent dryness
- Perimetry is done by the perimetrist not the perimeter. It is important that the patient is monitored throughout the test, and that realignment, rest breaks, reinstruction and reassurance be provided, if necessary
- Perimetrists should make a note of patient's co-operation, reliability and level of attention

- Some other potential sources of error include:
  - Wrong patient, wrong eye, wrong entry of date of birth
  - Inattention to the change in refraction of the patient over time
  - Performing the test in an overlit, noisy and crowded room can affect the thresholds of seeing.

SUGGESTED READING

1. Anderson DR, Patella VM. Automated static perimetry, 2nd edition. St Louis: Mosby; 1999.
2. Bengtsson B, Heijl A. False-negative responses in glaucoma perimetry: indicators of patient performance or test reliability? Invest Ophthalmol Vis Sci. 2000;41(8):2201-4.
3. Castro DP, Kawase J, Melo LA. Learning effect of standard automated perimetry in healthy individuals. Arq Bras Oftalmol. 2008;71(4):523-8.
4. Hong S, Na K, Kim CY, Seong GJ. Learning effect of Humphrey Matrix perimetry. Can J Ophthalmol. 2007;42(5):707-11.
5. Kutzko K, Brito C, Wall M. Effect of instructions on conventional automated perimetry. Invest Ophthalmol Vis Sci. 2000;41(7):2006-13.
6. Zalta AH. Lens rim artifact in automated threshold perimetry. Ophthalmology. 1989;96(9):1302-11.

Sources of Errors While Performing and Interpreting Tonometry

Nikhil S Choudhary, Paaraj Dave, Parul Ichhpujani

INTRODUCTION

Determination of the intraocular pressure (IOP) is a central feature in the diagnosis and management of the glaucomas. A true measurement of IOP requires a direct fluid connection to the anterior chamber, but since that is not possible in clinical settings, an indirect measurement of IOP is done by tonometry. Tonometry is the measurement of the IOP by relating a deformation of the globe to the force responsible for the deformation. Over the years, there has been a radical change in our approach to the measurement of the IOP.

GOLDMANN APPLANATION TONOMETER

Goldmann applanation tonometer (GAT) is the current standard against which all other tonometers are compared. GAT is based on the Imbert-Fick principle, which states that the pressure (Pt) inside a sphere is equal to the external force (W) necessary to flatten the surface divided by the area (A) of flattening.

$$Pt = W/A$$

How to Perform Applanation Tonometry using Goldmann Applanation Tonometer?

Before undertaking Goldmann applanation tonometry, following precautions need to be taken:
- Avoid tonometry in infected or injured eyes.
- Clean prism before every use.
- Wait adequately for the cleaned surface to dry.
- Disinfect prism before first use and when indicated.
- Replace prism every 2–3 years.
- Unused prism can be kept indefinitely.
- Verify prism for scratches/sharp edges (Fig. 14C.1) and cracks because scratches can injure cornea and disinfectant can get into hollow of cracks and can cause chemical injury to cornea.

Procedure and Instrumentation

Insert the prism into the tonometer holder, ensuring the 0° or 180° markings line-up with the white line on the bracket. GAT is usually mounted permanently on the slit lamp; if not, mount the instrument on the slit lamp (Fig. 14C.2). Swing the tonometer round to locate it centrally in the measuring position. Prism and the tonometer should get fixed in the notch:
- Increase the light source to maximum intensity with the cobalt blue filter on and the slit opened fully. It should illuminate the prism from the side at about 60°.
- Explain the procedure to the patient. Instill a drop of anesthetic into the eyes.
- Positioning and co-operation of the patient are vital. Ensure the patient is comfortable with the chin on the chin rest and forehead firmly against the forehead bar. Ask the patient to look straight ahead with eyes wide open.
- Advance the slit lamp toward the eye with the joystick. When the tip of the prism is within a centimeter or so of the cornea, use the joystick to gently bring the tip into contact with cornea under direct vision. The limbus will light-up when you have made contact.

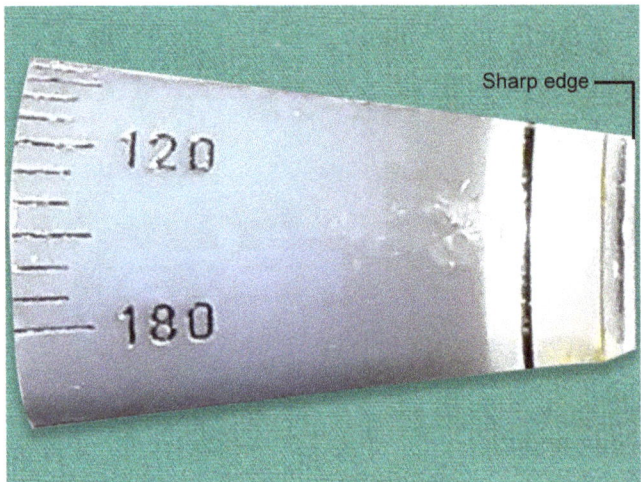

Fig. 14C.1: Tonometer tip with a sharp edge.

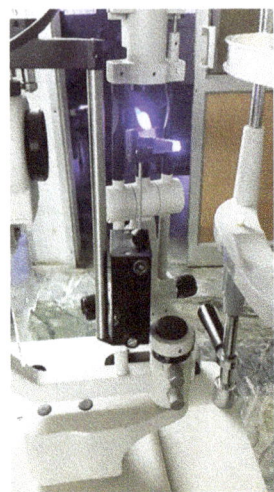

Fig. 14C.2: Applanation tonometer mounted on slit lamp.

- Look through the slit-lamp eyepiece (only one eyepiece, usually the left, is lined-up with the prism). You should see two semicircles of fluorescein shifted away from each other along the horizontal axis.
- Use the slit-lamp joystick to position the semicircles at the center of the prism. Now adjust the dial to alter the force on the prism and thus alter the overlap of the semicircles. The end point is regular pulsation of two semicircular rings of equal size the inner edges of which just interlock (Fig. 14C.3). These pulsations represent cardiac cycles. The correct value is the midpoint of this variation. The IOP in mm Hg is the value on the dial multiplied by ten.

Common Sources of Error and Ways to Avoid Them

- Patient should not hold breath during tonometry or have tight collar around neck. This can lead to overestimation of IOP.
- Patients are often unable to keep the eyes open without blinking, in which case you must gently hold open the lids with one hand. It is important not to apply any pressure to the globe, as this would increase the measured IOP. To avoid this, hold the lids against the orbital rim.
- Ensure the tonometer tip does not touch eyelashes. They are not anesthetized and this will induce blinking.
- Large overlapping semicircles, which do not pulsate and do not change size when the measuring dial is turned, indicate overapplanation (Fig. 14C.4). Ensure the slit lamp is not moved too far forward.

- The width of the fluorescein semicircles should be about one-tenth the diameter of the ring. A thin ring indicates insufficient fluorescein. This will underestimate the pressure. Ask the patient to blink or instill more fluorescein and try again.
- If there is too much fluorescein in the tear film or the prism touches the upper lid, a thick ring will be seen, resulting in overestimation of the pressure. Dry the prism and repeat.
- Inaccurate IOP readings can result from the presence of abnormal corneal thickness or corneal pathology. One may correct the measured IOP level for the pachymetry value of the patient using an appropriate correction formula.
- Repeating the measurement allows you to take an average to improve the accuracy.
- *Change in gaze*: IOP must be measured in primary gaze; IOP may be elevated in up-gaze (elevation of the eyes more than 15°).
- *Observer bias*: Expectations and digit preference for even numbers.

What to Do in a Patient with Marked Astigmatism?

- In patients with astigmatism of greater than 3D, the applanated area will be elliptical, not circular. This error can be avoided by applanation at 43° to the axis of the minus cylinder. This is done by lining-up the angle of the minus cylinder on the prism with the red mark on the prism holder (Figs. 14C.5A and B).

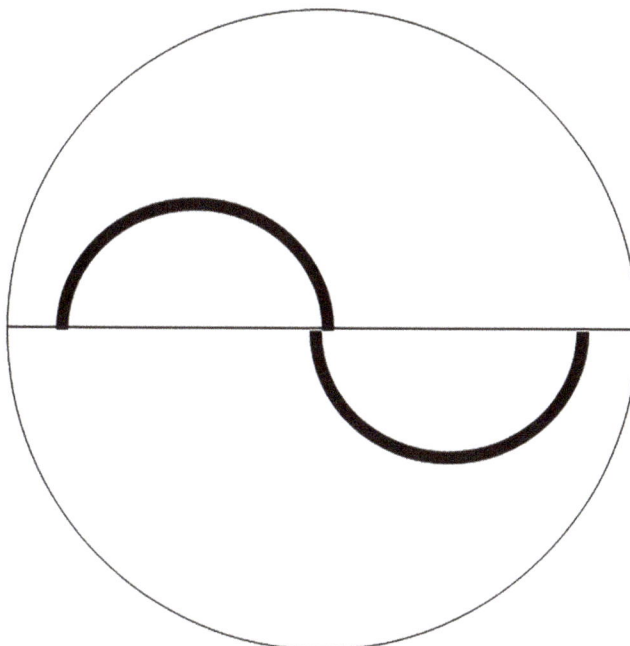

Fig. 14C.3: The recommended end point.

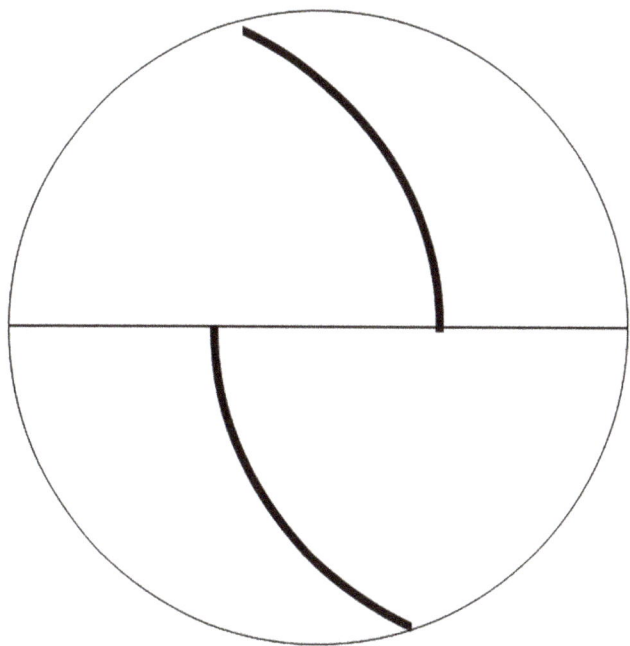

Fig. 14C.4: Overapplanation.

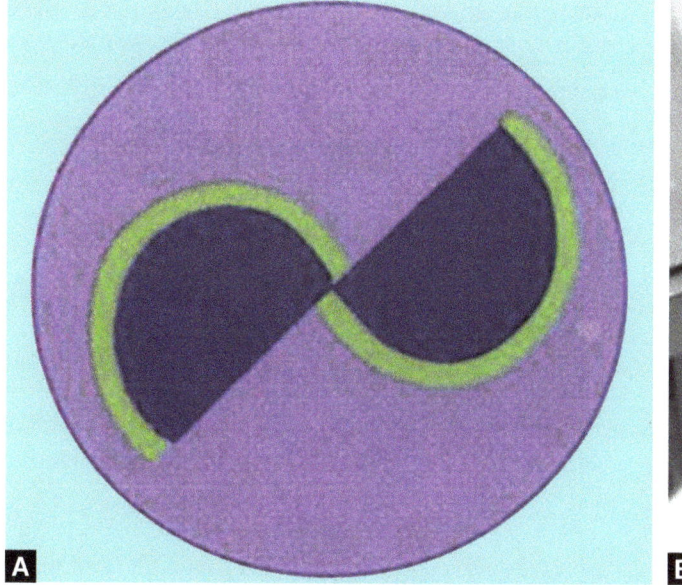

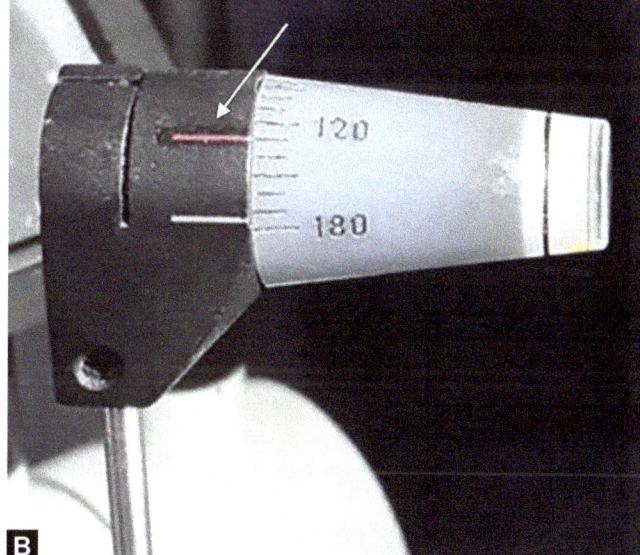

A **B**

Figs. 14C.5A and B: (A) Applanation tonometry in astigmatism; and (B) Arrow showing the red mark.

- One can also measure IOP in horizontal and vertical meridian and take average of these two readings as the final IOP
- Instead of using GAT for patients with marked astigmatism, you may consider using the Tono-Pen or a pneumotonometer, if a patient's cornea is significantly irregular (from refractive error, ectasia, scarring, etc.)

- For every three-diopter (3D) change in curvature, IOP increases by about 1 mm Hg as more fluid is displaced under steeper axis resulting in increased ocular rigidity
- Additionally, four-diopter (4D) with the rule astigmatism underestimates IOP and 4D against the rule astigmatism overestimates IOP.

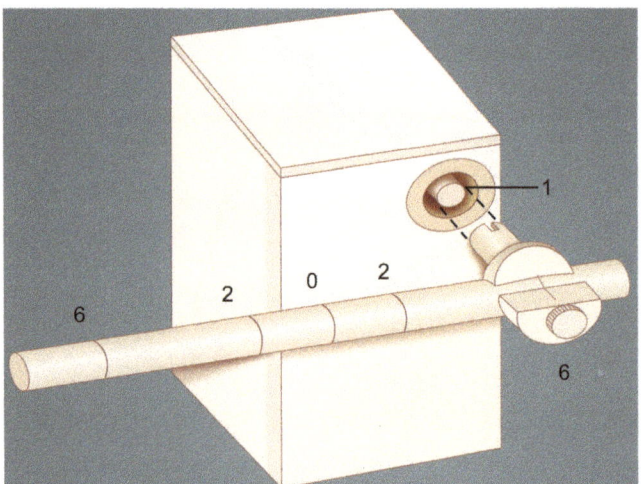

Fig. 14C.6: Calibration error check weight assembly.

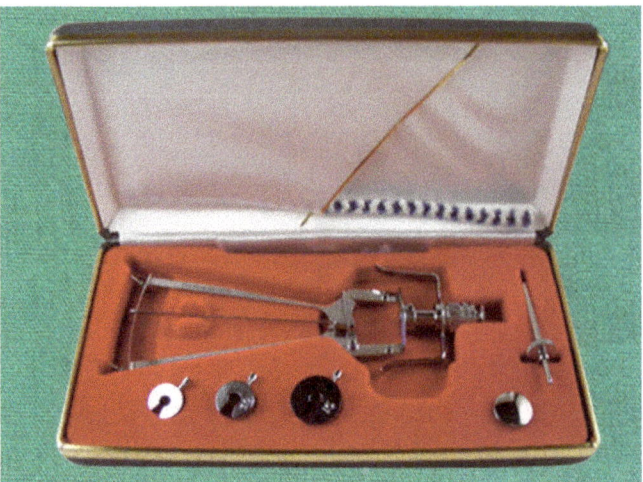

Fig. 14C.7: Schiotz tonometer.

How to Detect Calibration Error of the Goldmann Applanation Tonometer?

One must check the instrument for calibration error from time to time. This is done at dial position 0, 2 and 6 (0, 20 and 60 mm Hg equivalents) (Fig. 14C.6):

- Insert the prism in the holder and place the tonometer on the slit lamp
- At setting 0, if the dial position is moved to –0.05, the feeler arm should fall toward the examiner; if the drum is moved to position +0.05, the arm should fall toward the patient
- To check settings 2 and 6, the calibration error check weight bar provided by the manufacture is used
- The calibration error check weight bar has 5 markings on it. The central marking corresponds to level 0. Two on either side of it represent level 2 and the two outermost markings represent level 6. These markings correspond to 0, 20 and 60 mm Hg of IOP, respectively
- The calibration error checks weight bar and holder are fitted into the slot provided on the side of the applanation tonometer. After setting the mark on the weight bar corresponding to position 2 or 6 on the index mark of the weight holder, the measuring drum is rotated forward. The reading at which the feeler arm with the prism in place moves forward freely is recorded. The difference of this reading from the respective test position is the positive error at that level of testing. Similarly, on rotating the revolving knob in the reverse direction, the reading at which the feeler arm moves backward is noted. The difference between the latter

and the testing position is the negative error at that level of testing.

- The manufacturers of Haag-Streit GAT accept calibration errors within ±0.5 mm Hg at all levels of testing (0, 20 and 60 mm Hg). World Glaucoma Association accepts calibration error within ±1 mm Hg at all testing levels. On the other hand, the South East Asia Glaucoma Interest Group (SEAGIG) guideline is less stringent and recommends that the acceptable range of calibration error should progressively widen at the higher levels of error testing. By this guideline, the acceptable error could be within ±2 mm Hg at 0 mm Hg, ±3 mm Hg at 20 mm Hg and ±4 mm Hg at 60 mm Hg testing levels.
- If a GAT has unacceptable calibration error, the instrument should be sent to the manufacturer for rectification of the error. One should avoid estimating true IOP from a faulty GAT by applying a correction factor as the calibration error of GAT has high variability.

SCHIOTZ INDENTATION TONOMETER

In the developed world, Schiotz tonometer has become obsolete, but still many peripheral health facilities in developing countries use the Schiotz tonometer (Fig. 14C.7). This tonometer works on the basic concept of indentation tonometry. The body of the tonometer has a footplate, which rests on the cornea. A plunger moves freely (except for the effect of friction) within a shaft in the footplate and the degree to which it indents the cornea gives an estimate of the IOP.

How to Perform Indentation Tonometry using Schiotz's Tonometer?

With the patient in supine position and fixing on a target just overhead, the examiner separates the eyelids and gently rests the tonometer footplate on the anesthetized cornea in a position that allows free vertical movement of the plunger. When the tonometer is properly positioned, the examiner observes a fine movement of the indicator needle on the scale in response to the cardiac pulsations. The scale reading should be taken as the average between the extremes of these excursions. It is customary to start with the fixed 5.5 gram weight. However, if the scale reading is four or less, additional weight should be added to the plunger. A conversion table is then used to derive the IOP in mm Hg from the scale reading and plunger weight.

Sources of Errors with a Schiotz Indentation Tonometer

The accuracy depends on the assumption that all eyes respond the same way to the external force of indentation, which is not the case. The following are some of the more common variables that introduce potential for error:

- *Errors inherent to the instrument*: Difference in weights of the different parts, difference in the curvature, size and shape of the footplate, friction arising in movement of the plunger and the pointer on the scale
- *Ocular rigidity*: The instrument is grossly unreliable for IOP measurement-following glaucoma or vitreoretinal surgery or open-globe injuries due to low-scleral rigidity in these conditions
- Error due to blood volume alteration
- *Corneal influences*: Steeper or thicker cornea leads to a falsely high-IOP reading
- *Moses effect*: Cornea may mold into space between plunger and hole in tonometer footplate, pushing up the plunger and yielding a falsely high-IOP reading
- Parallax error in reading the scale
- Repeated tonometry causes underestimation of IOP, this effect most marked between first and second readings, but the trend continues through a number of repetitions
- Errors due to contraction of extraocular muscles tend to increase IOP
- Error due to accommodation, if the patient looks toward tonometer while reading is being taken. Contraction of ciliary muscle increases the facility of aqueous outflow by pulling on trabeculae.

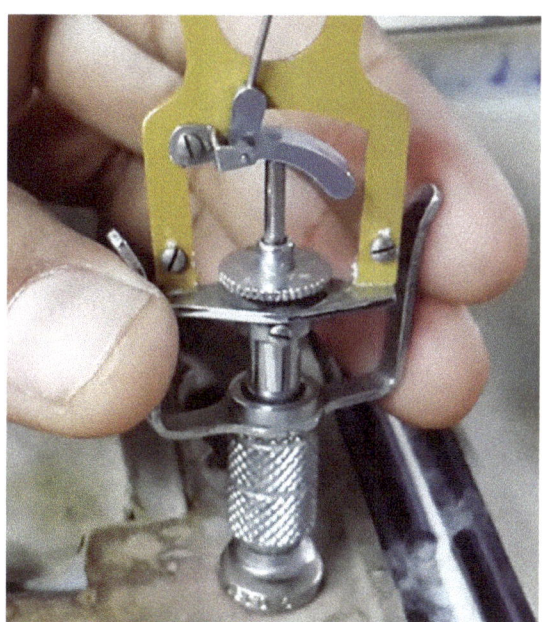

Fig. 14C.8: Checking for calibration error in Schiotz tonometer.

Pearls for the Care of Schiotz Tonometer

- Zero error must be checked before the day starts (Fig. 14C.8)
- For cleaning in between cases, sodium hypochlorite can be used to disinfect the tonometer
- Cleaning of barrel should be done daily to avoid plunger sticking to the barrel
- Storage must be done in dry, dust free environment with separable parts separated.

NONCONTACT TONOMETER

The noncontact tonometer (NCT) has three components mounted on a table (Fig. 14C.9):

1. *Pneumatic system*: Generates a puff of air whose force increases linearly with time, progressively flattening the cornea
2. *Alignment system*: Allows the operator to align the patients cornea
3. *The optoelectronic applanation monitoring system*: Consists of a transmitter, which directs a collimated beam of light at the corneal vertex and a receiver and detector, which accepts only parallel, coaxial rays reflected from the cornea. The undisturbed cornea reflects very few rays into the receiver, but a reduction of corneal curvature increases the number of rays that

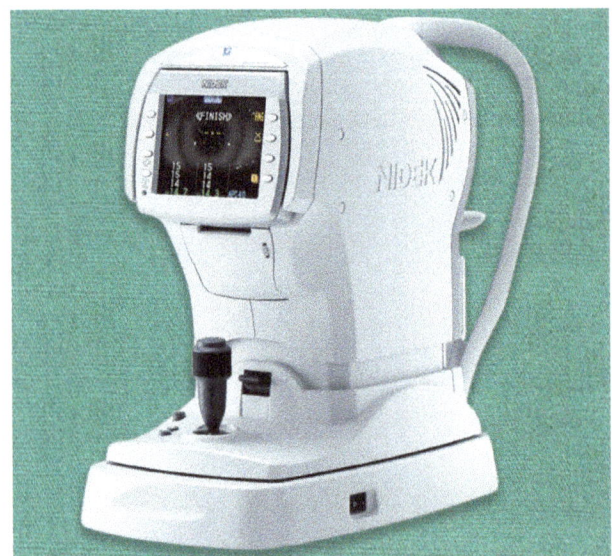

Fig. 14C.9: Noncontact tonometer.

are accepted and sensed, with the maximum occurring at the moment of applanation. An electronic clock measures the time from the ejection of the puff to the reception of the maximum number of rays in microseconds. The time interval is dependent upon the IOP with higher pressures requiring more time. Some newer machines directly measure the force of the air puff generated at the moment of applanation. The IOP reading is based on prior comparisons with the GAT.

How to Perform Noncontact Tonometry?

As the patients head is positioned on the chin rest, the pneumatic system generates a puff of room air that is triggered automatically when the cornea is properly aligned. The IOP is then shown on the digital display in mm Hg.

Sources of Errors with Noncontact Tonometer

Many patients need assistance for adequately opening their eye during tonometry. Small fissure sizes, dermatochalasis, long eyelashes, blepharospasm and the reflex or fear of an object close to the eye can all make obtaining a pressure reading difficult and artificially high. Instruct patients to keep both eyes open and concentrate on a distant target (such as a fixation light).

Intraocular pressure is an important element for glaucoma examination and it must be done carefully and accurately.

SUGGESTED READING

1. Choudhari NS, George R, Baskaran M, Vijaya L, Dudeja N. Measurement of Goldmann applanation tonometer calibration error. Ophthalmology. 2009;116(1):3-8.
2. Choudhari NS, Jadhav V, George R, Vijaya L. Variability in the calibration error of the Goldmann applanation tonometer. J Glaucoma. 2011;20(8):492-6.
3. Friedenwald JS. Some problems in the calibration of tonometers. Am J Ophthalmol. 1948;31(8):935-44.
4. Garway-Heath T, Kotecha A, Lerner F, et al. Measurement of intraocular pressure. In: Weinreb RN, Brandt JD, Garway-Heath DF, Medeiros FA (Eds). World Glaucoma Association: Intraocular pressure: Consensus Series-4, 4th edition. Amsterdam: Kugler publications; 2007. pp. 17-54.
5. Grafe M. The effect of corneal thickness on non contact tonometry. Klin Monbl Augenheilkd. 1991;199(3):183-6.
6. Popovich KS, Shields MB. A comparison of intraocular pressure measurements with the XPERT noncontact tonometer and Goldmann applanation tonometry. J Glaucoma. 1997;6(1):44-6.
7. South East Asia Glaucoma Interest Group. (2008). Asia Pacific Glaucoma Guidelines. [online] Available from http://www.icoph.org/dynamic/attachments/resources/asia-pacific_glaucoma_guidelines.pdf. [Accessed July, 2016].

Clinical Trials in Glaucoma

Suneeta Dubey, Madhu Bhoot, Nishtha Singh, Dushyant Sharma, Monica Gandhi

INTRODUCTION

There are numerous clinical trials in glaucoma, which provide adequate statistical power to address the issues relating to the treatment paradigms and natural history of glaucoma across the spectrum of glaucoma disease from ocular hypertension to advanced glaucoma. In depth knowledge of these evidence-based clinical trials is must for improvement in patient care and clinical outcomes. This chapter reviews these landmark clinical trials and highlights the clinical implications and practical usage of each study in a format which is easy to read and understand.

OCULAR HYPERTENSION TREATMENT STUDY

In the spectrum of glaucoma presentation, 4–7% are ocular hypertensives. There is no consensus on the efficacy of medical treatment in delaying or preventing the onset of primary open-angle glaucoma (POAG) among these individuals. With this rationale, the ocular hypertension treatment study (OHTS)[1,2] was designed to address the issue, whether the benefits of treatment outweigh the potential risks of long-term ocular hypotensive medication use in ocular hypertensives.

The study has been conducted in three phases. Phases 1 and 2 have been completed and phase 3 is in under planning.

Purpose

Phase 1

- To determine the safety and efficacy of topical ocular hypotensive medication in delaying or preventing the onset of POAG
- To identify baseline demographic and clinical factors which predict the risk of developing POAG.

Phase 2

- To compare the safety and efficacy of earlier versus later treatment in preventing POAG in individuals with ocular hypertension.

Methodology

The OHTS was a long-term randomized, multicentered clinical trial conducted on 1,636 patients age 40–80 years enrolled between 1994 and 1996. All patients had untreated intraocular pressure (IOP) of 24–32 mm Hg in one eye, 21–32 mm Hg in fellow eye with normal visual fields (VFs) and optic discs.

Considering the higher prevalence of POAG in African American races, it was made sure that at least 25% African American were enrolled in the study.

Ocular hypertension patients who were at a moderate risk of developing POAG were randomly assigned to either close observation only or a stepped medical regimen with the commercially available topical antiglaucoma drugs.

All the patients were followed for a period of 5 years with VF testing by Humphrey 30-2 every 6 months and stereoscopic disc photos annually. The end point of the study was the development of glaucoma, which was defined as the development of a reproducible VF abnormality or a reproducible clinically significant optic disc deterioration in one or both eyes that could be atributed attributed to POAG.

Results

Phase 1

- At the end of 5 years, the medication group had mean IOP reduction of 22.5 ± 9.9% as compared to 4.4 ± 11.6% in the observation group. The probability of development of POAG at the end of 5 years was 4.4% in the medication compared to 9.5% in the observation group thereby decreasing the incidence of POAG by 50% by starting medicines in ocular hypertensives
- On univariate analysis, the baseline factors which predict the development of POAG in ocular hypertensives were older age, race (African American), sex (male), higher IOP, larger vertical cup-to-disc (C:D) ratio, larger horizontal C:D ratio, greater pattern standard deviation (PSD), heart disease and thinner central corneal measurement. Where as on multivariate analysis only factors like older age, higher IOP, greater PSD, thinner central corneal thickness (CCT), larger vertical C:D ratio were found to contribute to a higher risk of glaucoma progression in ocular hypertensives.

Some additional results of the follow-up studies are:

- Ocular hypertension study was the first study which has laid emphasis on the role of CCT in glaucoma. Out of all the risk factors, thinner CCT (555 microns or less) had the maximum hazard ratio, i.e. they were at threefold higher risk of developing POAG irrespective of baseline IOP and vertical C:D ratio. CCT also influences the IOP measurements
- Due to availability of large database of VF, the OHTS group determined the reproducibility of retest in VF analysis. On retesting, abnormalities were not confirmed in 604 (85.9%) of the 703 originally abnormal and reliable VFs.

Phase 2

At the end of phase 1 of OHTS, the treatment group had a 50% less likelihood of developing POAG as compared to observation only group. However it did not answer when the treatment should be started and what are the risks of not starting treatment.

Phase 2 began in 2002, after 7.5 years of observation, and participants originally randomized to observation group were started on medication. Both the groups were followed-up and the development of POAG was compared at the end of 13 years.

Cumulative probability of developing POAG at 13 years was 22% in observation group (delayed treatment) and 16% in medications (early treatment) and no statistical difference in the risk of developing POAG in either group was noted. The delayed group had more eyes with structural and functional damage and more subjects with bilateral disease. Early treatment did delay the onset of POAG (6.0 vs 8.7 years) but the risk remains equal for both groups on long-term follow-up.

Conclusion

Starting IOP-lowering medication in ocular hypertensive patients is effective in reducing the risk of development of POAG by 50%. However, this does not imply that all borderline elevated IOP should receive treatment. Clinician should have an individual approach based on risk factors.

Phase 3 (In Planning)

With growing emphasis on evidence-based healthcare, OHTS phase 3 trial has been planned with the following aims:

- Find out if the incidence of glaucoma increases, decreases or stays the same over 20 years and how many people develop substantive VF loss as opposed to just preperimetric glaucoma
- Develop a 20-year prediction model for stratifying OHT patients by their risk of developing POAG
- Develop a model for predicting which OHT and early POAG patients will progress rapidly versus slowly.

EARLY MANIFEST GLAUCOMA TRIAL

The pathogenesis of POAG remains uncertain. A higher than average IOP often accompanies POAG and is considered to be a major risk factor for developing open-angle glaucoma (OAG). The goal of medical and surgical treatments for glaucoma is to reduce intraocular pressure. Although the association between IOP and glaucoma risk seems clear, the role of IOP reduction in preventing field loss is not well-established. This has led to controversies in glaucoma management and difficulties in defining indications for treatment, especially in early disease and in patients with moderately increased IOP. The Early Manifest Glaucoma Trial (EMGT) was designed to evaluate the efficacy of IOP-lowering treatment on the progression of POAG with moderately elevated and low-IOP values.[3]

Purpose

Primary Aim

- To compare the effect of immediate therapy to lower IOP, versus late treatment or no treatment on the progression of newly detected OAG, as measured by increasing VF loss and/or optic disc changes.

Secondary Aims

- To determine the extent of IOP reduction attained by treatment
- To explore factors that may influence glaucoma progression
- To describe the natural history of newly detected glaucoma.

Methodology

Early manifest glaucoma trial was a randomized controlled clinical trial consisting of 255 patients between age group of 50 and 80 years. All the patients had early glaucoma with mean deviation MD of less than equal to 6 dB and a median IOP of 20 mm Hg. The patients were identified by a population-based screening. Patients with IOP more than 30 mm Hg or advanced glaucoma were excluded.

Eligible patients were randomized evenly in control (n = 126) and treatment arm (n = 129). The treatment group received 360° trabeculoplasty and betaxolol 0.5% twice a day. Latanoprost 0.005% once a day was added, if IOP was more than 25 mm Hg checked in two consecutive visits for patients in treatment arm. In control group, latanoprost was added if the IOP was more than 35 mm Hg. Patients were followed for a minimum period of 4 years and maximum of 9 years to assess the development and progression of glaucoma. Study visits included VF analysis and IOP recording every 3 months and optic disc photographs done every 6 months.

Results

- After a median follow-up of 6 years the treatment decreased the IOP by 25% (5.1 mm Hg) and this was maintained throughout the follow-up

- Progression was seen in 62% of the control group participants compared to 45% of the treatment group. The treatment initiation delayed the progression by approximately 2 years.
- The risk of progression increased by 10% with each mm Hg higher baseline IOP, 3% per 1dB of worse MD, 1% per year of age.
- Factors associated with progression were higher baseline IOP, exfoliation, bilaterality of disease, worse MD, older age and frequent disc hemorrhage.

Conclusion

The benefits of IOP lowering were reiterated and the natural history of early glaucoma was highlighted.

The absolute risk reduction of 17% by starting early treatment and that for every 1 mm Hg decrease in IOP on follow-up reduced the risk of progression by 10% remain the major contribution of the study.

COLLABORATIVE INITIAL GLAUCOMA TREATMENT STUDY

Medications have been traditionally used as first-line therapy for glaucoma whereas recent reports suggest that more effective control of glaucomatous damage can be obtained by early or immediate filtration surgery. In addition, increased attention to the impact of therapy on health-related quality of life has added another consideration in deciding upon appropriate treatment of such patients. The collaborative initial glaucoma treatment study (CIGTS) was undertaken to evaluate the effect of trabeculectomy versus eye drops in newly diagnosed glaucoma patients and also used quality of life measures to assess the impact of these therapies on patients.

Purpose

To compare the effectiveness of standard medical therapy versus filtration surgery to treat newly diagnosed OAG.

Methodology

The CIGTS, a randomized, controlled clinical trial, conducted on 607 newly diagnosed OAG patients through 14 centers and community ophthalmologists in United States between 1993 and 1997. Patients aged between 25 and 75 years, IOP more than or equal to 20 mm Hg and evidence of optic nerve damage in one or both eyes were included in the study. Eligible patients were randomized to receive either a stepped medication treatment regimen or filtration surgery to control their OAG.

The patients in both groups were aggressively treated to lower the IOP to a predetermined individualized target based on the patient's baseline pretreatment IOP and VF score.

In the surgical arm, the patient underwent trabeculectomy within 14 days of randomization. If further treatment was required, argon laser trabeculoplasty (ALT) followed by medications and a repeat trabeculectomy with an antifibrotic agent was planned.

In the medical arm, patients received a stepwise regimen of topical medication, beginning with monotherapy. Additional medicines were added, if IOP remained uncontrolled followed by ALT and trabeculectomy.

Patients were followed every 6 months for a period of 5 years to look for any signs of intervention failure (failure to meet the target IOP or evidence of progressive VF loss or both). Patients were interviewed over phone to assess their health-related quality of life.

Results

At up to 5 years follow-up, both groups had substantial/sustained decrease in IOP with surgical group's IOPs 2–3 points lower than medication group. However, initially over first 3 years, surgical group had more VF and visual acuity (VA) loss. Difference disappeared after 4/5 years. Surgery group had more cataract extractions than the medical group. Both groups were satisfied with the quality of life associated with their treatment. Surgery group reported more eye symptoms over the first few years of follow-up. Medical group reported inconsistent systemic symptoms.

An IOP lowering of 30% or IOP in upper teens was found to prevent progression. The overall rate of progression was slightly higher in the medication group in terms of both VF loss and optic disc cupping (P = 0.007).

Conclusion

Strict IOP lowering by any means halts glaucoma progression. Overall, the QOL impact reported by the two treatment groups is remarkably similar, with relatively few significant study group differences observed after up to 5 years of follow-up in the CIGTS.

COLLABORATIVE NORMAL-TENSION GLAUCOMA STUDY

Normal-tension glaucoma (NTG) is a form of OAG characterized by optic nerve cupping and corresponding VF defects in patients with IOP measurements consistently below 21 mm Hg. The treatment for NTG has been the subject of intense debate for many years as there was no solid evidence to show that lowering eye pressure prevents continued VF loss. The collaborative NTG study was designed to find out whether IOP was involved in producing optic nerve damage and characteristic VF loss, even when the IOP was in the statistically normal range.[8,9]

Purpose

To evaluate the role of IOP control in preventing the progression in NTG.

Methodology

Collaborative NTG study (CNTGS) was a randomized controlled multicenter study conducted on 230 patients enrolled from 24 collaborating centers. Eligible patients were 20-90 years of age, with unilateral or bilateral NTG. A median IOP of 20 mm Hg or less in 10 baseline measurements along with definitive glaucomatous optic nerve head changes with corresponding visual field loss was the inclusion criteria. Patients with advanced damage were excluded. One eligible eye of the subject was randomized to either observation arm or the treatment arm. Treatment aimed at 30% reduction of IOP from baseline within 6 months and maintaining for 4 years by treatment with medication, laser trabeculoplasty or filtration surgery (no β-blocker and α-agonist in view of cardiovascular effects). In the observation arm the eye was followed without treatment until there was evidence of deterioration. Some eyes were randomized immediately, if the field defect threatened the point of fixation or there was previously documented progression of the disease. Other patients were randomized later; if there was VF progression, progression of optic nerve head (ONH) cupping, or a new disc hemorrhage.

Results

- Progression occurred in 35% in control arm versus 12% in treatment arm. Mean IOP was 16.0 mm Hg in control versus 10.6 mm Hg in treatment arm. This difference was not significant between the groups.
- Thirty percent lowering of IOP was achieved in half of the patients with only medications and laser treatment. Very few patients needed surgery.
- Eleven (14%) patients developed cataract in the control group as compared to 23 (38%) in the treatment group. The highest incidence of cataract was in patients who underwent filtration surgery.

- The study associated women, history of migraine and history of disc hemorrhages with greater risk of progression.
- Even in the control group, nearly 50% were stable at the end of follow-up.

Conclusion

The CNTGS concluded that IOP-lowering halts VF progression in majority of NTG patients. Adequate IOP lowering can be achieved by nonsurgical modalities. However, there are subgroups of patients who do not progress without treatment even up to 5 years.

ADVANCED GLAUCOMA INTERVENTION STUDY

In advanced glaucoma, filtration surgery is considered to be a viable option, as adequate IOP lowering with medication alone is difficult. A newer popular alternative in the form of ALT came into practice in 1980. However, the outcome with ALT was found to be variable in terms of IOP lowering and duration. Also, the effect varied in different races. Because success is limited and unpredictable, some patients, over time, may need to undergo a sequence of surgical interventions. Little was known about which sequence gives the best long-range outcome. Advanced glaucoma intervention study (AGIS) was designed to provide a comprehensive assessment of the long-range outcomes of medical and surgical management in advanced glaucoma.[10-13]

Purpose

To evaluate the outcomes of sequences of interventions involving trabeculectomy and ALT in eyes that have failed initial medical treatment for glaucoma.

Methodology

Advanced glaucoma intervention study is a multicenter, prospective, randomized study conducted at 11 centers on 789 eyes of 591 patients from April 1988 to November 1992. The study included phakic patients between 35 and 80 years with advanced POAG who were uncontrolled on maximum medical therapy. Patients were randomized into two intervention sequences.

1. Trabeculectomy was the first intervention. If this failed argon laser trabeculoplasty (ALT) was done and if ALT failed, a second trabeculectomy was offered. (TAT sequence)

2. The second intervention group followed the sequence of ALT first. If ALT failed, a trabeculectomy was done. This was followed by a second trabeculectomy if the first trabeculectomy failed. (ATT sequence)

All the second surgeries were supplemented with antimetabolites. Medical treatment was started as and when required in either group. Failing eyes were treated on clinician's discretion.

Patients were followed for a period of 5 years to determine functional loss in terms of VA, failure rate, complication rate and need of supplemental therapy. The follow-up schedule after the first intervention was of 1 week, 4 weeks and 3 months, 6 months and 6 monthly, thereafter. But after additional intervention, visits were scheduled at 1 week and 4 weeks.

Results

- Advanced glaucoma intervention study was one of the first National Institute of Health Sciences studies to determine a difference in treatment among racial groups. Results at the end of 7-year follow-up revealed that the response to sequences was different in different races. The African American benefited more with the laser first (LF) sequence with a decrease in vision of 28% as compare to a higher vision loss of 37% in the trabeculectomy first group
- The Caucasian American favored the LF for the initial 4 years but at the end of 7-year follow-up, vision loss was 31% with the trabeculectomy first as compared to a higher value of 35% in the LF sequence.
- On analyzing the association between IOP lowering and VF progression it was found that eyes with more than 17.5 mm Hg IOP showed greater VF deterioration in comparison to those with less than 14 mm Hg. When the IOP was maintained less than 18 mm Hg in all follow up visits, the increase in visual field defect score was negligible. And if this was maintained in less than 50% of their followup visits the worsening of the VF was more. The deterioration was more at 7 year as compared to 2 year follow up.
- Trabeculectomy increased the risk of cataract formation by 47% and the risk increased by 78% if the surgery was complicated. Increased age and diabetes were additional risk factors for cataract formation.
- Eyes with previous ALT were at a higher risk of bleb encapsulation
- Factors associated with failure of ALT were younger age and higher baseline IOP, where as diabetes and

postoperative complications were additional risk factors for the trabeculectomy failure

- Factors responsible for VF loss in both the groups were a decreased base line VF and decreased VA and male gender in ATT group and diabetes additionally in the TAT group. When studied the factors responsible for VA loss, a lesser baseline VA, older age along with lesser formal education were associated

- When these patients were followed-up under AGIS protocols for 10 years, the blacks still had better results with the ATT sequence and the whites with the TAT sequence. VA loss was less in both the races for ATT whereas IOP reduction was lesser in the TAT sequence. Failure rate of first intervention were lower for trabeculectomy as compared to trabeculoplasty.

Conclusion

Modifying treatment as per races in terms of starting with ALT in blacks and trabeculectomy in whites is beneficial. Maintaining an IOP lower than 18 mm Hg decreases VF progression significantly.

GLAUCOMA LASER TRIAL

Historically, the treatment of glaucoma is broadly either medical or surgical. The introduction of ALT enabled the ophthalmologist to interpose this treatment between medication and surgery with the hope that the pressure-lowering effect of the procedure would either postpone or obviate the need for surgery. The Glaucoma Laser Trial (GLT) was initiated to evaluate its IOP-lowering efficacy when used as a primary treatment option in POAG.[14,15]

Purpose

To assess the efficacy and safety of ALT as an alternative to treatment with topical medication for controlling IOP in patients with newly diagnosed, previously untreated POAG.

Methodology

The GLT, a multicenter, randomized clinical trial involving 271 patients was conducted on newly diagnosed POAG patients between February 1984 and April 1987. All patients were required to have IOP of at least 22 mm Hg in each eye and evidence of optic nerve damage in either eye. Each patient had one eye randomly assigned to ALT (the LF eye) and the other eye assigned to standard topical medication [the medication first (MF) eye]. The follow-up of GLT was up to 2 years.

Out of 271, 203 participated in the Glaucoma Laser Treatment Follow-up Study (GLTFS), with a median duration of follow-up being 7 years (maximum 9 years).

Argon laser trabeculoplasty was done in two sessions 1 month apart, 180° on each setting with 40–45 burns. Patients were followed-up for a period of 2 years for IOP, VF acuity, ONH assessment and any adverse events. Medication was initiated or changed for either eye as per the stepped regimen in case of inadequate IOP lowering, VF deterioration, optic disc worsening or any adverse events. If the IOP was still not successfully reduced, surgery or further laser treatment was done as per clinician's discretion.

Results

- At the end of 2 years of GLT, eyes in the LF group had a lower IOP by 2 mm Hg as compared to the MF group. This difference in IOP was seen even at the end of 9 years, in the GLTFS. There was also a 0.6 dB improvement in the VFs and less deterioration in the C:D in the eyes treated with ALT

- At all times during the follow-up period, more MF eyes than LF eyes required two or more medications to control IOP (P less than 0.001)

- Both groups had equal percentage of filtering surgery at the end of 9 years.

Conclusion

Initial treatment with ALT is at least as efficacious as initial treatment with topical medication. In the short-term, ALT provides good pressure control and has the advantage of postponing and/or reducing the inconvenience, and side effects associated with medications.

TRABECULECTOMY VERSUS TUBE STUDY

Glaucoma surgery is performed when further IOP reduction is needed despite the use of maximum-tolerated medical therapy and appropriate laser treatment. Despite the introduction of several new glaucoma operations in recent years trabeculectomy still remains the most commonly performed incisional procedure for the management of glaucoma. However, concern about bleb-related complications has contributed to an expanded use of tube shunts as an alternative to trabeculectomy even in nonrefractory glaucomas. Surveys have also indicated a lack of consensus regarding the best surgical approach for managing glaucoma in eyes with previous intraocular surgery. Until the Tube versus Trabeculectomy Study (TVT), there was little information comparing the two procedures.[16-18]

Purpose

This study was designed to answer the question of whether implantation of an aqueous drainage device or a trabeculectomy should be performed on patients who need glaucoma surgery and who have had previous cataract surgery or trabeculectomy.

Methodology

It was a multicenter randomized clinical trial, which included 17 clinical centers. Patients 18–85 years of age with uncontrolled glaucoma (IOP more than or equal to 18 mm Hg and less than or equal to 40 mm Hg on maximum-tolerated medical therapy) were enrolled in the study. The mean age of the study population was 71 years, and 53% were women. The baseline IOP was 25.3 ± 5.3 mm Hg (mean ± SD) on 3.1 ± 1.2 glaucoma medications (mean ± SD), and 81% of patients had POAG. Among enrolled patients, 44% had previously undergone cataract surgery, 35% trabeculectomy and 20% combined cataract and glaucoma surgery as the qualifying prior ocular surgery for entrance into the study. These patients were randomly assigned to treatment with a tube shunt or a trabeculectomy with mitomycin C (MMC). Patients in the tube group underwent placement of a 350 mm² Baerveldt glaucoma implant (BGI; Abbott Medical Optics, Santa Ana, California, USA) superotemporally with a complete restriction of flow at the time of implantation. Patients in the trabeculectomy group had a superior trabeculectomy with a standard dosage of MMC of 0.4 mg/mL for 4 minute. On each follow-up visit, patients were evaluated for IOP, VA, use of supplemental medical therapy, surgical complications, VFs, quality of life and failure (IOP more than 21 mm Hg or not reduced by 20%, IOP less than or equal to 5 mm Hg, reoperation for glaucoma, or loss of light perception vision).

Results

The TVT study enrolled 212 eyes of 212 patients between October 1999 and April 2004, randomising 107 in the tube group and 105 in the trabeculectomy group.

- Both surgical procedures produced a significant and sustained reduction in IOP. At 5 years, IOP (mean ± SD) was 14.4 ± 6.9 mm Hg in the tube group and 12.6 ± 5.9 mm Hg in the trabeculectomy group. The degree of IOP reduction was similar between the two treatment groups
- A significant reduction in the use of medical therapy was seen in both treatment groups. The number of glaucoma medications (mean ± SD) decreased from baseline by 1.8 ± 1.8 in the tube group and 1.7 ± 2.0 in the trabeculectomy group in patients who completed 5-year follow-up visits. A significantly greater use of supplemental medical therapy was observed in the tube group compared with the trabeculectomy group at all follow-up visits during the first 2 postoperative years. No significant difference in the mean number of medications was seen between treatment groups after 5 years of follow-up
- A significantly higher failure rate was seen in the trabeculectomy group than in the tube group after 5 years. Treatment failure had occurred in 24 patients (33%) in the tube group and 42 patients (50%) in the trabeculectomy group at 5 years (P = 0.034)
- Risk factor analysis for treatment failures was done by evaluating baseline demographic and clinical features and none of the baseline factors predicted failure for tube shunt surgery or trabeculectomy with MMC
- A higher rate of reoperation for glaucoma was observed in the trabeculectomy group compared with the tube group, the 5-year cumulative reoperation rate being 9% in the tube group and 29% in the trabeculectomy group (P = 0.025)
- Significant decreases in Snellen VA and Early Treatment of Diabetic Retinopathy Study (ETDRS) VA were observed in both treatment groups during 5 years of follow-up, 31 patients (46%) in the tube group and 33 patients (43%) in the trabeculectomy group had lost 2 or more Snellen lines from baseline. The most frequent causes of vision loss after 5 years were glaucoma, macular disease and cataract.

Conclusion

The TVT study supports the expanding use of tube shunts beyond the surgical management of refractory glaucoma. In eyes with previous cataract and/or glaucoma surgery, the TVT study found that tube shunt surgery had a higher success rate compared to trabeculectomy with MMC during 5 years of follow-up. The two surgical procedures were associated with similar IOP reduction and use of supplemental medical therapy at 5 years. The rate of reoperation for glaucoma was higher after trabeculectomy with MMC than tube shunt placement. Vision loss occurred at a similar rate after both procedures.

AHMED-BAERVELDT COMPARISON STUDY

Tube versus Trabeculectomy study validated the shift toward increased use of drainage implants, but literature was sparse as regards prospective studies comparing different implant designs. The two principal aqueous shunts in common use at the present time are the Ahmed glaucoma valve (AGV; New World Medical, Ranchos Cucamonga, CA) and the BGI (Abbott Medical Optics, Abbott Park, IL). Both the AGV and BGI share a common design consisting of a tube that shunts aqueous humor to an end plate located in the equatorial region of the eye. These shunts differ in two aspects. First, the AGV has a flow restrictor that limits flow through the device when the IOP becomes critically low in order to limit early hypotony without the need for an external ligation. Second, the end plates differ significantly in terms of the surface area of the plate; the surface area of the BGI (350 mm^2) is almost double that of the AGV (184 mm^2). The absence of a flow resistor also permits the BGI to have a lower IOP than the AGV. Ahmed-Baerveldt comparison (ABC) study is a randomized trial, which attempts to compare these two implants.

Purpose

This study was designed to compare the outcomes of the Ahmed FP7 glaucoma valve and the Baerveldt 101–350 glaucoma implant for the treatment of refractory glaucoma.[19,20]

Methodology

Investigators at 16 clinical centers in United States enrolled patients between 18 and 85 years of age inclusive, with inadequately controlled glaucoma despite maximum-tolerated medical therapy, with IOP greater than or equal to 18 mm Hg, and who had an aqueous shunt as the planned surgical procedure. Patients with primary glaucomas with a previous failed trabeculectomy or other intraocular surgery were included. Patients without previous intraocular surgery were also eligible, if they had secondary glaucomas known to have a high failure rate with trabeculectomy, such as neovascular, uveitic or iridocorneal endothelial syndrome-associated glaucoma.

A total of 276 patients were enrolled in this study between October 2006 and April 2008. 143 patients were randomized to the AGV and 133 patients were randomized to the BGI.

Patients were excluded if they lacked light perception vision, were unwilling or unable to give informed consent, lived out of the area and were expected to be unavailable for follow-up visits, had a previous cyclodestructive procedure or previous aqueous shunt implanted in the same eye, had a prior scleral buckling procedure or other external impediment to supratemporal drainage device implantation, had presence of silicone oil, had vitreous in the anterior chamber sufficient to require a vitrectomy, had uveitis associated with a systemic condition like juvenile rheumatoid arthritis, had nanophthalmos, had Sturge-Weber syndrome or other conditions associated with elevated episcleral venous pressure, or needed aqueous shunt surgery combined with other ocular procedures.

Results

- At 5 years, mean IOP was 14.7 ± 4.4 mm Hg in the AGV group and 12.7 ± 4.5 mm Hg in the BGI group (P = 0.015)
- The mean number of glaucoma medications in use at 5 years was 2.2 ± 1.4 in the AGV group and 1.8 ± 1.5 in the BGI group (P = 0.28)
- The cumulative probability of failure during 5 years of follow-up was 44.7% in the AGV group and 39.4% in the BGI group (P = 0.65). The number of subjects failing because of inadequately controlled IOP or reoperation for glaucoma was 46 in the AGV group (80% of AGV failures) and 25 in the BGI group (53% of BGI failures; P = 0.003)
- Eleven eyes in the AGV group (20% of AGV failures) experienced persistent hypotony, explanation of implant, or loss of light perception compared with 22 eyes (47% of failures) in the BGI group. Change in logMAR VA (mean ± SD) at 5 years was 0.42 ± 0.99 in the AGV group and 0.43 ± 0.84 in the BGI group (P = 0.97).

Conclusion

Similar rates of surgical success were observed with both implants at 5 years. The BGI produced greater IOP reduction and a lower rate of glaucoma reoperation than the AGV, but the BGI was associated with twice as many failures because of safety issues.

AHMED VERSUS BAERVELDT STUDY

Ahmed versus Baerveldt (AVB) study is another landmark randomized clinical trial involving the aforementioned tube shunts, which has provided useful information to assist in surgical decision.[21,22]

Purpose

This study also attempted to compare the aqueous drainage devices, Ahmed FP7 glaucoma valve and the Baerveldt 101-350 glaucoma implant for the treatment of refractory glaucoma.

Methodology

Patients were recruited from seven international clinical sites and treated by 10 surgeons between 2005 and 2009. Inclusion criteria required that patients be at least 18 years of age and have uncontrolled glaucoma refractory to medical, laser and surgical therapy. Eligible patients were randomized to undergo implantation of an Ahmed-FP7 valve or a Baerveldt-350 implant using standardized surgical technique, and were followed up for 5 years.

Results

- A total of 238 patients were enrolled and randomized; 124 received the Ahmed implant and 114 received the Baerveldt implant. Baseline characteristics were similar in both groups. Half the study group had secondary glaucoma, and 37% had previously failed trabeculectomy
- Mean IOP was 15.7 ± 4.8 mm Hg in the Ahmed group (49% reduction) and 14.4 ± 5.1 mm Hg in the Baerveldt group (55% reduction; P = 0.09)
- Mean number of glaucoma medications was 1.8 ± 1.4 in the Ahmed group (42% reduction) and 1.1 ± 1.3 in the Baerveldt group (65% reduction; P = 0.002). There was a moderate but similar decrease in VA in both groups (P less than 0.001)
- At 3 years, the cumulative probability of failure was 51% in the Ahmed group and 34% in the Baerveldt group (P = 0.03)
- The two groups had similar complication rates (52% Ahmed, 62% Baerveldt; P = 0.12); however, the Baerveldt group had a higher rate of hypotony-related vision-threatening complications (0% Ahmed, 6% Baerveldt; P = 0.005). More interventions were required in the Baerveldt group, although the difference did not reach statistical significance (38% Ahmed, 50% Baerveldt; P = 0.07). Most complications were transient, and most interventions were slit-lamp procedures.

Conclusion

Both devices were effective in reducing IOP and glaucoma medications. The Baerveldt group had a lower failure rate and required fewer medications than the Ahmed group after 3 years, but it experienced more hypotony-related vision-threatening complications.

REFERENCES

1. Kass MA, Heuer DK, Higginbotham EJ, et al. The Ocular Hypertension Treatment Study: a randomized trial determines that topical ocular hypotensive medication delays or prevents the onset of primary open-angle glaucoma. Arch Ophthalmol. 2002;120(6):701-13.
2. Gordon MO, Beiser JA, Brandt JD, et al. The Ocular Hypertension Treatment Study: baseline factors that predict the onset of primary open-angle glaucoma. Arch Ophthalmol. 2002;120(6):714-20; discussion 829-30.
3. Heijl A, Leske MC, Bengtsson B, et al. Early Manifest Glaucoma Trial Group. Reduction of intraocular pressure and glaucoma progression: results from the Early Manifest Glaucoma Trial. Arch Ophthalmol. 2002;120(10):1268-79.
4. Lichter PR, Musch DC, Gillespie BW, et al. CIGTS Study Group. Interim clinical outcomes in the Collaborative Initial Glaucoma Treatment Study comparing initial treatment randomized to medications or surgery. Ophthalmology. 2001;108(11):1943-53.
5. Janz NK, Wren PA, Lichter PR, et al. CIGTS Study Group. The Collaborative Initial Glaucoma Treatment Study: interim quality of life findings after initial medical or surgical treatment of glaucoma. Ophthalmology. 2001;108(11):1954-65.
6. Musch DC, Gillespie BW, Lichter PR, Niziol LM, Janz NK; CIGTS Study Investigators. CIGTS Study Group. Visual field progression in the Collaborative Initial Glaucoma Treatment Study the impact of treatment and other baseline factors. Ophthalmology. 2009;116(2):200-7.
7. Musch DC, Gillespie BW, Niziol LM, Lichter PR, Varma R; CIGTS Study Group. CIGTS Study Group. Intraocular pressure control and long-term visual field loss in the Collaborative Initial Glaucoma Treatment Study. Ophthalmology. 2011;118(9):1766-73.
8. Collaborative Normal-tension Glaucoma Study Group. Comparison of glaucomatous progression between untreated patients with normal-tension glaucoma and patients with therapeutically reduced intraocular pressures. Am J Ophthalmol. 1998;126(4):487-97.
9. Anderson DR; Normal Tension Glaucoma Study. Collaborative Normal-tension Glaucoma Study. Curr Opin Ophthalmol. 2003;14(2):86-90.

10. The AGIS Investigators. The Advanced Glaucoma Intervention Study (AGIS): 1. Study design and methods and baseline characteristics of study patients. Control Clin Trials. 1994;15(4):299-325.

11. The AGIS Investigators. The Advanced Glaucoma Intervention Study (AGIS): 4. Comparison of treatment outcomes within race: 10-year results. Ophthalmology. 2004;111(4):651-64.

12. The AGIS Investigators. The Advanced Glaucoma Intervention Study (AGIS): 7. Comparison of treatment outcomes within race. Seven-year results. Ophthalmology. 1998; 105(7):1146-64.

13. The AGIS Investigators. The Advanced Glaucoma Intervention Study (AGIS): 13. The relationship between control of intraocular pressure and visual field deterioration. Am J Ophthalmol. 2000;130(4):429-40.

14. Glaucoma Laser Trial Research Group. The Glaucoma Laser Trial (GLT): 2. Results of argon laser trabeculoplasty versus topical medicines. Ophthalmology. 1990;97(11):1403-13.

15. Glaucoma Laser Trial Research Group. The Glaucoma Laser Trial (GLT) and glaucoma laser trial follow-up study: 7. Results. Am J Ophthalmol. 1995;120(6):718-31.

16. Gedde SJ, Singh K, Schiffman JC, Feuer WJ; Tube Versus Trabeculectomy Study Group. The Tube Versus Trabeculectomy

17. Gedde SJ, Schiffman JC, Feuer WJ, et al. Treatment outcomes in the Tube Versus Trabeculectomy (TVT) Study after five years of follow-up. Am J Ophthalmol. 2012;153(5):789-803.e2.

18. Gedde SJ, Schiffman JC, Feuer WJ, et al. The Tube Versus Trabeculectomy Study: design and baseline characteristics of study patients. Am J Ophthalmol. 2005;140(2):275-87.

19. Budenz DL, Barton K, Gedde SJ, et al. Five-year treatment outcomes in the Ahmed Baerveldt comparison study. Ophthalmology. 2015;122(2):308-16.

20. Barton K, Gedde SJ, Budenz DL, Feuer WJ, Schiffman J; Ahmed Baerveldt Comparison Study Group. The Ahmed Baerveldt Comparison Study methodology, baseline patient characteristics, and intraoperative complications. Ophthalmology. 2011;118(3):435-42.

21. Christakis PG, Tsai JC, Zurakowski D, et al. The Ahmed Versus Baerveldt study: design, baseline patient characteristics, and intraoperative complications. Ophthalmology. 2011;118(11):2172-9.

22. Christakis PG, Tsai JC, Kalenak JW, et al. The Ahmed versus Baerveldt study: three-year treatment outcomes. Ophthalmology. 2013;120(11):2232-40.

Study: interpretation of results and application to clinical practice. Curr Opin Ophthalmol. 2012;23(2):118-26.

Basics of a Trial Design for Glaucoma

Shibal Bhartiya, Parul Ichhpujani

INTRODUCTION

The world of glaucoma management has been rapidly evolving over the last decade and promises to do so at an extraordinary pace in the days to come. It is only logical that newer modalities and techniques, both diagnostic and interventional, be tested per se, and against the accepted gold standard. Glaucoma trial design, thus, becomes a necessary tool in the serious glaucomatologists armamentarium in this era of evidence-based medicine (EBM).[1-9] It also helps the glaucomatologist in reviewing available literature better and helping him/her to chose what may be best relevant to his/her clinical practice. This chapter is majorly based on the World Glaucoma Association (WGA) guidelines for trial design, and the reader is advised to refer to the document available free online for clarifications and details.[1]

LEVELS OF EVIDENCE FOR CLINICAL APPLICATION (CHOOSING THE STUDY DESIGN)

Evidence-based medicine requires the integration of clinical judgment, recommendations from the best available evidence and the patient's values.[2-5] Figure 15B.1 describes the hierarchy of evidence and how the integration of this evidence can be used to formulate a grade of recommendation.

Meta-analyses of randomized-controlled trials in effect uses the data from individual randomized-controlled trials and statistically pool it.[6,7] This effectively increases the number of patients that the data was obtained from, thereby increasing the effective sample size. This, therefore, typifies the highest level of evidence.

Oxford Centre for Evidence Based Medicine recommends further classification of the *grade of recommendation* system (grades A to D) to the more-detailed levels of evidence (Box 15B.1 and Fig. 15B.1).[8,9]

- *Grade A*: Consistent randomized controlled clinical trial, cohort study, all or none, clinical decision rule validated in different populations.
- *Grade B*: Consistent retrospective cohort, exploratory cohort, ecological study, outcomes research, case-control study; or extrapolations from level A studies.
- *Grade C*: Case-series study or extrapolations from level B studies.
- *Grade D*: Expert opinion without explicit critical appraisal, or based on physiology, bench research or first principles.

DEFINITION OF DISEASE (TYPE AND SEVERITY)

The glaucoma must be defined on the basis of anatomy of the anterior chamber angle (i.e. open or closed angle); etiology (primary or secondary), age of onset, as well as structural (i.e. quantified by optic nerve head and retinal nerve fiber layer) and functional (i.e. quantified by visual field defects) state of disease (i.e. mild, moderate, severe) (Boxes 15B.2 and 15B.3).

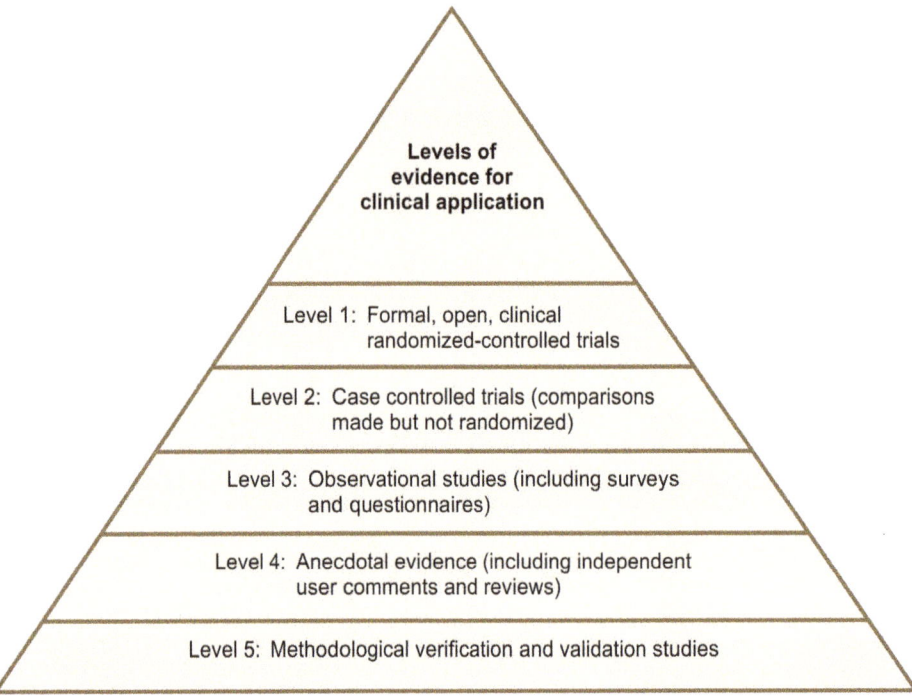

Fig. 15B.1: Levels of evidence for clinical application.

Box 15B.1: Levels of evidence for therapy/prevention, etiology/harm.

Level 1A
- Systematic review with *homogeneity* (*) of randomized control trials

Level 1B
- Individual randomized control trial with narrow *confidence interval* (studies with wide confidence interval should be tagged with a "-" at the end of their designated level)

Level 1C
- All or none (met when all patients died before Rx became available, but some now survive on it; or when some patients died before the Rx became available but none now die on it)

Level 2A
- Systematic review with homogeneity (*) of cohort studies

Level 2B
- Individual cohort studies; low-quality randomized control trials (e.g. less than 80% follow-up)

Level 2C
- *Outcomes* Research; ecological studies

Level 3A
- Systematic review with homogeneity (*) of case-control studies

Level 3B
- Individual case-control studies

Level 4
- Case series
    - Poor-quality cohort studies (failed to clearly define comparison groups and/or failed to measure exposures and outcomes in the same, objective way in both exposed and nonexposed individuals and/or failed to identify or appropriately control known confounders and/or failed to carry out a sufficient long and completely follow-up)
    - Poor-quality case-control studies (failed to clearly define comparison groups and/or failed to measure exposures and outcomes in the same, objective way in both cases and controls and/or failed to identify or appropriately control known confounders)

Level 5
- Expert opinion without explicit critical appraisal, or based on physiology, bench research or *first principles*

Note: (*) A systematic review free of worrisome variations in the directions and degrees of results between individual studies. Not all systematic reviews with statistically significant heterogeneity need be worrisome, and not all worrisome heterogeneity need be statistically significant. Studies displaying worrisome heterogeneity should be tagged with a "-" at the end of their designated level

Box 15B.2: Broad classification of glaucoma.

- *Congenital and developmental glaucoma*
  - Primary congenital glaucoma
  - Developmental glaucoma associated with systemic anomalies
- *Adult onset glaucoma*
  - Open-angle glaucoma
    - Primary open-angle glaucoma
      a. Juvenile open-angle glaucoma
      b. Primary adult onset open-angle glaucoma
      c. Normal-tension glaucoma
      d. Ocular hypertension
    - Secondary open-angle glaucoma
      a. Exfoliation
      b. Pigment dispersion
      c. Traumatic
      d. Lens-induced glaucomas
  - Angle-closure glaucoma
    - Primary angle-closure disease
      a. Primary angle-closure suspect (PACS)
      b. Primary angle closure (PAC)
      c. Primary angle-closure glaucoma (PACG)
      d. Acute attack of angle closure
    - Secondary angle-closure glaucoma
      a. Secondary angle-closure glaucoma with pupillary block
      b. Secondary angle-closure glaucoma with anterior pulling mechanism without pupillary block
      c. Secondary angle-closure glaucoma with posterior pushing mechanism without pupillary block
- Glaucomas associated with syndromes
  - Sturge-Weber syndrome

Box 15B.3: Broad classification for severity of glaucoma.

- *Mild*: Optic nerve abnormalities consistent with glaucoma but no visual field abnormalities on any white-on-white visual field test, or abnormalities present only on short-wavelength
- *Moderate*: Optic nerve abnormalities consistent with glaucoma and glaucomatous visual field abnormalities in one hemifield, and not within 5° of fixation
- *Severe*: Optic nerve abnormalities consistent with glaucoma and glaucomatous visual field abnormalities in both hemifields, and/or loss within 5° of fixation in at least one hemifield

DEFINITION OF DATA POINTS EVALUATED AND END POINT

The investigators must describe the data points, which will be evaluated in the course of trial, and pre-establish the criteria for success and failure for each of these.

Baseline Intraocular Pressure Measurement

The gold standard is Goldmann applanation tonometer (GAT) and any deviation from the use of GAT must be mentioned and the rationale for the same provided. Each GAT must be repeated once (in case reading within 2 mm of first) or twice (in case difference more than 2 mm) and the average noted. It is recommended to take the average of at least two readings, either on separate days or at least few hours apart, to establish IOP baseline. It is also recommended to consider recording diurnal variation of IOP when evaluating IOP change as a criterion for success. Central corneal thickness also should be recorded in order to validate GAT measurements.

Visual Acuity

Vision must be recorded (unaided and best-corrected visual acuity, refraction) under standardized conditions using Snellen chart or the Early Treatment Diabetic Retinopathy Study (ETDRS) chart at appropriate intervals. This is especially relevant in surgical trials, and in patients with coexistent cataract.

Visual Field

Investigators must recognize that standard-automated perimetry is essential to classify and monitor glaucoma

DEFINITION OF COHORT DEMOGRAPHICS

The investigators must describe the cohort demographics and criteria for both inclusion and exclusion of patients into the trial. The essential baseline data includes age, gender, ethnicity, systemic and ocular comorbidities as well as previous. A note must be made of all ocular and systemic concomitant medications.

In case, a patient is already on treatment for glaucoma, a washout period is recommended to ascertain intraocular pressure (IOP) baseline. It is important to remember that for glaucoma-surgical trials, previous surgeries for glaucoma and any other surgeries on the conjunctiva may confound the results of the surgical procedure being evaluated.

Table 15B.1: Recommended reporting durations.

	Pre-op	POD1	POW1	POM1	POM3	POM6	POY1	POM18	POY2	POY≥3
Ideal	1–7 d	1 d	7d	28–31 d	90–92 d	181–183 d	Ann. date	547–548 d	Ann. date	Ann. date
Preferred	0–21 d	1–2 d	4–11 d	21–42 d	77–106 d	161–204 d	334–387	486–609 d	669–822 d	±91 d
Acceptable	0–42 d	1–3 d	4–14 d	15–60 d	61–122 d	123–272 d	273–456 d	457–639 d	640–913 d	±181 d

(d: days; Ann date: Anniversary date; POD: Postoperative day; POW: Postoperative week; POM: Postoperative month; POY: Postoperative year).

progression. There are no standardized criteria for evaluating this; however, investigators may choose a protocol from any of the larger clinical trials for uniformity so that results may be compared across reported trials. Progression analysis softwares may help in this. It must be kept in mind that visual field progression is usually a slow process, and long-term follow-up is essential to achieve statistical significance.

Ocular Hypotensive Medication

Concomitant medication especially that for lowering IOP must be recorded. Each medication is counted as one, while oral acetazolamide is traditionally counted as two medications.

FOLLOW-UP AND REPORTING TIME WINDOWS

Studies, which are of a longer duration, provide more valuable information relevant to glaucoma practice. The minimum-recommended duration for a surgical trial is a year. Table 15B.1 shows the ideal, preferred and recommended durations for follow-up and reporting. It is important that the survival analysis (i.e. how many patients are still being followed-up) be represented while reporting at each point in time.

EVALUATION (CRITERIA FOR SUCCESS AND FAILURE)

For Diagnostic Modalities

The predictive values of the diagnostic modality must be compared with the gold standard. False-positive and false-negatives identified by the machine must be reported. When comparing measurements by two different instruments it must be kept in mind that a correlation alone is not sufficient, and a Bland-Altman plot with limits of agreement provides a better representation.

For Therapeutic Modalities (Surgical and Medical)

The success must be reported in terms absolute success (without any ocular hypertensive medication) or qualified success (with ocular hypertensive medication), based on the pre-established acceptable end points.

Failure may be defined as IOP above or below the acceptable limits of two consecutive visits. Loss of light perception, a vision loss attributable or glaucoma, or the need for a second glaucoma-surgical intervention, is considered complete failure.

Interventions, like suture adjustments, bleb needling or goniopuncture, may be considered as acceptable, if so mentioned in the pre-established protocol for evaluation.

The points to consider include:

- *Intraocular pressure*: The end point for success may be represented as a percentage drop from baseline and/or an absolute-accepted IOP (less than 21, 18, 15 or 12 mm Hg), or various acceptable highest levels of IOP. The lower limit for acceptable IOP is 6 mm of Hg, which is the accepted definition of hypotony. For non-penetrating glaucoma surgeries IOPs as low as zero may be considered acceptable, if not accompanied by any complications of hypotony.

Any evaluation of diurnal/short-term/long-term IOP fluctuation provides clinically relevant information.

- *Vision*: Decrease in visual acuity (in terms of lines lost; decrease in logMAR acuity when average visual acuity is reported) or progression of visual field defects must be reported. Usually change in mean deviation is reported to represent visual field changes, and this change must be repeatable (i.e. at least one more repeat field must show similar changes)

- *Decrease in ocular hypotensive medications*: The change in number of ocular hypotensive medications must be documented. The need for oral acetazolamide for achieving target IOP is usually considered a failure of the therapeutic intervention

- *Complications*: All complications, along with interventions, and the resultant outcomes, must be reported in the clinical trial. These include both minor adverse events and major ones.

ETHICAL CONSIDERATIONS

Randomization to Nontreatment Arm

When assigning any patient to the nontreatment arm of a study, the possible deleterious effects of the same must be kept in mind and clearly discussed with the patients. It is often better to have a crossover study design for the intervention, whenever possible.

Clear Definition of Acceptable Outcomes

A predeclared clear definition of outcomes makes evaluation of any innovation easy and transparent. Any complications also must be clearly documented and reported.

Informed Consent

A comprehensive, written, informed consent must be obtained from the subjects enrolled for the trial in their own language. The patient must be assured that denying enrollment will, in no way, influence his/her treatment plan at the facility, and that he/she can revoke consent at any point during the trial.

Approval from Institutional Review Board or Ethics Committee

A formal approval from the Institutional Review Board (IRB) or Institutional Ethics Committee (IEC) must be sought before commencement of a trial. In case the investigators do not have either of the two in the hospital, an independent Ethics Committee may be approached for approval. Manual of Procedures and Case Report Forms must be approved by the IRB/IEC. Any deviations from approved protocol, complications must be reported to the IRB/IEC.

Adherence to Tenets of Declaration of Helsinki

The 1958 declaration of Helsinki outlines the tenets of good clinical practice and patient rights. They must be adhered to strictly.

Declaration of Sources of Funding (Financial and Nonfinancial Support and Conflicts of Interest)

Given that both conflicts of interest and funding can lead to a bias in reporting, the same must be clearly declared and managed.

STATISTICAL CONSIDERATIONS

Calculation of Sample Size

The calculation of sample size is dependent on the variable under study and the expected change from the established gold standard. Appropriate sample size calculation is essential for establishing statistical significance. Most studies assume an alpha error of 0.05 for calculation of sample size; and acceptable power may be 80, 90 or 95% (less than 80% not acceptable).

Statistical Significance

The level of statistical significance for reporting success must be established beforehand (e.g. P less than 0.1, 0.01, 0.001, etc.).

Software for Data Analysis

The software used for data analysis must be mentioned clearly.

Randomization

Randomization lists may be developed prior to patient enrollment. In case of multicenter studies stratification of these lists may be carried out by the study statistician.

Data Analysis

Whenever possible, data analysis for all patients must be presented at all time points. In case of interventional trials, a survival analysis at each time point, mentioning clearly the number of patients represented is essential.

Eyes versus Patients

It is better to use data from only one eye of each patient to avoid confounding results due to patient factors. However, the decision to include both eyes may be made before patient enrollment, if so, preferred by the investigator.

Interim Analysis and Stopping Rules

These must be predetermined especially with respect to safety criteria. This is especially relevant in studies in which the patient enrollment would continue even after some data may be available for interim analysis.

Data Representation

A graphical representation, along with tabulation of actual numerical data is essential for clear communication of results of the trial.

For survival analysis, a Kaplan-Meier survival curve or Cox Regression time to failure method are preferred. This can be supplemented with a proportion of treatment failures in each group.

For comparing agreement and/or repeatability of diagnostic modalities, a Bland-Altman plot along with limits of agreement must be plotted. Specific IOP or mean deviation may be represented as a scatterplot with clear symbols for pre- and postintervention values. Appropriately positioned horizontal lines may indicate the acceptable IOP levels.

Box plots that show median values as well as the appropriate percentiles (25/75 better than 5/95) are preferred over bar charts depicting mean and standard deviations.

Risk rations and multivariate analysis with 95% confidence intervals may be calculated with or without important covariates and represented.

■ SPECIAL CONSIDERATIONS

Methods of Economic Evaluation of Glaucoma

Economic evaluation of glaucoma intervention (diagnostic test, medical or surgical intervention or therapy) comprises analysis of the cost of the intervention with respect to the benefits of the intervention, as compared to pre-existing, validated intervention. Any modality must be so evaluated so as to allow patients, doctors and policy makers to make a judicious choice.

The various modalities of doing so include:

- *Cost minimization analysis*: This is used to compare the cost of treatment when alternative therapies have demonstrably equivalent clinical effectiveness. Since equal efficacy and equal tolerability is already demonstrated, a common efficacy denominator is not required

- *Cost benefit analysis*: This assigns a monetary value to the measure of effect and, therefore, is less used in evaluation of health economics of glaucoma interventions since it is difficult to monetize the effects of a health-related intervention

- *Cost-effectiveness analysis*: This compares the relative costs and outcomes of two or more courses of action. Cost-effectiveness analysis typically expressed in terms of a ratio where the denominator is a gain in health from a measure (years of life, sight-years gained) and the numerator is the cost associated with the health gain. The most commonly used outcome measure is quality-adjusted life years (QALY).

Other related measures include:

- *Incremental cost-effectiveness ratio*: This represents the resources that must be spent to gain one unit of effectiveness. It is the ratio between the difference in costs and the difference in benefits of two interventions

- *Cost-utility analysis*: This estimates the ratio between the cost of the glaucoma intervention and the benefit it produces in terms of the number of years lived in full health by the patient. Hence, it can be considered a special case of cost-effectiveness analysis.

Methods of Quality of Life Assessments

Investigators may include quality of life (QoL) assessments as part of the larger clinical trial, or separately to evaluate a particular intervention. Validated questionnaires may be either self-administered or by the investigator. The National Eye Institute Visual Function Questionnaires (NEI-VFQ) (51 points) and NEI-VFQ-25 (with 25 points) remain the benchmark against which new glaucoma QoL are compared. Both are fully validated and widely used tools that allows vision-dependent tasks to be assessed. The NEI-VFQ-25 is an improved version of NEI-VFQ, and takes roughly 5 minutes to use. However, the lack of visual field consideration is a major drawback.

Few available methods for assessing QoL include:

- Generic instruments, i.e. not disease state specific. [Medical outcomes study short form-36 (SF-36),[10] sickness impact profile (SIP)][11]

- *Vision-specific instruments*: [VF-14,[12] NEI-VFQ,[13] NEI-VFQ-25,[14] activities of daily vision scale (ADVS)][15]

- *Glaucoma-specific instruments*: [Glaucoma symptom scale (GSS),[16] comparison of ophthalmic medication for tolerability (COMTOL),[17] glaucoma QoL-15 (GQL-15),[18] symptom impact glaucoma score (SIG) and glaucoma health perceptions index (GHPI)][19]

REFERENCES

1. World Glaucoma Association. (2008). Guidelines on Design & Reporting Glaucoma Trials. [online] Available from http://www.worldglaucoma.org/guidelines-on-design-reporting-glaucoma-trials/. [Accessed July, 2016].

2. Sackett DL, Rosenberg WM, Gray JA, Haynes RB, Richardson WS. Evidence based medicine: what it is and what it isn't. BMJ. 1996;312(7023):71-2.

3. Sackett DL, Richardson WS, Rosenberg WM, Haynes RB. Evidence Based Medicine: How to practice and teach EBM, 1st edition. New York: Churchill Livingstone; 1997.

4. Atkins D, Best D, Briss PA, Eccles M, Falck-Ytter Y, Flottorp S, et al. Grading quality of evidence and strength of recommendations. BMJ. 2004;328(7454):1490.

5. Phillips B, Ball C, Sackett DL, Badenoch D, Straus S, Haynes B, et al. Centre for evidence-based medicine. Oxford-centre for evidence based medicine: GENERIC; 1998. Levels of evidence and grades of recommendation.

6. Atkins D, Eccles M, Flottorp S, Guyatt GH, Henry D, Hill S, et al. Systems for grading the quality of evidence and the strength of recommendations I: critical appraisal of existing approaches The GRADE Working Group. BMC Health Serv Res. 2004;4(1):38.

7. Sackett DL, Haynes RB, Guyatt GH, Tugwell P. Clinical epidemiology: a basic science for clinical medicine, 2nd edition. Boston: Little, Brown and Company; 1991.

8. A guide to the development, implementation and evaluation of clinical practice guidelines. NHMRC. 1999.

9. Levels of Evidence. (2009). Centre for Evidence Based Medicine. [online] Available from www.cebm.net. [Accessed July, 2016].

10. Ware JE, Gandek B. Overview of the SF-36 health survey and the international quality of life assessment (IQOLA) project. J Clin Epidemiol. 1998;51(11):903-12.

11. Bergner M, Bobbit RA, Carter WB, Gilson BS. The sickness impact profile development and final revision of a health status measure. Med Care. 1981;19(8):787-805.

12. Steinberg EP, Tielsch JM, Schein OD, Javitt JC, Sharkey P, Cassard SD, et al. The VF-14: an index of functional impairment in patients with cataract. Arch Ophthalmol. 1994;112(5):630-8.

13. Mangione CM, Lee PP, Pitts J, Gutierrez P, Burry S, Hays RD. Psychometric properties of the National Eye Institute Visual Function Questionnaire (NEI-VFQ). Arch Ophthalmol. 1998;166(11):1496-504.

14. Mangione CM, Lee PP, Pitts J, Gutierrez PR, Spritzer K, Burry S, et al. Development of the 25-item National Eye Institute Visual Function Questionnaire. Arch Ophthalmol. 2001;119(7):1050-8.

15. Mangione CM, Phillips RS, Seddon JM, Lawrence MG, Cook EF, Dailey R, et al. Development of the Activities of Daily Vision Scale: a measure of visual functional status. Med Care. 1992;30(12):111-26.

16. Lee BL, Gutierrez P, Gordon M, Wilson MR, Cioffi GA, Ritch R, et al. The Glaucoma Symptom Scale. A brief index of glaucoma-specific symptoms. Arch Ophthalmol. 1998;116(7):861-6.

17. Barber BL, Strahlman ER, Laiboritz R, Goess HA, Reines SA. Validation of a questionnaire for comparing the tolerability of ophthalmic medication. Ophthalmology. 1997;104(2):334-41.

18. Nelson P, Aspinall P, Papasouliotis O, Worton B, O'Brien C. Quality of life in glaucoma and its relationship with visual function. J Glaucoma. 2003;12(2):139-50.

19. Janz NK, Wren PA, Lichter PR, Musch DC, Gillespie BW, Guire KE. Quality of life in newly diagnosed glaucoma patients: the Collaborative Initial Glaucoma Treatment Study. Ophthalmology. 2001;108(5):887-97.

Index

Page numbers followed by *f* refer to figure and *t* refer to table.